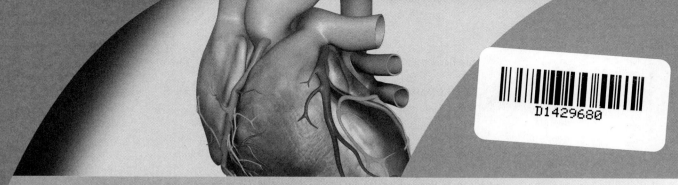

Essentials of Public Health Biology

A Guide for the Study of Pathophysiology

Constance Urciolo Battle, MD

Adjunct Professor
Department of Prevention and Community Health
School of Public Health and Health Services

Clinical Professor of Pediatrics
Children's National Medical Center
School of Medicine and Health Sciences

The George Washington University
Washington, DC

JONES AND BARTLETT PUBLISHERS
Sudbury, Massachusetts
BOSTON   TORONTO   LONDON   SINGAPORE

World Headquarters

Jones and Bartlett Publishers
40 Tall Pine Drive
Sudbury, MA 01776
978-443-5000
info@jbpub.com
www.jbpub.com

Jones and Bartlett Publishers
Canada
6339 Ormindale Way
Mississauga, Ontario L5V 1J2
Canada

Jones and Bartlett Publishers
International
Barb House, Barb Mews
London W6 7PA
United Kingdom

Jones and Bartlett's books and products are available through most bookstores and online booksellers. To contact Jones and Bartlett Publishers directly, call 800-832-0034, fax 978-443-8000, or visit our website www.jbpub.com.

Substantial discounts on bulk quantities of Jones and Bartlett's publications are available to corporations, professional associations, and other qualified organizations. For details and specific discount information, contact the special sales department at Jones and Bartlett via the above contact information or send an email to specialsales@jbpub.com.

This publication is designed to provide accurate and authoritative information in regard to the subject matter covered. It is sold with the understanding that the publisher is not engaged in rendering legal, accounting, or other professional service. If legal advice or other expert assistance is required, the service of a competent professional person should be sought.

Production Credits
Publisher: Michael Brown
Production Director: Amy Rose
Associate Editor: Katey Birtcher
Editorial Assistant: Catie Heverling
Production Editor: Tracey Chapman
Marketing Manager: Sophie Fleck
Cover Design: Kristin E. Ohlin
Photo Researcher: Lee Michelsen
Assistant Photo Researcher: Meghan Hayes
Composition: Auburn Associates, Inc.
Cover Image: © MedicalRF.com/age fotostock
Printing and Binding: Malloy, Inc.
Cover Printing: John Pow Company

Library of Congress Cataloging-in-Publication Data
Essentials of public health biology : a guide for the study of pathophysiology / [edited by] Constance Urciolo Battle.
    p. ; cm. — (Essential public health)
 Includes bibliographical references and index.
 ISBN-13: 978-0-7637-4464-9 (pbk.)
 ISBN-10: 0-7637-4464-6 (pbk.)
1. Public health. 2. Health promotion. 3. Medicine, Preventive. I. Battle, Constance Urciolo. II. Series.
 [DNLM: 1. Public Health. 2. Health Promotion. 3. Preventive Medicine. WA 100 E785 2009]
 RA425.E744 2009
 362.1—dc22

                                                    2008009984

6048
Printed in the United States of America
12 11 10 09 08   10 9 8 7 6 5 4 3 2 1

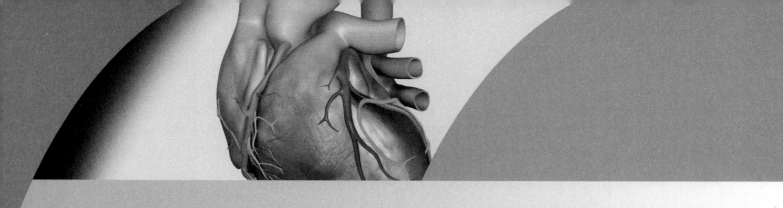

Dedication

TO MY BEST TEACHERS
with appreciation

Ursula, Bill, and Christopher and Susan
who taught me more than anyone about life
and
Raphael G. Urciolo, PhD
and
Vera Marie DeWolff, O.S.U.

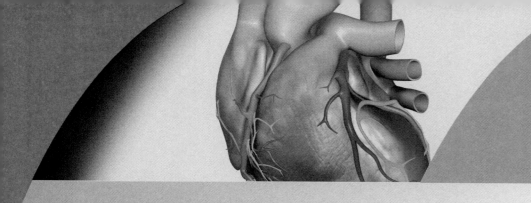

Acknowledgments

Assistant Editor
Adella Brown, BS
School of Public Health and Health Services
The George Washington University
Washington, DC

Special Thanks to
William S. Battle, PhD
New York, NY

Cynthia Kahn, MLS, MPH, AHIP
Reference and Instruction Librarian
Himmelfarb Health Sciences Library
The George Washington University Medical Center
Washington, DC

Kristina Krupincza, BS
School of Public Health and Health Services
The George Washington University
Washington, DC

Raluca Popovici, MPH
School of Public Health and Health Services
The George Washington University
Washington, DC

Jane Watkins, MAR
Decatur, IL

Tareq A. Yousef, BS
School of Public Health and Health Services
The George Washington University
Washington, DC

- All my past and present GWU undergraduate students in public health who have taught me about learning public health biology.
- Adella Brown and Phyllis O. Brown, who made this book possible. Adella worked on the project from beginning to completion and was involved in every part of the preparation.
- Raluca Popovici, who filled in gaps at critical stages and located references.
- Ayman El-Mohandes, who provided a friendly atmosphere and support.
- Richard Riegelman for his vision, critical thinking, synthesis, and collegiality.

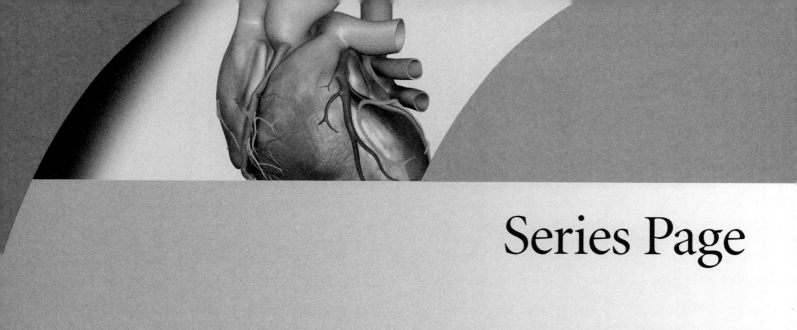

Series Page

See **www.jbpub.com/essentialpublichealth** for the latest information on the series.

Texts in the Essential Public Health Series:

Essentials of Public Health—Bernard J. Turnock, MD, MPH

Essentials of Environmental Health—Robert H. Friis, PhD

Essentials of Health Policy and Law—Joel B. Teitelbaum, JD, LLM, and Sara E. Wilensky, JD, MPP
       With accompanying *Essential Readings in Health Policy and Law*

Essentials of Global Health—Richard Skolnik, MPA

Case Studies in Global Health: Millions Saved—Ruth Levine, PhD, and the
       What Works Working Group

Essentials of Health Behavior: Social and Behavioral Theory in Public Health—Mark Edberg, PhD
       With accompanying *Essential Readings in Health Behavior*

Essentials of Biostatistics—Lisa Sullivan, PhD
       With accompanying Workbook: *Statistical Computations Using Excel*

Epidemiology 101—Robert H. Friis, PhD

Essentials of Infectious Disease Epidemiology—Manya Magnus, PhD, MPH
       With accompanying *Essential Readings in Infectious Disease Epidemiology*

Essentials of Public Health Economics—Diane Dewar, PhD

Essentials of Public Health Biology: A Guide for the Study of Pathophysiology—Constance Urciolo Battle, MD

Essentials of Evidence-Based Public Health— Richard K. Riegelman, MD, MPH, PhD

About the Editor:

Richard K. Riegelman, MD, MPH, PhD, is a professor of Epidemiology-Biostatistics, Medicine, and Health Policy and founding dean at The George Washington University School of Public Health and Health Services in Washington, DC.

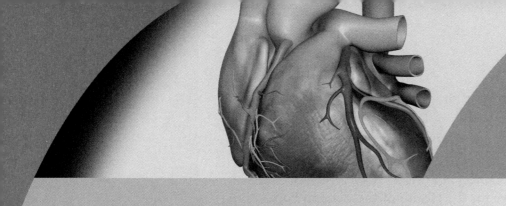

Contents

Part III Concepts of Pathophysiology 223

Chapter 16 Immunizations and Immunity 225

Chapter 17 Inflammation: Understanding Its Role in Acute and Chronic Disease 239

Chapter 18 Why We Stay Well: Stress, Allostasis, and Scientific Integrative Medicine 253

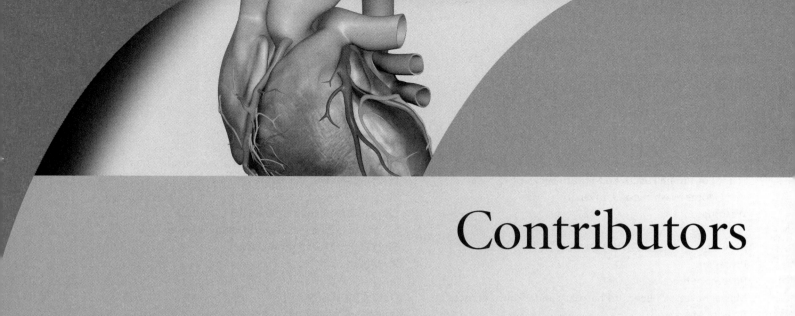

Contributors

Dale Avers, PT, DPT, PhD
Director
Transitional Doctor of Physical Therapy Program
Assistant Professor
Physical Therapy
SUNY Upstate Medical University
Syracuse, NY

Lawrence M. Barat, MD, MPH
Malaria Advisor
U.S. Agency for International Development
Washington, DC

Christopher J. Battle, BA
Clinical Research Coordinator
The Innovative Clinical Research Center
Alexandria, VA

Harolyn M.E. Belcher, MD, MHS
Neurodevelopment Pediatrician
Director of Research
Kennedy Krieger Institute
Family Center
Baltimore, MD

Yanis Ben Amor, PhD
Associate Research Scientist
The Earth Institute
Columbia University
New York, NY

Mary Beth Bigley, DrPH, MSN, ANP
Assistant Professor
Nursing Education
The George Washington University
Washington, DC

Richard A. Billingsley, RN, MSN, MSLS
Adjunct Professor/Coordinator
Information and Instruction
Himmelfarb Health Sciences Library
The George Washington University Medical Center
Washington, DC

Ami Shah Brown, PhD, MPH
Director of Vaccine Operations
Human Hookworm Vaccine Initiative
Assistant Professor
Microbiology, Immunology, and Tropical Medicine
The George Washington University and the Sabin
   Vaccine Institute
Washington, DC

Christina L. Catlett, MD
Associate Director
The Johns Hopkins Office of Critical Event Preparedness
   and Response
Baltimore, MD

James F. Cawley, MPH, PA-C
Professor and Interim Director
Physician Assistant Program
Professor of Prevention and Community Health
School of Public Health and Health Services
The George Washington University
Washington, DC

Judy Cheng, PharmD, MPH, FCCP, BCPS
Professor
Pharmacy Practice
Massachusetts College of Pharmacy and Health Sciences
Boston, MA

Vincent A. Chiappinelli, PhD
The Ralph E. Loewy Professor
Chair
Pharmacology and Physiology
The George Washington University Medical Center
Washington, DC

John M.P. Cmar, MD
Associate Program Director
Johns Hopkins University/Sinai Hospital Program in
    Internal Medicine
Faculty
Divisions of Internal Medicine and Infectious Diseases
Sinai Hospital of Baltimore
Baltimore, MD

Lawrence J. D'Angelo, MD, MPH
Chief
Division of Adolescent and Young Adult Medicine
Director
Burgess Clinic and HIV Services
Children's National Medical Center
Professor of Pediatrics
Medicine, Prevention, and Community Health and
    Epidemiology
The George Washington University
Washington, DC

Ayman El-Mohande
Prevention and Community Health
School of Public Health and Human Services
The George Washington University
Washington, DC

Mark S. Elliott, PhD
Associate Professor
Biochemistry and Molecular Biology
The George Washington University Medical Center
Washington, DC

Frances F. Fiocchi, MPH, DrPH (Cand.)
School of Public Health and Health Services
The George Washington University
Washington, DC

Daniel J. Foley, MS
Epidemiologist
Substance Abuse and Mental Health Services Administration
U.S. Department of Health and Human Services
Rockville, MD

Julia B. Frank, MD
Associate Professor of Psychiatry
Director of Medical Student Education Psychiatry
Psychiatry and Behavioral Sciences
School of Medicine and Health Sciences
The George Washington University
Washington, DC

David S. Goldstein, MD, PhD
Chief
Clinical Neurocardiology Section
Division of Intramural Research
National Institute of Neurological Disorders and Stroke
National Institutes of Health
Bethesda, MD

Tenagne Haile-Mariam, MD
Assistant Professor
Emergency Medicine
School of Medicine and Health Sciences
The George Washington University
Washington, DC

Victoria A. Harden, PhD
Director, Emerita
Office of NIH History
U.S. National Institutes of Health
Bethesda, MD
Scholar in Residence
American University
Washington, DC

Katrina D. Hawkins, MD
Resident in Medicine
Internal Medicine
The George Washington University Medical Center
Washington, DC

Peter J. Hotez, MD, MPH, PhD
President
Sabin Vaccine Institute
Walter G. Ross Professor and Chair
Microbiology, Immunology, and Tropical Medicine
The George Washington University
Washington, DC

Stephen D. Hursting, PhD, MPH, RD
Professor and Margaret McKean Love Chair
Nutrition, Cellular, and Molecular Sciences
University of Texas at Austin
Professor
Carcinogenesis
University of Texas M. D. Anderson Cancer Center
Austin, TX

Cynthia Rose Kahn, MTLS, MPH, AHIP
Reference and Instruction Librarian
Himmelfarb Health Sciences Library
The George Washington University Medical Center
Washington, DC

Michelle M. Kalis, PhD
Professor of Pharmacology
Vice President for Academic Affairs/Provost
Massachusetts College of Pharmacy and Health Sciences
Boston, MA

Karen L. Kemmis, PT, DPT, MS, CDE
Physical Therapist
Physical Medicine and Rehabilitation
SUNY Upstate Medical University
Syracuse, NY

Paul L. Kimmel, MD
Professor
Medicine
The George Washington University Medical Center
Washington, DC

Patricia S. Latham, MD
Associate Professor of Pathology and Medicine
School of Medicine and Health Sciences
The George Washington University
Washington, DC

Jackie A. Lavigne, PhD, MPH
Chief
Office of Education
Division of Cancer Epidemiology and Genetics
National Cancer Institute
National Institutes of Health
Bethesda, MD

Geoffrey S.F. Ling, MD, PhD
Professor and Vice-Chair
Neurology
Uniformed Services University of the Health Sciences
Bethesda, MD

Joseph D. McInerney, MA, MS
Executive Director
National Coalition for Health Professional Education
    in Genetics
Lutherville, MD

Mary Pat McKay, MD, MPH
Associate Professor
Emergency Medicine and Public Health
Director, Center for Injury Prevention and Control
The Ronald Reagan Institute of Emergency Medicine
The George Washington University
Washington, DC

Richard V. Milani, MD
Vice-Chairman
Cardiology
Director
Non-Invasive Laboratories
Ochsner Heart and Vascular Institute
Ochsner Clinic Foundation
New Orleans, LA

Veronica Miller, PhD
Executive Director, Forum for Collaborative HIV Research
Research Professor
Prevention and Community Health
School of Public Health and Health Services
The George Washington University
Washington, DC

Wayne C. Miller, PhD
Professor
Exercise Science
School of Public Health and Health Services
The George Washington University
Washington, DC

Matthew Mintz, MD
Associate Professor of Medicine
School of Medicine and Health Sciences
The George Washington University
Washington, DC

Randall K. Packer, PhD
Professor of Biology
Biological Sciences
The George Washington University
Washington, DC

David M. Parenti, MD
Professor
Medicine, Microbiology, Immunology, and Tropical Medicine
Division of Infectious Diseases
The George Washington University Medical Center
Washington, DC

Pamela Zubow Poe, PhD, MA
Research Scientist
Health Promotion Research Center
University of Washington
Seattle, WA

Raluca Popovici, MPH
School of Public Health and Health Services
The George Washington University
Washington, DC

Sudhindra Pudur, MD, MBBS
Fellow
Renal Diseases
The George Washington University Medical Center
Washington, DC

Sophia Raff, MPH
Executive Coordinator
Medicine, Microbiology, Immunology, and Tropical Medicine
The George Washington University Medical Center
Washington, DC

Ronald G. Riechers, II, MD
Assistant Professor
Neurology
Uniformed Services University of the Health Sciences
Bethesda, MD

Sabrina Roundtree, MPH
Public Health Practitioner
Morgan State University
Baltimore, MD

Richard H. Schlagel, PhD
Elton Professor of Philosophy Emeritus
Philosophy
The George Washington University
Washington, DC

Christopher Scott, IV, MS
Medical Student
School of Medicine and Health Sciences
The George Washington University
Washington, DC

Sylvia Silver, DA
Associate Dean for Health Sciences
Professor
Pathology
The George Washington University Medical Center
Washington, DC

Gary L. Simon, MD, PhD
Walter G. Ross Professor of Medicine
Director
Division of Infectious Diseases
Vice Chairman
Medicine
The George Washington University School of Medicine
Washington, DC

Carol A. Smith, MS
Assistant Professor
Pathology
Clinical Laboratory Science Program
The George Washington University
Washington, DC

E. Richard Stiehm, MD
Professor
Pediatrics
University of California, Los Angeles School of Medicine
Los Angeles, CA

Elaine J. Sullo, MLS, MAEd, AHIP
Reference and Instruction Librarian
Himmelfarb Health Sciences Library
The George Washington University Medical Center
Washington, DC

Brian A. Szekely, BA, MS (Cand.)
Biomedical Science and Pathobiology
Virginia Polytechnic Institute and State University
Blacksburg, VA

Michael J. Tabacco, MS, DDS
Assistant Clinical Professsor of Prosthodontics
Restorative Dentistry
School of Dentistry, University of Maryland
Baltimore, MD

Mellen Duffy Tanamly, MSPH
Adjunct Assistant Professor
Prevention and Community Health
School of Public Health and Health Services
The George Washington University Medical Center
Washington, DC

Elizabeth Tedrow, BS
Resource Development Coordinator
Self Reliance Foundation
Acesso Hispano
Washington, DC

Cynthia M. Tracy, MD
Professor of Medicine
Associate Director of Cardiology
Director of Electrophysiology
Medicine
The George Washington University Medical Center
Washington, DC

Michele N. Wagner, MPH
National Sleep Foundation
Washington, DC

Daniel Webb, MPH
School of Public Health and Health Services
The George Washington University
Washington, DC

Jennifer A. Weber, RD, MPH
Manager, National Nutrition Policy
American Dietetic Association
Washington, DC

Patience H. White, MD, MA
Chief Public Health Officer, Arthritis Foundation
Professor of Medicine and Pediatrics
Division of Rheumatology
The George Washington University Medical Center
Washington, DC

Tareq A. Yousef, BS
School of Public Health and Health Services
The George Washington University
Washington, DC

Special Contributions

Joseph F. Pauley, B.S.Ed.
Adjunct Professor, Education Leadership Program
George Mason University
President, Process Communications, Inc.
Potomac, MD

Richard A. Billingsley, RN, MSN, MSLS
Adjunct Professor/Coordinator
Information and Instruction
Himmelfarb Health Sciences Library
The George Washington University Medical Center
Washington, DC

Kristina Krupincza, BS
School of Public Health and Health Services
The George Washington University
Washington, DC

Daniel Adam Lyons, BS, BA
University of Missouri–Columbia
Kansas City, MO

Tareq A. Yousef, BS
School of Public Health and Health Services
The George Washington University
Washington, DC

Daniel Webb, MPH
School of Public Health and Health Services
The George Washington University
Washington, DC

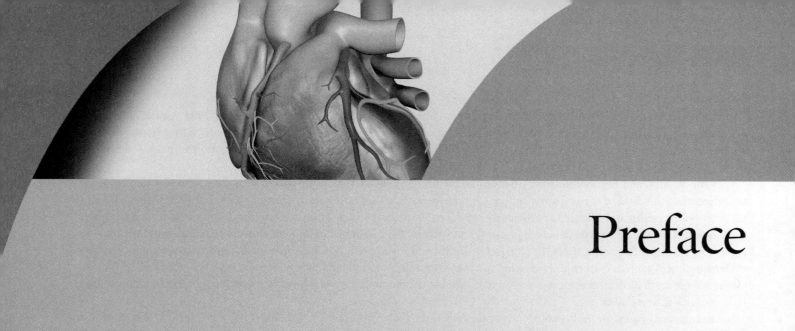

Preface

- Why this textbook?
- Background
- Purpose for (or of) compiling this book
- Overview
- The compilation and editing process
- The contributing authors
- Ancillaries

Understanding how and why illness and the manifestations of a disease occur and incorporating this knowledge into public health decision-making is the very essence of public health practice.

WHY THIS TEXTBOOK?

Excellent pathophysiology textbooks abound in multiple editions, aimed mainly at nursing, exercise science, and health science students. Almost any one of these two dozen or so comprehensive texts could be utilized effectively by instructors educating students in the basic scientific concepts, mechanisms, and principles of human biology.

None of these two dozen U.S. major texts, however, places pathophysiology within the context of the disciplines and profession of public health. This textbook is a science-based biology and clinical guide book that can stand alone or can be used by instructors as an adjunct to their favorite pathophysiology textbook.

BACKGROUND

There are three important characteristics of students today who choose to pursue the study of public health. *First*, even at the undergraduate and graduate levels, they have recognized and acknowledged with Thomas Friedman that the world is indeed flat.[1] These students understand that the great changes taking place in our time due to advances in technology and communication put people all over the globe in touch as never before with both positive and negative consequences. This global awareness draws them to undertake studies in public health.

In 2003, the Institute of Medicine, in *Who Will Keep the Public Healthy? Educating Public Health Professionals for the 21st Century*, recommended that **all** undergraduate students should have access to education in public health, not just dedicated public health majors and master's students.[2] In fact, the *second* aspect of note is that today, undergraduate students across the country and from all sorts of majors and schools are seeking to elect a course or two in public health out of conviction or curiosity.[3–5]

The *third* aspect is that today's public health students do not come to this study with clinical backgrounds as once was the case. Consequently, the study of biology is essential now.

Biology (and other closely related sciences) is the foundational discipline for a public health practitioner. A basic understanding of the essentials of public health biology is the *sine qua non* for the introductory student as the cornerstone upon which rest all the other five core discipline areas (biostatistics, epidemiology, environmental health sciences, health policy and management, and social and behavioral sciences).

Turnock, Afifi, and Breslow maintain that one of the unique characteristics of public health study, and one that continues to differentiate this field of study from other social movements or social action, is its grounding in science.[6,7] The relationship between public health and science is particularly clear for the medical and physical sciences that govern our understanding of the biological aspects of humans, microorganisms, and vectors. This relationship also governs the risks present in our physical environment. Turnock further states that the public health and science connection is true for the other sciences that affect our understanding of human culture and behavior and thereby influence health and illness, namely, the social sciences.[6] It is necessary to appreciate that anthropology, sociology, and psychology help us to understand **how** human culture and behavior profoundly influence health and illness.

The purpose of a major multiyear project of the American Society of Zoology, *Science as a Way of Knowing*[8] was to provide background materials to those who taught introductory biology courses, for they have both the responsibility and opportunity to prepare students to function in a world that is dominated by science and technology. The study of biology as a science for public health students is a *way of knowing*, of understanding, of learning to think critically, and of going deeper, and of preparing one's self to ask and finally to address complex interdisciplinary questions. These processes help public health practitioners recognize flaws in their thinking about biological information.

Through a comprehensive, multidisciplinary effort, the Association of Schools of Public Health's Education Committee has produced a document outlining the core Master's of Public Health *competencies*.[9,10] The final set, updated in 2007, included the five core disciplines mentioned earlier and added a second group of integrated and interdisciplinary cross-cutting set of overall competency domains that included public health biology.[11] Further, public health biology illustrative **sub-competencies** were posted in June 2007.[12]

Thus, in the past as well as today, through multidisciplinary effort, the field of public health has been rooted in science. Public health is a scientific endeavor that begins by understanding its own biological and molecular context.

PURPOSE FOR (OR OF) COMPILING THIS TEXTBOOK

The intent of this book is to present a dynamic approach to the study of biology rather than to impart a static body of knowledge. I will not dare to suggest that facts are not essential, nor would I ever go so far as Samuel McChord Crothers did.[13] In a chapter entitled, "The Anglo-American School of Polite Unlearning," he stressed the importance of unlearning. The idea was whimsically carried forward by Russell Backer in an essay in which he suggested founding a University of Un-Learning and proposed that a Non-Bachelor of Un-Arts would be awarded to students who clearly manifested their ignorance of factual knowledge.[14] Baker points to the importance of an *approach* to learning rather than rote memorization. My intention with this textbook is to provide an approach to the study of the biology of public health that goes way beyond memorizing facts.

In a critical look at our future, Sterling points to a speech given almost two hundred years ago by Ralph Waldo Emerson, who said that a scholar has the obligation to "organize knowledge into verifiable, sensible, and schematic fashion."[15,16] Likewise, students of public health have the same obligation to organize their knowledge of biology in a verifiable, sensible, and schematic fashion so that they can convey it to others in a variety of settings.

My goal in writing this book both for the student and the instructor is to create a bridge between the study of biology and the study of public health biology.

Components of the approach that I have included are:

- Applying principles of biology to issues of public health
- Developing critical thinking skills
- Rooting information in a historical perspective
- Emphasizing an integrative approach to the study of biology
- Recognizing how changes in the individual manifest themselves across the human lifespan
- Considering biologists' proximate and evolutionary causes of diseases[17]
- Assessing the impact of scale: looking at things from the next largest frame of reference and the next smallest
- Envisioning the next fifty years: What are the unintended consequences of what we do or fail to do today?

- Analyzing not only the causes of disease but also the evolution of our understanding of those causes
- Appreciating that there is also an evolution of our understanding of what public health is, can do, and can do potentially

OVERVIEW

[Essentials] of Public Health Biology augments teaching pathophysiology by contextualizing it within a broad public health framework and perspective. It is appropriate for introductory students in public health at both the undergraduate and graduate levels. It also can be used by any undergraduate student interested in exploring the underpinnings of public health.

This book is organized into six units. The first unit addresses the underlying concepts of health and disease, using some alternate or different ways of looking at the different layers of complexity. The second unit addresses outcomes and applications of human behavior. The third unit addresses alterations in body physiology and pathophysiology that result from disease or injury. The fourth unit is devoted to the topic of infectious diseases, both the future as well as the past of public health. The fifth unit addresses the chronic diseases that have gained ascendancy since the mid-1950s. The sixth and final unit addresses some necessary professional skills for practitioners of public health.

Insofar as possible, each chapter addresses the following:

- significant or startling facts
- history/overview/introduction
- basic science facts/key concepts review
- case studies: scenario, defining the issues, patient's understanding
- clinical and public health perspectives
- questions for further research, study, reflection, and discussion
- exercises/activities
- Healthy People 2010
- key terms
- references
- resources
- cross references to other chapters

A major overarching theme is an emphasis on the comparison between the clinical perspective and the public health perspective, between medicine and public health. Other themes, explicit or embedded in most chapters, include: fundamental, indispensable biological facts; major issues and challenges to the health of the public; developmental perspectives across the lifespan; historical perspectives; Healthy People 2010 objectives; and childhood origins of adult diseases.

Two sections of each chapter in particular (**Basic Science Facts/Key Concepts Review** and **Public Health Perspective**) will be a useful summary/review for master's degree students in public health who are preparing for the certifying examination. These students are also encouraged to review the study guides on the Web site of the National Board of Public Health Examiners available in 2008.[18] The competencies and sub-competencies developed by the ASPH Education Committee can be found in the **Ancillaries** to this book for instructors and students. A grid prepared for this textbook for all introductory students is also posted on the Web site to assist students in focusing on the important biological aspects of public health.

THE COMPILATION AND EDITING PROCESS

It has been said that the process of compiling a book teaches the editor most of all. I have learned a great deal from this project. Working with sixty-five authors of forty-five chapters was an enriching experience for me. Intending that their individuality be allowed to shine through these pages, I provided only the format for each chapter and made only one request, namely that the authors adhere to it insofar as was feasible. I further intended that the wide variety of subjects be juxtaposed to demonstrate their essential similarities and complementarities in moving the student from conceptualizing the field of biology to conceptualizing the field of public health biology. One editor recently tried this technique with a novel by passing his book through the hands of fifteen Irish authors, each of whom contributed one chapter of the book.[19] As he did, I tried to keep the flow cohesive throughout. My textbook also has a strong central plot line, advancing smoothly from section to section: it is critical to study biology as an underpinning to studying the field of public health. Once students understand biology, they must make the shift to grasping the elements of public health biology. My strongest wish is that this textbook will assist students by informing their decision-making as they take their next step toward their public health practice.

THE CONTRIBUTING AUTHORS

The levels of education of the authors range from undergraduate and master's level students (the target audiences) all the way to senior researchers with dual doctoral degrees. The contributing authors gave generously of their time and effort because of their conviction of the importance of understanding the biological basis of disease, and they made great effort to distill their vast knowledge and experience. For all this work I am grateful. The totality of their work sends the student to the next level with a strong foundation.

I have taught the Biologic Basis of Disease, a foundational course in the public health curriculum at the School of Public Health and Health Services of The George Washington University, to introductory students for the past five years. For over two decades, I served as the medical director and CEO of a 130-bed hospital for severely disabled children from birth to age 21. At this hospital, I attempted to provide the best outcomes for conditions that were the result of public health failures: prematurity, environmental exposures, nutritional deficiencies, intentional and unintentional injury, poisoning, infectious diseases, and many others. I realized that I was working on the wrong end of health care: how much better for these vulnerable children if their conditions had been prevented in the first place.

ANCILLARIES

Jones and Bartlett Publishers offers additional online supplements to assist instructors and aid students in mastering public health biology. These materials are available for download from the text's web site: http://www.jbpub.com/essentialpublic health/battle/.

Instructors, please contact your sales representative to learn more.

Online Resources:

___

FOR INSTRUCTORS:

- **Instructor's Manual** is provided as a text file and contains a sample syllabus, weekly homework assignments and samples, a list of my epigraphs (encapsulating my teaching philosophy) to the course that I teach, and teaching suggestions.
- **Major Integrating Homework Assignments and Samples:**
  - Critical thinking exercises
  - Understanding disease causation exercise
  - Essay topics and student samples
  - PowerPoint presentation of Mind Mapping and exercises
  - Miscellaneous exercises that suggest varied ways of thinking
  - Suggested interdisciplinary questions
- **Test Bank** is available as a text file. Multiple choice questions are provided for most chapters, where appropriate.
- **Answer Keys/Instructor's Guidelines** for each chapter's three levels of questions.
- **Answer Keys/Instructor's Guidelines** for each chapter's exercises/activities.
- **PowerPoint Lecture Outline Slides Presentation Packet** provides lecture notes for each applicable chapter. These materials can be customized by the instructor.
- **Informatics: Additional Overarching Exercises with Guidance for Instructors for Parts 1 through 5 and PowerPoint Lecture on Informatics.** This material provides instructors with additional strategies and exercises for their students to use for each section of the book. This material will reinforce and enrich the development of student skills in learning where and how to search for professional information beyond the exercises in each individual chapter.
- **Core Competencies in Public Health Biology:**
  - **Association of Schools of Public Health**
    - Masters Degree in Public Health Core Competency Development Project Version 2.3
    - Public Health Biology Illustrative Sub-Competencies

- ○ Student Perceptions of Why it is Important to Study Public Health Biology
- ○ **Cross Reference Grid Between Chapters and Competencies**

FOR STUDENTS:
- **Core Competencies in Public Health Biology:**
  - ○ **Association of Schools of Public Health**
    - – Masters Degree in Public Health Core Competency Development Project Version 2.3
    - – Public Health Biology Illustrative Sub-Competencies
  - ○ **Cross Reference Grid Between Chapters and Competencies**

Constance Urciolo Battle, MD
School of Public Health and Health Services
The George Washington University
Washington, DC

REFERENCES

1. Friedman TL. *The World Is Flat: A Brief History of the Twenty-First Century.* New York: Farrar, Straus and Giroux; 2006.
2. Institute of Medicine. *Who Will Keep the Public Healthy? Educating Public Health Professionals for the 21st Century.* Washington, DC: National Academics Press, 2003:144.
3. Riegelman RK. Undergraduate public health education: supporting the future of public health. *J Public Health Manage Pract* 2007;13:237–238.
4. Wahl PW. Public health education in the 21st century: topics and trends. *Public Health Rep* 2007;122:828–831.
5. Riegelman RK, Albertine S, Persily NA. *The Educated Citizen and Public Health: A Consensus Report on Public Health and Undergraduate Education.* Council of Arts and Science, October 2007.
6. Turnock BJ. *Public Health: What It Is and How It Works.* Sudbury, MA: Jones and Bartlett; 2004:19.
7. Afifi AA, Breslow L. The maturing paradigm of public health. *Ann Rev Public Health* 1994;15:223–235.
8. American Society of Zoologists. *Science as a Way of Knowing.* VII Centennial meeting, Boston; December 1989.
9. Association of the Schools of Public Health. MPH Core Competency Development Project. Version 2.3 Introduction to the Model. Available at http://www.asph.org/document.cfm?page=851. Accessed May 29, 2008.
10. Association of the Schools of Public Health. MPH Core Competency Development Project. Version 2.3 Competency Resources. Available at http://www.asph.org/document.cfm?page=935. Accessed May 29, 2008.
11. Association of the Schools of Public Health Education Committee. Master's degree in public health core competency development project. Version 2.3. Available at http://www.asph.org/userfiles/version2.3.pdf. Accessed May 29, 2008.
12. Association of the Schools of Public Health. Public Health Biology Illustrative Sub-competencies. Available at http://www.asph.org/document.cfm?page=928. Accessed May 29, 2008.
13. McChord Crothers S. *Among Friends.* New York: Houghton Mifflin; 1910:25–63.
14. Selles R, Quealy G, O'Connell B, Mahoney S, Leopold AK, eds. *Fifty Things to Do When You Turn Fifty.* New York: Sellers Publishers, Inc.; 2005.
15. Sterling B. *Tomorrow Now: Envisioning the Next 50 Years.* New York: Random House; 2003:48.
16. Sacks KS. *Understanding Emerson: "The American Scholar" and His Struggle for Self-Reliance* (chapt 1). Princeton, NJ: Princeton University Press.
17. Nesse RM, Williams GC. *Why We get Sick: The New Science of Darwinian Medicine.* New York: Vintage Books; 1994:6–7.
18. National Board of Public Health Examiners. Available at http://www.publichealthexam.org/. Accessed May 29, 2008.
19. O'Connor J, ed. *Yeats Is Dead! A Mystery by 15 Irish Writers.* New York: Alfred A Knopf; 2001.

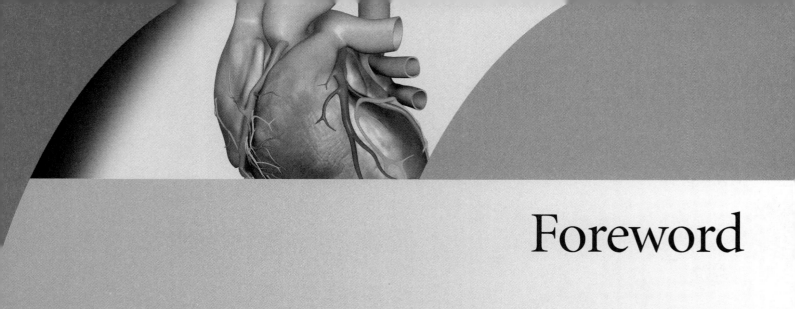

Foreword

This textbook is intended to assist students in public health in their understanding of the pathogenesis of various disease conditions and to identify critical points at which such pathogenesis could either be prevented or interrupted. Infectious, nutritional, metabolic, genetic, and environmental risks are examined as they may compromise human health independently or in combination. The impact of such risks on various organ systems is discussed, including multi-organ system involvement in complex disease models.

The impact of public health as a discipline is measured by its success in promoting health and preventing illnesses and their complications. This discipline engages a variety of professional and technical skills toward a common goal. The efficacy of public health interventions, at an individual or community level, whether biological, psychosocial, or behavioral in nature, is directly influenced by the depth of understanding of the origins, natural history, and clinical manifestations of disease. Professionals in all of the domains of public health must be conversant in the various health risk models in order to maximize the link between health policy, intervention program, and health outcome.

Dr. Battle, as an editor to this text, has assembled a formidable list of authors with a wide spectrum of experience and significant professional credibility. They have contributed knowledge and personal expertise to a comprehensive list of topics that integrate the concepts mentioned above. I wish the reader of this text enjoyment and success and I feel confident that the content will forward your careers in the field.

Ayman El-Mohandes, MBBCh, MD, MPH
Professor and Chairman of Prevention and Community Health
School of Public Health and Health Service
The George Washington University
Washington, DC

Prologue

Essentials of Public Health Biology is a unique contribution to the Essential Public Health series. Dr. Battle has built upon her extensive teaching experience to extend the series in an important new direction. *Essentials of Public Health Biology* reconnects public health with its biological roots and builds its future foundations. During the late 1900s and first half of the 20th century, public health was an applied laboratory science closely connected with the biological revolution that transformed science and society. Infectious diseases, nutritional diseases, and understanding of human growth and development provided the biological underpinnings for public health applications that transformed and extended life so dramatically in the century before World War II.

The last half of the 20th century, with its miracle cures and other temporary triumphs, took public health away from a focus on biology. The 21st century is rapidly bringing public health back to biology not only in infectious diseases, nutrition, and human growth and development but also in genetics, cognitive sciences, and a range of other areas that are now ready for applications that respond to new needs and new opportunities.

Connecting biology and public health is especially important for two groups of students who increasingly make up a clear majority of public health students: undergraduate students and masters degree students pursuing the core competencies. The undergraduate public health movement began in response to the Institute of Medicine's recommendation that " . . . *all* undergraduates should have access to education in public health." Taking the "all" seriously has meant that public health must be seen as essential to becoming an educated citizen. Connecting biology and public health is central to the development of educated citizens who can understand and address today's and tomorrow's public health issues.

The re-incorporation of biology into graduate public health education has received a recent boost from the designation of public health biology as a cross-cutting competency by the Association of Schools of Public Health and the formal incorporation of public health biology into the certifying examination of the National Board of Public Health Examiners. Dr. Battle's book provides a useful framework for exploring these competencies. In addition, she has provided guidance for graduate students who wish to use the *Essentials of Public Health Biology* as a key component of their preparation for the certifying examination.

Take a look at the impressive range of topics and the equally impressive array of authors who have contributed to this book. Dr. Battle has done a service to students by gathering together these authors and structuring their contributions in a consistent and accessible manner. The *Essentials of Public Health Biology* fulfills a key role in the Essential Public Health series. I am confident that you, like Dr. Battle's students, will find it useful whether you are an undergraduate beginning your study of public health or a graduate student stepping back and putting it all together.

Richard K. Riegelman, MD, MPH, PhD
Series Editor—Essential Public Health

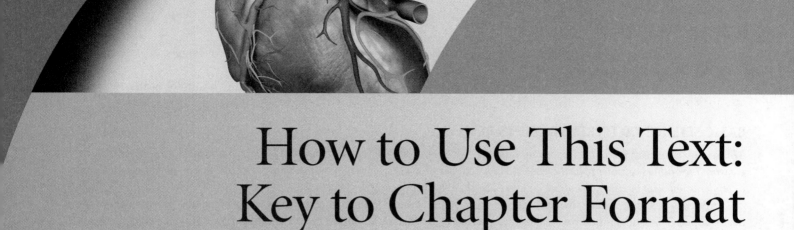

How to Use This Text: Key to Chapter Format

Insofar as possible, the chapters follow the format outlined below. Chapter 31, Avian and Seasonal Influenza, by Cmar and Simon, is used as an example. Italicized explanations are provided for each section.

CHAPTER TITLE

BOXED FACT

Each chapter begins with a salient, significant, or startling fact which stresses the public health importance of this topic.

> The first pandemic clearly consistent with influenza occurred in 1580, which spread from Asia to Europe via North Africa, resulting in over 8,000 dead in Rome and near-total mortality in several Spanish cities.[1]

LEARNING OBJECTIVES

The author lists learning objectives:

By the end of this chapter, students will be able to:

- Understand the basic science topics relevant to the public health ramifications of a possible influenza pandemic, especially:
    - the role of antigenic drift and shift in pandemic influenza
    - the use of antiviral medications for treatment and prophylaxis of influenza
    - the role of vaccines in the prevention of influenza infection
- Identify both important clinical features and public health concerns in a real-world case involving a possible influenza outbreak.

HISTORY/OVERVIEW/INTRODUCTION

Included in this section is a brief notation of important, relevant historical facts; or major public health milestones; or general survey of the topic; or a preliminary discussion.

As illustrated by the above fact, influenza has been a persistent global threat to human life and health for nearly 500 years. The 1918 influenza pandemic killed 50 to 100 million people worldwide, and over 549,000 in the United States alone . . . .

BASIC SCIENCE FACTS/KEY CONCEPTS REVIEW

This section is an overview of the important material and/or one aspect of the topic, including charts, pathways, and schemata. It covers what the authors consider to be the essential information for students to retain. In most instances, this section will be a supplement as students will also be using one of the major textbooks of pathophysiology.

Influenza has long been associated with issues of public health. Indeed, in many ways it represents the prototypical public health concern. Seasonal influenza, an illness associated with substantial morbidity and significant mortality, is a predictable and persistent threat to both individual well-being and societal resources . . . .

CASE STUDY

This section tells the story of a patient indicating sex, race, age, and occupation. It also defines the issues and describes what the patient and family understand.

Scenario

Mr. A is a 35-year-old man of Vietnamese descent who presented to his outpatient physician with a three day history of cough, fever, and myalgias. He is physically fit, with no past medical history, and currently takes no medications or supplements . . . .

Defining the Issues

There are several issues presented in this scenario. Mr. A was unwilling to engage in routine health care, and so neither received a seasonal influenza vaccination, nor sought medical advice prior to travel back to Vietnam . . . .

Patient's Understanding

Mr. A's understanding of the medical issues involved in this case is quite poor. He is concerned with supporting his family over his own personal health and appears to have little insight into the fact that he may be infected with a communicable disease that he could easily transmit to both his family and to the students with whom he works . . . .

CLINICAL PERSPECTIVE FOR THE INDIVIDUAL PATIENT AND THE HEALTHCARE PROVIDER

In this section, the author will include considerations about diagnosis and various intervention levels that can be tried in the present as well as what might have worked earlier or prevented the condition. Levels of prevention: 1, 2, 3.

Level of Intervention Now

Mr. A has an illness that is clinically consistent with influenza. Excluding other possible infectious etiologies, there are two options that might be considered relative to this episode, namely, seasonal influenza or avian influenza . . . .

Potential Level Earlier

Mr. A has had symptoms for three days. Therapy should be simply supportive because he is well beyond the 24-hour window in which antiviral therapy with oseltamivir could alter the course of his disease . . . .

PUBLIC HEALTH PERSPECTIVE FOR THE HEALTH OF THE GENERAL POPULATION AND OF HIGH RISK GROUPS

This section contrasts the public health perspective from the clinical perspective and includes what can be done to promote, protect, and maintain health and to prevent disease, injury, and disability in the population through organized community effort.

Mr. A's cousin, immediate family, and the students and their family members who were potentially exposed in the dormitory constitute high risk groups in this scenario . . . .

KEY TERMS

Key terms are listed and defined in the chapters as well as in the Glossary at the end of the book.

Biology/Clinical/Scientific Terms

Antigenic Drift: Minor genetic changes to circulating influenza viruses that occur seasonally and cause small, localized outbreaks of varying severity and extent.

Public Health Terms

Pandemic Influenza: Influenza virus that has spread to cause epidemic disease on a continental or worldwide level, regardless of source (i.e., avian).

QUESTIONS FOR FURTHER RESEARCH, STUDY, REFLECTION, AND DISCUSSION

For the Individual Student

*The purpose of these questions is to motivate the student to seek additional or deeper information about the material in the **Basic Science Facts/Key Concepts Review** section.*

In order to answer these questions, it may be necessary to research the primary literature.

- What are other described varieties of **avian influenza** beyond H5N1 that have caused outbreaks in humans, and what have been the impacts of those outbreaks?

For Small Group Discussion

These questions allow students to delve into the Case Study and assure that the small group understands the causes and the multiple implications and ramifications on the patient and the family microcosm.

- Discuss practical ways for public institutions to encourage someone in Mr. A's situation to practice meticulous hand hygiene and to appropriately cover coughs/wear a mask to prevent transmission of influenza to others.

For Entire Class Discussion

*Through these **Public Health Perspective** questions, the class will consider the impact of individual illnesses/diseases on the population and the impact of major crises/epidemics resulting from this condition on the health of the present and future populations, on national resources, and services available or needed.*

- Discuss options for companies, both in terms of sick leave policy and providing **barrier precautions** (masks, gloves, etc. . .) to employees, in order to responsibly prevent transmission of influenza in an outbreak or pandemic setting among its employees, without penalizing said employees through compulsory leave without pay or possible termination of employment.

EXERCISES/ACTIVITIES

This section includes any additional activities outside the classroom, including field trips (to agencies, health clinics, and national/international organizations), group research, role playing, and development of presentations for the entire class, which could add to the understanding of the group and the class.

Each class member should assume the role of one of the people involved in the case above, from the following list: Mr. A, Mr. A's girlfriend, the physician, a college student, a parent of one of the students, and Mr. A's cousin . . . .

HEALTHY PEOPLE 2010

This section lists what the author considers to be the most important relevant indicators, focus areas, goals, or objectives in Healthy People 2010.

Healthy People 2010

Indicator: Immunization

Focus Area: Immunization and Infectious Diseases

Goal: Prevent disease, disability, and death from infectious diseases, including vaccine-preventable diseases.

Objectives:

14-1. Reduce or eliminate indigenous cases of vaccine-preventable diseases

14-29. Increase the proportion of adults who are vaccinated annually against influenza and ever vaccinated against pneumococcal disease

REFERENCES AND RESOURCES

*These two sections include the **References** (specific citations) and **Resources** recommended for further exploration.*

RESOURCES

Belshe RB. The origins of pandemic influenza—lessons from the 1918 virus. *N Engl J Med* 2005;353:2209–2211.

Centers for Disease Control. Avian Influenza (Bird Flu). (2007). Available at http://www.cdc.gov/flu/avian/. Accessed May 29, 2008.

CROSS REFERENCES

This section indicates any other topics addressed in this textbook that might add to the students' understanding of the disease or condition discussed in this chapter.

Behavioral Determinants of Health

Information-Seeking Strategies in Public Health

The Public Health Triad

About the Author

Constance Urciolo Battle, MD, has been an Adjunct Professor of Prevention and Community Health in the School of Public Health and Health Services since 2003 and a Clinical Professor of Pediatrics in the School of Medicine and Health Sciences at The George Washington University and a member of the academic staff at Children's National Medical Center since 1977. In 2006–2007, Dr. Battle served as Director of the Undergraduate Program in Public Health. Dr. Battle has formerly served as President of the Medical School Alumni Association, President of the George Washington Alumni Association, as well as a Trustee of the University.

Dr. Battle was Chief Executive Officer and Medical Director of the Hospital for Sick Children in Washington, DC, from 1973–1995. The Hospital, which was founded in 1883, is one of approximately twenty hospitals in the country dedicated to pediatric rehabilitation and transitional care and the only hospital of its kind in the metropolitan Washington area. During Dr. Battle's administration, the Hospital kept pace with the latest technology and became a model for other pediatric facilities that provide care to children with disabilities, developmental delays, and chronic illness.

After receiving an undergraduate degree in chemistry from Trinity College, Dr. Battle graduated from The George Washington University School of Medicine and Health Science. She completed her internship and residency in pediatrics at Rochester General and Strong Memorial Hospitals of the University of Rochester in New York. In 1972, she was awarded a Health Services and Research Fellowship from the U.S. Department of Health, Education and Welfare for study at the Center of Health Administration Studies of the University of Chicago's Graduate School of Business. During 1993–1994, Dr. Battle was a fellow in the Creating Healthier Communities Fellowship of the Healthcare Forum. Her fellowship project, which focused on HIV/AIDS adolescent mothers and their children, evolved into the Minority Adolescent Community Initiative (MACI), a collaborative effort between the National Institutes of Health and the Hospital for Sick Children. Dr. Battle was appointed the Principal Investigator of the MACI Project.

Throughout her career as a physician, Dr. Battle has focused on pediatric and adolescent health care for children with disabilities or chronic illness and she is active in many professional organizations that advocate on their behalf. Dr. Battle completed a two-year term as President of the Association for the Care of Children's Health, an international membership and advocacy group that is dedicated to psychosocially sound, developmentally appropriate, and family-centered health care for children. She served on both the Section for Rehabilitation Hospitals and Related Institutions and on the Governing Council of the Section for Rehabilitation Hospitals and Programs of the American Hospital Association and she also served as chairman of the Scientific Review Board of Children's Hospice International, which developed guidelines for pediatric hospice care. She is a member of the Children with Disabilities Section of the American Academy of

Pediatrics and was elected to the Governing Council of the Section of Maternal and Child Health of the American Hospital Association. As President of the DC Hospital Association, Dr. Battle worked closely with District of Columbia hospital administrators to address the profound changes that confront healthcare.

During 1997, Dr. Battle served as Interim Director of the Child Development Center of the Department of Pediatrics of the Howard University School of Medicine. Before returning to The George Washington University in 2003, she served as Executive Director of the Foundation for the National Institute of Health. Currently, Dr. Battle is a consultant for the Multidisciplinary Team for the Infants and Toddlers Program at the Lt. J.P. Kennedy Institute, in Washington DC. In 2005 and 2008, Dr. Battle received the Excellence in Teaching Award for The George Washington University's Undergraduate Public Health Program.

The Alumni Volunteer Award of The George Washington University Alumni Association and the President's Medal for Distinguished Community Service of The Catholic University of America have acknowledged Dr. Battle's many years of service to the community. In 1993, she was named a Washingtonian of the Year by *Washingtonian* magazine. She was included in an exhibition at the National Library of Medicine: Changing the Face of Medicine, Celebrating America's Women Physicians. The exhibition ran from 2003–2005 before traveling around the country.

Dr. Battle is the mother of three children: Ursula, Bill, and Christopher. Her leisure activities include travel, music, reading, and philately.

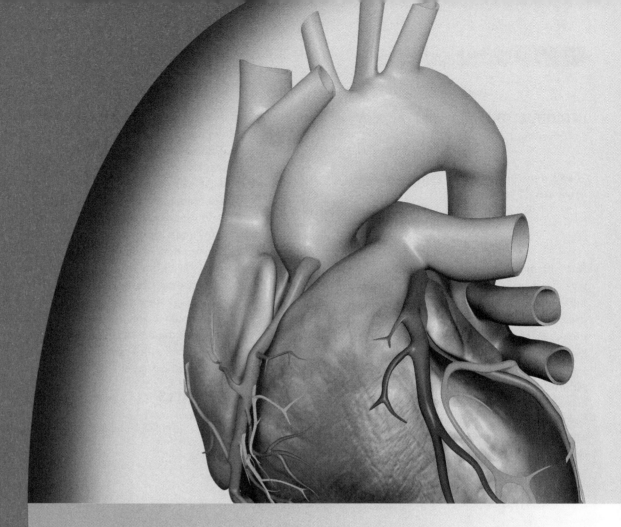

PART I

Concepts of Health and Disease in Public Health

INTRODUCTION

Constance Battle

"I seek a method by which teachers teach less and learners learn more."[1]

—Johann Amos Comenius (1592–1670)
Author of the first illustrated textbook and
father of modern education

Part I attempts to make sure that education occurs by illustrating diverse ways for students to explore assorted themes around the science of human life on earth. By no means all-inclusive, these six chapters suggest additional or alternate ways to approach learning biology as a preparation for understanding health and disease.

The book begins as it should with history, with one philosopher-historian's insistence that science is **the** way of knowing. A second chapter maintains that students must go beyond biology to its fundamental level: to biochemistry. Three other chapters address the interactive and relative contributions of human genetics, individual behaviors, and the constantly changing environment—all major areas of inquiry for biologists. The interactions among germs, genes, geography, and human behavior have resulted in a marked increased in life expectancy over the last century, addressed in the chapter on aging. Finally, the remaining two chapters suggest new ways of thinking about disease causation: some diseases ameliorate others and some diseases are drug-induced.

In summary, these six chapters address several of the main disciplines that, when combined, reveal different interpretive, contributory approaches to understanding biological sciences, medical science, disease causation, science of ecology, science of epidemiology, the study of history, and the behavioral sciences.

I encourage you to read these chapters as Francis Bacon would have you do: "read not to contradict and confute; nor to believe and take for granted; nor to find talk and discourse; but to weigh and consider."[2]

REFERENCES

1. Comenius JA. *Opera Didactica Omnia*. Amsterdam, NL; 1657.

2. Bacon F. Of Studies. In: Pitcher J, ed. The Essays of Francis Bacon. New York: Penguin Group; 1625.

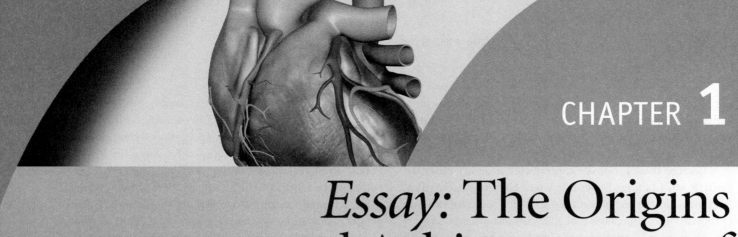

CHAPTER 1

Essay: The Origins and Achievements of Modern Science

Richard H. Schlagel

There is no human endeavor, whether it be artistic, musical, literary, political, or legal, more important than the acquisition of knowledge. Even morality depends upon understanding the principles, choices, and consequences of ethical behavior. The only reliable means so far for attaining knowledge is the scientific method. It has lifted humanity from a state of complete ignorance to some understanding of the universe and control of events.

For primitive humans, the causes of nearly everything were unknown: the origin and order of the universe; the nature of human conception and embryological development; the structure and function of our organs; the explanation of fire, lightning, and thunder; the nature of matter, energy, and chemical processes; the cause of diseases, plagues, and other natural disasters; the formation of the earth's topology; how inherited characteristics are acquired and transmitted, and so forth. Lacking more effective explanations, humans created mythical narratives to account for phenomena, such as Prometheus bringing fire or Zeus throwing thunderbolts, or they adopted as a model of explanation the most familiar form of causality, that human acts are intentional, willed, or commanded. Thus, phenomena were intentionally caused by "evil spirits," "demons," "guardian angels," or "deities," and supplications in the form of human or animal sacrifices were common.

THE GREEKS

The one ancient society capable of piercing the veil of myth and casting aside anthropomorphism was the ancient Greeks, who eventually sought natural, as opposed to supernatural, explanations. In the sixth century BC, Anaximander began the tradition with his theory that the present universe arose from a previous state of chaos by a process of "separation," not by an act of god. Subsequent Greek theories foreshadowed later developments of science: the Pythagorean claim that the numerical harmonies underlying the musical scale also generated the order of the cosmos; Empedocles' doctrine that fire, earth, air, and water constituted the four basic elements of the universe—factitiously referred to as the Greek Periodic Table—and that land creatures evolved from sea urchins; believing that the four elements were not sufficient to explain the great diversity of things, Anaxagoras declared that in its original state, "All things were together, infinite in respect of both number and smallness." To avoid the paradox of elements being both infinitely large and infinitely small, Leucippus and Democritus introduced the theory that matter consists of indivisible atoms, whose deterministic interactions cause the diversity in the universe which itself was eternal, infinite, and composed of endless solar systems.

Although Plato did not believe an exact knowledge of the Receptacle or imperfect world of becoming was possible, his pupil Aristotle created one of the most enduring and comprehensive cosmologies and theories of explanation in history. His organismic cosmology culminating in the Prime Mover and explanatory framework of substance and form, the four causes, and syllogistic reasoning dominated Western thought from the 13th through the 17th centuries. The influence of Greek astronomers is evident in Copernicus' justification of his defense of heliocentrism by citing Greek forerunners: Proclus, who held that the earth revolved around a central fire analogous to heliocentrism; Heraclides, who argued that it was simpler to attribute the apparent diurnal rotation of the whole universe from east to west to the rotation of the smaller earth from west to east; and Aristarchus, who first proposed the heliocentric system in the second century BC.

Because these proposals contradicted ordinary observations, it was Claudius Ptolemy, a Greco-Roman who lived in Alexandria in the second century AD and whose geocentrism comprised a complex system of epicycles and equants "to save the phenomena," who was the leading astronomer until Copernicus. Other innovations were Euclid's geometry so essential to astronomical calculations and Archimedes' "method of exhaustion" that anticipated modern differential calculus in computing the rate of change of a function with respect to an independent variable.

Another area where the Greeks made outstanding contributions was medical science. While the practice of medicine in other societies at that time generally relied on magical potions, mysterious remedies, or superstitious rituals in the hope of curing wounds, illnesses, or diseases, the Greeks advanced the science of medicine by empirical research. As Morris Cohen and I. E. Drabkin assert in their excellent book, *A Source Book in Greek Science*, "Although reason and observation were not absent from pre-Hellenic medicine, it was among the Greeks that rational systems of medicine developed largely free from magical and religious elements and based on natural causes."

Hippocrates of Cos, the founder of the tradition, is called the Father of Medicine. Among its contributors was Aristotle, whose treatises on the history, parts (describing vivisection of animals), and generation of animals were extremely influential, and Herophilus, who lived in the latter part of the fourth century BC and advocated the humoral theory. Herophilus was famous for his investigations of the eye, brain, and nervous and vascular systems. His younger contemporary, Erasistratus of Ceos, is known particularly for his anatomical and physiological research, and his theories of digestion, blood flow, and the causes of disease. Asclepiades of Bithynia worked mainly in the first century BC and, like Erasistratus, rejected the humoral theory for a mechanistic-atomic theory, which maintained that health depended upon the harmonious status of the corpuscles throughout the body. Finally, the Greco-Roman Galen in the second century AD is considered the greatest physician of antiquity. His influence extended to that of Vesalius and Fabricius in the 16th century.

THE POST HELLENIC WORLD: THE MIDDLE AGES

This great legacy of Greek scientific research ended about the second century AD and was not carried on by the Romans, who did not produce a single outstanding mathematician or scientist. With the transfer of the seat of the Roman Empire to Constantinople by the Emperor Constantine in the fourth century AD, subsequently making Christianity with its other-worldly orientation the dominant religion of Byzantium, there was no interest in scientific inquiry throughout the Medieval Period. As St. Augustine (Bishop of Hippo and early Church Father of the fourth and fifth centuries) declared: "Nothing is to be accepted except on the authority of Scripture, since greater is that authority than all powers of the human mind."

It was the Muslim Empire that was largely responsible for the preservation of Greek manuscripts and the continuation of scientific research from the 9th to the 12th centuries in places like Aleppo, Damascus, Babylon, and Cordoba. This preservation was due to the prophet of Islam, Muhammad's declaration that one can learn of Allah by studying his manifestations in nature as well as by revelation. Creation of the Baghdad Academy of Science by the Caliph Al-Mamun, with its collection of Greek philosophical, mathematical, and scientific manuscripts, centered scientific research in the Middle East, attracting scholars from India, Persia, and Syria. Yet it was the Arabs at this time who were the main contributors.

To mention a few, the first half of the ninth century included al-Kindi, known as the Arabic "philosopher King," and the famous Arabic mathematician, al-Khwarizmi. Al-Kindi, who taught in Bagdad, is known for his treatises on meteorology, geometrical optics, and physiology, while al-Khwarizmi gave to the West a treatise on *Algebra* (*al-jabr*), so crucial for formulating mathematical equations, the word 'algorithm,' and the so-called "Arabic numerals" that he had derived from the Hindus. Al-Battani, the greatest of the Arabian astronomers, lived in the second half of the ninth century and is known for his precise measurements of the obliquity of the ecliptic, the precession of the equinoxes, and the orbital motions of the sun and the moon. Ptolemy's book, the *Almagest*, derived its name from al-Battani's Arabic version.

Al-Farabi, who worked in Aleppo and Damascus in the early tenth century, is known as the "second Aristotle" for having translated his *Organon* into Arabic, introducing syllogistic reasoning into Arabic scientific inquiry, and for his refinement of Aristotle's distinction between the material and formal causes in medical research. A scholar of the early eleventh century especially renowned in the West is the Persian scholar Ibn Sina (or Avicenna), whose *Cannon of Medicine* integrating the medical investigations of Aristotle, Galen, and the Arabs was one of the most influential medical works of the late Middle Ages and early Renaissance. His famous book on philosophy, *Healing*, interpreted Aristotle as a Neoplatonist. The last Arabic scientist to be mentioned was not from the Arabic Near East but was born in Cordoba in the twelfth century. Though his Arabic name is Ibn Rushd, he is commonly known as Averroës and, like Avicenna, wrote a series of commentaries on Aristotle from a Neoplatonic perspective.

THE RENAISSANCE

Beginning in the 13th century after their translation into Latin, it was the dissemination throughout Europe of Greek texts from the Arabic schools of Cordoba in Spain and Salerno in Italy that contributed to the renewal of scientific research in the West; this lasted during the 14th and 15th centuries. While important contributions to experimental science were made by Robert Grosseteste, Roger Bacon, Erazmus Witelo, and others during these two centuries, it is convenient to date the beginning of modern science with the publication of Copernicus' *De Revolutionibus orbium coelestium* in 1543 because it marks a dramatic transition to the modern worldview.

Influenced by his Greek predecessors, Copernicus believed that a sun-centered planetary system offered a simpler, more exact, and more harmonious system of the universe than geocentrism. Having the same vision, Johannes Kepler used Tycho Brahe's astronomical data to drive his three astronomical laws replacing Aristotle's uniform circular motions of the planets with *elliptical orbits* whose nonuniform revolutions was swifter at the perihelion than the aphelion. Undergoing a remarkable intellectual development, his final conception was that the heavens resembled "a kind of clockwork" that runs on purely physical laws. It was Kepler's third law, that "*the ratio which exists between the periodic times of any two planets is precisely the ratio of the 3/2th power of the mean distances of the spheres themselves,*" which suggested to Newton that the strength of the gravitational force decreases with the 3/2 power of the distance from the sun.

Although the works of both Copernicus and Kepler challenged Aristotle's cosmological system, they were not influential enough to pose a serious threat to his authority. Thomas Aquinas' 13th century synthesis of Aristotle with Christianity revised the worldview and provided the theoretical foundation of Christianity. Thus, it was the authority of the Catholic Church plus the fact that Aristotle's cosmological system seemed at the time to be in agreement with ordinary experiences and common sense beliefs that made it such a lasting system. For example, it does appear that the earth is stationary in the center of the universe; that all the heavenly bodies revolve around the earth; that the natural motion of the celestial bodies is uniform, circular, and eternal while natural terrestrial motion is vertical, accelerating downward proportional to the weight of objects to the earth's center, or the "unnatural or violent" motion of projectiles. Thus, revolving is inherent to the celestial realm while a state of rest is normal for the terrestrial world. Conceiving the celestial heaven as composed of a weightless, incorruptible aither, while the terrestrial world consists of the four elements, fire, earth, air, and water, with contrasting motions and properties, reinforced the distinction between the two realms.

It was this distinction that Galileo refuted with his new telescopic observations: that the surface of the moon with its observable craters and canyons resembles the earth, not celestial bodies; that Mars' orbital distances from the earth vary and therefore could not be circular; that the satellites of Jupiter, the rings of Saturn, the phases of Venus, and the sun spots were discoveries not mentioned by Aristotle; that Venus and Mercury were seen to revolve around the sun, not the earth; and that new comets were observed in the celestial world, contradicting Aristotle's belief that the heavens were immutable.

While these unique telescopic observations tended to refute Aristotle's cosmological system, Galileo still had to rebut the arguments supporting geocentrism, which he did brilliantly in his *Dialogues Concerning the Two Chief World Systems* published in 1632. For instance, how could the earth, a stationary material body, exist and revolve in the celestial realm? Why do we not feel the motion of the earth if it has a diurnal rotation and annual revolution around the sun? Why does the sun appear to rise in the east and set in the west if the earth rotates in the opposite direction? If the earth rotates on its axis, why does an object thrown vertically upward fall straight down, rather than at a removed distance, because during its trajectory the earth would have rotated beneath it? These objections were rebutted by Galileo by showing that they were relative to the perspective of someone on the earth, and not absolute. If one views the planetary system from the perspective of an orbiting earth, as required by heliocentrism, the objections fade away. As Einstein noted, his theories of relativity began with Galileo.

Despite the new telescopic evidence and credibility of his arguments, the Commission of the Inquisition under Pope Urban VIII forced Galileo to recant on his knees his belief in the heliocentric system. It challenged the authority of the Church that endorsed geocentrism. Yet after recovering from the trial he wrote his last book, *Dialogues Concerning Two New Sciences*, describing his earlier experiments with falling objects, incline planes, and projectiles. This work also proved his laws of motion, that in a vacuum similar objects would fall with the same velocity regardless of their weights, in contrast to Aristotle's theory that free falling objects accelerate with the squares of the times. He also explained that the trajectory of projectiles is parabolic and described his conception of the true method of scientific inquiry. Thus, Galileo achieved his objectives of demolishing Aristotle's system, freeing science from the authority of the Catholic Church, and demonstrating the use of experimentation and mathematics in scientific inquiry, illustrating how science has had to rectify erroneous beliefs due to the naturally limited and distorted perspective of human beings.

Galileo's eradication of Aristotle's organismic cosmology led to Newton replacing it with an entirely new framework: mechanistic materialism. This consisted of the concepts of mass, motion, and forces of attraction, repulsion, and gravity operating within the absolute frameworks of space and time. While the latter were disproved by Einstein's general theory of relativity, they still apply to velocities insignificant compared to that of light. Newton's *Principia Mathematica*, considered the greatest scientific treatise ever written, describes all the various kinds of motions in Volume I, while Volume II, *The System of the World*, presents his celestial mechanics and terrestrial motions based on his laws of motion, especially the universal law of gravitation and equation $F = ma$. His *Opticks* presents his prism experiments showing that ordinary light is composed of a spectrum of color-rays that he interpreted mainly as corpuscular. Newton created differential calculus and even constructed a reflecting telescope entirely by himself. Because of his genius as a theoretical physicist, experimentalist, and mathematician, he could be considered the greatest scientist who ever lived.

THE 18TH AND 19TH CENTURIES

The last sections of this chapter describe the main scientific advances that were a legacy of prior scientific developments. In the late 18th century, two major investigations pertained to electricity and the explanation of combustion. The name "electric" comes from the Greeks who first identified it, but its properties were not fully discovered until the 18th century when Franklin introduced the distinction between positive and negative charges. In the late 19th century Faraday demonstrated that a moving electric current generates a magnetic field, while a change in the magnetic field generates an electric current, thus discovering electromagnetism. Then Maxwell devised the equations describing the spatial structure of the magnetic field and how it changes with time. Experimenting with light in the early 19th century, Fresnel and Young discovered the diffraction patterns of light that led them to reintroduce the wave theory. After Foucault and Fizeau had measured the finite velocity of light and Hertz found it to be the same as the propagation of electromagnetic waves, it too was identified as electromagnetic in one of the grand unifications of science.

Other developments in the late 18th century were the explanation of combustion and the discovery of oxygen. Priestly had detected a gas that was extremely inflammable but had misinterpreted it as "dephlogisticated air." It was Lavoisier who correctly identified it and named it "oxygène" after experi-

ments meticulously weighing the ingredients. He proposed a definition of "element," and showed that it was possible to identify particular gases and determine their proportion by weight in the compounds. He found that ordinary air is composed mainly of nitrogen and oxygen with some carbon dioxide and water vapor, and that water consists of two parts hydrogen and one part oxygen. Thus, Lavoisier's experiments foreshadowed the development of modern chemistry and atomism.

The 19th century is noted for three critical scientific developments. It is difficult to accept today that the adherents of the three Abrahamic religions believed that the universe was created by God in six days about six thousand years ago; that all the myriad genera and species were created in their present forms; that Adam and Eve were the progenitors of the human race tainted by Eve's disobedience, which so angered God that He destroyed all living creatures in the great Deluge except Noah, his family, and pairs of each genera and species, which were preserved in the Ark; and that it was this Deluge that formed the earth's topology.

Scientific disclosures in the 19th century, however, refuted each of these claims.

Geologists' discovery of strata in the earth's surface indicated a much longer history. Paleontologists' uncovering of fossilized remains of earlier creatures showed that genera and species were not immutable but had evolved in prehistory. During his trip to the Archipelago Islands, Charles Darwin observed the great diversity of species despite their being too distant from the mainland for any interbreeding. He suggested that, rather than being specially created, living creatures had evolved, a finding supported by his familiarity with animal breeding and awareness that the earliest stages of mammalian embryological development were similar despite their later diverse characteristics, thus implying they had a common ancestry.

Refuting current beliefs about the Deluge, a young Swiss naturalist, Louis Agassiz, stunned a meeting of Natural Sciences in Switzerland in 1837 by endorsing glaciation as the cause of the earth's geological formations. Although most in the audience had seen glaciers in the Alps, they could not imagine they were the cause. Only after an American sea captain and polar explorer brought back from Greenland exact sketches of its enormous size were they largely persuaded. Then a convincing explanation of the origin of the story of the Deluge emerged when two geologists, William Ryan and Walter Pitman, proposed in their book, *Noah's Flood*, that the Black Sea was formed about 7,800 years ago, at about the time when the Old Testament was formulated. According to their account, melting glaciers caused the Mediterranean Sea to rise and overflow the Bosporus Strait, flooding the Black Sea and "covering thousands of square miles of dry land . . . killing thousands of people and billions of land and sea creatures." Recently, additional confirmation was provided by a team of deep-sea explorers led by Robert D. Ballard. Based on radioactive dating of mollusk shells, they found evidence of a huge flooding about 7,500 years ago (the same time alluded to by Ryan and Pitman) along with locating the submerged pre-flood shoreline that also had been predicted. These discoveries are too convergent to be coincidental, indicating that these ancient legends often have some factual basis.

The third remarkable advance in the 19th century was an affirmation of the Ancient Greek doctrine of atomism with the development of the atomic-molecular theory and chemistry. As indicated previously, Lavoisier had identified individual gases as well as a number of compound gases, such as nitric oxide, carbon dioxide, and mercury oxide, but questions remained concerning the *number and weights* of the atoms comprising the various gases and molecular compounds. These questions were first answered by John Dalton, who is credited with laying the foundations for modern physical meteorology as well as modern atomism.

Dalton envisioned an entirely new conceptual framework in which the components of every sample of a substance such as water or salt contain "*ultimate particles*" (like hydrogen and oxygen) that "*are perfectly alike in weight, figure, etc.*," ensuring their uniformity. Consequently, all chemical investigations have as their objective to determine "*the relative weights of the ultimate particles, both of simple and compound bodies,*" along with "*the number of simple elementary particles which constitute one compound particle*" (i.e., molecule), such as H_2O, NaCl, or HCl. He also introduced "the rules of greatest simplicity" for arranging them and the first Atomic Table of twenty known elements was established, with individual symbols and weights relative to hydrogen taken as 1; this eventuated in the Periodic Tables of Mendeleev and Meyer. The Periodic Table was refined later in the century, owing to the theory of valences, of complex chemical structures and their chemical bonds, and the creation of organic chemistry.

THE MODERN WORLD

It was in 20th century that more advances were made in scientific inquiry than in all past history, of which only a brief summary can be given here. At the turn of the century, discoveries of subatomic particles such as electrons, protons, and neutrons, along with radiation, indicated that atoms, rather than being indivisible, had a composite structure that explains their physical properties and interactions. Then in 1900, Max Planck's investigation of blackbody radiation creating quantum mechanics opened up a whole new field of scientific inquiry. This resulted in Einstein's 1905 paper on the photoelectric ef-

fect introducing light quanta and Werner Heisenberg's injecting an element of uncertainty or indeterminacy in the measurement of the properties of light and other subatomic phenomena in 1925. The discovery of subatomic particles (to which he contributed) enabled Ernest Rutherford to depict the structure of the atomic nucleus and Niels Bohr to construct the Saturnian model of the atom, contributing to the explanation of radiation and chemical properties.

In 1905, in "*l'anno mirabile*," Einstein published five revolutionary papers including one on Brownian motion, one on the photoelectric effect just mentioned, and one on the special theory of relativity containing his famous equation, $E = mc^2$. Then in 1915 he published his general theory of relativity, describing the four-dimensional manifold of space-time that is fundamental to modern cosmology. Predicting that light would be curved in a strong gravitational field like the sun, this was confirmed four years later. In the 1920s, Edwin Hubble's telescopic observations revealed millions of galaxies beyond our Milky Way, along with the "red shift" in the light waves from outer space that implied an inflationary expansion of the universe. In 1927, the Belgian priest, Georges Lemaître, posited that if the universe were expanding it must have had a beginning. This phenomenon was coined the "Big Bang" by Fred Hoyle; it allowed astrophysicists finally to resolve the controversy over the age of the universe, computing it to have occurred about 14.7 billion years ago. The expansionary theory was firmly substantiated in 1965 when Arno Penzias and Robert Wilson of the Bell Laboratories discovered the background radiation left over from the Big Bang.

Then in 1938–1939 Otto Hahn announced his experiments injecting slow-moving neutrons into the nucleus of uranium, which created two units of barium and released a tremendous energy. Lisa Meitner and her nephew Otto Frisch interpreted these experiments and named the action *atomic fission*. This led to the building of the atomic bomb and nuclear reactors, confirming the structure of the atomic nucleus.

There were major advances in pharmacology, health care, and medicine beginning with the discovery of penicillin in 1929, followed by the polio vaccine created in 1954 by Dr. Jonas Salk, along with organ transplants and computed axial tomography (CAT) scans. But the major achievement was Watson and Crick's discovery in 1953 of DNA and the deciphering of the genetic code announced in 1993. This was revolutionary because, instead of treating the adverse consequences of genetic defects, one now would be able to eliminate their genetic causes by locating and removing or altering the defective gene that produced them. In addition, the recent breakthrough technology of creating stem cells (without destroying human embryos) by injecting retroviruses into skin cells in the future will allow for the replacement of any damaged tissue in the human organism.

Finally, tremendous advances in technology are exemplified in the development of nuclear reactors, computer science, and space explorations with the stunning lunar landing in 1969 along with the future expectations of landing on Mars. It is fair to say that whatever advances have been made in health care, standards of living, and enlightenment can be attributed to the achievements of science. And thus ends our odyssey through the history of science.

RESOURCES

The background research, along with bibliographical references to the original sources, and cited quotations can be found in my two volume work: *From Myth to Modern Mind: A Study of the Origins and Growth of Scientific Thought,* Vol. I, *Theogony through Ptolemy,* and Vol. II, *Copernicus through Quantum Mechanics* (New York: Peter Lang Publishers, Inc.; 1995, 1996). Also, they can be found in my upcoming book entitled, *Seeking the Truth: How Science Contested Revelation and Faith as the Basis of Belief.*

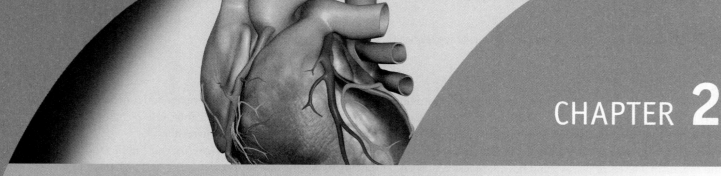

CHAPTER 2

Essay: Biochemistry: A Foundation for Health Sciences

Mark S. Elliott

Congratulations on your choice to study Health Sciences and Public Health issues. It is my fervent hope that this course of study will aid in providing you a productive and satisfying professional niche in the wide field of population health. As you focus on the biological basis of disease presented in this text and associated course work, I encourage you to remain aware of the underlying fundamentals involved in supporting these fields of work.

Professional healthcare workers are a curious breed. Not that they are "odd" mind you (except maybe some surgeons); they are curious intellectually. In order to be effective as a healthcare worker, you must stay current in the rapid developments of your chosen field. Education is a constant, and you must maintain a constant commitment to your education in order to remain professionally viable. That "something happens" requires nothing more than an act of faith. Asking "why something happens" requires an education. The very best students and professionals have an intrinsic desire to understand why things work the way they do. I find this characteristic progressively waning in the classroom demeanor of the more recent student classes. "Is this going to be on the test?" which implies that if it isn't on the test, I have other things I'd rather be doing. Where is the curiosity to know and understand what is going on? Curiosity may well have killed a cat or two, but curiosity may also save your patients and clients. Nurture your curiosity! Actively pursue your education!

Ask questions; questions that probe various levels of understanding. We are all familiar with innocent young children asking fundamental questions such as, "Why is the sky blue?" or "Why does Sparky (the family dog) scratch behind his ears all the time?" Do we answer these questions at their fundamental level, explaining the electromagnetic spectrum of visible light and its interaction with the electron orbital structure of molecular nitrogen, or that mange is an inflammatory skin disease, or flea saliva can initiate hyperimmune responses in some dogs? Doubtful. We judge the intellectual level of our students', patients', or clients' questions and interpret the response they require and respond in the most appropriate context. Frequently they trundle off completely satisfied with the answers that, "The sky is blue because blue is God's favorite color" (or so they say it is in Carolina), or "Sparky is just itchy." Clear meaning. Totally understood. However, your students, patients, and clients may be a bit more sophisticated and educated than to settle for such banal responses. What do you do when a patient, a person, or a group of family members is standing before you asking questions, desperately trying to understand why you are giving their son or daughter methotrexate and 5-fluorouracil, or why a newly married couple should seriously consider never ever having children for fear of some mystically fatal genetic disease they have a 50-50 chance of passing on to their offspring. Yes, curiosity may well have killed a cat or two, but your curiosity may also aid your patient's need to know what is happening to him or her.

My point here is that biochemistry is of critical importance for understanding public health issues at their most fundamental level. This essay is a reminder, a nudge towards a notion, that in your chosen public health field, the more you are motivated into understanding your discipline at deeper levels, the closer you are going to get to the fundamentals of *Biochemistry*. Of course, this can be frightening, a core science course that actually has the always feared "*Chemistry*" term in its title. But if you, your patients, clients, and consultants have curiosity, biochemistry is where to go to look for the deep answers explaining what is going on at the molecular, cellular, and organismal levels of disease, and how the social and societal issues of these diseases are manifest at their most fundamental levels. Depending on your level of interest and concern, and that of your patients and clientele, there are different levels of depth to generate the satisfactory answer. But I encourage you to cultivate your own curiosity, your insatiably inquisitive need to know the causation disease at deeper levels of understanding, if for no other reason than to educate and communicate with an emotionally concerned and typically fearful population. *Fight fear with knowledge.* You, the public health practitioner, need to know your fundamental biochemistry in order to explain disease states, drug treatments, likely outcomes, side effects, probabilities of genetic susceptibility, and to be prepared for the rapidly arriving era of personal molecular medicine. How are you going to explain "23andMe" (time to go "Google") to a concerned group of individuals (genetic counselors, lawmakers, and attorneys involved in medical ethics and personal privacy) if you "don't get" DNA. It's easy to spell, but difficult to fathom without some biochemical education. Biochemistry forms a foundation supporting all other health science disciplines. You'd better have a friction grip on the basic principles of biochemistry because as a professional, you are going to be questioned by the public.

For example, in this book there are a slew of well-written chapters from experts in their fields. All of these authors are trying to give you a perspective on their expertise in the context of public health concerns. But, after enjoying this course and the no doubt scintillating lectures therein, are you ready—totally prepared—to answer the questions of an 18 year old pondering the realities of undergoing a preemptive double mastectomy because a gene screen came up "funny," or explaining to an entire African village of rural poor people that over half of them will be dead in two years from a viral epidemic? Knowledge and education may not cure the disease, but knowledge and education do alleviate the fears and comfort to a degree, the angst of not knowing. You must approach this as a teacher and in this quest; a little fundamental biochemistry is your friend.

Let us look at a few of these chapters from the perspective of a student, patient, or client who might be inquisitive enough to crave knowledge at a deeper level. Chapter 25 on **HIV Biology** speaks to viruses and species-specific interactions and receptors on CD4 cells. The chapter goes on to discuss DNA and RNA viruses and protein coats and the *pol, env,* and *gag* genes, reverse transcriptase, testing technologies (ELISA), drug interventions, and toxic consequences. What are all these things? Can you ef-

fectively describe these, their importance and function to a person recently diagnosed with HIV? You can explain these things with a little background in biochemistry.

In a lovely Chapter 3 on **Genetics and Public Health**, the history of genetic disease, predictability, and pedigrees, mutations and disease, genetic factors in drug reactions through pharmacogenomics, genetic testing and counseling with all the social, psychological, ethical, and legal question pertaining there unto are elegantly discussed. But what are the diseases discussed at the molecular level, the mutations, the damaged DNA and its repair, the gene expression phenomena? What are *BRCA1* and *BRAC2* and how do they work in breast cancer as suggested in the chapter? How do genetics and public health lead us into the realm of personalized medicine and the place for commercial genetic testing services like "23andMe"? You can help explain some these things with a little background in biochemistry.

Chapter 11 about **Exercise** speaks to activity as the cure for obesity as opposed to drug interventions; a very common-sense approach dealing with social and psychological issues and balancing caloric intakes with metabolic rates. But, how are amphetamines and fen-phen working? What are they doing to me? What are the heart, kidney, and diabetes ramifications of exercise versus the lack thereof? What are metabolic rates, and how are they controlled? What about the dynamics of metabolism for carbohydrates and fats that are the essence of energy metabolism in exercise? Can you answer basic questions regarding these issues to a person coming off a minor heart attack who is now on an adjusted diet with exercise in order to strengthen his or her recovering heart muscle? Yup! You can answer a great number of these questions with a little background in biochemistry.

Chapter 17 on **Inflammation** speaks to cellular responses from neutrophils, monocytes, and macrophages and their interactions with cytokines and chemoattractants. Cytoskeletal actin-myosin filaments, the enzymology of proteases, peroxidases, and hydroxyl free radicals from lysosomes, and the actions of anti-inflammatory agents such as antihistamines, steroids, aspirin, and other nonsteroidal anti-inflammatory drugs (NSAIDs) are discussed in the global context of the biology of inflammation. But an individual comes to you with a case of arthritis in both knees and this person has read the same book chapter you just did, only this person wants to know what all these confounding factors are really doing in his poor aching knees. Can you answer these questions? You can give it a pretty good shot with a little background in biochemistry.

What about the Chapter 13 on **Smoking and Nicotine Addiction**? Can you explain to a three pack-a-day smoker what addiction is at the molecular level, so that he or she might begin to understand better what he or she already knows physically and socially: "I'm an addict. I can't stop. Why?"

And finally, after reading through **Avian and Seasonal Influenza**, Chapter 31, can you explain to your friends how it would only take four point mutations in a relatively benign flu virus strain commonly found in Mallard ducks (they're so cute in those little farm ponds *all over the country!*) in order to change the virus into a super-virulent form that could conceivably kill two thirds of the earth's human population in just a couple of months (getting even with a few duck hunters there)! Yup, you need to know some biochemistry! But where to look?

Here's a revelation for you: Biochemistry is part of the real healthcare world. You have a professional need to know some fundamental biochemistry in the context of public health issues in order to be an effective provider. There are widespread negative perceptions and myths about biochemistry courses. These stem entirely from lack of practical applications presented in the old texts and the old ways of presenting materials (Oh no! Not another pathway!). Yet every medical, epidemiological, physiological, dietary and nutritional, or other health-related application can find its fundamental root explanation in biochemical principles. Presented in these practical contexts, biochemistry can be damn fascinating. You do not have to change your major; you can take a biochemistry survey course or simply get yourself involved in your own self-motivated adult education. Biochemistry is such a rapidly developing field that the textbooks can barely keep up with the basics. These are important reference sources to be sure, but the real fun in discovery is personally motivated exploration guided by an appropriate mentor, a current library, and a fast Internet connection.

The Wheel of Science

Pictured is one of my favorite opening lecture slides. I use it to give my class a perspective on the position of biochemistry in the "Great Wheel of Science." Biochemistry sits right on the cusp of the differentiation between the physical science world and the biological science world. As the sciences are developed, they each feed, support, and form a foundation for development and applications in the next level of science. So if you put Health Science–related fields somewhere on the wheel in the Biology, Sociology, Psychology region, we can see that working back for fundamental understanding of core principles for any given medical phenomena requires Biochemistry and Molecular Biology as a foundation. Simple! Right?

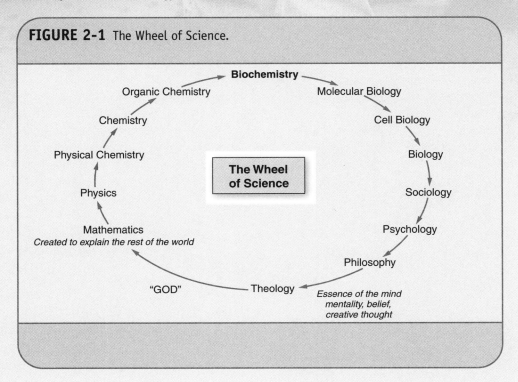

FIGURE 2-1 The Wheel of Science.

Primary modern educational resources are electronic, digital databases, Web sites, and assorted resources through on-line computers. Libraries with journals and textbooks are regularly used but these sources are augmented with extensive electronic resources. Why? Because you can search for anything from your home, office, or library using an on-line computer. It's a target rich environment that is so nearly instantaneously available, it's ridiculous. All you need is motivation and curiosity, and you can discover the answers to almost any health-related questions. If you answer a man's question, it will keep him happy for a few minutes. But if you give him a laptop computer and a WiFi uplink, he'll leave you alone for weeks! This is one of the major principles of adult learning: with enough internal motivation an adult will marshal resources to support his or her own educational quests. The teacher merely becomes the guide to facilitate the journey along the path to understanding. Fortunately, we still get a paycheck.

For an additional major resource, check this: http://www .ncbi.nlm.nih.gov/! It is the World Wide Web (www.) site for the National Center for Biotechnology Information (ncbi.) at the National Library of Medicine (nlm.) at the National Institutes of Health (nih.) supported by your United States Government (.gov). They have *everything*, including some very useful site maps and tutorials on how to use their vast information services to educate both yourself and others. It is a very powerful research and reference tool. You can search topics directly, find primary research literature, general reviews, search genome and proteome databases for disease linkages, or scan electronic textbooks on a vast number of health science–related topics, including biochemistry. And all of this is free, free, FREE! Your tax dollars are at work, finally generating something useful from Washington (well, Bethesda actually).

This Web site provides access to the mountains of available data, but *not* the level of understanding. You must be able to synthesize your own clear picture or interpretation of what the data actually mean. Hence, you have a need for a relevant education and background in biochemistry and its applications to your chosen public health field. Finally, a warning: if you rely on the Internet as your sole source of information, you could be led astray. There are problems with the less authoritative Web sites, so you must use good professional and educated judgment in interpreting information from your sources.

Today's learning is obsolete tomorrow. Learning is a constant active process. The best healthcare workers must maintain their knowledge base at the forefront, cutting-edge, in order to remain an effective professional for society. So, curiosity may well have killed a cat or two, but curiosity can serve to push on into deeper levels of understanding for the molecular mechanisms that drive the disease, its potential treatments and possible cures. And the foundation of that understanding ultimately involves knowledge and application of biochemistry. Amen, see ya' around the lab.

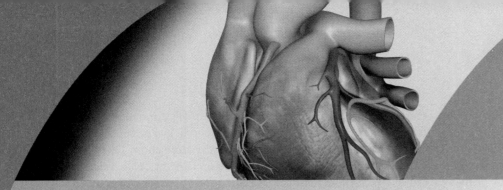

CHAPTER 3

Genetics and Public Health

Joseph D. McInerney

Infectious disease, long a focus of public health professionals, is a battle between two variable genomes: that of the host and that of the pathogen. Sometimes there actually are three genomes involved, as in the case of malaria, when an insect vector transmits the infectious organism to its human host. Many people would not normally view infection as genetic, which serves as a reminder that the distinction between 'genetic' and 'non-genetic' disease is somewhat artificial.

J.D. McInerney

LEARNING OBJECTIVES

By the end of this chapter, the student will be able to:

- Define genetics and its relationship to the health of individuals and populations.
- Recognize the benefits and risks of incorporating genetics perspectives into public health.
- Describe major differences between single-gene and common, complex disorders.
- Describe several different types of genetic testing and important issues related to each.
- Define major ethical, legal, and social implications of genetics as applied in the clinical setting and in public health.
- Apply genetics perspectives to a hypothetical public health campaign to screen for risk of colorectal cancer (CRC).

HISTORY

Genetics is the study of inherited biological variation, and it is instructive to view the history of the discipline in the context of insights into the sources and nature of that variation.

- Charles Darwin recognized that variation is the rule, not the exception, in the living world. Inherited variation in populations of organisms is a central aspect of his revolutionary theory of **evolution** by natural selection, elaborated in 1859 in *On the Origin of Species by Means of Natural Selection, or the Preservation of Favoured Races in the Struggle for Life*. Darwin realized that without variation among organisms there could be no differential selection. He died, however, unable to identify where that variation resides or how it is transmitted intact from one generation to the next.

- Gregor Mendel, a Darwin contemporary, uncovered the answers to both questions as a result of his famous experiments on pea plants. He demonstrated the presence of "factors"—what we now call *genes*—that carry hereditary information from generation to generation and contribute to the differences in appearance of individual organisms. Mendel, known as the father of genetics, established the basic laws of inheritance, including the laws of **segregation** and **independent assortment**. He published his important work in 1865, to resounding silence. No one really understood the implications of what Mendel had done, and it appears that Darwin was unaware of this now-classic paper.

- In 1900, three botanists working independently on plant hybridization rediscovered Mendel's paper and recognized its importance. That began the growth of **genetics** as a discipline.

- Three years later, Walter Sutton and Theodore Boveri, working independently and building on the knowledge of chromosome behavior during meioses, proposed that the genetic material is carried on the chromosomes, thus establishing the chromosome theory of inheritance. During the next several decades, biologists combined chromosome theory with intensive research on a variety of experimental organisms to provide many significant insights into the transmission and nature of genes. Although the terms "**gene**" and "genetics" quickly made their way into the scientific lexicon, the nature of the genetic material remained a mystery until the middle of the century. Of the major biological macromolecules, only protein seemed to have the ability to harbor the variation required of the molecule of heredity.

- In 1944, Oswald Avery, Colin MacLeod, and Macklyn McCarty demonstrated in research on bacteria that genetic information is carried by **DNA**. In 1952, Alfred Hersey and Martha Chase, using investigations in viruses, confirmed that DNA is the genetic material.
- Nine years after Avery's discovery, James Watson and Francis Crick published their famous double-helix model of DNA, which indicated that variation is encoded in the sequence of four bases in the DNA molecule: A-adenine, T-thymine, C-cytosine, and G-guanine. They further demonstrated that A always pairs with T and C always pairs with G. This model implied a copying mechanism for the genetic material and sparked the growth of molecular biology.
- In 2003, 50 years after the publication of the Watson-Crick Model, an international consortium completed work on the **Human Genome Project** (HGP), which specified the complete sequence of all 3.2 billion base pairs in the human **genome**. It now is possible to elaborate human variation at the level of individual base pairs of DNA. Equally important, other teams have sequenced the genomes of many other species (including microbial, insect, plant, reptilian, and mammalian species), allowing structural and functional comparisons of species across evolutionary history. The completion of the HGP represents an extraordinary amount of progress in a century and a half—about six human generations—from the time of Darwin and Mendel.
- During the last five decades, the application of genetics to health and disease has grown enormously, encompassing, for example, classic "genetic diseases" such as cystic fibrosis and Huntington disease, common diseases such as cancer and diabetes, and the application of genetic variation to the selection and dosing of medications.

BASIC SCIENCE FACTS/KEY CONCEPTS REVIEW

DNA is the universal information molecule for all life on Earth. The information is organized digitally as As, Ts, Cs, and Gs. The ability to analyze and manipulate this information has enormous implications for our understanding of personal and public health. Human DNA is organized into about 20,000 genes, which specify the production of proteins. Most DNA (about 95 percent, in fact) is not translated into protein. This untranslated material sometimes is referred to as "junk DNA," but continuing research shows that some of it does have a function, often in gene regulation. Human DNA is carried on 23 pairs of chromosomes; one pair of each is of maternal origin, the other paternal. One of the pairs, designated X and Y, are the sex chromosomes. Human females have an XX chromosomal constitution, males XY. A small amount of additional genetic material, about 16,000 base pairs, is carried in the mitochondria of human cells. Some of this material has implications for health and disease.

Many biomedical scientists believe that continuing advances in genetics and genomics will transform health care through a combination of technological innovations and conceptual insights that will improve our understanding of the causes of disease and of basic disease processes, thereby improving diagnosis, treatment, and prevention. The time frame for this transformation varies depending on the prognosticator, from a hopeful five years to a more sobering two decades or more. In reality, no one knows because, as in all sciences, the ever-changing creative mix of ideas and techniques in genetic medicine produces a level of complexity that makes prediction risky at best, much as the emergent properties of organisms remind us that we cannot predict the characteristics of living things simply by examining their constituent parts, molecular or otherwise.

Genetics and Common Disease

No matter how long the putative transformation of health care takes, it will not truly be transformative until genetics has something compelling to contribute to our understanding of the diseases that constitute the major portion of the healthcare burden worldwide. The historical focus of genetic medicine was relatively rare single-gene disorders such as cystic fibrosis and sickle cell disease, and chromosomal disorders such as Down syndrome, categories of disease primarily involving obstetrics and pediatrics. The effect of this history was to leave the impression that genetics is not relevant for the vast majority of diseases or other disciplines.

As Figure 3-1 demonstrates, however, virtually all diseases have a genetic basis, including those that occupy the day-to-day activities of primary care providers and public health professionals. In addition, as treatment for classic "genetic diseases" has improved, some affected individuals are living well beyond childhood, and the healthcare community

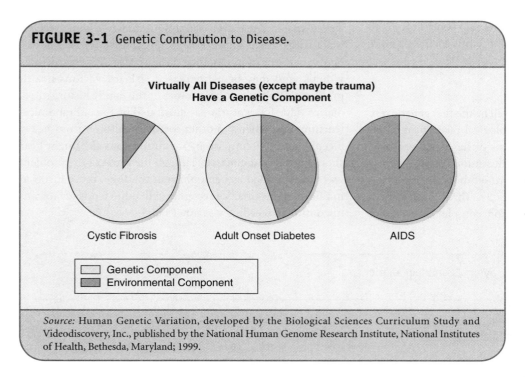

FIGURE 3-1 Genetic Contribution to Disease.

Virtually All Diseases (except maybe trauma) Have a Genetic Component

Cystic Fibrosis

Adult Onset Diabetes

AIDS

☐ Genetic Component
■ Environmental Component

Source: Human Genetic Variation, developed by the Biological Sciences Curriculum Study and Videodiscovery, Inc., published by the National Human Genome Research Institute, National Institutes of Health, Bethesda, Maryland; 1999.

is struggling with the transition of care from pediatrics to specialties such as internal medicine and family medicine. Many adult-medicine practitioners are unfamiliar with these disorders, and often are unprepared to manage such patients. In addition, more children with genetic and chromosomal disorders are beginning to outlive their parents. Some of those children will not be fully functional adults and will require ongoing support, creating financial challenges for parents and public health agencies.

Recent studies based on genomic analysis[1–5] show that genetics increasingly will provide insights into genetic contributions to the common chronic diseases that constitute the major causes of mortality and morbidity worldwide: heart disease, cancer, diabetes, mental illness, and other disorders (including infection) that many people do not generally categorize as "genetic." In fact, one might envision a time when the phrase "genetic disease" disappears from our lexicon and we no longer ask ourselves, "Is this disease ge-

netic?" but ask instead, in recognition that all disease has a genetic basis: "What is the role of genetic variation in the onset and expression of this disease?"

Common, complex disorders, which are becoming the focus of genetically based health care, result from the interactions of multiple genes and multiple environmental factors. As Table 3-1 indicates, these diseases differ from single-gene disorders in some critical ways. Among the most important differences for the clinician and public health professional is the pattern of occurrence of disease in a family history. Whereas single-gene disorders follow classic, predictable patterns of Mendelian inheritance (that is, the phenotype segregates in the pedigree) common disorders generally do not follow such patterns. Instead, they cluster, or aggregate, in unpredictable ways because of the complex combination of genetic and environmental factors that precipitate disease. This makes the familial nature of the disease in question more difficult to recognize if one is not looking for it. Aggregation, which

TABLE 3-1 A Comparison of Complex and Single-Gene Disorders

Characteristics	Complex	Single-Gene
Gene(s)	**segregates**	**segregates**
Disorder	**aggregates**	**segregates**
Gene products involved	multiple	primarily one
Role of environment	important	often overridden by effect(s) of gene mutation
Age at onset	older	younger
Risks for relatives of probands	smaller, less predictable	larger, more predictable
Healthcare burden	high	low
Selection against	low	high

Source: Courtesy of the National Coalition for Health Professional Education in Genetics (NCHPEG). Available online at http://www.nchpeg.org

signals multiple genetic and environmental contributions to disease, also makes risk assessment for family members more difficult, because the pattern is not predictable.

Family History

A medical family history may very well be the first genetic test. A family history documents the biological relationships and medical histories of a patient and his or her **first-, second-, and third-degree relatives**. When this information is represented in diagram form with standard symbols and terminology, it is called a pedigree. Figures 3-2 through 3-4 show pedigrees for single-gene and common, complex disorders, as well as standard pedigree symbols.[6] A pedigree is an excellent way to organize health information because it is easier to recognize patterns of inheritance, and therefore to identify individuals who may be at increased risk for various health problems. People have been aware of the family history's predictive value for centuries, as illustrated by the old rabbinical teaching that when a mother lost two children from heavy bleeding after circumcision, any future sons she might bear should not be circumcised. Though the cause of the problem was not identified as hemophilia at the time, those involved in this religious practice recognized that the tendency toward uncontrolled bleeding was inherited.

FIGURE 3-2 Standard Pedigree Symbols and Explanations.

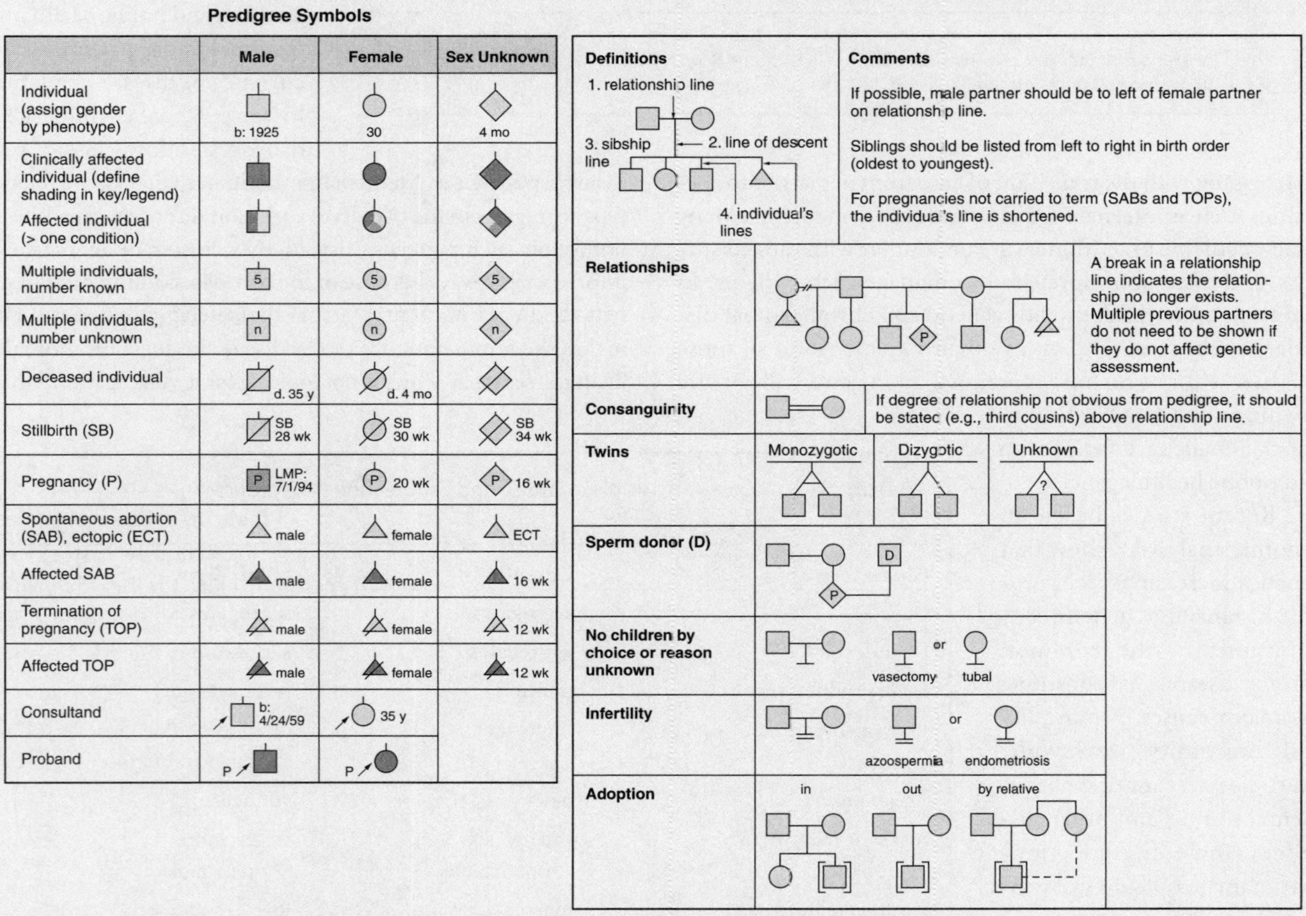

Source: From Bennett, et al. Recommendations for standardized human pedigree nomenclature. *American Journal of Human Genetics* 1995;56:745–752.

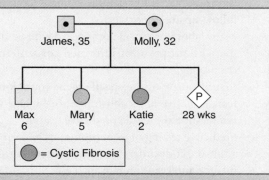

FIGURE 3-3 Pedigree Showing Autosomal Recessive Inheritance. Note that Katie's parents are unaffected carriers.

James, 35   Molly, 32

Max 6   Mary 5   Katie 2   P 28 wks

⬤ = Cystic Fibrosis

Source: Courtesy of the National Coalition for Health Professional Education in Genetics (NCHPEG). Available online at http://www.nchpeg.org. Accessed March 10, 2008.

Knowledge of a patient's family history has long been recognized as beneficial for diagnosis and treatment of relatively uncommon single-gene disorders, such as cystic fibrosis, fragile X syndrome, Huntington disease, familial hypercholesterolemia, and other disorders inherited in classical Mendelian patterns.[7] More recently, family history has been shown to be a major risk factor for more common chronic diseases such as cardiovascular disease, diabetes, several cancers, osteoporosis, and asthma.[7,8] Therefore, inclusion of family history collection and interpretation in general health care is increasingly becoming standard of care. For example, in its Medical Genetics Core Educational Guidelines for Family Practice Residents, the American Academy of Family Physicians recommends that its members have the knowledge and skill to prepare and interpret a family history pedigree. The American College of Obstetricians and Gynecologists also lists health status of the patient's family as part of the screening that should take place during assessments in primary and preventive care.

At a minimum, taking a family history requires a pen or pencil, a piece of paper, and a small amount of time. Time, however, is a valuable commodity in the current healthcare environment. Therefore, providers may choose to decrease the time spent actually taking the family history by having patients complete questionnaires and other forms prior to the appointment. The U.S. Surgeon General has produced "My Family Health Portrait," an online tool that allows anyone with Internet access to prepare a personalized, printable family health history. This secure tool is available in English and Spanish on the Internet (https://familyhistory.hhs.gov/, accessed March 10, 2008).

Although time is limited, the initial 10 to 20 minutes a provider spends gathering family history information might actually decrease the amount of time spent on unnecessary testing, procedures, and visits, which saves the provider and the patient time and money in the long run. For example, studies have demonstrated that using family history as a screening tool for conditions such as colorectal cancer,[9] cardiovascular disease,[10] and thrombophilia[11] is more cost-effective than population screening for the same conditions.

Table 3-2 lists some "red flags" in a family history that should alert the health professional to consider more in-depth investigation of genetic factors.

Genetic Testing

Genetic testing is one of the most obvious and practical applications of genetics and genomics for clinicians and public health professionals. Data show that during the last 14 years there has been a steady increase in the number of tests being offered and a more gradual, but still steady, increase in the number of

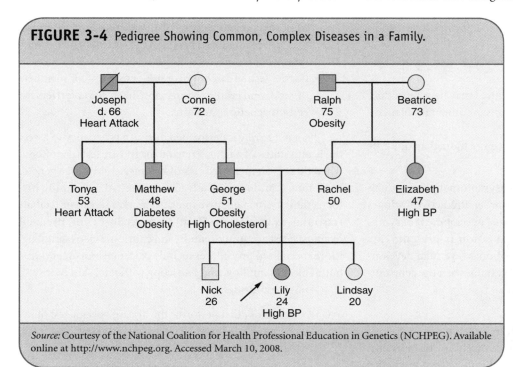

FIGURE 3-4 Pedigree Showing Common, Complex Diseases in a Family.

Joseph d. 66 Heart Attack   Connie 72   Ralph 75 Obesity   Beatrice 73

Tonya 53 Heart Attack   Matthew 48 Diabetes Obesity   George 51 Obesity High Cholesterol   Rachel 50   Elizabeth 47 High BP

Nick 26   Lily 24 High BP   Lindsay 20

Source: Courtesy of the National Coalition for Health Professional Education in Genetics (NCHPEG). Available online at http://www.nchpeg.org. Accessed March 10, 2008.

TABLE 3-2 Genetic Red Flags in a Family History

- Multiple affected individuals
- Early age at onset of disease
- Severe disease
- Presence of disease in the less-frequently affected sex, e.g., breast cancer in a male
- Recurrence of disease
- Presence of disease despite preventive measures
- Multifocal disease

labs providing such tests (www.genetests.org; accessed March 10, 2008). As of August 2007, GeneTests, a comprehensive database on genetic testing, reported that there were 620 laboratories providing clinical testing for 1,134 diseases (www.genetests.org). Gudgeon et al.[12] reported "an annual rate of increase (for genetic tests) of about 25 percent between 1996 and 2006." The following information describes the major categories of genetic tests.

Diagnostic testing is used to confirm or rule out a known or suspected genetic disorder in a symptomatic individual.

Points to consider:

- Diagnostic testing is appropriate in symptomatic individuals of any age.
- Confirmation of a diagnosis may alter medical management for the individual.
- Diagnostic testing of an individual may have reproductive or psychosocial implications for other family members as well.
- Establishing a diagnosis may require more than one type of genetic test.

Predictive testing is offered to asymptomatic individuals with a family history of a genetic disorder. Predictive testing is of two types: presymptomatic (eventual development of symptoms is certain when the gene mutation is present; e.g., Huntington disease) and predispositional (eventual development of symptoms is likely but not certain when the gene mutation is present; e.g., breast cancer).

Points to consider:

- Predictive testing is medically indicated if early diagnosis allows interventions that reduce morbidity or mortality.
- Even in the absence of medical indications, predictive testing can influence an individual's decisions about major life-defining matters such as education, marriage, career choices, and child bearing.
- Because predictive testing can have psychological ramifications, careful patient assessment, counseling, and follow-up are important.
- Many laboratories will not proceed with predictive testing without proof of informed consent and genetic counseling.
- Identification of the specific gene mutation in an affected relative or establishment of linkage within the family should precede predictive testing.
- Predictive testing of asymptomatic children at risk for adult-onset disorders is strongly discouraged when no medical intervention is available.

Carrier testing is performed to identify individuals who have a gene mutation for a disorder inherited in an **autosomal recessive** or **X-linked recessive** manner. Carriers usually do not have symptoms related to the gene mutation. Carrier testing is offered to individuals who have family members with a genetic condition, family members of an identified carrier, and individuals in ethnic or racial groups known to have a higher carrier rate for a particular condition.

Points to consider:

- Identifying carriers allows reproductive choices.
- Genetic counseling and education should accompany carrier testing because of the potential for personal and social concerns.
- Molecular genetic testing of an affected family member may be required to determine the disease-causing mutation(s) present in the family.
- Carrier testing can improve risk assessment for members of racial and ethnic groups more likely to be carriers for certain genetic conditions.

Prenatal testing is performed during a pregnancy to assess the health status of a fetus. Prenatal diagnostic tests are offered when there is an increased risk of having a child with a genetic condition resulting from advanced maternal age, family history, ethnicity, or suggestive multiple marker screen or fetal ultrasound examination. Routine procedures for prenatal diagnostic test are amniocentesis and chorionic villus sampling. More specialized procedures include placental biopsy, periumbilical blood sampling, and fetoscopy with fetal skin biopsy.

Points to consider:

- A laboratory that performs the disease-specific test of interest must be identified before any prenatal diagnostic test procedure is offered.
- All prenatal diagnostic tests carry associated risks to the fetus and the pregnancy; therefore, informed con-

sent is required, most often in conjunction with genetic counseling.

- In most cases, specific gene mutation(s) must be identified in an affected relative or carrier parent(s) before prenatal diagnosis using molecular genetic testing is possible.
- Prenatal testing for adult-onset conditions is controversial. Individuals seeking prenatal diagnosis for these conditions should be referred to a professional trained in genetic counseling for a complete discussion of the issues.

Preimplantation testing (preimplantation genetic diagnosis) is performed on early embryos resulting from in vitro fertilization to decrease the chance of a particular genetic condition occurring in the fetus. It generally is offered to couples who have a high probability of having a child with a serious disorder. Preimplantation testing provides an alternative to prenatal diagnosis and termination of affected pregnancies.

Points to consider:

- Preimplantation testing is performed at only a few centers and is available only for a limited number of disorders.
- Preimplantation testing is not possible in some cases because of difficulty in obtaining eggs or early embryos and problems with DNA analysis.
- Because of possible errors in preimplantation diagnosis, traditional prenatal diagnostic methods are recommended to monitor these pregnancies.
- The cost of preimplantation testing is very high and usually is not covered by insurance.

Newborn screening identifies individuals who have an increased chance of having a specific genetic disorder so that treatment can begin as soon as possible.

Points to consider:

- Newborn-screening programs are usually legally mandated and vary from state to state.
- Newborn screening is performed routinely at birth, unless specifically refused by the parents in writing.
- Screening tests are not designed to be diagnostic but to identify individuals who may be candidates for further diagnostic tests.
- Many parents do not realize that newborn screening has been done (or which tests were included), even if they signed a consent form when their child was born.
- Education is necessary in the wake of positive screening results to avoid misunderstandings, anxiety, and discrimination.

The American College of Medical Genetics (ACMG) directs the National Coordinating Center for the Regional Genetics and Newborn Screening Collaboratives. The center serves "to improve the working relationships among public health, specialists, and primary care providers in order to improve access to genetic services in communities." The ACMG Web site (see Resources) has additional details of interest to public health professionals.

Genetic testing of minors (generally defined by state law as children under the age of 18) has been controversial, often placing parents who want genetic testing for their children in conflict with health professionals who believe that a genetic test confers no medical benefit to the child.

Points to consider:

- whether the test is for diagnosis/current management versus future susceptibility,
- the benefits and harms of the test to the child,
- the decision-making capacity of the child,
- the availability of interventions to improve health/reduce risk based on test results, and
- the best interest of the child versus needs/interest of parents.

Although predictive testing of minors is not recommended for adult-onset disorders for which there are no preventive measures and no treatment in childhood, clinicians may interpret clinical situations differently. Many ethicists and clinicians consider the status of older, mature adolescents who have not yet reached 18 years of age on a case-by-case basis.

Possible **benefits** of testing a minor for susceptibility to a disease of adulthood include:

- intervening to reduce risk;
- reducing anxiety if the test is negative;
- preparing for future if the test is positive;
- screening for early detection if the test is positive;
- considering the potential impact on reproductive decisions;
- reducing uncertainty;
- influencing career/lifestyle choices.

Possible **risks** of testing a minor for susceptibility to a disease of adulthood include:

- worry/anxiety if the test is positive;
- alteration of self-image;
- altered family relationships;
- stigmatization by family/friends/others;
- potential for genetic discrimination;
- influence on career/lifestyle choices;
- adoption of unhealthy lifestyle/behaviors if the test is negative.

In 1995, the American Society of Human Genetics and the American College of Medical Genetics published a joint report on genetic testing in minors. The report takes a cautious view of such testing, noting that, "timely medical benefit to the child should be the primary justification for genetic testing in children and adolescents." (The complete report is available online at: http://www.ashg.org/genetics/ashg/pubs/policy/pol-13.htm; or in print: Points to consider: ethical legal and psychosocial implications of genetic testing in children and adolescents. *Am J Hum Genet* 1995;57:1233–1241.)

In summary, professionals who receive requests for presymptomatic, predictive genetic testing of minors must carefully weigh benefits and harms to the child against the wishes of the parents and families. Because genetic testing has the potential for great benefit and great harm, discussions with parents should include psychosocial, reproductive, and medical aspects, and the potential effects on their children. These issues will increase in frequency with the increased availability of predictive tests.

Direct-to-consumer (DTC) genetic testing, among other online delivery of health-related services, has been enabled by the growth of the Internet and World Wide Web. A January 2007 position statement by the American Society of Human Genetics identifies some of the benefits and pitfalls of this type of testing:

> Proponents of DTC testing cite benefits that include increased consumer access to testing, greater consumer autonomy and empowerment, and enhanced privacy of the information obtained. Critics of DTC genetic testing have pointed to the risks that consumers will choose testing without adequate context or counseling, will receive tests from laboratories of dubious quality, and will be misled by unproven claims of benefit[13] (the complete statement is available at http://www.pubmedcentral.nih.gov/articlerender.fcgi?artid=1950839, accessed March 10, 2008)

Among the problematic aspects of DTC genetic testing are the uneven regulatory landscape for such tests and the often-unsupported claims of benefit that accompany promotion of such tests on the Internet. These are fruitful areas of investigation for students and health professionals interested in public health issues related to genetics and genomics.

Genetic Services and Counseling

Genetic services generally are provided by teams of specialists trained and board certified in genetics as MDs, PhDs, or masters-level specialists. The latter category, classified as genetic counselors, comprises specialists trained in more than 40 accredited programs in the United States and several other countries. Genetic services generally are associated with tertiary care facility settings in large urban or suburban settings and are not evenly distributed nationally. One can find counseling services and genetic counselors through the National society of Genetic Counselors (NSGC) or the American College of Medical Genetics (see Resources).

As genetics begins to make its way into mainstream health care, more clinicians and public health professionals will need to know how to provide basic information and counseling about genetically based diseases. Those professionals should be mindful, however, of the limits of their expertise and be prepared to refer to specialized genetic services as necessary. The National Coalition for Health Professional Education in Genetics (NCHPEG) has produced a set of core competencies in genetics for health professionals. The competencies document is available from NCHPEG's Web site (see Resources).

Early in the history of the discipline, most genetic counseling revolved around issues related to reproductive planning or to undergoing a prenatal genetic test. Because such matters are intensely personal, genetic counseling was and continues to be generally non-directive; that is, the counselor provides information and support, but does not seek to impose a course of action on the patient. As genetics continues to contribute to our understanding of common disease, however, counseling may need to become more directive. Consider, for example, a predictive genetic test that indicates increased risk for early onset heart disease. In this case, it might be quite appropriate for the clinician to be directive about lifestyle modifications that can help to forestall the onset of disease.

According to NSGC,
Genetic counseling is the process of helping people understand and adapt to the medical, psychological, and familial implications of genetic contributions to disease. This process integrates the following:

- Interpretation of family and medical histories to assess the chance of disease occurrence or recurrence
- Education about inheritance, testing, management, prevention, resources, and research
- Counseling to promote informed choices and adaptation to the risk or condition

(adapted from the National Society of Genetic Counselors Available at http://www.nsgc.org/consumer/definition.cfm; accessed March 10, 2008.)

Exhibit 3-1 NCHPEG's Core Competencies in Genetics for Health Professionals, September 2007

Baseline Competencies

At a minimum, each healthcare professional should be able to:

a. examine one's competence of practice on a regular basis, identifying areas of strength and areas where professional development related to genetics and genomics would be beneficial.
b. understand that health-related genetic information can have important social and psychological implications for individuals and families.
c. know how and when to make a referral to a genetics professional.

1. KNOWLEDGE

All health professionals should understand:

1.1 basic human genetics terminology.
1.2 the basic patterns of biological inheritance and variation, both within families and within populations.
1.3 how identification of disease-associated genetic variations facilitates development of prevention, diagnosis, and treatment options.
1.4 the importance of family history (minimum three generations) in assessing predisposition to disease.
1.5 the interaction of genetic, environmental, and behavioral factors in predisposition to disease, onset of disease, response to treatment, and maintenance of health.
1.6 the difference between clinical diagnosis of disease and identification of genetic predisposition to disease (genetic variation is not strictly correlated with disease manifestation).
1.7 the various factors that influence the client's ability to use genetic information and services, for example, ethnicity, culture, related health beliefs, ability to pay, and health literacy.
1.8 the potential physical and/or psychosocial benefits, limitations, and risks of genetic information for individuals, family members, and communities.
1.9 the resources available to assist clients seeking genetic information or services, including the types of genetics professionals available and their diverse responsibilities.
1.10 the ethical, legal, and social issues related to genetic testing and recording of genetic information (e.g., privacy, the potential for genetic discrimination in health insurance and employment).
1.11 one's professional role in the referral to or provision of genetics services, and in follow-up for those services.

2. SKILLS

All health professionals should be able to:

2.1 gather genetic family history information, including at minimum a three-generation history.
2.2 identify and refer clients who might benefit from genetic services or from consultation with other professionals for management of issues related to a genetic diagnosis.
2.3 explain effectively the reasons for and benefits of genetic services.
2.4 use information technology to obtain credible, current information about genetics.
2.5 assure that the informed-consent process for genetic testing includes appropriate information about the potential risks, benefits, and limitations of the test in question.

3. ATTITUDES

All health professionals should:

3.1 appreciate the sensitivity of genetic information and the need for privacy and confidentiality.
3.2 seek coordination and collaboration with an interdisciplinary team of health professionals.

Competencies that delineate the components of the genetic-counseling process are not expected of all healthcare professionals. Health professionals should, however, be able to facilitate the genetic-counseling process and prepare clients and families for what to expect, communicate relevant information to the genetics team, and follow up with the client after genetic services have been provided. Those health professionals who choose to provide genetic-counseling services to their clients should be able to perform all components of the process, as delineated at http://abgc.iamonline.com/english/View.asp?x=1529 (accessed March 10, 2007).

Source: Courtesy of the National Coalition for Health Professional Education in Genetics (NCHPEG). Available online at http://www.nchpeg.org

Pharmacogenomics

Archibald Garrod, one of the pioneers of human genetics, noted in 1930 that human beings and experimental animals responded differently to the same medications: "Every drug which has a definite physiological action acts as a poison when taken in excessive doses, but in different individuals and in animals of different species the dose per kilogram needed for the production of such effects differs somewhat widely. The same is true of children and adult men and women respectively, as witness the well-known tolerance by children of belladonna, and their relative intolerance of opium."[14]

Many factors influence an individual's response to medications, including diet, other medication, and general health status. Individual genetic differences, however, are among the most important factors in variations from person-to-person, and can even influence to efficacy of vaccines for major public health problems such as measles, polio, influenza, and hepatitis.[15] Many of the genetic variants involved are part of the cytochrome P450 system in the liver, and research indicates that the recently discovered phenomenon of copy number variants—variations among individuals in the number of certain genes—also can affect the efficacy of medications.[16] Under identical dosage for given drug, individual genetic variation can result in

- slow metabolism of the drug, leading to toxic levels of the drug or its byproducts;
- intermediate metabolism, resulting in a steady and safe level that has the intended therapeutic effect;
- ultra-rapid metabolism, which clears the drug from the system so quickly that it never achieves the intended therapeutic effect.

The study of genetic factors that directly influence a person's reaction to medications is called **pharmacogenetics**. In the broader sense, **pharmacogenomics** is the application of genomic information (all human genes and their interactions relevant to drug response) and technology in drug development and therapy.

The published literature indicates that adverse drug responses (ADRs) are responsible for 6.7 percent of unintentional injuries that lead to hospitalization, with a fatality rate of 0.32 percent.[17,18] If those estimates are correct, there are more than 2.2 million serious ADRs in hospitalized patients (not including ADRs in ambulatory settings), causing more than 106,000 deaths annually. These data rank ADRs as the fourth leading cause of death, which is ahead of pulmonary disease, diabetes, AIDS, pneumonia, accidents, and automobile deaths.[19]

ADRs have a significant impact on our aging population as well, with more than 350,000 ADRs reportedly occurring in U.S. nursing homes each year.[20] The risk for ADRs is compounded as the number of medications increases, as demonstrated by a random chart review of 283 emergency-department patients over age 65. That review found that the number of medications per patient ranged from zero to 17 and averaged 4.2 per individual. ADRs in this population accounted for 10.6 percent of all emergency visits.[21]

The U.S. Food and Drug Administration is developing regulations for pharmacogenetic testing, and it is likely that many drug labels ultimately will carry recommendations for the clinician to conduct such testing before specifying medication and dosage. The hope is that this approach will supplant the traditional method of "start low and go slow," whereby clinicians adjust drugs and dosage until the patient achieves the desired result. Pharmacogenetic testing should increase the likelihood that a clinician will prescribe the correct drug, at the correct dose, for the correct patient each time.

The exact number of ADRs in the United States per year is not certain, but it is clear that ADRs represent a largely preventable public health problem. The use of pharmacogenetic testing to identify individuals who are susceptible to ADRs could result in a significant reduction of healthcare costs.

Ethical, Legal, and Social Implications (ELSI)

Funding for the Human Genome Project, which began in 1989, was accompanied by the recognition that the ethical, legal, and social implications of human genome research (**ELSI**) would be important in the consideration of new genetic tests, treatments, and technologies. Most of the ELSI issues that arise in a genetic context (i.e., privacy, discrimination, and autonomy) are already familiar to clinicians and public health professionals. Some issues, however, are unique to genetics because by definition, genetic information relates not only to a patient but also to a family, and in some cases an ethnic group and a population. The idea that genetic information is unique and deserving of special attention is an ongoing policy debate that is being considered in national and state legislatures as well as in states devising their state public health plan for genetics.

The paragraphs below review some ELSI issues as they arise in the course of providing care in a genetics context for individuals or populations.

Access to and insurance coverage of genetic services, tests, and technologies. Public health agencies attempt to assure the provision of health care when it is otherwise unavailable. The potential health benefits of genetics can be achieved only with appropriate access to genetic counseling, genetic risk assessment, genetic testing services (when applicable), and health management based on genetic risk status. Genetic services are currently funded by individual patients and by private and public organizations including Medicaid, Children with Special Health Care Needs (CSHCN), Title V, state tax revenues, and insurers. Public health providers, primary care practitioners, and genetics professionals must work together to improve the genetics services infrastructure so that more communities can be reached. Some issues related to access to acute services follow.

- Some genetic tests and technologies are not covered routinely by insurance, especially when they are new or their clinical utility has not been established; Medicaid does not cover many genetic tests.
- Genetic tests may be covered under individual consideration, especially if they are determined to be medically necessary.
- Tests may not be covered if they are being performed only to provide information for another family member. For example, Medicare will not cover genetic testing of an older cancer survivor to determine if she carries a *BRCA1/2* mutation to facilitate testing her daughter, unless testing the Medicare beneficiary herself is a medical necessity.
- Most consultations with clinical geneticists are covered by third-party payers, including Medicaid; genetic counseling is not covered uniformly.
- Many genetic tests are expensive, reducing access to them by indigent or medically underserved populations.

Informed consent. The two major components of informed consent are disclosure and autonomy. Many ethicists and policy makers suggest that some or all genetic tests should be performed only after obtaining informed consent because the results have implications for family members and future children as well as for the patient requesting the information. Some states have laws that require informed consent for genetic testing.

Informed consent is justified especially for the following:

- Tests that provide predictive rather than diagnostic information. Diagnostic tests are part of routine medical care, and the results are used to guide treatment of the patient. Tests for susceptibility to a disorder provide a probability of developing a condition, and the uncertainty of the information may be a burden rather than a benefit to some patients, especially when primary prevention is unavailable.
- Tests that document susceptibility to a disorder for which there are no proven risk-reduction interventions. Unless there are options for reducing risk, being identified as at increased risk may not be beneficial. This is the rationale for policies that discourage genetic testing for risk of Alzheimer disease.

Disclosure refers to the process of informing patients about the risks, benefits, limitations, and alternatives of undergoing a procedure or test. Disclosure may be verbal or facilitated by educational materials. When detailed information is being provided to patients, especially when there is uncertainty about the meaning of the results, most genetics professionals agree that the results should be provided face-to-face, regardless of whether the test result is positive or negative.

Autonomy, which refers to an individual's ability to make decisions without undue influence of others, may be affected by the following:

- Influence or even coercion by providers, family members, or others. Family members, for example, may have an interest in or opinion about testing a relative, and coercion may occur if the mutation status of an affected family member is needed to facilitate genetic testing of unaffected relatives.
- The patient's or provider's perceived role in decision-making. Some patients want the provider to make decisions for them, and most want to know the provider's recommendation and consider it as a part of their decision. A minority want to make all decisions without knowing their provider's opinion.
- Complexity of the decision. For complex decisions, patients are more likely to want input from others, including providers and family members. Because of uncertain implications of many genetic tests, and the frequent lack of interventions to modify risk, patients consider any decisions about genetic tests to be complex.

Genetic discrimination. The use of genetic information by third parties to discriminate could involve an individual, a family, or a population. Genetic discrimination against an individual can relate to insurance (health, life, disability) and employment. Few well-documented cases of genetic discrimination exist, but it is clear that fear of genetic discrimination can prevent some patients from seeking risk assessment, consultation, or genetic testing. State-level protections against genetic discrimination are uneven, and Congress has debated comprehensive federal legislation several times in recent years without final passage (see the Genetic Information Nondiscrimination Act). There is considerable hope that the Act will pass and that the President will sign it into law before the end of 2008.

Privacy/disclosure of genetic information. Most families readily share information with relatives. However, some patients will not want to share personal medical information with their family members. If genetic testing is being considered, the provider should include a discussion of the implications of

CASE STUDY

Scenario

Maria is a 32-year-old married mother of a six-year-old daughter and a three-year-old son. She is seeing her family physician, Dr. Yashida, because of concern about breast cancer in her family. Maria wants to know if she is at risk and, if so, whether there is anything she can do to prevent the disease. Dr. Yashida collects a three-generation family history that shows the following:

- Maria's mother was diagnosed with breast cancer at the age of 47.
- One of Maria's maternal aunts was diagnosed with breast cancer at the age of 43.
- Maria's mother died at age 75, but the cause of death is unclear.
- Maria has a 29-year-old sister, reported to be healthy.

Before proceeding, construct a pedigree that displays the available information and consult the "red flags" discussed in Table 3–2 to determine whether there is reason for concern about Maria.

Defining the Issues

- About 5% to 10% of breast cancers among women result from inherited mutations in genes known as *BRCA1* and *BRCA2*. These genes also are associated with ovarian cancer. (Men can develop breast cancer, too. Check the red flags to see what that might indicate.)
- Women who carry any of these variants have a lifetime risk as high as 85% for breast cancer and more than 40% for ovarian cancer by age 70.
- Genetic testing is available for the mutations in these genes.
- Personal and/or family history of breast cancer diagnosed before age 50 is one of the indications for genetic testing.

Patient's Understanding

Maria has a general sense that she may be at increased risk for breast cancer. The literature indicates that most people overestimate their risks for disease. Dr. Yashida must take time to review Maria's family history with her and to explain the implications of that history for Maria's risk of breast cancer. She also must explain the indications for testing, the different types of tests that are possible, and when each is indicated.

CLINICAL PERSPECTIVE FOR THE INDIVIDUAL PATIENT

Level of Intervention Now

Maria clearly meets the criteria for *BRCA1/2* testing, and Dr. Yashida should discuss that with her. This discussion should be comprehensive, including the meanings of positive and negative results, the management options in each case, the potential implications for family members, the costs of the tests, and the nature of insurance coverage. Ultimately, Dr. Yashida should elicit formal informed consent from Maria before ordering the test, and he should be prepared to provide appropriate education and counseling when the test results arrive. He also should be prepared to refer Maria to a genetics specialist before or after testing if he is uncertain of his ability to render these services effectively.

The test selected for Maria will depend on a number of factors. For example, it is more informative to test an affected person first to determine the specific mutation in the family. Maria's mother is deceased, and the clinician should ask whether it is possible to test Maria's aunt. If that is not possible, the lab will perform a more comprehensive test on Maria's DNA. In addition, if Maria is of Ashkenazi Jewish extraction, the lab will perform tests that look for *BRCA1/2* variants that are common in that population.

Once the test results are available, Dr. Yashida will discuss appropriate management options with Maria. For example, if the test is positive, they can discuss more intensive surveillance (self-exam, clinical exam, mammography, MRI) begun at an earlier age, and potential chemoprevention. If the test is negative, Maria should maintain a standard level of surveillance appropriate to all women. Note that a negative test does not guarantee that Maria will not develop breast or ovarian cancer, which might arise for reasons unrelated to *BRCA1/2* mutations.

Maria also should understand that her test results have implications for other members of her family, including her sister, and she should be encouraged to share the test results with them. If the test is positive, Maria's daughter and son are at risk (50% each) to carry the mutation in question, and Maria should be prepared to discuss testing with them at the appropriate time.

Knowing Test Results Earlier

If Maria had raised her concerns earlier with her provider, she might have had earlier access to genetic testing for *BRCA1/2* variants, which could have led to earlier appropriate management. If Maria were so inclined, she also would have been able to inform her family members earlier, which would have allowed them earlier access to their own testing (if appropriate) and to related management options.

test results for other family members in the informed-consent process. Once information (family history or genetic-test result) is obtained, the provider and the patient should discuss who might benefit from the information and why, and the patient should be encouraged to share the information.

Duty to inform. Duty to inform refers to an obligation held by an individual (patient or provider) to inform a third party (e.g., biological relative) of a potential risk. For example, if a patient is found to carry an inherited mutation that increases cancer risk, the patient or even the healthcare provider may have a duty to inform biological relatives that they might carry the mutation.

Because warning a third party of a risk against a patient's wishes would mean breaching patient confidentiality, there are likely to be only a few situations where the provider might incur a duty to warn:

- the risk of harm is high (e.g., if a relative has a strong likelihood of carrying mutation that is highly likely to cause disease);
- the potential harm from not being warned is great (e.g., the relative could become seriously ill or die); and
- steps could have been taken to mitigate the risk of harm (effective intervention would avert the possible serious consequences of carrying the mutation).

PUBLIC HEALTH PERSPECTIVE FOR THE HEALTH OF THE GENERAL POPULATION AND OF HIGH RISK GROUPS

How does genetics—"a science of the individual"[22]—find a home in public health, a discipline that by definition focuses on populations? Of course, the two fields cannot remain separate because populations are comprised of individuals, and the seeming separation disappears when one recognizes that the two fields employ complementary perspectives. As Johns Hopkins physician and geneticist Barton Childs observed, "The public health person will assert, 'This (dietary component, environmental exposure, behavior, etc.) is a risk factor'; and the geneticist will respond, 'Yes, but for whom?'" Insights from genetics will continue to inform public health as it becomes increasingly possible to stratify individual and population risks on the basis of biology, in concert with traditional public health approaches that stratify risks on the basis of exposure or behavior. Conversely, genetics will benefit from public health insights about the best ways to structure population-based research and to introduce new services, interventions, and educational efforts to the public.

Among the most obvious areas for collaboration is the investigation of whether individual knowledge of genetic susceptibility to disease results in behavior change, but many other areas are ripe with possibility. A 2006 article by Burke et al.[23] makes the case for a new "evaluation process, based in ongoing integration of knowledge within and across multiple disciplines (including ELSI) to determine the outcomes, both health-related and social, of new genome-based applications." The Genome-based Research and Population Health International Network (GRAPH *Int*) now exists to promote the necessary international and interdisciplinary collaborations.

The marriage of genetics and public health is still in its infancy, and specialists in both fields are addressing the scientific and technological challenges associated with this burgeoning field, including the identification of genetic contributions to complex disease and the application of genetic approaches in a public health context. Many of the related efforts are coordinated by the National Office of Public Health Genomics, at the U.S. Centers for Disease Control and Prevention. For example, the office directs the Human Genome Epidemiology Network (HuGENet), and has developed a set of competencies in genomics for public health professionals. In addition, the American Public Health Association (APHA) is developing a new forum on genomics to serve as a locus for activities of APHA members interested in this area (see www.aphagenomics forum.org; accessed March 10, 2008).

KEY TERMS

Biology Terms

Alleles: Alternate versions of the same gene. A gene might have multiple alleles, but each individual can have only two different alleles for any given gene.

Autosomal Dominant Trait: A trait that is carried on an autosome (a non-sex chromosome) and requires only one copy of the associated allele for expression of the phenotype.

Autosomal Recessive Trait: A trait that is carried on an autosome (a non-sex chromosome) and requires two copies of the associated allele for expression of the phenotype.

Chromosomes: Thread-like structures in the nucleus of a cell that are made of DNA and structural proteins. Human cells other than egg and sperm normally have 46 chromosomes (23 pairs). Egg and sperm cells have 23 chromosomes each.

DNA (deoxyribonucleic acid): The universal genetic material; the information molecule that carries hereditary information from one generation of cells to the next and from one generation of individuals to the next. Genes are made of DNA, which is the molecular basis of heredity.

ELSI: Acronym for "ethical, legal, and social implications" of human genome research. The ELSI program began as a central component of the Human Genome Project (q.v.), with the goal to support research and education about the applications of knowledge derived from research in genetics and genomics. The term ELSI now has come to signify any such category of issues, even if they are not directly related to the Human Genome Project.

Evolution: The change in gene frequencies in populations of organisms over time, potentially leading to the production of new species. Evolution helps to determine the genetic structure of human populations, thereby helping to determine the nature and extent of disease in those populations.

First-Degree Relatives: Parents, siblings, children.

Gene: A segment of DNA that contains instructions for making a specific protein or proteins required by the body. Genes are found in succession along the length of chromosomes. Human beings have about 20,000 genes.

Genetics: The branch of science concerned with the means and consequences of inherited biological variation.

Genetic Counseling: "The process of helping people understand and adapt to the medical, psychological and familial implications of genetic contributions to disease. This process integrates interpretation of family and medical histories to assess the chance of disease occurrence or recurrence, education about inheritance, testing, management, prevention, resources and research, counseling to promote informed choices and adaptation to the risk or condition." (From the National Society of Genetic Counselors)

Genome: All of the DNA of a given organism. One speaks, for example, of the human genome or the mouse genome.

Genomics: The study of whole genomes, usually focusing on extensive DNA sequences.

Genotype: The genetic constitution of an organism or cell; the set of alleles inherited at a locus.

Human Genome Project: The effort, completed in 2003, to determine the sequence of all 3.2 billion base pairs of human DNA. The results of the project are deposited in public databases that are accessible to all interested parties.

Independent Assortment: The principle that different genes (and versions of genes, i.e., alleles) are distributed independently into egg and sperm. Independent assortment explains why it is possible to look like a certain family member, but not to have the same medical conditions or traits, and vice versa.

Mendelian Inheritance: Relating the principles of heredity first described by Gregor Mendel in 1865. Mendelian (single-gene) traits follow well-defined patterns of inheritance.

Pedigree: A diagram showing the genetic relationships between members of a family that is annotated with relevant medical information. Pedigrees are used to visualize inheritance patterns and to aid in diagnosis and risk assessment.

Pharmacogenetics: The study of genetic factors that directly influence a person's reaction to medications.

Pharmacogenomics: The application of genomic information (all human genes and their interactions relevant to drug response) and technology in drug development and therapy.

Phenotype: The physical expression of a trait or disease.

Second-Degree Relatives: Grandparents, grandchildren, nieces, nephews, aunts, uncles, half siblings.

Segregation: The distribution of chromosomes during the formation of an egg or sperm. Each person has two versions of each chromosome, but can only contribute one of each pair to an egg or sperm cell.

Third-Degree Relatives: First cousins, great-grandchildren, great-grandparents.

X-Linked Trait: A trait that is carried on the X chromosome; that is, not on an autosome.

Public Health Term

Public Health Genetics: Application of knowledge from genetics and genomics, in the context of the principles of public health, to improve the health of populations.

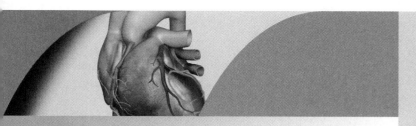

Questions for Further Research, Study, Reflection, and Discussion

For the Individual Student

In order to answer these questions, it may be necessary to research the primary literature.

- How does comparative genomics—the ability to compare the genome of *Homo sapiens* to the genomes of other species—improve our understanding of health and disease?
- Define the following terms with respect to genetic testing:
  - Analytic validity
  - Clinical validity
  - Clinical utility
- What percentage of their genes do the following people share, on average?
  - First-degree relatives
  - Second-degree relatives
  - Third-degree relatives

For Small Group Discussion

- Explain how progress in genetics can help public health professionals stratify risk on the basis of biology, as contrasted with stratification of risk on the basis of exposure to environmental variables.
- Assume that Maria, the patient in the Case Study scenario, tests positive for one of the *BRCA1/2* variants. Maria's sister (a first-degree relative) is at risk for carrying the variant and would benefit from testing. Dr. Yashida explains that Maria should share this test result with her sister, but Maria says she and her sister do not get along and refuses to share the information. How should the provider respond?
- Discuss the difference between relative and absolute risk.

- Investigate the concept of "penetrance" in genetics and discuss its impact on risk assessment.
- Research shows that many people have trouble understanding statements of risk and probability. Investigate and discuss this research literature and suggest the best method(s) for communicating risk statements to patients.

For Entire Class Discussion

- Should all students in public health be required to take course work in human and clinical genetics? If yes, what is the best way to integrate that instruction into the curriculum? If not, justify your opinion (see Chen LS, Goodson P. Public health genomics knowledge and attitudes: a survey of public health educators in the U.S. *Genet Med* 2007;9:496–503).
- Should the federal government regulate direct-to-consumer genetic tests? Defend your position.
- Explore the ways in which research in genetics and genomics has influenced thinking about race in the scientific and clinical communities. Should race be a variable in the clinical setting and in biomedical research?
- Some commentators are concerned that the costs of genetically based health care will limit access to care for those who cannot afford it, exacerbating already serious health disparities. How might society ensure equal access to this care?
- The most significant contributions to mortality and morbidity are diseases that result from a combination of genetic and environmental variables. Given the current limitations of genetically based interventions for common disease, should public health policy focus instead on reducing exposure to the environmental factors that contribute to disease and assign genetics a lower priority?
- Many developing countries are still struggling with infectious diseases such as malaria and with the inability to provide safe drinking water to their populations. Should international public health agencies concentrate on those needs and eschew genetically based care?

EXERCISE/ACTIVITY

- CDC notifies Congress that the morbidity and mortality related to colorectal cancer are issues in need of federal regulation. Congress issues a mandate that allows funding for demonstration programs. The state director of public health asks your group to design a demonstration program that incorporates genetic perspectives, with the following goals:

  ○ reduce the morbidity and mortality associated with colorectal cancer by a certain percentage, *and*
  ○ determine whether knowledge that one has an inherited risk for colorectal cancer is a motivating factor for screening and health-promoting behaviors.

REFERENCES

1. Bowcock AM. Genomics: guilt by association. *Nature* 2007:447:645–646.

2. Diabetes Genetics Initiative of Broad Institute of Harvard and MIT, Lund University, and Novartis Institutes of BioMedical Research, Saxena R, Voight BF, et al. Genome-wide association analysis identifies loci for type 2 diabetes and triglyceride levels. *Science* 2007;316:1331–1336.

3. Helgadottir A, Thorleifsson G, Manolescu A, Gretarsdottir S, Blondal T, et al. A common variant on chromosome 9p21 affects the risk of myocardial infarction. *Science* 2007;316:1491–1493.

4. Wellcome Trust Case Control Consortium. Genome-wide association study of 14,000 cases of seven common diseases and 3,000 shared controls. *Nature* 2007;447:661–678.

5. Zuchner S, Roberts ST, Speer MC, Beckham JC. Update on psychiatric genetics. *Genet Med* 2007;9:332–340.

6. Bennett RL. The family medical history. *Prim Care Clin Office Pract* 2004;31:479–495.

7. Guttmacher AE, Collins FS, Carmona RH. The family history—more important than ever. *N Engl J Med* 2004;351:2333–2336.

8. Yoon PW, Scheuner MT, Peterson-Oehlke KL, Gwinn M, Faucett A, Khoury MJ. Can family history be used as a tool for public health and preventive medicine? *Genet Med* 2002;4:304–310.

9. Ramsey SD, Burke W, Pinsky L, Clarke L, Newcomb P, Khoury MJ. Family history assessment to detect increased risk for colorectal cancer: Conceptual considerations and a preliminary economic analysis. *Cancer Epidemiol Biomarkers Prev* 2005;14(11 Pt 1):2494–2500.

10. Rumboldt M, Rumboldt Z, Pesenti S. Premature parental heart attack is heralding elevated risk in their offspring. *Coll Antropol* 2003;27:221–228.

11. Wu O, Robertson L, Twaddle S, Lowe G, Clark P, Walker I, Brenkel I, Greaves M, Langhorne P, Regan L, Greer I. Screening for thrombophilia in high-risk situations: a meta-analysis and cost-effectiveness analysis. *Br J Haematol* 2005;131:80–90.

12. Gudgeon JM, McClain MR, Palomaki GE, Williams MS. Rapid ACCE: Experience with a rapid and structured approach for evaluating gene-based testing. *Genet Med* 2007;9:473–478.

13. Hudson K, Javits G, Burke W, Byers P, et al. ASHG statement on direct-to-consumer genetic testing in the United States. *Am J Hum Genet* 2007;81: 635–637.

14. Garrod A. *The Inborn Factors in Disease*. Oxford, UK: Oxford-Clarendon Press; 1931.

15. Kimman TG, Vandebriel RJ, Hoebee B. Genetic variation in response to vaccination. *Comm Genet* 2007;10:201–217.

16. Ouahchi K, Lindeman N, Lee C. Copy number variants and pharmacogenomics. *Pharmacogenomics* 2006;7:25–29.

17. Budnitz DS, Pollock DA, Weidenbach KN, et al. National surveillance of emergency department visits for outpatient adverse drug events. *JAMA* 2006;296:1858–1866.

18. Lazarou J, Pomeranz B, Corey PN. Incidence of adverse drug reactions in hospitalized patients: a meta-analysis of prospective studies. *JAMA* 1998;279:1200–1205.

19. United States Food and Drug Administration. Center for Drug Evaluation and Research. Available at http://www.fda.gov/cder. Accessed March 10, 2008.

20. Gurwitz JH, Field TS, Avorn J, et al. Incidence and preventability of adverse drug events in nursing homes. *Am J Med* 2000;109:87–94.

21. Kohl CM, et al. Polypharmacy, adverse drug-related events, and potential adverse drug interactions in elderly patients presenting to an emergency department. *Ann Emerg Med* 2001;38:666–671.

22. Childs B, Weiner C, Valle D. A science of the individual: implications for a medical school curriculum. In: Chakravarti A, Green E, eds. *Annual Review of Genomics and Human Genetics*. Palo Alto, CA: Annual Reviews; 2005.

23. Burke W, Khoury MJ, Stewart A, Zimmern RL. The path from genome-based research to population health: development of an international public health genomics network. *Genet Med* 2006;8:451–458.

RESOURCES

American College of Medical Genetics: http://www.acmg .net//AM/Template.cfm?Section=Home3

American Society of Human Genetics: http://www.ashg.org/ genetics/ashg/ashgmenu.htm

GeneTests: http://www.genestar.org/

National Coalition for Health Professional Education in Genetic (NCHPEG): http://www.nchpeg.org/

National Human Genome Research Institute: http://www .genome.gov/

National Office of Public Health Genomics, Centers for Disease Control and Prevention: http://www.cdc.gov/genomics/

National Society of Genetic Counselors: http://www.nsgc.org/

Genome projects of the U.S. Department of Energy Office of Science: http://genomics.energy.gov/

ACKNOWLEDGMENTS

Portions of this chapter were extracted or adapted from the following programs developed by the National Coalition for Health Professional Education in Genetics:

- Core Competencies in Family History for Health Professionals
- Core Competencies in Genetics for Health Professionals
- Core Principles in Genetics for Health Professionals
- Genetics and Common Disease: Implications for Primary Care and Public Health Providers
- Genetics and Major Psychiatric Disorders
- Genetics in the Physician Assistant's Practice
- Genetics in the Practice of Speech-Language Pathology & Audiology
- Genetics, Race, and Health Care: What We Know and What It Means for Your Practice

CROSS REFERENCES

All chapters

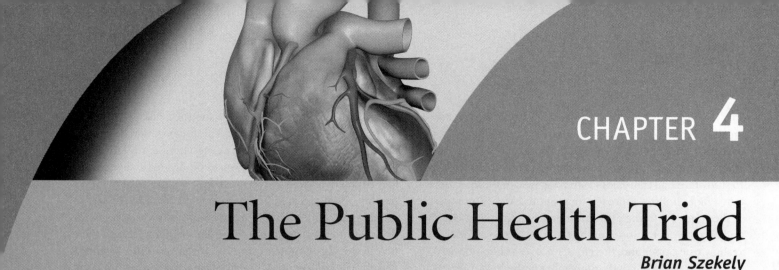

CHAPTER 4

The Public Health Triad

Brian Szekely

Modification of natural habitats by humans is a leading cause of emerging zoonoses. The new "habitat" is used mostly by livestock that are in close proximity to wild species possibly harboring disease. Modification of rainforests to pasture thereby increases the chance for zoonotic disease transmission to occur. It is the proximity of humans to infected domesticated and/or wild animals that perpetuates the spread of the **pathogen**.[1]

LEARNING OBJECTIVES

By the end of this chapter, the student will be able to:

- Explain the public health triad and discuss why and how we study it.
- Discuss how conservation biology is directly tied to public health.
- Demonstrate how we are contaminating the planet's resources, and what can we do, if anything, to offset these actions.
- Discuss how we are altering infectious disease transmission.
- Define **biodiversity**, and discuss why it is so important to the future of the planet.

INTRODUCTION

This chapter serves as an introduction to the public health triad and the emerging field of **conservation medicine**. The public health triad involves studying the interactions among humans, animals, and the environment. Conservation medicine practitioners study these interactions in order to solve global and micro-scale health problems. The topic of zoonoses—diseases transmitted between humans and animals—is one of high importance to the public health triad. Presently, zoonoses account for nearly 75% of emerging infectious diseases worldwide.[2]

Preventable human behavior has been attributed to some of these outbreaks and is discussed throughout the chapter. In addition, several current ecological problems are caused by some of the same human actions. An overview is provided on how we are misusing man-made products and natural resources shown by their local and global consequences. Human behavior can negatively affect the health of the environment and the animals that are sustained by that environment.

Additionally, human behavior can lead to *human*-related health problems, which is an obvious concern for the health and well-being of the planet. If the stewards of the planet are in trouble, what does that say for the planet as a whole? Other topics discussed include the need to decipher relationships between environmental issues and human and animal health in the hope to promote a sustainable future. Furthermore, the implications of biodiversity reduction and their associated loss of **biologically active substances** are explained.

BASIC SCIENCE FACTS/KEY CONCEPTS REVIEW

What Is The Public Health Triad?

The public health triad (or simply, the triad) describes the interactions among humans, animals, and the environment using health-related consequences. The triad attempts to fuse scientific disciplines to characterize public health issues, as all forms of life on earth are extremely interactive. To understand each role the triad plays in any given health problem, one must take a theoretical "step back" to gain the right perspective. Rarely is only one aspect of the triad involved in a public health crisis; usually all three play a role. Confounding factors affect disease epidemics, extraordinary ecological phenomena, the extinction of an uncommon species, or the changing of our atmosphere. To study the triad translates to studying ALL of these factors to gain a more holistic approach to health research. The concept of the triad is a frame of mind more than anything else. By studying the interactions among the triad, we have the ability to show true causes and, therefore, uncover real solutions.

One example of how each member of the triad interacts is how the poor maintenance of livestock or agricultural fields by humans can aid in the spread of many animal and human diseases. Over the past several years, a number of different bacterial outbreaks have plagued vegetable growers in the western United States. Many believe that the contamination was due to the poor maintenance of livestock in the immediate or adjacent area.

Also, the overuse of petroleum products has led to the increase of carbon dioxide (CO_2; a greenhouse gas) in the atmosphere,[3] which in turn enhances the greenhouse effect that is associated with global warming. Another instance is human's previous use of chlorofluorocarbons (CFCs), which were proven to be a cause of reducing ozone in the Earth's stratosphere. This reduction allowed more direct sunlight (UVB in particular) to enter the earth's atmosphere, and in turn could have made more people at risk for nonmelanoma skin cancer and plays a major role in malignant melanoma development.[4] In addition, the hole in the ozone layer, concentrated mostly over the Antarctic, increases melting of the polar ice caps that alters weather patterns, increases flooding incidence, and destroys wildlife habitat.[5] These human, animal, and environmental problems caused by human's use of a dangerous chemical made the international community pass the Montreal Protocol in 1989. The phasing out of several groups of halogenated hydrocarbons, including CFCs, was implemented.

The health of the planet and its resident can benefit if we humans strive to determine relationships among the fields of human, animal, and environmental health, rather than trying to separate them. All of the above examples illustrate a point. Human behavior (possibly preventable) has negatively affected the health of the triad. Each aspect of the triangle is inexplicitly linked to the other. What happens to one no doubt can affect the rest. That is the core concert of the triad (Figure 4-1).

One organization that sees the benefit of these three disciplines working together is the World Health Organization (WHO). WHO openly and strongly stresses the cooperation between human, veterinary, and environmental public health professionals and refers to the term "public health triad" throughout its Web site.

Established in 1948, WHO is the specialized agency for health under the United Nations. This organization deals with all aspects of health, including everything from emerging infectious diseases and nutrition, to biodiversity, alcoholism, and ethics. In addition to trying to link all aspects of the triad together, WHO recognizes that these links are much tighter in developing nations. Human populations in these areas work directly with animals for transportation, agriculture, and their own food supply much more often than in industrialized nations. Horses are used instead of cars, tractors are used for draught power, and their meats aren't cut and sealed in plastic wrap and waiting at the grocery store. The connections among humans, animals, and the environment are impacted to a greater extent by those relying on the rawest natural resources, of which most reside in underdeveloped or developing nations. One way that these close conditions can negatively affect public health is the increased incidence of zoonotic transmission.

Zoonoses

Many historical and current human diseases originated from animal hosts. A handful of these zoonoses and their hosts are: the plague (rodents), anthrax (cattle, sheep, goats, and other herbivores), epidemic typhus (rodents), tuberculosis (mainly cattle), Lyme disease (**vector borne** from rodents and deer), West Nile fever (vector borne from birds and some other small mammals), Ebola virus (undetermined animal reservoir), avian influenza (birds), severe acute respiratory syndrome (SARS; possibly several animal hosts including cats and ferrets but currently undetermined). The proximity of humans to animals harboring such diseases is a large factor for the emergence of these zoonoses. Humans who work with or live near animal species are at a much greater risk of contracting and perpetuating zoonoses as well as starting new epidemics. As humans expand their range into wild animal habitat, we are documenting the emergence of more zoonoses. We are also documenting the reemergence of zoonoses that were thought to have been controlled, such as bovine tuberculosis in Great Britain.[1]

Bovine Tuberculosis in Great Britain

Bovine tuberculosis (bTB), caused by the bacteria *Mycobacterium bovis*, has the greatest host range out of all TB organisms, being able to infect all warm-blooded vertebrates.[6] During the 1930s, a large portion of dairy cows were infected with *M. bovis* in Great Britain. This became a major public health concern because people drank the raw milk from infected cows, which increased the spread of the disease to include high density urban areas. Approximately 2,500 people

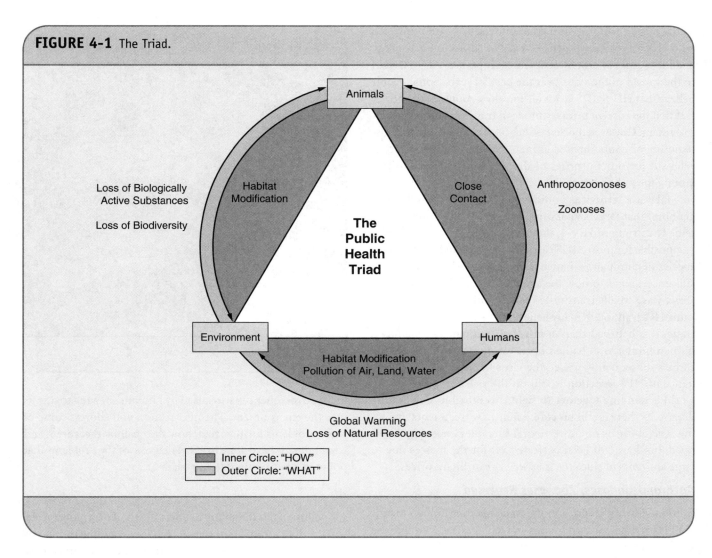

FIGURE 4-1 The Triad.

The Public Health Triad

Animals

Humans

Environment

Habitat Modification

Close Contact

Anthropozoonoses

Zoonoses

Loss of Biologically Active Substances

Loss of Biodiversity

Habitat Modification
Pollution of Air, Land, Water

Global Warming
Loss of Natural Resources

Inner Circle: "HOW"
Outer Circle: "WHAT"

died per year from bTB during the 1930s in Great Britain.[6] The disease was spread among cattle due to large numbers being closely confined and in poorly ventilated cowsheds, an ideal environment for this airborne disease. bTB is primarily transmitted through the exchange of respiratory secretions between infected and noninfected humans or animals. Over the subsequent 50 years, the voluntary and eventual compulsory testing and slaughter program helped to reduce the incidence of bTB and TB in humans to a very low level by 1980. However, there has been a rise in bTB incidence in the past 15 years and it is currently one of the most difficult animal health problems facing the farming industry in Great Britain. A long-term epidemiological study in Woodchester Park in southwest England shows the rise having been attributed to badgers, one of the natural reservoirs of the disease. Less than adequate cattle farming practices bring badgers into close contact with these domesticated species, increasing the risk of disease trans-

mission to cattle[7] and ultimately to humans. Constant surveillance, routine testing, and effective barriers for badgers are some ways that can lessen the incidence rate of bTB. However, time and money are not always available to the farmer, and TB-infected badgers can contaminate cattle either by infecting their food supply or by direct contact.[8] Therefore, many factors (cultural, financial, environmental, and biological) are affecting the rate of disease transmission of bTB in England. Public health officials are still figuring out the best course of action for curbing this **zoonosis**.

Human Immunodeficiency Virus (HIV) and Acquired Immune Deficiency Syndrome (AIDS)

One of the most devastating epidemics of the 21st century, HIV/AIDS has killed more than 25 million people since it was first recognized in 1981. HIV/AIDS infects children under the age of 15 EVERY MINUTE OF EVERY DAY, while over 90%

of the more than 5 million children who have been infected with HIV were born in Africa.[9] Lack of education, resources, and the nonuse of prophylactics in many parts of Africa has led to the spread of the virus over the past 30 years. Some people believe that HIV/AIDS is not technically a zoonosis, due to the fact that the current primary mode of transmission is human-to-human. However, the disease has been attributed to the mishandling of contaminated animal products and therefore is relevant for our purposes of demonstrating relationships among the public health triad.

HIV is a retrovirus (which integrates itself into the host genome) that targets vital organs related to the immune system. The origin of HIV-1, the more common, virulent strain responsible for most AIDS cases, has been accredited to a subspecies of chimpanzee native to west equatorial Africa.[10] It is still uncertain as to how the simian immunodeficiency virus (SIV) was actually transmitted to humans (which in turn became HIV), although many believe it was due to the bushmeat trade. It is believed that an infected chimpanzee killed by a human hunter who had an open wound when handling the carcass subsequently passed the virus to other humans. Incidence of HIV infection is still on the rise and much of the world is banding together to fight this horrible, debilitating disease, as there is still no cure. Many new treatments involving several forms of antiretroviral therapies are being developed, but have not been perfected yet for the masses due to large amounts of side effects as well as exorbitant prices.

Anthropozoonoses: Zoonoses Reversed

Additionally, anthropozoonotic transmission (human to animal) is a serious concern in zoos and national parks around the world. Certain "harmless" human sicknesses (such as the common cold) can be lethal in a novel host, a non-human primate for example. Tanzanian National Parks (TANAPA) require tourists and researchers to wear masks in Mahale National Park (and others) when viewing chimpanzees, specifically to cut down on possible diseases transmission from humans to the endangered population of wild chimpanzees of the region (Figure 4-2).

Zoonoses pose an obvious threat to both human and animal health. It is difficult to discuss the topic without taking the time to talk about its relation to the environment, specifically in the form of **habitat modification** (discussed below in the section entitled *Land*).

Pollution of Air, Water, and Land: How Humans Affect the Environment

Health of the triad is also linked to the changes in chemistry of earth's air, water, and land. Many diseases and negative eco-

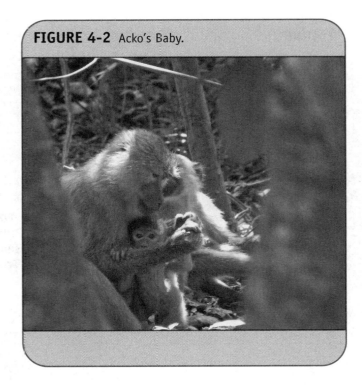

FIGURE 4-2 Acko's Baby.

logical consequences are caused by humans spewing toxicants into the environment. The next section will address some of these problems for the triad, how they can be measured, and what humans have done to alleviate some of the problems that pollutants have caused to the triad.

Air

Air pollution has the ability to affect the triad on a global scale, as hazardous air pollutants have been seen traveling thousands of miles and having a severe impact on Earth's atmosphere along the way. Pollution was first seen as a problem in the air within urban environments during the mid to late 1800s. Most of the pollutants at this time were soot consisting of sulfur dioxide (SO_2), volatile organic compounds (VOCs) such as benzene and toluene, and nitrogen oxides (NO_x), all from the burning of fossil fuels. By the mid 1900s, the effects of these pollutants were known to be lethal in urban centers where a large amount of factories produced such pollutants. To correct this problem in some areas, newer smokestacks were built taller and away from city centers. These actions helped the local residents of the city, but overall, the region was affected by an increase in acid rainfall as more of the pollutants were able to react with water, oxygen, and other chemicals naturally in the atmosphere. Pollution as well as the deposition of acidified rain can damage forests and lakes, which can increase the amount of fish kills in a particular area as well as have serious impacts on human health.

Air pollution is known to increase the risk of chronic respiratory disease and lung cancer, damage the liver and kidneys, generate reproductive complications, and can also exacerbate other existing health conditions for the triad. The Environmental Protection Agency (EPA) has estimated that with the full implementation of the Acid Rain Program (Title IV under the Clean Air Act) by 2010, the public health benefits will be valued at $50 billion annually due to decreased mortality, hospital admissions, and emergency room visits alone.[11] The goal of the Acid Rain Program is to reduce annual SO_2 emissions 10 million tons below 1980 levels. This goal is to be carried out by the stricter regulations set on fossil fuel–fired power plants.

The most common chemicals found in the air today that are considered pollutants are still SO_2, VOCs, and NO_x; however, ground level ozone, carbon monoxide, and lead have been added in recent years.[12] Lately, more and more research is being published about the effect of increased CO_2 levels in the atmosphere, which contributes to global warming. Therefore, CO_2 has become a much more common air pollutant than in the past due to its higher-than-natural concentration in the atmosphere. Nearly all of these compounds are generated from the burning of fossil fuels from such activities as driving cars and trucks, electricity production from coal, manufacturing chemicals, and other large-scale industrial processes.

Air pollution in the United States is regulated by the EPA, and guidelines pertaining to air quality are outlined in the Clean Air Act. Under this law, first passed in 1970, the EPA set limits to how much of a pollutant can be in the air. Permits are now being issued to larger sources of air pollution that detail how much of and what type of pollutant may be expelled into the atmosphere based on how it affects humans, animals, and the environment. Economic incentives are being issued by the EPA for clearing the air of toxicants. One example of such an incentive is how gasoline refiners can receive credits if the gasoline they produce is cleaner than required. Those credits may then be used in place of paying a fine when their gasoline doesn't meet EPA's standards.[13] However, industrialized cities are by no means the only areas feeling health effects from air pollution. Air pollution is affecting the triad on a *global* scale. Mean temperatures worldwide are rising, mainly due to air pollution caused by human actions (Figure 4-3).

Global Warming: Human-Induced Air Pollution Has Its Consequences

Increased levels of greenhouse gases (CO_2, water vapor, methane, and ozone) in the air are caused by the combustion of fossil fuels and the changes of land use by humans.[14] The "greenhouse effect" is a natural, essential process that warms the earth enough to make it suitable for life. Without it, the Earth's surface would be approximately 33°C colder.[15] It is the "enhanced greenhouse effect" that is contributing to the warming of the planet. More and more greenhouse gases are being expelled into the air due to the increased amount of carbon products that humans are using, which allows increased trapping of heat that is radiated from the earth's surface. The topic of whether global warming was even occurring has been debated since the 1970s. Within the past few years, more information has been brought into the public eye and to the desks of politicians (most scientists in the field have agreed with the theory for a number of years now). Finally, most of the world believes that global warming is occurring and that humans are playing an active role in the cause of this trend. It has been strongly speculated that due to human behaviors, increases in global mean temperature can influence disease transmission. Could driving to work every day be a biological basis for perpetuating disease?

Many disease-harboring parasites and vectors are affected by rainfall, humidity, and temperature. Temperature extremes may kill *Anopheles* mosquitoes (a species that carries malaria in Africa), but a slight increase in temperature from 19°C to 21°C shortens the interval between blood meals (the gonotrophic cycle). It can also increase their pace of development, thereby infecting more people at a faster rate.[16] Malakooti's group have

FIGURE 4-3 Communicating with the Author's Laboratory: Bush2Base.

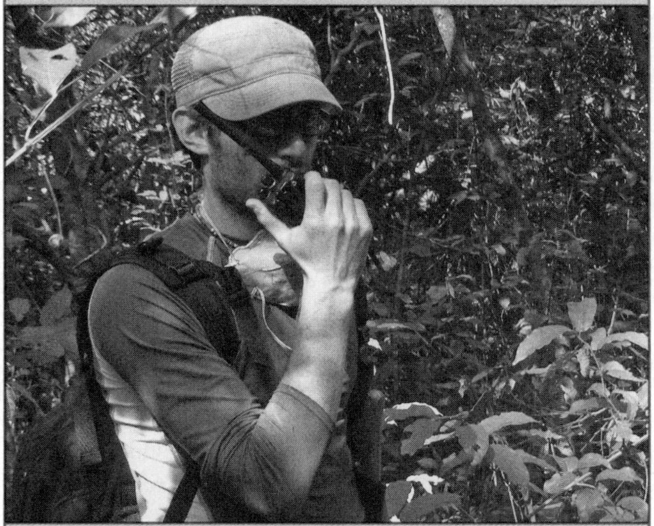

documented the emergence of epidemic malaria in a highland area of Kenya traditionally thought to be free of the disease due to its high altitude.[16] Warmer mean temperatures have caused the expansion of the "mosquito line," and these vectors are spreading disease at elevations they have never survived at in the past. Additionally, the rate of dengue virus replication in *Aedes aegypti* mosquitoes increases directly with temperature in the laboratory, and it was also found that epidemics of Saint Louis encephalitis virus and West Nile virus may be influenced by climatic factors.[17] The chemistry of the atmosphere is changing in part due to human activity. Some consequences of the shift in chemistry are serious and already causing problems for the health of the planet. If we don't have air in our lungs, in a sense, what do we have?

Water

Safe accessible water is a cornerstone for maintaining nearly all life on Earth. Potable drinking water is a necessity for the health and well-being of humans and animals. Water can be contaminated with a seemingly endless array of chemicals from a number of different sources, both natural and **anthropogenic**. The erosion of certain rock formations during natural flow and percolation of groundwater can lead to the buildup of minerals, some of which are radioactive. The prolonged exposure of drinking water contaminated with these minerals increases the risk of cancer to humans. The EPA also regulates water quality within the United States under the Clean Water Act (formerly known as the Federal Water Pollution Control Act Amendments of 1972). The Act allowed the EPA to set up standards for discharging any pollutant into waters of the United States. Point sources (PSs) such as industrial complexes, toxic waste sites, and manufacturing plants play a role in water contamination. The mishandling of harmful chemicals by both consumers and workers at the plants can aid this type of pollution. Some of the implications associated with the release of dangerous chemicals (VOCs, pesticides, and heavy metals) into the drinking water supply include chronic and acute health problems such as: cancer, damage to the immune system, liver and kidney disease, birth defects, and disorders of the nervous system. Nonpoint source (NPS) pollution comes from rainfall or snowmelt that travels over the ground and carries away pollutants for final deposition in lakes, ponds, rivers, wetlands, and underground sources of drinking water that can affect a large number of people simultaneously. NPS toxicants include: fertilizers, pesticides, oil and toxic chemicals from urban runoff, and improper management of animal by-products. Everything from cancer and birth defects to skeletal fluorosis has been attributed to contaminated waters. Nearly all of the water pollution discussed above is due to the poor containment of dangerous

chemicals by humans, thereby negatively affecting the triad once again.

Water can be contaminated with infectious disease particles also. Transmission of parasites such as *Crytosporidium* as well as bacterial and viral infections (*Escherichia coli* and hepatits A, respectively) can be spread by infected water. Waterborne infectious diseases are a major global problem, as it is estimated that nearly 1 million deaths worldwide are due to waterborne bacterial infections alone, caused by large poorly functioning municipal water distribution systems.[18] The amount of fresh water available is dwindling as the human population grows. If we don't find ways to use it more wisely, another one of life's necessities will slowly vanish.

Land

Healthy plant growth and food production rely on the health of the soil in which the organism grows. Land contamination therefore has the ability to affect the food chain, which has an obvious application to public health. **Biomagnification**, the accumulation of a substance (in this case, a pollutant) up the food chain is one clear example of how higher trophic levels can be in serious danger. For example, land can be polluted with a hazardous chemical such as a harmful pesticide, which seeps into the soil and eventually resides in a plant to be eaten by a consumer, such as a cow. Granted, maybe only a trace amount of pollutant is within each blade of grass. But, if a cow eats nearly 40 pounds of grass a day, the concentration of pesticide within the cow will slowly rise, making it unfit to be eaten by humans. This is another case where humans are

Habitat Modification: Human Population Needs More Land. Who Suffers?

1. Can cause a loss of flood control as trees and other vegetation are uprooted.
2. Can cause a loss of beneficial species from which prescription drugs and vaccines are developed.
3. Can help to spread disease (zoonoses in particular) as more people are exposed to new arthropods harboring infections.
4. Slash and burn habitat modification can aid in the release of greenhouse gases that contribute to global warming.
5. Can cause ecological imbalances where there is a boom or bust of a certain species, which can negatively affect the food chain.

negatively affecting the environment. However, in this instance, a food-animal's health is put in jeopardy, which in turn could negatively affect the health of the humans who eat it. It comes full circle very quickly, and therefore affects us ALL. Additionally, the use of pesticides can have other affects on the triad. Certain pests may become resistant to pesticides. Consequently, the more robust species survive. After several instances of spraying ineffectively, a farmer may have to spray more often and in higher doses. But spraying massive amounts of pesticides on crops has its price. Some acute dangers to humans include headaches, dizziness, nausea, and fatigue. Long-term exposure through the food we eat can cause cancer, endocrine disruption, and multiple chemical sensitivity (MCS; a medical condition characterized by the body's inability to tolerate relatively low amounts of chemicals). Pesticides also can harm the environment. Beneficial insects, worms, and soil microorganisms may be killed from pesticides, in turn harming the plants that we are trying to protect in the first place. Essential plant nutrient concentration may be affected, causing too little or too much nutrient uptake by the plant roots.

Contamination of our air, water, and land is a considerable threat to the triad, causing acute health complications as well as diseases. It is imperative that we not lose sight of the larger goal to protect the planet by acting in a sustainable manner. Pollution is inevitable; however, the contents of the pollution and how we are disposing or recycling them make a large difference.

The term *habitat modification* is used instead of the word *deforestation* at times, but the term generally means the addition or subtraction of plants, animals, or man-made products to an ecosystem by humans. As human population is on the rise, the need for land is also growing. Cattle pasture remains the dominant land use once forests are cleared in the most heavily deforested state of Mato Grosso in Brazil.[19] Rainforests that are modified to developed, agricultural or pasture land pose a twofold environmental complication: first, the loss of flood and erosion control can be significant, while the loss of plant and animal species affects the health of the ecosystem from the bottom up (in terms of the food chain, otherwise known as trophic levels). Second, if livestock is transported to the new pasture land, and wild animals also have a chance to fill a new niche in the recently cleared habitat, potential zoonoses threaten the local human population simply due to their close proximity to both wild and domestic animals.

Some land clearing practices are affecting the triad negatively, such as *slash and burn*, where forests are clear cut and burned, leaving fairly less fertile soil behind. This technique has been used for thousands of years. However, much more time between burnings was allotted in the past so the forest could recover properly. A farmer now may repeatedly slash and burn, thereby leaving plots completely infertile. Much of the infertility comes from the loss of natural fertilizers. Under ideal conditions, decaying biomass such as animal waste, fruit, and leaves are quickly reabsorbed once returning to the forest floor. However, mismanaged farmland can lead to a loss of plant and animal species in the area, which translates to a loss of nutrients in the soil. The farmer then simply moves his garden plot to another area and starts again.

Many natural systems in these areas are becoming out of balance due to the loss of species caused by their destruction of habitat and food supply. This imbalance can cause droughts, floods, a boom or bust in a certain population of animals or plants, and the emergence of infectious diseases, all of which have a major effect on public health.

Increased Disease Occurrence

Infectious diseases can arise when rainforests and other habitats turn into pasture/cropland or are cut for the logging industry, for example, when loggers invade a particular forest and find themselves in close proximity to disease-causing agents. Mayaro and Oropouche virus infections in Brazilian woodcutters in recent years are due to exposure to new arthropods and the viruses they carry.[20] Mayaro and Oropouche viruses are nonfatal mosquito-borne diseases that are commonly mistaken for dengue fever. Large outbreaks have occurred throughout Amazonia, with more cases seen every year. While loggers are venturing into newly acquired forests, these workers may not be given the necessary education or equipment (mosquito nets, insect repellant, sufficient clothing) to ward off the arthropods and the emerging infectious diseases they carry. Consequently, after areas have been cleared, more land is available for domesticated or wild animals to spread disease and expand their range as discussed earlier. It is simply the closer proximity of wild and domestic animals that aid pathogens to "jump" species. A pathogen that has a regulated life cycle (typically low virulence) within one host may not be the same in another closely related host and might be lethal to the new host harboring such a novel pathogen. This poses problems for domestic animals as well as wildlife and of course humans.

Yellow Fever

Yellow hemorrhagic fever is caused by an arbovirus found in South America, Africa, and the Caribbean. It is transmitted between humans and some new world primates, with mosquitoes being the primary vector. In South America, sporadic infections occur almost exclusively in forestry and agricultural workers.[21] Monkeys, infected by mosquitoes carrying the disease, pass the virus on to other mosquitoes, which in turn can infect humans entering tropical forests. Urban yellow fever results when travelers and workers from rural and forested areas harboring the disease venture into major cities. Therefore, an increase in workers entering tropical forests (for deforestation activities or otherwise) provides an increased chance for urban yellow fever epidemics to occur once the workers return to their city centers. Also, varying cultural and political facets prolong the problem, as many high-risk undeveloped and developing countries are ill-equipped to distribute vaccinations and educate the public.

Reduction in Biodiversity: Humans May Be the Cause of Species Loss

The last great extinction event took place 65 million years ago at the end of the Cretaceous period with the demise of the dinosaurs and the subsequent radiation of small mammals. An extinction event describes the rapid loss (a relative term here, as some extinction events lasted more than 10 million years) of a large number of species. Using the fossil record to determine such extinction events, the remains of a certain taxonomic class (mammals, reptiles, fish, etc.) are no longer present and are therefore considered to have gone extinct. The largest of such extinction events (The Late Devonian extinction) occurred 360 million years ago, with nearly 70% of all species going extinct.

Some biologists refer to the present time period as "the sixth extinction" as more species are being recorded to have gone extinct every year. Humans are continuing to destroy other species at an astonishingly faster rate than the previous five extinction events.[22] Evolutionary and geological scientists have described human activity to result in species extinction rates to be anywhere from 100 to 10,000 times the pre-human rate, although these numbers are still highly debated. The loss of biodiversity is largely due to the decline of sustainable habitat from human encroachment (increase in pasture, agricultural, and developed land to support the growing human population).

Humid tropical forests are the location of almost half of all species in the world.[23–25] The largest area of such forests is in the Amazon rainforest of Brazil. Between 1990 and 2005, 42 million hectares (approximately the size of California) of forest were cleared. Scientists are now gathering and analyzing current rates of deforestation, which appear to be slowing down due to the increased awareness of the effects of deforestation.[26] This corresponds to nearly a 20% reduction of the Amazon rainforest since 1970, when scientific land destruction research in Brazil first began. Many highly specific arthropod species are only found on several hectares of forest and nowhere else in the world. If their habitat is destroyed or modified, these species could be lost forever. Humans are squandering the opportunity to learn from and develop the species we are eradicating through habitat modification.

Loss of biodiversity negatively affects both our physical health and our ability to enjoy the natural world. Although not all humans are emotionally enriched by spending time close to nature, many people enjoy hunting, gardening, fishing, and camping. Whether or not someone enjoys being outdoors, there are large consequences to our *physical* health by the reduction in biodiversity. We risk the loss of biologically active substances (BAS) that are used to treat diseases in animals and humans, as well as other environmental health crises.

Loss of Prescription Medication and Vaccines

BAS affects the metabolic activity of living cells and therefore is extremely valuable to medical and pharmaceutical sciences. Over the past several millions of years, species have developed highly specific BASs that are of great use to humans to directly fight disease or gain knowledge through medical models to combat disease. It is no wonder that natural products have been the ultimate source of medicines for thousands of years, but you may not know that they are still the primary source for which new prescription drugs are designed.[27] With each species that goes extinct, we are risking the loss of cures for such diseases as AIDS, cancer, human to human avian flu (if it ever mutates), and many more.

The top two selling prescription drugs for the year 2005 in the United States are the cholesterol-lowering drugs atorvastatin and simvastatin, both of which are synthetically modified versions of a fungal-derived chemical.[28] Additionally, aspirin, codeine, morphine, colchicine (anti-tumor), (l)-dopa, vincristine (anti-tumor), quinine (anti-malarial) as well as approximately **75% of the top 20 hospital drugs** (mostly antibiotics) and approximately **20% of the top 100 most widely prescribed drugs** are derived from natural sources.[29,30]

Taxol

Taxol is a cancer fighting compound that works in a significantly different way from other chemotherapeutic techniques, in that it prevents cell division specifically by inhibiting disassembly of the mitotic spindle.[31] Taxol is extracted from the Pacific yew, once discarded as a trash tree during logging of old growth forests in the Pacific Northwest.[22] In early clinical trials, taxol was able to induce remission in cases of advanced ovarian cancer that were unresponsive to other treatments.[32] After recognition of the importance of the Pacific yew, many environmental campaigns used the tree to save ancient forests in Washington state, Oregon, and northern California. The possible cure for ovarian and breast cancer was overlooked for many years. Now, the Pacific yew is not only able to help save

CASE STUDY
Love Canal

Love Canal, located in Niagara Falls, New York, was named after William T. Love, who had a vision of creating a modern community. He thought that by creating a canal between the upper and lower Niagra Rivers, power could be generated to run the industry and homes in the immediate area. Alternating current was the invention that allowed electricity to travel large distances, but by 1910, Love's vision faded away. A partially built canal was all that could be seen in the area. The site was sold to the City of Niagara Falls in 1920 to be used as a municipal waste disposal site. Love Canal was such a fitting place as there was an unpopulated surrounding area and a large hole existed already. In 1942, Hooker Chemical and Plastics (HCP) expanded use of the site and buried more than 20,000 tons of chemicals over the following 10 years.[33] The site was reportedly covered with several feet of dirt in 1953 and subsequently sold to the Board of Education for one dollar. The deed spoke of a "warning" of the chemical wastes under the site; however, the Board of Education and the local residents were not fully aware of the consequences they could face in the future. Some also believe that other options should have been entertained by the Board of Education and the town before building a school on a known chemical waste disposal site.

From the mid 1950s through the 1970s, residents of Niagara Falls complained of unfamiliar odors and actual substances coming from the ground, which were covered with earth and clay by city workers. More and more complaints were being filed every year, and cancer and birth defects began to be more prevalent within the community. In 1978, President Carter declared a federal emergency and permanently relocated 239 families who lived in the first two rows of homes that surrounded the landfill. Several other evacuations occurred throughout the following two years. Blood tests conducted by the EPA in 1979 concluded that the residents of Niagara Falls had chromosomal damage and were at risk for genetic disorders, cancer, and reproductive complications, in part due to the chemical dioxin from the hazardous waste. The unmistakable and serious health effects associated with the mishandling of toxic waste prompted President Carter to sign the Comprehensive Environmental Response, Compensation, and Liability Act (CERCLA) in 1980. One of the first impacts of CERCLA was the prompt relocation of all residents who wished to be relocated out of the small Niagara Falls community. A large impact that CERCLA had on the nation was the charging of very high taxes on the chemical and petroleum industries to create a "Superfund," the act's more commonly used name. Superfund would be used to clean up the nation's poorly maintained hazardous waste sites that posed a current or future threat to human health, animals, or the environment. Nearly $1.6 billion was collected in only 5 years under Superfund, for use in cleaning up Love Canal among several other sites.[34] New sites are found every year, and superfund is now beginning to struggle as more and more serious risk sites are found, which are called National Priorities List (NPL) sites. Most cleanup processes are anything but fleeting, and as each site requires long-term monitoring, more money is needed all the time. Currently, the EPA has more proposed NPL and other sites than there are funds available to start work.

Human's mishandling of hazardous chemicals at Love Canal caused severe public health concerns and made the public aware some of the dangers associated with less than adequate disposal practices. Despite that the story of Love Canal examined environmental contamination as a serious public health problem in the United States, dangerous chemicals and other hazardous materials are still being deposited into the environment irresponsibly. Some offenders continually fail to see connections between polluting the environment and the associated health risks. Humans are surely part of the problem, but we also are the only ones that can actually be a part of the solution. Sadly, many people know the risks associated with polluting the earth but either do not care or do not want to pay the costs associated with disposing various materials according to law. Others simply are not aware of the "big picture" of how pollution can be a serious problem for the triad, which unknowingly includes the polluters themselves and generations to come.

cancer patients, but it is also used to help save old growth forests, which are a much-needed natural resource. Old growth forests tend to be an extremely biodiverse area that in turn could host many more beneficial substances like taxol. Pharmaceutical companies, non-profit organizations, and many scientific researchers are continuing to scour the earth for more BASs, as the need for newer drugs, vaccines, and medical models is ever-growing.

CONCLUSION

Ultimately, the need for more interactions to be described among humans, animals, and the environment is great. Knowing the effects of altering earth's atmosphere, waterways, and land is inherent to our future as a species and—more importantly—of the planet. Is there a "point of no return" with regards to deforestation, and, if so, have we already passed that point? Can we reverse global warming? Why do zoonoses account for nearly 75% of emerging infectious diseases? Should air pollution standards be raised in certain areas? Researching these and other interactions among the triad will enable us to preemptively strike against threats to public health such as environmental contamination and the spread of disease. Additionally, the research of vital biochemical pathways can be performed that may lead to new vaccines and prescription drugs.

Throughout the chapter, we have demonstrated that some ecological and disease-related problems are caused by humans. A portion of these problems can be solved by knowing the consequences of our actions to us and the rest of the triad. William Karesh, in an interview with National Geographic, summed up the public health triad succinctly: "It's not about wildlife health or about human health or about livestock health. There's really just one health—the health and balance of ecosystems throughout the planet."[33] Therefore, the more connections we can describe, the more preventative measures can be taken to protect public health.

Environmental causes of health problems include both natural and anthropogenic forces. Most of these causes are understudied, complex, and found all over the globe. Conservation medicine practitioners form interdisciplinary panels to study these environmentally related health problems. Teams are formed by vastly diverse types of researchers including: epidemiologists, microbiologists, environmental engineers, anthropologists, veterinarians, and public health scientists. The goals of the teams are twofold: to improve overall ecosystem health and tackle the social and environmental problems that are causing disease or other complications for the triad. The Consortium for Conservation Medicine is a unique collaborative institution that strives to understand the link between anthropogenic environmental change, the health of all species, and the conservation of biodiversity.[35] Several schools of public health, including Johns Hopkins University and the University of Pittsburg, as well as the United States Geological Survey National Wildlife Center, are key partners in CCM. This is one of many organizations dedicated to conservation medicine and the public health triad.

As several billion more people will populate the earth this century, more land will be deforested, more raw materials consumed, more pollutants created, and more stresses will be put on the environment. Demands for clean air, water, and useable land will increase during this time as well. A change of thought must be embraced within the global community. Although people believe that we are the most important species, we are merely one among millions, and our health and welfare depend on the strength of our environment and all the species it contains.

KEY TERMS

Anthropogenic: Ideas, actions, products, or effects that are caused or produced by humans.

Anthropozoonosis (pl. anthropozoonoses): Infectious diseases that can be transmitted from humans to animals.

Biodiversity: The number, variety, and range of different organisms (and their genes) located within an ecosystem.

Biomagnification: The accumulation of an element or compound up the food chain

Biologically Active Substance (BAS): A substance that has the ability to alter a biological function of an organism.

Conservation Medicine: A dynamic biological discipline that describes the relationships among human-induced environmental impact, public health, and the conservation of endangered species or ecosystems.

Habitat Modification: The addition or subtraction of plants, animals, or man-made products to an ecosystem that is performed by humans.

Pathogen: An infectious biological agent that causes disease.

Vector Borne Diseases: Infectious diseases, both bacterial and viral that are transmitted via an arthropod.

Zoonosis (pl. zoonoses): Infectious diseases that can be transmitted from animals to humans.

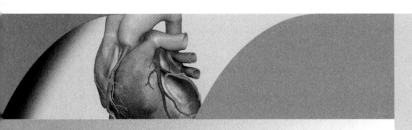

Questions for Further Research, Study, Reflection, and Discussion

For the Individual Student

In order to answer these questions, it may be necessary to research the primary literature.

List 4 problems associated with habitat modification.

- What is non-point source (NPS) pollution? How can it affect public health?
- What is WHO, and what is its purpose?
- What percent of emerging infectious diseases are zoonotic? Name some of the reasons why that percentage is so high.
- What is the CCM? What are their conservation goals, and how are they achieved?
- How are slash and burn farming techniques bad for the triad?

For Small Group Discussion

- Should Superfund have been passed earlier than 1980? If so, then why and when?
- Who are all the parties to blame for Love Canal, and why?
- Under Superfund, chemical and petroleum industries were taxed very heavily. Should any other industry or group be taxed with such harshness? If so, then why?

For Entire Class Discussion

- Why is biodiversity important to our physical and mental health?
- First, what defines a species? Next, what species are most important for the health and well-being of the planet? Should ALL species on the planet be conserved if they are all potentially useful? Which ones could we do without?
- What is the biggest environmental threat that leads to an increase in disease occurrence? Nuclear waste, air pollution, industrialization, urbanization, land modification, poor farming practices? Think of more causes and write them down. Split into a group of five to six, and have each person research one threat outside of class. Make your case to the rest of the group about why your threat is the most severe.

EXERCISES/ACTIVITIES

- Go to your local zoo. If there is no zoo in the area, you may go to a zoo's Web site, although this is not preferred.
- Find at least three animals at the zoo that are endangered or threatened. Write down why each species is at risk for extinction. There should be a placard with this information near each exhibit.
- Once you've fully enjoyed your visit to the zoo, now it's time to do some research. Determine the niche of each species (how it interacts with the other species in its environment). Is it a top predator, a scavenger, a bottom-feeder? What purpose does it serve for the surrounding environment? Determine if the animal has a mutually beneficial species associated with it. For example, several bird species will perch themselves on large mammals like buffalo, which are a source of ticks and other arthropods. The birds get a meal, while the large mammals get groomed and subsequently have fewer disease outbreaks.
- Now, focus on one species in particular. List as many effects as possible that would arise from that animal's extinction. Are any biological active substances associated with the animal or animals similar to it? Does another species rely on it for survival? Try to think from as many different angles as possible. What might happen to the triad and why?
- Write a one page summary of what would happen to the world if your species went extinct.

REFERENCES

1. Chomel BB, Belotto A, Meslin FX. Wildlife, exotic pets, and emerging zoonoses. *Emerg Infect Dis* 2007;13:6–11.

2. World Health Organization (2007). *Veterinary public health.* Available from http://www.who.int/zoonoses/vph/en/. Accessed March 17, 2008.

3. Haines A, Pats JA. Health effects of climate change. *JAMA* 2004; 291:99–102.

4. United States Environmental Protection Agency. *The Effects of Ozone Depletion.* (2006). Available from http://www.epa.gov/ozone/science/effects.html. Accessed March 17, 2008.

5. Natural Resource Defense Fund. *Issues: Global Warming.* Available at http://www.nrdc.org/globalWarming/qthinice.asp#4. Accessed March 17, 2008.

6. The Department for Environment, Food and Rural Affairs *Bovine TB. What is Bovine Tuberculosis?* (2007). Available at http://www.defra.gov.uk/animalh/tb/aboutb/index.htm. Accessed March 17, 2008.

7. Delahay RJ, Cheeseman CL, Clifton-Hadley RS. Wildlife disease reservoirs: the epidemiology of *Mycobacterium bovis* infection in the European badger (*Meles meles*) and other British mammals. *Tuberculosis* 2001;81:43–49.

8. Garnett BT, Delahay RJ, Roper TJ. Use of cattle farm resources by badgers (*Meles meles*) and risk of bovine tuberculosis (*Mycobacterium bovis*) transmission to cattle. *Proc Natl Acad Sci U S A* 2002;269:1487–1491.

9. UNAIDS–Joint United Nations Programme on HIV/AIDS. Available at http://data.unaids.org/pub/EPISlides/2007/2007_epiupdate_en.pdf. Accessed March 17, 2008.

10. Gao F, Bailes E, Robertson DL, Chen Y, Rodenburg CM, Michael SF, Cummins LB, Arthur LO, Peeters M, Shaw GM, Sharp PM, Hahn BH. Origin of HIV-1 in the chimpanzee *Pan troglodytes troglodytes. Nature* 1999;397:436–441.

11. United States Environmental Protection Agency. The Effects of Acid Rain (updated June 2007). Available at http://www.epa.gov/acidrain/effects/health.html. Accessed March 17, 2008.

12. United States Environmental Protection Agency. *What are the 6 Common Air Pollutants?* (updated July 2007). Available at http://www.epa.gov/air/urbanair/index.html. Accessed March 17, 2008.

13. United States Environmental Protection Agency. *The Plain English Guide to the Clean Air Act* (updated June 2007). Available at http://www.epa.gov/air/caa/peg/. Accessed March 17, 2008.

14. Intergovernmental Panel on Climate Change Fourth Assessment Report. *Climate Change 2007: Impacts, Adaptation and Vulnerability Summary for Policy Makers.* Available at http://www.ipcc.ch/pdf/assessment-report/ar4/wg2/ar4-wg2-spm.pdf. Accessed March 17, 2008.

15. Lloyd SA. The Changing Chemistry of Earth's Atmosphere. In: Aron JL, Patz JA. *Ecosystem Change and Public Health. A Global Perspective.* Baltimore, MD: The Johns Hopkins University Press; 2001:188–227.

16. Malakooti MA, Biomndo K, Shanks GD. Reemergence of epidemic malaria in the highlands of western Kenya. *Emerg Infect Dis* 1998;Oct-Dec:4(4).

17. Haines A, Pats JA. Health effects of climate change. *JAMA* 2004;291:99–102.

18. Centers for Disease Control and Prevention. *Preventing Bacterial Waterborne Diseases* (2005). Available at http://www.cdc.gov/ncidod/dbmd/diseaseinfo/waterbornediseases_t.htm. Accessed March 17, 2008.

19. Morton, DC, Defries RS, Shimabukuro YE, Anderson LO, Arai E, Bon Espirito-Santo FD, Freitas R, Morisette J. Cropland expansion changes deforestation dynamics in the southern Brazilian Amazon. *Proc Natl Acad Sci U S A* 2006;103:14637–14641.

20. Murphy FA. Emerging zoonoses. *Emerg Infect Dis* 1998;4:429–435.

21. Centers for Disease Control and Prevention. *Yellow Fever* (updated November 2007). Available at http://www.cdc.gov/ncidod/dvbid/yellowfever/. Accessed March 17, 2008.

22. Chivian E. Environment and Health: 7. Species loss and ecosystem disruption—the implications for human health. *CMAJ* 2001;164:66–69.

23. Myers N. *The Primary Source: Tropical Forests and Our Future.* New York, NY: Norton; 1992.

24. Pimm SL. *The World According to Pimm: A Scientist Audits the Earth.* New York, NY: McGraw-Hill; 2001.

25. Ferraz G, Russel GJ, Stouffer PC, Bierregaard RO Jr, Pimm SL, Lovejoy TE. Rates of species loss from Amazonian forest fragments. *Proc Natl Acad Sci U S A* 2003;100:14069–14073.

26. National Aeronautics and Space Administration. Earth Observatory. *Causes of Deforestation.* Available at http://earthobservatory.nasa.gov/Library/Deforestation/deforestation_update3.html. Accessed March 17, 2008.

27. Grifo F, Rosenthal J. *Biodiversity and Human Health.* Washington, DC: The Island Press; 1997.

28. Young RN. Importance of biodiversity to the modern pharmaceutical industry. *Pure Appl Chem* 1999;71:1655–1661.

29. Gwynn J, Hylands PJ. Plants as a source for new medicines. *Drug Discovery World* 2000:Summer:54–59.

30. Wright AE. *Ocean Explorer Explorations.* Biological Diversity Equals Chemical Diversity—The Search for Better Medicines (revised July 2005). Available at http://oceanexplorer.noaa.gov/explorations/02sab/background/biodiversity/biodiversity.html. Accessed March 17, 2008.

31. Cowden CJ, Paterson I. Cancer drugs better than taxol? *Nature* 1997;387:238–239.

32. McGuire WP, Rowinsky EK, Rosenshein NB, Grumbine FC, Ettinger DS, Armstrong DK. Taxol: a unique antineoplastic agent with significant activity in advanced ovarian epithelial neoplasms. *Ann Intern Med* 1989;111:273–279.

33. Gibbs LM. *History: Love Canal: the Start of a Movement.* (2002). Lessons from Love Canal, A Public Health Resource. Available at http://www.bu.edu/lovecanal/main.html. Accessed March 17, 2008.

34. United States Environmental Protection Agency (1990). *The Environmental Protection Agency: A Retrospective* (updated November 2007). Available at http://www.epa.gov/history/topics/epa/20a.htm. Accessed March 17, 2008.

35. Consortium for Conservation Medicine: Core Values. *Top News Stories.* Available at http://www.conservationmedicine.org/core.htm. Accessed March 17, 2008.

CROSS REFERENCES

Infectious Disease Chapters

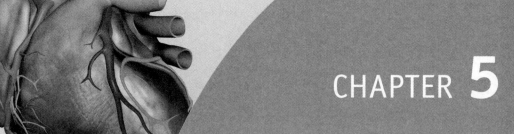

CHAPTER 5

Epidemiological and Public Health Perspectives on Aging in America

Daniel Foley

- The "baby boom" generation, those born 1946 to 1964, is projected to number roughly 70 million or one-in-five persons in our population by the year 2030.[1]
- Less than 5 percent of the elderly population is institutionalized in nursing homes.[2]
- One in ten community-dwelling people over 65 years of age requires help performing basic activities of daily living (ADLs) such as bathing, dressing and using the toilet.[2]
- Four out of five men over 70 years of age still drive, including half of those over the age of 85.[3]
- Three out of four deaths are persons over 65 years of age.[4]
- Alzheimer's disease is the 7th leading cause of death in this country.[5]

LEARNING OBJECTIVES

By the end of this chapter, the student will be able to:

- Estimate the number and growth of the elderly population in the United States.
- Define "instrumental and basic activities of daily living" as measures of disability.
- Cite several common "geriatric conditions."
- Describe typical dying trajectories among older people.
- Discuss the importance of maintaining physical and mental well-being with aging.

HISTORY

Over the last century, the public health burden from morbidity and mortality has shifted substantially from **acute** and **in-**fectious disease to **chronic** disease and with it, marked increases in **life expectancy**. In 1900, only 4 percent of the U.S. population was over 65 years of age compared with approximately 13 percent today and an estimated 20 percent projected for the year 2030. Much of the nation's gain in life expectancy was achieved in the first half of the 20th century, increasing from around 50 years of age in 1900 to 68 years of age by 1950. This nearly 20-year increase in life expectancy over a period of just 50 years stemmed mainly from public health initiatives to improve sanitation, living conditions, and infectious disease control, which greatly reduced infant and childhood mortality rates. In the second half of the century, however, life expectancy only increased by 10 more years mainly through marked reductions in mortality rates from heart disease and cerebrovascular disease, the leading causes of death among middle-aged and older adults. Some demographic projections suggest that today's life expectancy of 78 years may increase to 85 to 87 years by the middle of this century.[6] By 2030, less than 25 years from now, the "baby boom" generation (those born 1946 to 1964) is projected to number roughly 70 million (one-in-five persons in our population) and many of them are expected to survive past 85 years of age (the "oldest old" age group). Consequently, public health policy and planning at the federal, state, and local level are beginning to focus on ways to lessen the burden and costs of aging-related morbidity and mortality in light of this "graying of America" (Figure 5-1).

BASIC SCIENCE FACTS/KEY CONCEPTS REVIEW

Comorbidity and Disability

Older people often have several coexisting health problems. The type, number, duration, and severity of these problems

FIGURE 5-1 The 10 Leading Causes of Death as a Percentage of All Deaths: United States, 1900 and 2004.

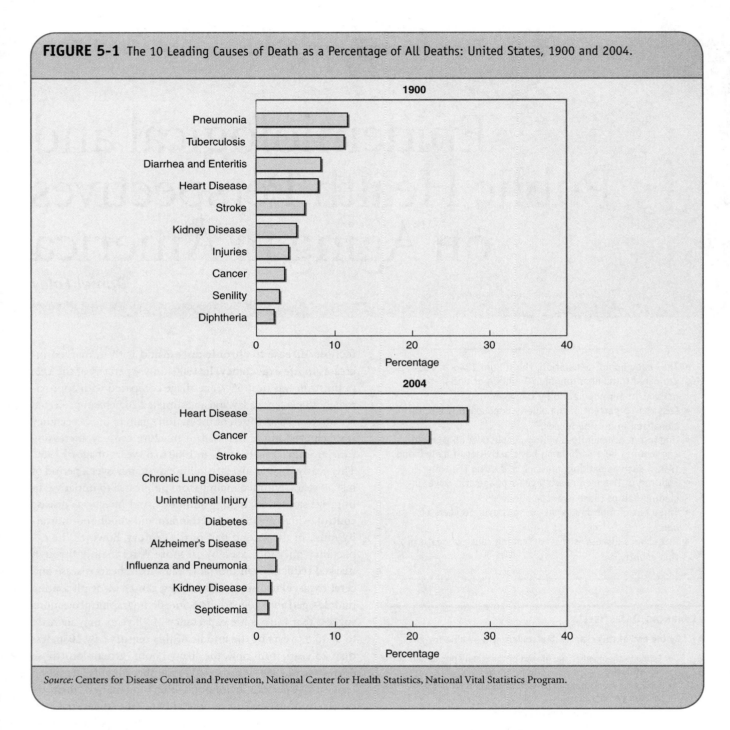

Source: Centers for Disease Control and Prevention, National Center for Health Statistics, National Vital Statistics Program.

may have an impact on longevity and maintenance of independence. Analyses of comorbidity can assess the additive or multiplicative effect of more than one chronic condition or impairment on the risks of mortality, loss of functioning, and use of health services.[7] In 1980, the World Health Organization published the International Classification of Impairments, Disabilities, and Handicaps, a manual of classification of the consequences of disease positing that diseases cause impairments that in turn cause disabilities and handicaps.[8] This codification represented a growing biomedical focus on the epidemiology of aging and disability mainly from the impact of **comorbidity**. It also marked a time of debate on the prospects for an aging society, so elegantly viewed as "two metaphors of ageing" in a 1985 commentary by Jacob Brody[9]:

Oliver Wendell Holmes, American physician-poet, likened human ageing to the obsolescence of a "one-hoss shay":

Have you heard of the wonderful one-hoss shay,
That was built in such a logical way
It ran a hundred years to a day,
And then, of a sudden, it...

You see, of course, if you're not a dunce,
How it went to pieces all at once,
All at once, and nothing first,
Just as bubbles do when they burst.
End of the wonderful one-hoss shay.
Logic is logic. That's all I say.

In stark contrast are W.B. Yeats' lines in the poem, "Sailing to Byzantium":

Consume my heart away; sick with desire
And fastened to a dying animal
It knows not what it is.

At issue was the prospect of a compression of comorbidity and a rectangularization of the survival curve. Conceivably, this could be achieved through an increased postponement of the onset of chronic disease over a relatively fixed lifespan in which the mean age at death would approach and stabilize at approximately 85 years. In contrast, there was also the prospect that gains in life expectancy would be accompanied by increased years of coping with comorbidity and disability. This debate compelled epidemiologists and other health scientists to assess the quality of those added years of life and thus began investigations of **active-life expectancy** or that portion of total-life expectancy free from disability. The studies generally were based on a standardized clinical measure of age-related disability referred to as the index of **activities of daily living (ADLs)**, developed in 1963. This index assessed a patient's basic need for assistance in bathing, dressing, eating, transferring from bed to chair, and using the toilet. Studies of active life expectancy readily showed that socioeconomic factors and health behaviors not only decreased total life expectancy, as expected, but also significantly increased the average number of years dependent in ADLs.[10] Fortunately, nationally representative epidemiological studies of aging have shown that since 1980, there has been a significant decline in the prevalence of disability in ADLs that lends support for a compression of comorbidity.[11] Unfortunately, more recent epidemiological studies of the baby boom generation are showing that epidemic increases in the prevalence of obesity and associated morbid-

ity among them (e.g., diabetes and obstructive sleep apnea) may significantly lower population projections for life and active life expectancies, thus raising the prospect of a decompression of comorbidity.[12,13]

Prevalence rates for common chronic diseases among older persons range from 10 to 50 percent; these diseases include stroke, chronic bronchitis, emphysema, diabetes, cancer, heart disease, arthritis, and hypertension. In addition, over one third report trouble with hearing and nearly one fifth report trouble with vision as sensory impairments. One in seven people over 65 years of age has clinically relevant symptoms of **depression** and a similar number have moderate or severe **memory impairment**.[2] With comorbidity being so common especially among the "oldest old," nearly 20 percent of men and 33 percent of women over 65 years of age have disease-related physical impairments.[2] In addition, many of them are dependent on **polypharmacy** that involves taking multiple prescribed and over-the-counter (nonprescription) drug products, which can be costly and increase risk for adverse drug reactions, especially when adding new medications or changing current dosing or brand (Figure 5-2).

In 1969, age-related disability was further conceptualized and operationalized through an index of **instrumental activities of daily living (IADLs)** that assessed abilities in self-maintaining tasks such as using the telephone, getting to places beyond walking distance, grocery shopping and preparing meals, doing housework or handyman work, doing laundry, taking medications, and managing money. This index further established a continuum or range of functioning and disability in the elderly population. In general, less than 5 percent of the elderly population is institutionalized and about one in ten noninstitutionalized older adults need assistance in basic ADLs, and roughly one in five requires assistance with IADLs. The inclusion of ADL and IADL assessments in community-based epidemiological studies of aging has shown a substantial public health burden from comorbidity and common geriatric conditions such as **incontinence**, **hip-fracture**, and **dementia** as regards to their impact on functional health, quality of life, and risk for institutional long-term care (Figure 5-3).

Given the projected growth of the elderly population, the clinical and public health promotion of preventive healthcare needs is extensive. It includes **primary prevention** of incident diseases and geriatric conditions, **secondary prevention** through early detection, treatment and management of prevalent and recurrent conditions, and **tertiary prevention** in reducing the impact of comorbidity on physical functioning, disability (e.g., ADL and IADL limitations), institutionalization and premature death (Figure 5-4).[14]

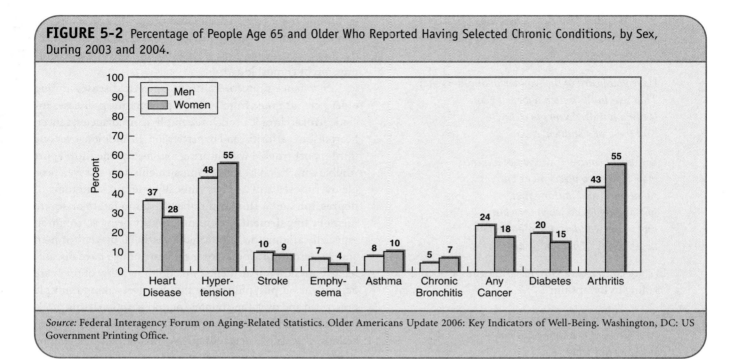

FIGURE 5-2 Percentage of People Age 65 and Older Who Reported Having Selected Chronic Conditions, by Sex, During 2003 and 2004.

Source: Federal Interagency Forum on Aging-Related Statistics. Older Americans Update 2006: Key Indicators of Well-Being. Washington, DC: US Government Printing Office.

Comorbidity and Mortality

But in this world nothing can be said to be certain, except death and taxes.

Benjamin Franklin
Letter to Jean Baptiste Le Roy (1789)

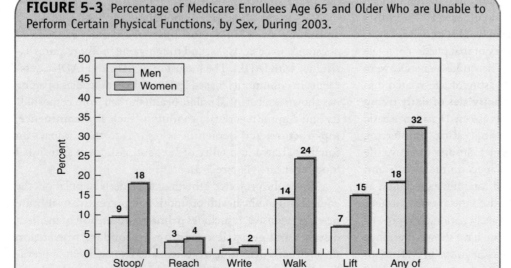

FIGURE 5-3 Percentage of Medicare Enrollees Age 65 and Older Who are Unable to Perform Certain Physical Functions, by Sex, During 2003.

Source: Federal Interagency Forum on Aging-Related Statistics. Older Americans Update 2006: Key Indicators of Well-Being. Washington, DC: US Government Printing Office.

In 2006, the United States reached the demographic milestone of having a population of 300 million people. Yet, nearly two and a half million persons died that year and three out of four of them were aged 65 years or older. Half of these deaths were from diseases of the heart (27 percent) and malignant neoplasm (23 percent). Other leading causes of death (ranging from 3 to 6 percent of all deaths for each cause) included cerebrovascular diseases, chronic lower respiratory diseases, accidents (unintentional injury), diabetes mellitus, Alzheimer's disease, and influenza and pneumonia. Since 1980, death rates for diseases of the heart and cerebrovascular diseases (stroke) in people 65 years of age and older have declined by roughly one third compared with a 40 percent increase in the death rate for diabetes mellitus and a 60 percent increase in the rate for chronic lower respiratory diseases. Additionally, the mortality rate for Alzheimer's disease rose dramatically during this period because of the increased recognition and acceptance by health

FIGURE 5-4 Progression of Preclinical Stages to Clinical Stages of Chronic Conditions, Diseases, and Disabilities of Aging.

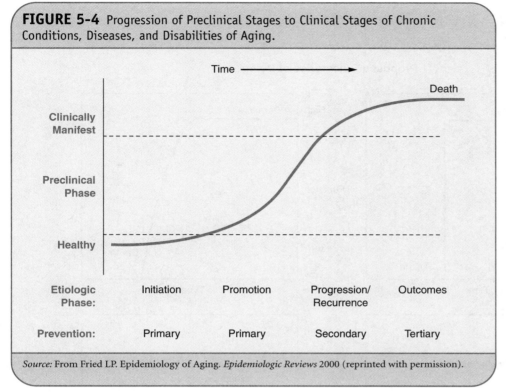

Source: From Fried LP. Epidemiology of Aging. *Epidemiologic Reviews* 2000 (reprinted with permission).

that sudden death and cancer-related terminal illness were more characteristic of younger-aged elderly decedents with fairly robust functioning up to the last month(s) of life. In contrast, organ failure and frailty-related trajectories of dying were associated with substantial dependency in basic ADLs in their final year of life (Figure 5-5).[17]

Currently, 28 percent of decedents are over 85 years of age. As more persons are expected to survive into their eight and ninth decades of life, this age group likely will increase as a proportion of all deaths in the future. Consequently, the quality of death among older persons is gaining as much attention as the quality of life by health professionals and policymakers including appropriateness of care and patient choices or "advance directives" for end-of-life care.[18] Continued public financing, primarily from tax revenues, of the federal Medicare and Medicaid Programs to meet the projected acute and long-term care needs of the aging baby boom generation, including terminal care, remains one of the most challenging issues for the future of public health and the economy (Figure 5-5).[16]

Comorbidity and Public Health Safety

Freedom's just another word for nothin' left to lose.

Janis Joplin
"Me and Bobby McGee,"
Lyrics, 1971 album, "Pearl"

Currently, one of the most pressing issues in the field of public health and aging is the effects of comorbidity on physical, cognitive, and sensory functioning that impairs driving skills. Four out of five men 70 years of age and older continue to drive, including half of those over age 85, though a higher proportion may have a valid license.[3] In contrast, only half of women age 70 and older drive, including just one in five over age 85. This lower prevalence of driving among the current generation of elderly women reflects a more traditional history of never learning to drive compared with women in the baby boom generation, who are as likely to be driving as men.

professionals that Alzheimer's disease causes death, particularly in those over 85 years of age, one of the fastest growing segments of our population today.[15] Since 1990, the age-adjusted death rate from Alzheimer's disease rose from 3 deaths per 100,000 population and the 11th leading overall cause of death to 22 deaths per 100,000 population and now the 7th leading overall cause of death.

In general, about half of older decedents die in a hospital and one-quarter die in a nursing home and the remaining one-quarter in a private residence. Although transitions usually occur among these settings, especially in the last year of life, approximately 70 percent of elderly decedents make only one transition to or from a health facility in their last three months of life.[4] Among the "oldest old," a large portion of the last three months of life are spent in a nursing home. Persons turning 65 years of age today are forecasted to need long-term care for three years, on average, over a remaining life-expectancy of about 17 years for men and 20 years for women.[16]

Empirical data from large cohort studies that included assessment of ADLs in the last year of life supported a clinical scheme that described four typical dying trajectories associated with comorbidity and patterns of functional decline occurring over the last year of life.[17] These trajectories were sudden death, cancer death, death from organ failure, and frailty. Roughly 80 to 90 percent of elderly deaths are estimated to conform to these functional trajectories. Findings showed

FIGURE 5-5 Theoretical Trajectories of Dying.

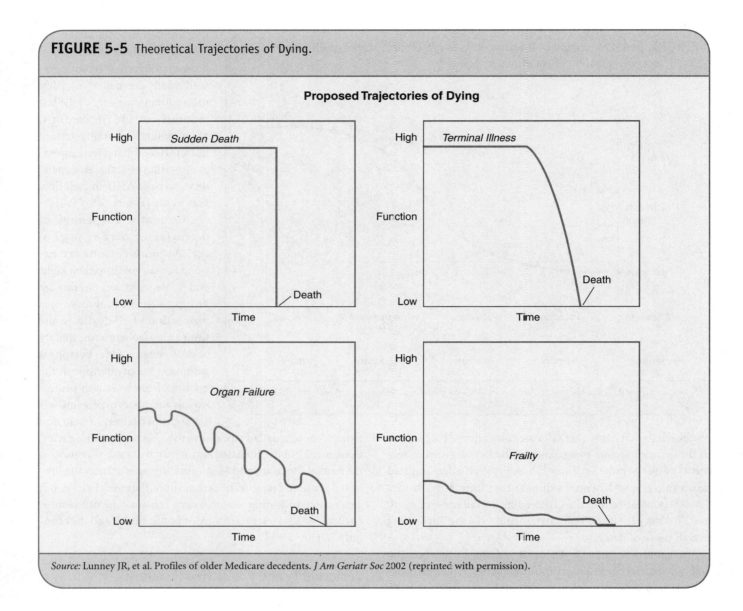

Source: Lunney JR, et al. Profiles of older Medicare decedents. *J Am Geriatr Soc* 2002 (reprinted with permission).

Consequently, the population of older drivers will increase substantially in the future from both the aging of the population and from higher rates of driving among women turning 65 years of age. It is expected that by 2030, the prevalence of driving among older women may be comparable to the current prevalence of driving among older men (Figure 5-6).

Older drivers have nearly a threefold increased risk of crashing per mile driven compared with middle-aged drivers. However, they have far less exposure and, on average, drive approximately one-third the average annual number of about 15,000 miles driven by middle-aged drivers. With their reduced exposure, older drivers have an annual crash risk of 3 to 5 percent that is comparable to middle-aged drivers and results in similar rates for their automobile insurance. Overall,

this crash risk reflects experience and sound judgment as regards their privilege to drive. However, older drivers involved in crashes are more vulnerable to serious injury and three times more likely to die from a crash even after controlling for severity.[3]

The driving life expectancy of men and women in their early seventies is approximately 11 more years, as many continue to drive into their ninth decade of life, a "decade of reckoning" as regards their continued ability to drive. Because of differences in life expectancy, women who stop driving will need approximately 10 more years of assistance from family members or public and private transportation services, on average, to meet their mobility needs compared with 7 years for men.[3]

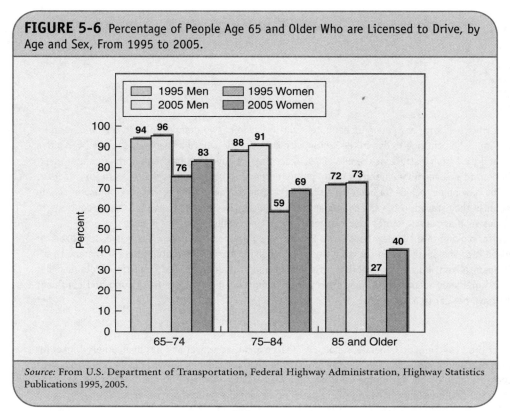

FIGURE 5-6 Percentage of People Age 65 and Older Who are Licensed to Drive, by Age and Sex, From 1995 to 2005.

Source: From U.S. Department of Transportation, Federal Highway Administration, Highway Statistics Publications 1995, 2005.

one should stop driving. Improvements in driving-simulation technology also may offer more opportunities in establishing the criteria for continued safe driving and to meet the rising demand for older driver assessments.

Unsafe driving among older adults is most strongly related to the onset of dementia, which greatly reduces an older person's ability to drive. In a large study of incident dementia over a period of three years among men 75 years of age and older, 78 percent were still driving in the absence of cognitive impairment.[20] By comparison, the age-adjusted rate of driving declined to 62 percent among those who developed poor cognition but did not meet clinical criteria for a diagnosis of dementia, to 46 percent among those who met criteria for a diagnosis of very mild staged dementia, and to only 22 percent among those with a diagnosis of mild staged dementia. Virtually all the drivers who developed moderate staged dementia over the three-year period of surveillance had stopped driving. Those who continued to drive with poor cognition or dementia were more likely to have good vision and good physical functioning, which also suggest the importance of these factors in the maintenance of driving skill.[20]

SUMMARY

In addition to increased demand for healthcare services, the aging baby boom generation likely will spur demand for other non-medical services such as affordable and suitable transportation and housing options. Each year, hundreds of thousands of older people quit driving and must seek alternatives for their transportation needs. This change in status can create unforeseen economic and social burdens that need to be addressed in the same way that people are encouraged to think about planning for retirement and end-of-life care. For many older persons, the decision to stop driving may be a sentinel for stepped up need with assistance in their other IADLs and subsequently basic ADLs. Physicians and transportation officials may have to step up their presence in regulating the privilege to drive among older persons. Many older persons retire in communities that are not well suited for "aging in place" and

When older persons stop driving, it is usually from poor health and oftentimes with encouragement from spouses and other family members, although some may stop driving because of costs as well. About 5 percent of drivers 70 years of age and older stop driving each year, currently about 1 million persons, and must turn to others for assistance in meeting their transportation needs.[3] This difficult transition has been linked to depression and social isolation especially among those with no other driver in the household. In rural and suburban areas that do not offer mobility options, driving cessation is associated with increased risk of placement in long-term care institutions.[19]

Fears of social isolation, of being a burden on family members, and lack of alternative transportation may compel some people to continue driving beyond their ability to drive safely. Therefore, physicians and other health professionals (i.e., occupational and physical therapists) are being educated about ways that they can help older drivers and their family members assess driving skills and the need for driving cessation. However, there are no standardized clinical screening tools that establish minimum levels of sensory, cognitive, and physical functioning required for safe driving. Initiatives to develop such driver assessment tools are under way and may further assist state licensing agencies, health professionals, family members, and drivers themselves in determining when

CASE STUDY
Scenario

Ms. Betty is an 83-year-old widow who lives with her youngest daughter, son-in-law, and two granddaughters. She and her husband raised three daughters and a son, who continue to live in the region with their families. Until a year ago, she had lived alone for about 10 years since her husband died from a stroke at the age of 79. A developer's buyout in her neighborhood and a week-long experience of needing daily help to recover from cataract surgery prompted her and her youngest daughter to join finances and buy a larger home together. The new home included a bedroom suite on the ground floor with a private bathroom, so she no longer needed to climb stairs. Because they stayed in the same familiar neighborhood, Ms. Betty felt she was able to continue to safely drive to all her familiar places such as church, stores, doctors, restaurants, and family and friends' homes.

However, about one month after moving into the new house, Ms. Betty tripped and fell over a box and was hospitalized for over a week with a severely bruised hip. She spent nearly six more weeks in a nursing home undergoing physical therapy to regain her ability to walk. While hospitalized, Ms. Betty experienced delirium and this undiagnosed condition prolonged her post–acute-care rehabilitation. She gradually recovered though after returning home but no longer felt strong and confident enough to resume driving, so she gave her car to a grandson.

Defining the Issues

Ms. Betty quit smoking shortly after the 1964 Surgeon General's Report on tobacco and lung cancer and has been a non-drinker for most of her life. Though somewhat overweight since mid-life (mostly around the hips and thighs), she maintains a healthy, well-balanced diet. Ms. Betty often cooks her own dinner during the week because she eats much earlier than the rest of the family and goes to bed earlier, usually by 9 pm. She sleeps well but must use the bathroom once or twice a night and experiences anxiety about possibly tripping or falling again in her haste. Ms. Betty currently is taking six prescription medications for anxiety, depression, hypothyroidism, high cholesterol (hypercholesterolemia), fluid retention (edema), and hay fever (allergic rhinitis). She also takes folic acid, vitamin E, zinc, and calcium as nutritional supplements. Her past medical history includes gastric ulcers and diverticulitis, but she feels fortunate in having no history of high blood pressure, heart disease, or diabetes as with many of her friends. However, because of recent problems in her balance, gait, memory, and continence, her physician has recommended that she undergo a series of tests, including a brain scan, for a possible diagnosis of normal pressure hydrocephalus (NPH).

Patient's Understanding

Though she gets out from time to time, Ms. Betty misses her independence from when she lived alone and the level of activity and socialization with her friends that she enjoyed while still able to drive. Of her group of eight long-time friends of similar ages, only one continues to drive and they often discuss their options when she can no longer provide transportation to social events.

Although she feels financially secure from the profit of selling her home, Ms. Betty worries that her declining health will overburden her daughter's family, as her daughter and son-in-law both work full-time and must tend to many afterschool and weekend activities for their daughters who are attending middle school. Ms. Betty is increasingly asking her other children for help in meeting doctor visits and other transportation needs. Her daughter and son-in-law increasingly have to assist Ms. Betty in instrumental activities including transportation, light housework, laundry, and assistance in managing her medications and finances especially now that Ms. Betty is showing more signs of forgetfulness. She stills bathes and dresses herself but realizes these activities are becoming more difficult and tiresome. A diagnosis of NPH may explain her recent problems, but she fears the possibility that treatment may require surgery and she doesn't want to be hospitalized again and become delirious.

CLINCIAL PERSPECTIVE FOR THE INDIVIDUAL PATIENT
Level of Intervention Now

Presently, Ms. Betty is receiving assistance from her daughter's family in some of her instrumental activities of daily living. Her relatively few chronic conditions are manageable and responding to medication but the recent onset of major geriatric problems that include walking disability, incontinence and poor memory may be more difficult to treat and manage in the absence of NPH. In addition, Ms. Betty's mental health is clinically significant in that she is having more difficulty falling asleep (insomnia) due to increased worries over her health and frequent awakenings to void urine (nocturia). The loss of sleep in relation to her depression, anxiety, and nocturia may necessitate a daily schedule for a short nap to overcome excessive daytime sleepiness, physical fatigue, reduced alertness, and importantly risk of falling.[21] Should Ms. Betty become hospitalized again, she may need monitoring for a recurrent episode of delirium, an increasingly recognized geropsychiatric condition that occurs frequently among admitted patients over 80 years of age.

Overall, the clinical perspective is that Ms. Betty is suffering from memory problems and frailty in old age, and is at risk for increased caregiver support and ultimately end-of-life care. Frailty in late life is a relatively new area of focus in clinical geriatrics and geriatric epidemiology.[14,22] Although there is no consensus on a gold-standard definition, widely accepted indicators of frailty include unintentional weight loss, slow walking speed, self-reported exhaustion, low energy expenditure, and muscular weakness.[22]

Shortly after Ms. Betty's discharge and recovery from her fall nearly a year ago, she and her daughter decided to prepare advance directives for her end-of-life-care. In addition, with the assistance of an attorney, Ms. Betty legally assigned powers of attorney for healthcare and financial decision-making to her daughter should she become incapacitated or otherwise unable to make decisions for herself. The hospital discharge planner recommended that they contact their local office of the area agency on aging for information and guidance on this matter as well as for additional information about caregiver support and long-term care services in the area.

Potential Level Earlier

Without successful primary, secondary, and tertiary prevention of Ms. Betty's preclinical and diagnosed chronic diseases and geriatric conditions, she may become increasingly frail. In addition, continued decline in her cognitive functioning may warrant further neurological assessment for Alzheimer's disease, the most common cause of cognitive impairment in persons over 80 years of age and for which an early diagnosis may provide for more effective treatment and long-term care (LTC) services for patients and their families.

Ms. Betty and her daughter often discuss the level of difficulty she has in performing her ADLs, particularly bathing and dressing as these are more apparent than her using the toilet or feeding herself. Her daughter has received an abundance of information regarding home-based care and services available in the vicinity including various support group programs from the area agency on aging. However, Ms. Betty's health insurance does not include reimbursement for non-medical home-based long-term care supportive services for which they seek assistance and so costs, especially for daily caregiver support, have been a factor in their discussions. Of concern to Ms. Betty's family is that she spends too much time alone at home while others are at work and school. Reluctantly, Ms. Betty has agreed to her daughter's wish that she try out attending an adult day care center a few days a week.

PUBLIC HEALTH PERSPECTIVE FOR THE HEALTH OF THE GENERAL POPULATION AND OF HIGH RISK GROUPS

Ms. Betty and her family are experiencing the realizations of aging, disability, and caregiver(s) burden. She is one of approximately 11 million men and women in the country currently over the age of 80 who face an uncertain future about their well-being and multiple life-threatening illnesses. In the United States, an 80-year-old person has a life expectancy of approximately nine additional years and an active-life expectancy of about six additional years, with the remaining years requiring assistance with basic ADLs.[10]

"The most recent White House Conference on Aging in 2005 (a decennial affair first held in 1961 and again in 1971, 1981, and 1995) was mandated to focus on the aging baby boom generation and carried the theme, "The Booming Dynamics of Aging: From Awareness to Action."[23] The top recommendations by the conference delegates focused on reauthorizing the Older Americans Act (#1) and strengthening and improving the Medicaid (#4) and Medicare (#5) programs. In addition, the delegates gave priority to developing a coordinated long-term care strategy (#2) including non-institutional LTC (#7) and the workforce as regards training (#6) and recruitment (#9). Importantly, the development of transportation options (#3) and improved responsiveness to mental illness (#8) were high priorities as well.[23]

The Older Americans Act, first authorized in 1965, created the Administration on Aging to facilitate federal grant support to the States to develop State Units on Aging and Area Agencies on Aging for community planning and services programs as well as for research, demonstration, and training projects in the field of aging. In 2004, programs under the Older Americans Act provided for approximately 143 million home-delivered meals, 105 congregate meals, 19 million hours of personal care and homemaker services, and 38 million rides, with a budget of over $1.3 billion.[23] These programs generally target low-income and rural dwelling elderly persons with the greatest social and economic need. The reauthorization of the Older Americans Act in 2006 continued the funding of existing services and also funded a pilot program, Choices for Independence, as a demonstration project to promote consumer-directed and community-based long-term care options.

In 2005, the United States spent roughly 2 trillion dollars on health care, representing over $6,500 per person and 16 percent of the nation's gross domestic product as measures of the nation's economy. Nearly one third of the total healthcare expenditures were public spending on the Medicare and Medicaid programs, $342 billion and $313 billion, respectively. Medicaid, a shared federal and state program to insure low-income residents, spends nearly 40 percent of its revenue on long-term care services, the program's largest category of expenditures, including nearly 20 percent on nursing home care. In contrast, Medicare, a federal program to insure aged and disabled residents, spends less than 10 percent of its revenue on long-term care services, as its largest category of expenditure is for hospital care at nearly 40 percent.[24]

Expenditures on prescription drugs is one of the fastest growing segments of these programs and will continue, especially from enactment of the Medicare Part D benefit that provides coverage for prescription medication among those enrolled in the Medicare program. On average, persons over 65 years of age fill over 30 prescriptions annually at a per capita cost of approximately $1,800.[2] Drug discovery by the pharmaceutical industry has remarkable potential for improvement in the quality of life of older adults especially in finding successful treatments for Alzheimer's disease. In addition, there is great demand for improved psychopharmacology for older adults as anxiety, depression, delirium, and psychotic and behavioral disturbance, especially in association with Alzheimer's, disease, are particularly burdensome to patients, caregivers, and their families. Hence, the number 8 priority resolution of the WHCOA delegates was to improve recognition, assessment, and treatment of mental illness and depression among older Americans.

The projected growth in healthcare services necessary to address the needs of the aging baby boom generation in the years ahead will require a substantial growth in the healthcare workforce to meet this challenge. For example, the number of jobs for home health aides and medical assistants is projected to grow by over 50 percent. In addition, the ethnic and racial composition of this emerging workforce may differ substantially from the majority of persons seeking their care and this has implications for sustaining a high quality of care. Similarly, the changing ethnic and racial composition of the elderly population itself also has implications for disparities in healthcare delivery. These issues have raised the importance of "cultural competency" in healthcare delivery. According to the Office of Minority Health in the Department of Health and Human Services:

"Cultural and linguistic competence is a set of congruent behaviors, attitudes, and policies that come together in a system, agency, or among professionals that enables effective work in cross-cultural situations. Because health care is a cultural construct, arising from beliefs about the nature of disease and the human body, cultural issues are actually central in the delivery of health services treatment and preventive interventions. By understanding, valuing, and incorporating the cultural differences of America's diverse population and examining one's own health-related values and beliefs, health care organizations, practitioners, and others can support a health care system that responds appropriately to, and directly serves the unique needs of populations whose cultures may be different from the prevailing culture." [25]

With unprecedented demand for healthcare services from a rapidly growing patient population, more age-related disparities in access and treatment may arise from a limited or inadequate number of professionals in the healthcare workforce specializing in geriatrics. This may be especially true in the delivery of quality behavioral-health care for mental and substance-use conditions among them.

must seek out more "livable" communities that provide an infrastructure of community-based services.

Can the economy sustain the projected growth in expenditures for healthcare and retirement benefits associated with public funding of the Medicare, Medicaid, and Social Security programs, especially in meeting the LTC needs of an aging populace? Are the boomers themselves adequately prepared for the cost of aging (pensions, LTC insurance, assets and savings)? These are some of the important questions facing the nation and the field of aging and public health. Furthermore, in addressing the policy committee for the 2005 WHCOA, Dr. Paul Hodge, Director of the Harvard Generations Policy Program, succinctly noted that, "America's graying will transform politics, retirement systems, health care systems, welfare systems, labor markets, banking and stock markets. It will force a re-thinking of social mores and prejudices, from issues of age/gender discrimination in the job market to end-of-life care. Whether that transformation is positive or negative will depend on planning and preparation that must begin today."[21]

In fact, America is not alone in this regard as many nations worldwide must grapple with the social, economic, and political demands of their aging populations (Figure 5-7).

KEY TERMS

Active-Life Expectancy (also, Disability-Free Life Expectancy): The average number of years an individual is expected to live free of disability if current patterns of mortality and disability continue to apply.

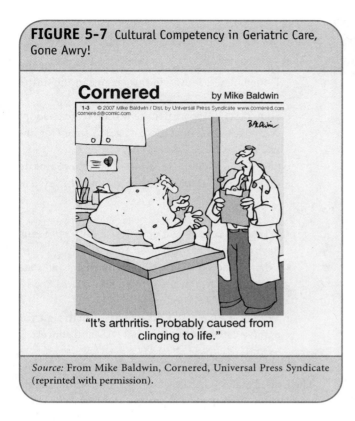

FIGURE 5-7 Cultural Competency in Geriatric Care, Gone Awry!

Cornered by Mike Baldwin

1-3 © 2007 Mike Baldwin / Dist. by Universal Press Syndicate www.cornered.com
cornered@comic.com

"It's arthritis. Probably caused from clinging to life."

Source: From Mike Baldwin, Cornered, Universal Press Syndicate (reprinted with permission).

Activities of Daily Living (ADLs): A scale to score physical ability/disability based on responses to questions about mobility and self-care; used to measure outcomes of interventions for various chronic disabling conditions such as arthritis.

Acute: Referring to a health effect (or exposure), with sudden onset, often brief; sometimes loosely used to mean severe.

Chronic: Referring to a health-related state (or exposure), lasting a long time. The U.S. National Center for Health Statistics defines a "chronic" condition as one of three months' duration or longer.

Comorbidity: Disease(s) that coexist(s) in a person in addition to the index condition.

Dementia: An organic mental disorder that results in permanent or progressive loss of intellectual abilities such as impairment in memory, judgment, and abstract thinking, and changes in personality.

Depression: A mental state or chronic mental disorder characterized by feelings of sadness, loneliness, despair, low self-esteem, and self-reproach; accompanying signs include psychomotor retardation (or less frequently, agita-

tion), withdrawal from social contact, and loss of appetite and insomnia.

Hip fracture: A break near the top of the femur where it angles into the hip socket of the pelvis.

Incontinence: The lack of voluntary control of excretory functions.

Infectious Disease (also, Communicable Disease): An illness due to a specific infectious agent or its toxic products that arises through transmission of that agent or its products from an infected person, animal, or reservoir to a susceptible host, either directly or indirectly through an intermediate plant or animal host, vector, or the inanimate environment.

Instrumental Activities of Daily Living (IADLs): A scale of activities related to independent living that includes preparing meals, managing money, shopping for groceries or personal items, performing light or heavy housework, and using a telephone.

Life Expectancy (also, Expectation of Life): The average number of years an individual of a given age is expected to live if current mortality rates continue to apply.

Long-Term Care (LTC): Services, care, or items (such as assistive devices), including disease prevention and health promotion services, in-home services, and case management services intended to assist individuals in coping with, and to the extent practicable, compensate for functional impairments in carrying out activities of daily living.

Memory Impairment: A neuropathological state indicative of some kind of disease process or toxic exposure affecting the brain such that memory loss has progressed to such an extent that normal independent function is impossible.

Primary Prevention: Protection of health by personal and communal efforts, such as enhancing nutritional status, immunizing against communicable diseases, and eliminating environmental risks, such as contaminated drinking water supplies.

Secondary Prevention: A set of measures available to individuals and communities for the early detection and prompt intervention to control disease and minimize disability, for example, by the use of screening programs.

Tertiary Prevention: Consists of measures aimed at softening the impact of long-term disease and disability by eliminating or reducing impairment, disability, and handicap; minimizing suffering; and maximizing potential years of useful life.

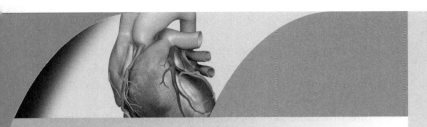

Questions for Further Research, Study, Reflection, and Discussion

For the Individual Student

In order to answer these questions, it may be necessary to research the primary literature.

- Identify a developing nation that has experienced a rapid increase in its life expectancy over the last few decades (comparable to the U.S. experience in the first half of the 20th century). Write a brief report on the demographic, social, economic, and political changes that occurred over this time.
- Acquire an IADL and ADL assessment form from the Internet, interview a frail older adult or their caregiver (i.e., conduct a proxy interview), and summarize their IADL/ADL needs in a case report. During the assessment, try to determine and document which diseases or geriatric conditions are causing the functional impairments.

For Small Group Discussion

- What is the prevalence of institutional LTC (i.e., nursing home care) for men and women 65 to 74, 75 to 84, and 85 years of age and older in the United States? How will this change in the future and why?
- Should State Department of Motor Vehicles adopt cognitive testing (and at what age) to screen for unsafe drivers?
- Should physicians be required to report unsafe drivers to the Department of Motor Vehicles?

For Entire Class Discussion

- What impact will the diabetes/obesity epidemic have on aging in the United States?
- What impact(s) will the growth in federal and state spending on health and retirement welfare benefits have on the U.S. economy?
- Will "Big Pharma" find effective treatment for aging-related illness, especially AD and cancer?

ACTIVITY/EXERCISE

The United States is hardly the only nation with an aging population. Organize into groups and research which other countries in the world have an aging population. What policies have those governments put into place to prepare for the growing numbers of elderly? In your group's opinion, which of those policies might work in the United States? Prepare a presentation of your group's research findings, and present it to the class.

Healthy People 2010

Indicators: Access to Health Care, Mental Health, Injury, and Violence

Focus Areas:

- Access to Quality Health Services
- Disability and Secondary Conditions
- Injury and Violence Prevention
- Mental Health and Mental Disorders
- Vision and Hearing

Goals:

- Improve access to comprehensive, high-quality healthcare services.
- Promote the health of people with disabilities, prevent secondary conditions, and eliminate disparities between people with and without disabilities in the U.S. population.
- Reduce injuries, disabilities, and deaths due to unintentional injuries and violence.
- Improve mental health and ensure access to appropriate, quality mental health services.
- Improve the visual and hearing health of the Nation through prevention, early detection, treatment, and rehabilitation.

Objectives:

1-15. Increase the proportion of persons with long-term care needs who have access to the continuum of long-term care services.

6-1. Include in the core of all relevant Healthy People 2010 surveillance instruments a standardized set of questions that identify "people with disabilities."

6-13. Increase the number of Tribes, States, and the District of Columbia that have public health surveillance and health promotion programs for people with disabilities and caregivers.

15-27. Reduce deaths from falls.

15-28. Reduce hip fractures among older adults.

18-14. Increase the number of States, Territories, and the District of Columbia with an operational mental health plan that addresses mental health crisis interventions, ongoing screening, and treatment services for elderly persons.

28-7. Reduce visual impairment due to cataract.

28-13. Increase access by persons who have hearing impairments to hearing rehabilitation services and adaptive devices, including hearing aids, cochlear implants, or tactile or other assistive or augmentative devices.

REFERENCES

1. Hobbs F, Damon BL. Bureau of the Census, U.S. Department of Commerce. Current population reports. (Special studies series P-23, no. 190). 65+ in the United States. Washington, DC: US GPO, 1996 (revised 1999). Available at http://www.census.gov/prod/1/pop/p23-190/p23-190.html. Accessed March 17, 2008.

2. Federal Interagency Forum on Aging-Related Statistics. Older Americans Update 2006: Key Indicators of Well-Being. Federal Interagency Forum on Aging-Related Statistics. Washington, DC: US Government Printing office (May 2006). Available at http://www.agingstats.gov/agingstatsdotnet/main_site/default.aspx. Accessed March 17, 2008.

3. Foley DJ, Heimovitz HK, Guralnik JM, Brock DB. Driving life expectancy of persons aged 70 years and older in the United States. *Am J Public Health* 2002;92:1284–1289.

4. Brock DB, Foley DJ. Demography and epidemiology of dying in the U.S. with emphasis on deaths of older persons. *Hospice J* 1998;13:49–60.

5. Centers for Disease Control and Prevention. National Center for Health Statistics. *Deaths: Final Data for 2004.* Available at http://www.cdc.gov/nchs/products/pubs/pubd/hestats/finaldeaths04/finaldeaths04.htm. Accessed March 17, 2008.

6. Wilmoth JR. Demography of longevity: past, present and future trends. *Exp Gerontol* 2000;35:1111–1129.

7. Cornoni-Huntley JC, Foley DJ, Guralnik JM. Co-morbidity analysis: a strategy for understanding mortality, disability and use of health care facilities of older people. *Int J Epidemiol* 1991;20 (Suppl 1): S8.

8. World Health Organization. *International Classification of Impairments, Disabilities, and Handicaps.* Geneva: World Health Organization; 1980.

9. Brody JA. Prospects for an ageing society. *Nature* 1985;315:463–466.

10. Ferrucci L, Izmirlian G, Leveille S, Phillips CL, Corti M, Brock DB, Guralnik JM. Smoking, physical activity, and active life expectancy. *Am J Epidemiol* 1999;149:645–653.

11. Manton KG, Gu X, Lamb VL. Change in chronic disability from 1982 to 2004/2005 as measured by long-term changes in function and health in the U.S. elderly population. *Proc Natl Acad Sci U S A* 2006;103:18374–18379.

12. Reynolds SL, Saito Y, Crimmins EM. The impact of obesity on active life expectancy in older American men and women. *Gerontologist* 2005;45:438–444.

13. Jagger C, Goyder E, Clarke M, Brouard N, Arthur A. Active life expectancy in people with and without diabetes. *J Public Health Med* 2003;25:42–46.

14. Fried LP. Epidemiology of aging. *Epidemiol Rev* 2000;22;95–106.

15. Foley DJ, Brock DB, Lanska DJ. Trends in dementia mortality from two National Mortality Followback Surveys. *Neurology* 2003;60:709–711.

16. Kemper P, Komisar HL, Alecxih L. Long-term care over an uncertain future: what can current retirees expect? *Inquiry* 2005/2006;42:335–350.

17. Lunney JR, Lynn J, Foley DJ, Lipson S, Guralnik JM. Patterns of functional decline at the end of life. *JAMA* 2003;289:2387–2392.

18. Foley DJ, Miles TP, Brock DB, Phillips C. Recounts of elderly deaths: endorsements for the patient self-determination act. *Gerontologist* 1995;35:119–121.

19. Freeman EE, Gange SJ, Munoz B, West SK. Driving status and risk of entry into long-term care in older adults. *Am J Public Health* 2006;96: 1254–1259.

20. Foley DJ, Masaki KH, Ross GW, White LR. Driving cessation in older men with incident dementia. *J Am Geriatr Soc* 2000;48:928–930.

21. Foley DJ, Vitiello MV, Bliwise DL, Ancoli-Israel S, Monjan AA, Walsh JK. Frequent napping is associated with excessive daytime sleepiness, depression, pain, and nocturia in older adults. *Am J Geriatr Psychiatry* 2007;15: 344–350.

22. Espinoza SE, Fried LP. Risk factors for frailty in the older adult. *Clin Geriatr* 2007;15:37–44.

23. 2005 White House Conference on Aging. Final Report. Available at http://www.whcoa.gov/about/about.asp#report. Accessed March 17, 2008.

24. U.S. Census Bureau. *Statistical Abstract of the United States: 2006* (125th ed). Washington, DC: USCB; 2006.

25. U.S. Department of Health and Human Services. The Office of Minority Health. *What is cultural competency?* Available at http://www.omhrc.gov/templates/browse.aspx?lvl=2&lvlID=11. Accessed March 17, 2008.

WEB RESOURCES

Hobbs F, Damon BL. Bureau of the Census, U.S. Department of Commerce. Current population reports. (Special studies series P-23, no. 190). 65+ in the United States. Washington, DC: US GPO, 1996. Available at http://www.census.gov/prod/1/pop/p23-190/p23-190. html.

Centers for Disease Control and Prevention. Achievements in public health, 1900–1999: Control of infectious diseases. *Morbid Mortal Wkly Rep* 1999;48:621–629. Available at http://www.cdc.gov/mmwr/preview/mmwrhtml/mm4829 a1.htm.

National Center for Health Statistics. *Health, United States, 2005, With Chartbook on Trends in the Health of Americans.* Hyattsville, Maryland; 2005:167. Available at http://www.cdc.gov/nchs/products/pubs/pubd/hus/2010/2010.htm# hus05.

NCHS Deaths: Final Data for 2004. Available at http://www.cdc.gov/nchs/products/pubs/pubd/hestats/final deaths04/finaldeaths04.htm.

Hoyert DL, Rosenberg HM. Mortality from Alzheimer's disease: An update. National Vital Statistics Reports; vol 47 no. 20. Hyattsville, Maryland: National Center for Health Statistics. 1999. Available at http://www.cdc.gov/nchs/data/nvsr/nvsr47/nvs47_20.pdf.

American Medical Association, National Highway Traffic Safety Administration, U.S. Department of Transportation. Physician's Guide to Assessing and Counseling Older Drivers. 2003. Available at http://www. nhtsa.dot.gov/People/injury/olddrive/OlderDriversBook/.

PRINT RESOURCES

Dubinsky RM, Stein AC, Lyons K. Practice parameter: risk of driving and Alzheimer's disease. *Neurology* 2000;54: 2205–2211.

Fries JF. Aging, natural death, and the compression of morbidity. *N Engl J Med* 1980;303:130–135.

Guralnik JM, Land KC, Blazer D, Fillenbaum GG, Branch LG. Educational status and active life expectancy among older blacks and whites. *N Engl J Med* 1993;329:110–116.

Inouye SK, Bogardus ST, Charpentier PA, Leo-Summers L, Acampora D, Holford TR, Leo M, Cooney LM. A multicomponent intervention to prevent delirium in hospitalized older patients. *N Engl J Med* 1999;340:669–676.

Institute of Medicine. *Approaching Death: Improving Care at the End of Life.* Washington, DC: National Academy Press; 1997.

Katz S, Branch LG, Branson MH, Papsidero JA, Beck JC, Greer DS. Active life expectancy. *N Engl J Med* 1983;309: 1218–1224.

Katz S, Ford AB, Moskowitz RW, Jackson BA, Jaffe MW. Studies of illness in the aged. The index of ADL: a standardized measure of biological and psychosocial function. *JAMA* 1963;185:914–919.

Lantz MS. The impaired older driver: when is it time to stop? *Clin Geriatr* 2007;15:17–20.

Lantz MS. Problems with polypharmacy. *Clin Geriatr* 2002;10:18–20.

Lawton, MP, Brody, EM. Assessment of older people: self-maintaining and instrumental activities of daily living. *Gerontologist* 1969;9:179–186.

Lee HC, Lee AH. Identifying older drivers at risk of traffic violations by using a driving simulator: a 3-year longitudinal study. *Am J Occup Ther* 2005;59:97–100.

Lunney JR, Lynn J, Hogan C. Profiles of older Medicare decedents. *J Am Geriatr Soc* 2002;50:1108–1112.

Murtaugh CM, Spillman BC, Warshawsky MJ. In sickness and in health: an annuity approach to financing long-term care and retirement income. *J Risk Insurance* 2001; 68:225–254.

Time Magazine. "Special report: America at 300 million." October 30, 2006; Vol. 168, No.18.

CROSS REFERENCES

Alzheimer's Disease

Drug-Induced Disease and Safe Medication Use

Pathophysiology of Injury

The Science of Sleep

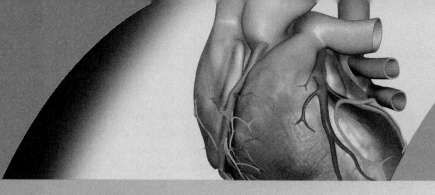

CHAPTER 6

Drug-Induced Diseases and Safe Medication Use

Michelle Kalis
Judy Cheng

According to an estimate by the Institute of Medicine (IOM), four out of five adults in the United States will use prescription medications, over-the-counter drugs, or dietary supplements in any given week. Almost one third of adults will take five or more different medications. With the increase in the number of medications on the market and the complexity of the healthcare system, between 44,000 and 98,000 people die in hospitals annually due to preventable medical errors, and the associated cost was estimated to be as much as $29 billion.[1] Medication errors leading to adverse drug events and drug-induced diseases are now the fourth leading cause of death in this country.[2]

LEARNING OBJECTIVES

By the end of this chapter, the student will be able to:

- Describe the prevalence of drug-induced diseases and medication errors in the United States and their impact on population health.
- Describe possible causes of medication misadventures (both drug-induced diseases and medication errors).
- Describe and discuss recommendations made by Institute of Medicine to prevent medication errors.
- When given a patient case, discuss approaches that can minimize medication misadventures.

INTRODUCTION

Drug-induced disease is defined by Tisdale and Miller[3] as, "an unintended effect of a drug that may result in morbidity or mortality with symptoms sufficient to prompt a patient to seek medical attention and/or require hospitalization." An **adverse drug event** (ADE) is defined as "an untoward effect or outcome associated with use of a drug."[4] All drugs are associated with some degree of risk of an adverse event that may be enhanced in patients with specific risk factors. In addition, the inappropriate handling and usage of medications may lead to medication errors and contribute to the occurrence of drug-induced diseases or ADEs.[5] Adverse drug events became a focus of public policy debate following the publication of the Institute of Medicine's (IOM) report entitled, *To Err Is Human: Building a Safer Health System.*[1] With the increase in the number of medications on the market and the complexity of the healthcare system, medication errors leading to ADEs and drug-induced diseases are now the fourth leading cause of death in this country.[2] This chapter discusses the mechanisms of drug-induced diseases and causes of medication errors as well as the role of pharmacists and other healthcare providers in minimizing these events.

HISTORY

Numerous examples of public health issues occur as the result of appropriate or inappropriate use of prescription and over-the-counter medications. The Food, Drug, and Cosmetic Act of 1938 was passed in the aftermath of the death of more than 100 persons due to the consumption of an elixir of a previously safe and effective antibiotic (sulfanilamide). The new formulation had not been tested for toxicity, and it was subsequently determined that the elixir contained a toxic chemical in its formulation.[6] This event provided the impetus to have the previously contentious Food, Drug, and Cosmetic Act passed by the legislature to help ensure the safety of medications.

One of the most notorious pharmacological agents is thalidomide.[7] Thalidomide was used in Europe and Canada in the 1960s to treat morning sickness during pregnancy.[8] However, children born to women who had taken thalidomide were born with serious limb deformities. The drug was subsequently banned worldwide, and the agent was determined a potent teratogen. Fortunately, the agent was never approved for use in the United States by the Food and Drug Administration (FDA) based upon concerns over the agent's safety in humans. The FDA concern was not related to birth defects but another side effect of the drug. The Kefauver-Harris amendment, which required the FDA to approve new drugs only after they have been proven both safe and effective, was passed as a result of the foreign experience with thalidomide.

An interesting twist to the story of thalidomide is its reintroduction into medical practice in the late 1990s when it was approved for use in treating the symptoms of leprosy.[9] The approval came with strict limitations on the prescribing and dispensing of the agent. Only physicians and pharmacists registered with the manufacturer could prescribe and dispense the agent, and strict criteria for its use in female patients were detailed (e.g., negative pregnancy test). The use of thalidomide has been expanded to other conditions including muscle wasting associated with HIV infections and multiple myeloma.

More recently, the increased risk of cardiovascular events associated with a group of new agents used to treat arthritis (the cyclo-oxygenase-2 [COX-2] inhibitors) demonstrates that despite improved regulations and clinical research, the drug approval process cannot prevent or predict all potential public health risks associated with drug therapy. In addition, as described below, the work done by the IOM and others in the past two decades has focused on the public health impact of drug therapy.

Pharmacists have the primary responsibility for dispensing medications and ensuring appropriate drug use. In recent years, with the increase in awareness of the impact of drug-induced diseases on society, pharmacists' role in public health has continued to expand. In 2004, leaders within the profession published a revised set of educational outcomes for pharmacy education in three main categories: Provision of Pharmaceutical Care, Systems Management, and Public Health.[10] The role of pharmacists in public health is to "promote health improvement, wellness, and disease prevention in cooperation with patients, communities, at-risk populations, and other members of an interprofessional team of healthcare providers."[10] Subsequently in 2006, the Accreditation Council for Pharmacy Education (ACPE) adopted the same professional competencies and outcome expectations in its revised accreditation standards.[11] Several main areas where pharmacists can impact public health include: patient education, therapeutic drug monitoring, disease prevention and detection, and enhancing immunizations.[12,13] Most importantly, pharmacists' collaboration with patients, communities, and other healthcare and public health providers can lead to the establishment of an error-proof system that will effectively reduce drug-induced diseases and ADEs.

BASIC SCIENCE FACTS/KEY CONCEPTS REVIEW

Epidemiology of Drug-Induced Diseases and Medication Errors

The IOM reported that between 44,000 and 98,000 people die in hospitals annually due to preventable medical errors, with an associated estimated cost as much as $29 billion.[1] Various studies have examined the issue and reported that between 0.2% and 22% of hospital admissions are drug-related.[14,15] Since 1971, the Consumer Product Safety Commission has been utilizing the National Electronic Injury Surveillance System to track injuries from consumer products. A pilot project was initiated in 2002 to determine if the system could track ADEs that occur in outpatient settings.[16] In 1998, the FDA began monitoring ADEs via the **Adverse Drug Event Reporting System** (also known as MedWatch). A review of the database from 1998 to 2005 reported a 2.6-fold increase in serious ADEs and a 2.7-fold increase in deaths attributed to reported ADEs.[17] The World Health Organization (WHO) reported that between 7% and 10% of patients in acute care settings experience an ADE, and many of them are preventable.[18] WHO called for additional research on preventable ADEs, especially in developing countries.

Although studies on ADEs have many limitations and assessment of the exact extent of drug-related hospital admissions is difficult, these studies provide important insights. First, the determination of a drug-induced ADE needs to be made with consideration of the following: 1) timing of the event with regard to exposure to the drug; 2) previous description of the noted effect as a result of the drug's administration; 3) evidence of exposure to an excessive quantity of the drug; 4) alternative causes for the observed effects; 5) dissipation of the observed effect when the drug is discontinued; and 6) reappearance of the observed effect if the drug is re-administered.[4] Second, the studies have identified the drug classes most commonly associated with adverse events, including antidiabetics, cardiovascular agents, antipsychotics, gastrointestinal agents, analgesics (specifically non steroidal anti-inflammatory agents [NSAIDs]), anticonvulsants, chemotherapeutic agents, corticosteroids, and antibiotics.[5] The most common types of ADEs reported to the FDA during the period from 1969 to 2002 include ineffective drug, skin reactions, headache, nausea, itching, fever, and difficulty breathing.[19] The same report also provided a list of more than 50 drugs removed from the market from 1964 to 1993 due to safety concerns. More common than drug removal once potential ADEs are recognized, reported strategies effective to minimize future risk include changes in dosing guidelines, changes in product labeling, letters of warning sent to healthcare providers, public health advisories, and restrictions on prescribing and/or distribution.[19]

Although many drug-induced diseases and ADEs may be considered unpredictable, epidemiological data allow the identification of high risk patient groups, drug classes (see above), or situations to help target interventions to prevent ADEs. Patient populations reported to have high incidence of ADEs include elderly patients, patients receiving multiple drugs, and patients with specific disease states such as kidney, liver, or heart disease.[20] The most likely approach to decrease ADEs is by the collaborative efforts of healthcare professionals and patients to improve the systems for drug ordering, dispensing, and administration.[20] In a study evaluating the impact of patient counseling, pharmacists counseling patients prior to hospital discharge lowered the incidence of preventable ADEs following discharge.[21]

Mechanisms of Drug-Induced Diseases

Whether due to errors or unpreventable, adverse drug reactions can be classified as **type A** (common, predictable, and generally related to the pharmacological effect of the agent) and **type B** (uncommon, unpredictable, and generally not related to the pharmacological effect).[22] Type A reactions are generally an extension of the desired therapeutic effect. For example, an agent used to treat hypertension might cause dizziness in a patient as a result of excess blood pressure lowering. A patient who becomes dehydrated (possibly due to the use of a diuretic) would have an increased risk of dizziness. Therefore, a complete understanding of the pharmacology of a drug can help to predict the types of adverse effects that can occur and the patient population that might be at greatest risk. The sensitivity of individual patients can be assessed by understanding that alterations in a patient's sensitivity to a drug can occur as the result of concurrent disease states.[23] In addition, alterations in the ability of patient's body to handle the drug (e.g., altered liver metabolism or renal elimination) can result in higher or lower than expected plasma concentrations of the drug. Interactions with other drugs and/or food can also change drug response and contribute to ADEs.[23] Pharmacists can play a vital role in relating specific patient situations to the potential for adverse drug events and preventing or minimizing the occurrence of these events.

Type B reactions are not an extension of the normal therapeutic effect. For example, allergic reactions associated with penicillin and other antibiotics are examples of a type B reaction.[22] These reactions are more difficult to predict and can often result in serious adverse consequences. However, complete patient histories may help to predict potential allergic reactions to agents with a similar chemical structure.

CASE STUDIES
Causes of Medication Errors and Adverse Drug Events

As previously mentioned, although some ADEs are unavoidable, many are preventable. Many ADEs are due to errors occurring throughout the drug utilization system. In addition to understanding the mechanism of drug-induced diseases and avoiding the use of certain medications in patients at high risk for developing ADEs to those medications, effective prevention of potential ADEs due to medication errors also requires understanding the system of drug utilization and examination of causes of medication errors.

Case 1

A patient returned an incorrectly dispensed prescription to the pharmacy. An internal review determined that the pharmacist involved in dispensing the prescription had conducted a final check of the prescription by reviewing and analyzing the content of the prescription container and reviewing the information on the prescription label. He verified the contents of the prescription bottle and label with information that was on the written prescription (with some difficulty due to poor handwriting on the original prescription). He also verified the contents of the prescription bottle with the contents of the original bulk container. But the pharmacist did state that he was routinely pulled away from the final check process by the pharmacy staff to either answer the telephone or attend to the needs of other customers.

Case 2

A 60-year-old patient was prescribed an antibiotic for her sore throat. Three days after taking the antibiotic, the patient did not feel better so she went back to her physician. Her physician wrote her a prescription for a different antibiotic and told her to try the new one instead. She filled the prescription and took the new antibiotic together with the old one, according to the instructions on both bottles. Another three days later, the patient started complaining of severe diarrhea (a side effect of taking too many antibiotics). She went back to her physician who told her that she was not supposed to take the two antibiotics together. The new prescription was supposed to replace the old treatment.

Case 3

An 80-year-old patient (80 kg) was taken to the emergency department from a nursing home for treatment of severe infection leading to low blood pressure. Among other intravenous fluids and medications, dopamine 15 micrograms/kilogram/minute (μg/kg/min) was ordered to treat the persistent low blood pressure. Over the next hour, the physician continued to increase the dose of dopamine as the patient demonstrated no response. Arrangement was made for the patient to transfer to the intensive care unit. When the transport team arrived, one of the nurses noticed that the dopamine dose had been programmed into the intravenous drug infusion pump as μg/kg/HOUR, not μg/kg/MINUTE.

CLINICAL PERSPECTIVE FOR THE INDIVIDUAL PATIENTS

The cases above are examples of medication errors that occur in different healthcare settings. At first glance, it may be easy to assume that each of the above incidents were errors caused by the pharmacist (case 1), the doctor (case 2), and the nurse (case 3). However, there are really multiple system errors that caused each of these events to take place. Medication errors, "near misses," or adverse drug events are usually caused by a convergence of multiple contributing factors. Table 6-1[24] summarizes common causes of medication errors or adverse drug events.

Medication misadventures usually begin with incomplete or unavailable patient information (e.g., demographics, medical history, and drug or food allergies). This information is essential for physicians and other healthcare professionals to optimize drug therapy, allowing them to avoid duplicate therapies, missing therapies, and drug interactions. Incomplete availability of patient information, unfortunately, occurs commonly in clinical practice, especially when patients seek medical care from multiple providers and do not keep a complete medical record for themselves, and/or there is a delay or miscommunication of information among providers. Also, when patients have prescriptions filled from multiple pharmacies, communication among pharmacies is rare, making it very difficult for the pharmacists to ensure that the therapy is optimal.

Errors also can occur during the medication dispensing and administration process. Despite the effort put forth by the FDA during the drug approval process, many medications still have names that sound alike and physically look alike, even though the drugs may be used for different therapeutic purposes. The similar names and physical features increase the risk of dispensing and administering the wrong medication, leading to potentially severe health consequences. The 2007 National Patient Safety Goals Hospital Program identified a list of sound-alike and look-alike medications and advised appropriate system changes needed to prevent errors.[25] Examples included Zantac®, a medication used to prevent stomach upset and Zyrtec®, a medication that is used to prevent allergy symptoms, runny nose, and watery eyes; Prilosec®, a medication used to prevent stomach acid reflux and Prozac®, an antidepressant.

Poorly handwritten prescriptions and those phoned in to the pharmacy by the physician can be confusing because of sound-alike names or transcription errors, both of which can cause dispensing errors. Many symbols and abbreviations commonly used in prescription writing can be dangerous because they can be easily confused or misinterpreted. For example, the abbreviations Q.D. (once daily), Q.I.D. (four times daily), and Q.O.D. (every other day) can look alike, especially if the prescription contains poor handwriting. Similarly, a dose of ".5 mg" can be interpreted as 5 mg instead of 0.5 mg; alternatively, a dose of "5.0 mg" can be interpreted as 50 mg instead of 5 mg. Therefore, on written prescriptions, one should always use leading zeros, but not trailing zeros.[24]

Environmental factors and distractions that can trigger slips and lapses in performance are other common causes of errors. For example, noise and interruptions can lead to transcription errors when receiving a verbal prescription; multitasking can divide a pharmacist's attention. Stress and fatigue (often related to understaffing) are other factors that make it difficult, if not impossible, to work with one's usual capability. Poor lighting and excessive heat or cold make it difficult to concentrate, increasing the risk of errors.

Even if patients receive the appropriate medications, once patients leave a healthcare setting, numerous opportunities for medication errors can occur. The most important contributing factors in these situations are patients' or caregivers' failure to read or

TABLE 6-1 Common Contributing Factors of Medication Errors

At Inpatient or Outpatient Healthcare Settings	At Home
Incomplete patient information • medical and medication history • laboratory test results • allergies	Patient failing to read or understand labeling and/or product information **Drug-drug, drug-food, or drug-herbal supplements interactions**
Unavailable drug information • drug contraindications • concomitant medications • duplicate prescriptions • drug interactions • miscommunication of drug orders	Non-adherence • prescription not filled or refilled • wrong dose, wrong time of administration • improper administration • ineffective transcultural communication
Written prescriptions • look-alike names • sound-alike names • misuse of decimal points and zeroes • inappropriate abbreviations • misuse of metric and apothecary measures • ambiguous or incomplete orders • poor prescription handwriting	Lost to follow-up • patients change healthcare providers
Environmental factors and distractions • noise, interruptions • transcription errors • multitasking • fatigue • work overload • poor lighting • stocking and storage problem (e.g., two drugs that look alike stored next to each other)	

Source: Reprinted with permission from the Massachusetts Medical Society. Chase BA, Bennett NL. Medication safety, systems and communications. (2006). Available at http://www.massmed.org/Content/NavigationMenu2/ MedicationSafetySystemsandCommunication/CourseInformation/default.htm. Accessed March 18, 2008.

understand labeling or product information and patient non-adherence to treatment. The National Adult Literacy Survey estimated that 90 million Americans (approximately half of the adult population) lack the necessary literacy skills to function effectively in the healthcare environment.[26] The IOM cited over 300 studies that revealed that limited health literacy resulted in patients being less knowledgeable about their disease states, more likely to have poorer health outcomes, and more likely to be hospitalized.[27] Furthermore, studies have shown that patients with inadequate health literacy have more difficulty using medications properly.[28–31] Therefore, it is important for healthcare professionals to be sensitive about whether or not the drug information provided to patients is easy to read and understand. One study recommends that brochures be written at or below the 6th-grade reading level.[32] Misunderstanding medication usage instructions can lead to wrong dose, wrong administration time, and improper method of administration, which may lead to drug interactions and ADEs.

Non-adherence to therapy is another major problem. If patients do not adhere to their treatment or decide not to refill their prescriptions, thus missing doses, or deliberately do not follow the instructions, ADEs may occur. Factors causing non-adherence include patient's disease states, age, number of medications prescribed, lack of appreciation of their disease state, and economic constraints. Differences in cultural beliefs also can lead to medication non-adherence.

Cultural diversity adds multiple levels of complexity to effective communication and delivery of safe healthcare. The need for healthcare providers to be culturally competent is reflected in the increased diversity of the American population. The U.S. Census Bureau estimated that, as of 2000, approximately 11% of the people living in the United States were born in other countries.[33] Language barriers are the most obvious transcultural issue adding to the complexity of treating non-English-speaking patients. Other factors, including different health belief models, social styles and moral values, religious beliefs and practices, and in some cases economic considerations, also affect how patients understand their treatment and their ability to adhere to their therapies, thus affecting their risk of experiencing ADEs. People have diverse beliefs about health and disease prevention, which may have nothing to do with objective measures or medical judgment. People also have different attitudes about how to deal with illness. These different factors will affect a patient's ability to cope with disease and comply with physician interventions, including medication use.

Chronic medical conditions pose a great challenge to continuity of care and patient safety, especially in elderly patients. Patients with chronic conditions are likely to be on multiple medications and to be seen by a number of different healthcare providers. These circumstances increase the likelihood of an error with serious clinical consequences. The difficulty of providing continuity of care and assuring patient safety is compounded if the patient changes health plans or employers or if the patient moves to a different state. People who are unemployed, uninsured, homeless, elderly, or live alone are particularly vulnerable to breaks in the continuity of care, thus increasing the risk of experiencing ADEs.

PUBLIC HEALTH PERSPECTIVE FOR THE HEALTH OF THE GENERAL POPULATION AND OF HIGH RISK GROUPS

Preventing Drug-Induced Diseases and Medication Errors

The common initial reaction when a medication misadventure occurs is to identify and blame someone. However, as discussed in the previous section, ADEs rarely are caused by human errors alone. A convergence of multiple factors usually leads to these events. Blaming an individual does not change these other factors and the same error is likely to recur. Preventing errors and improving safety for patients requires a system approach in order to modify the conditions that contribute to errors. Only when the system is thoroughly evaluated can the root cause of errors be identified and the system modified to prevent future occurrences. Systems, including the healthcare system, consist of many parts that can be grouped under the broad categories of Design, Equipment, Procedures, Operators, Supplies, and Environment (DEPOSE).[34] For example, the safety of administering a new medication depends on how well the new substance was tested before being marketed (Design). Safety also depends on how well the drug is manufactured and packaged (Equipment), whether its prescribing criteria have been properly established (Procedure), whether it is given to patients correctly and effectively (Operator), whether supplies are reliable and consistent over time (i.e., if the patient refills his/her prescription: Supply), and whether the situations in which it is given to those who need it allow proper administration (Environment).[34] Weaknesses in the structure of an organization, such as faulty information management, ineffective personnel training, or a faulty drug labeling and distribution system, as discussed in the previous section, are factors contributing to drug mishaps. Each factor alone may cause latent, subtle failures that do not lead to severe adverse outcomes.[35]

The consequences are hidden and only become apparent when the factors occur in a specific sequence. Therefore, providing an optimal level of medication safety requires recognition and correction of the latent failures in the system.

Institute of Medicine Recommendations for Reducing Medication Errors

Starting in 2001, the IOM began publishing a series of reports on quality in healthcare, which raised public awareness of medical and medication safety.[36] The publication entitled *Crossing the Quality Chasm* defined four important aspects of medication safety: 1) Errors are common and costly. 2) Systems cause errors. 3) Errors can be prevented and safety can be improved with proper system modification; and 4) Medication-related adverse events are the single leading cause of injury among all medical errors.[36] In 2004, Congress mandated that the Center for Medicare and Medicaid Services sponsor the IOM to conduct a comprehensive study of drug safety and quality issues in order to provide recommendations of system-wide changes. Based on the findings of the study, the following recommendations were published in *Preventing Medication Errors*.[37]

1. Evaluate the structure of the medication use process and implement safety measures. This recommendation suggests that the system should be restructured in a way to empower patients to self-manage their medication regimen. After all, patients are ultimately the final checkpoint before any medication is administered. Patients should be told that they have the right to ask and to expect healthcare providers to provide them adequate information to understand the rationale for the use of drug therapy. Patients should be taught that they are responsible for their own treatment, which may be a change of culture and belief for many patients, as they often view themselves as passive witnesses to their healthcare. However, for patients to be able to understand their disease states in order to ask the right questions, it is also very important that individual health professionals and the public health system work to improve the health literacy level of patients. Providing more patient education to improve the level of understanding of their medication therapy is essential. Patients who ask questions if they believe that they do not completely understand something should prompt healthcare professionals to recheck the medications and potentially prevent medication errors. Simple questions such as, "What drug is this?"; "Why am I taking it?"; and "What is it used for?" can raise awareness and increase detection of potential errors. The National Patient Safety Foundation introduced the "Ask Me 3" campaign to specifically address this issue.[38]

Another method to empower patients being implemented by health institutions is a **medication reconciliation** system, as recommended by the Joint Commission, the accreditation body for healthcare institutions.[25] Medication reconciliation is a process that identifies, maintains, and updates the most accurate list of all medications (including non-prescription medications, herbals, and alternative medicines) that patients are taking, including dosage and route of administration. The purpose of medication reconciliation is for hospitals to ensure that patients will be able to continue all the necessary medications when they transfer from one setting to another and from admission to discharge. It also allows the hospital to modify and streamline the patient's therapy prior to hospital admission, to ensure that their medications are most appropriate for their disease states and to prevent any potential drug-drug, drug-food, and drug-herbal interaction. In addition, once patients are ready to be discharged, the patients are provided a list of their updated medications to be taken to their primary physician and local pharmacist. Patients who are capable also can be taught to update the list as the regimen changes, so no matter where they go to receive their healthcare in the future, they will be able to provide their healthcare providers the most up-to-date list of medications.

Medication consultations that include teaching patients what the drugs are used for, therapeutic outcomes or potential side effects to anticipate, and important drug-drug and drug-food interactions, should routinely be available to patients at key points in the medication use process, such as when a patient is admitted and discharged from a hospital or when receiving medication at a pharmacy. Repetition of information at multiple points will reinforce information and help patients to better understand their regimen. Pharmacists play a pivotal role in educating patients regarding their medications.[37]

2. Enhance consumer-oriented drug information resources and establish standards affecting drug-related healthcare in-

formation technology. Three out of four Americans have Internet access and frequently resort to the Internet for health information.[39] However, not all medication information available on the Internet is accurate and unbiased. In addition, direct-to-consumer advertising has been used more frequently by pharmaceutical industries to raise consumers' awareness of their products. Most often, patients do not have adequate skills to differentiate credible versus non-credible information. Therefore, the IOM recommended that medication leaflets distributed by pharmacies be standardized and written at appropriate consumer reading levels.[37] It also recommended that the National Library of Medicine be developed into the chief Internet resource for consumers to ensure that patients receive accurate, understandable, and unbiased drug and medical information.

3. All healthcare organizations should make available to providers important patient information and decision-support tools in electronic forms.

Specific recommendations by the IOM in this category include making effective use of technologies to maintain an accessible,[37] comprehensive information base as well as using technologies to assess safety through active monitoring. To be able to prescribe the most appropriate regimens for patients and administer them appropriately, healthcare providers need access to certain types of patient demographic information as well as drug reference sources to guide them to dose and monitor therapy optimally. This information needs to be readily available during patient encounters for prescribing or dispensing medications. In addition, to truly be able to identify factors that contribute to ADEs in any system, better monitoring systems are needed. Currently, there is too much reliance on spontaneous reporting of ADEs. Most healthcare providers lack incentives to take extra time out of their busy schedules to report adverse events. The current system results in an inability to provide a sense of the magnitude of the problem with medication safety.

The IOM proposed that by 2008, all prescribers have plans in place to e-prescribe (computerized physician order entry) and by 2010, write all prescriptions and have pharmacists receive all prescriptions electronically.[37] E-prescribing not only minimizes errors due to poor handwriting, it also allows linkages built in the system so drug information sources or medication utilization guidelines can be made readily available at the time when physicians are prescribing. In addition, using other technology such as automated prescription dispensing systems that identify medications by bar code also will minimize dispensing errors. Prescribing and dispensing medications in this manner allow each step of the process to be captured and traced, making possible a continuous monitoring process to ensure safe medication use. Reports can be generated for any adverse drug events (instead of relying on healthcare providers to voluntarily report the events). A 1998 study demonstrated that implementation of a computerized prescribing system (even one with very limited reference support) resulted in an 83% reduction in overall medication error rate. The cost of each preventable adverse drug event was approximately $6,000.[40] In addition, another study performed in the same institution indicated that the implementation of a bar coding system for medications reduced dispensing errors by 31% and the potential adverse drug event ("near miss") rate by 63%.[41]

4. Better labeling of drug products.

The IOM recommended that the FDA develop standards and guidelines for the pharmaceutical industry for proper drug labeling and packaging as well as work with pharmaceutical industry to develop a strategy for expanding unit-of-use packaging (i.e., each package contains one dose unit).[37]

The government and pharmaceutical industry should work together to standardize drug nomenclature in order to reduce the number of sound-alike medications on the market. It is confusing enough to patients that each medication has at least three official names, the chemical name, **generic name**, and **brand name**. If a drug is manufactured by multiple different companies, there may be multiple brand names. Other strategies to reduce the risk of errors with drugs having names that sound alike or physical appearance that look alike include always telling the patient or caregiver what the drug is for and why it is being prescribed, and always referring to the drugs by both generic and brand names. If prescription information is communicated over the telephone, the name of the drug should be spelled to the receiving party. The person receiving the information should repeat the information back to the person who gives the information.

5. Establish better methods of communications.

In order to improve patient communication, multiple methods to overcome obstacles to communication need to be implemented concurrently. Language barrier is probably the most immediate challenge in providing safe and effective medical care for people of different cultures. Access to translators is the first step toward overcoming this barrier. A medical facility with a multicultural staff would be ideal, or medical translators may be available in the community for a fee. Another method to improve communication beyond language barriers is the practice of active listening. Often people tend to see or hear what they expect, and not what's really there or said. This increases the risk of slips and lapses due to biases. Active listening means seeking verification from the speaker that the listener heard what the speaker actually said and understood what they actually meant. Doing so is a good method to intercept errors rooted in slips and lapses, and it also may help to uncover and correct mistakes.

Effective communication by healthcare professionals ensures that patients receive the message being delivered. Healthcare professionals take certain information and terminology for granted and do not realize that patients may not interpret the information in the same manner. Follow-up is an important strategy to ensure that the message was understood and to ensure continuity of care. Having nurses or pharmacists make follow-up telephone calls to patients to make sure that patients are adhering to the medication regimen may reduce the risk of medication misadventures and prevent patients from "falling through the cracks" of the healthcare system.

Every time a patient is transferred from one healthcare setting to another and eventually to home, there are opportunities for miscommunication, especially oral miscommunication. Therefore, effective communication between healthcare providers is as important as effective communication between providers and patients in terms of minimizing medication errors. Systems should be in place so that every time a patient is transferred to a different setting, complete medical information follows that patient. As previously mentioned, in 2005, JCAHO adopted medication reconciliation as part of its National Patient Safety Goal,[42] which requires healthcare institutions to implement a process for obtaining and documenting a complete list of the patient's current medications upon admission to the organization. This process includes a comparison of the medications the organization provides to those on the list the patient provides on admission. In addition, JCAHO recommends placing the medication list in a highly visible location in the patient's chart. When information is transmitted from one setting to another, confirmation of transmission is an important follow-up step. Effective communication between the support staff and/or between the hospital and outpatient setting is critical. When a chart has been faxed or e-mailed to the primary care office, for example, it is important to assure that the transmission was received and communicated to the patient's physician. The use of electronic medical records, which can be made accessible to the patient's physician, is one method to guarantee that the follow-up loop is completed.

Electronic medical records have a tremendous potential for alleviating the difficulties of continuity of care for patients because they permit rapid, seamless communication and easy retrieval. As mentioned previously, automatic checking for potential drug interactions and allergies is one benefit of electronic prescribing systems, which can be integrated with an electronic medical records system. Potential barriers to widespread adoption of electronic medical record system include the cost of establishing and maintaining the system and ensuring patient privacy.

6. Government should provide adequate funding to develop a broad research agenda on safe and appropriate medication use, especially evaluating error prevention strategies. Currently, the federal government has no allocated funding dedicated to research relating to safe medication use. However, in order to ensure that all the other recommendations made by IOM,[37] especially those relating to the use of technology and system changes, are having a positive impact on appropriate medication use and are money well-spent, the Congress needs to invest in research. The IOM recommended an annual budget of $100 million to support government agencies such as the Agency on Healthcare Research and Quality to perform research on reducing medication errors.[37]

7. Use incentives to motivate the adoption of safe practices and ensure that providers have needed competencies. Implementing system changes requires initial financial and human resource investment, although eventually money may be saved as the incidence of medication errors is reduced. Early financial incentives may facilitate the initial implementation process. Accreditors of professional education also should continue to ensure that healthcare professionals dealing with medication utilization have the appropriate training to maintain an appropriate level of competence. This is particularly important for those in specialty areas who are working with medications that are prone to errors. For example, prescribers of oncology medications and pharmacists performing medication order reviews on oncology drugs need to have appropriate skills to perform these specific tasks.

Role of Public Health Providers in Preventing Medication Errors

Interdisciplinary Collaborations

Because ADEs due to errors can occur at every step of the prescribing, dispensing, and administration process, the only successful way to minimize errors is for healthcare professionals, healthcare management staff, and patients to work as an interdisciplinary team to streamline the medication utilization process. Establishing a culture of safety is essential. The team must develop a "no blame" attitude. The goal should be to perfect a system so that it will be safe for every patient, every time, while making it easy for caregivers to do the right thing and impossible to do the wrong thing.

Identifying errors is the first step to correcting the errors. Institutions should form a specific committee to oversee medication safety, as suggested as part of the Joint Commission National Patient Safety Goal described earlier in the chapter. This committee should be composed of members from all disciplines, including staff with information technology expertise. The active involvement of information technology staff is particularly crucial if the changes involve effective use of new technology. Healthcare professionals also can educate each other and provide a safety net (e.g., double checking) for each other in order to improve safe medication use. With input from all disciplines, standardized policies and guidelines can be developed and implemented in order to enhance patient safety.

Role of Pharmacists

Because pharmacists maintain the inventory of medications, review prescriptions, and dispense medications, pharmacists have an important role in ensuring safe medication use. The IOM made specific recommendations on the role of pharmacists in monitoring the incidence and reducing the frequency of medication misadventures.[37] Pharmacies should develop a mechanism to regularly evaluate the medical literature and reports of drug misadventures and be proactive in preventing similar errors. Working with other health professionals to adopt computer physician order entry and bar-code medication administration in order to verify accurate prescribing, dispensing, and administration of medications also allows close monitoring of error frequencies and near misses, so improvements can be made to the drug distribution system. Pharmacists should develop stronger initiatives to report errors to external reporting programs like the Institute for Safe Medication Practices, which monitors patterns of medication misadventures to identify widespread problems. Pharmacists should actively monitor patients for medication side effects and recommend appropriate management and follow-up should side effects occur. When filling a prescription, pharmacists should review the patients' medication profile routinely and review different treatment options to determine if the medication on the prescription is the most appropriate therapy for the patient.

Because IOM's 2006 recommendations heavily focused on empowering patients to be in charge of their own medication use, patient education is crucial.[37] Pharmacists play a pivotal role in educating patients, not only about the drugs, but also about medication error prevention. Pharmacists should always discuss with the patient the purpose of the medication, when and how to take the medication, what to expect in terms of therapeutic effects and side effects, and what to do if adverse events occur. The final step in these discussions should be pharmacists verifying that the patient understood the information.

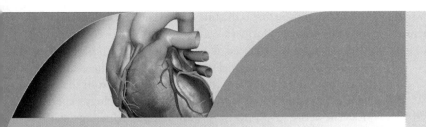

Questions for Further Research, Study, Reflection, and Discussion

For the Individual Student

In order to answer these questions, it may be necessary to research the primary literature.

- What are the two types of ADEs? What are the differences between them?
- List each category of provider involved in the supply of pharmaceuticals to patients? How might each type of provider cause an ADE? What steps could they take to reduce ADEs?
- List the categories of drugs most commonly involved in ADEs. Postulate some of the biological and public health factors that might contribute to the frequency of the ADEs with these agents.

For Small Group Discussion

- Please evaluate the three cases described in this chapter under "Causes of Medication Errors and Adverse Drug Events" and describe what may have gone wrong in the system to bring on the errors. Suggest how future errors similar to these may be avoided.
- Recall/share with the class any incident encountered (whether it happened to yourself, a family member, or friend) with the healthcare system, where an error occurred or almost occurred ("near miss"). Discuss what might have contributed to the error or near miss. Is there any possible solution to prevent similar errors in the future?

For Entire Class Discussion

- Patient non-adherence to medication regimens and differences in cultural belief are two important potential causes of medication errors discussed in the chapter. Aside from not fully understanding the instructions on how to take the medications, what are other important reasons that may lead to patients not adhering to their medication regimens? Describe some examples of cultural beliefs that may lead to patients purposely not adhering to their medication regimens. What methods can healthcare professionals and public health providers use to improve the situation?

EXERCISE/ACTIVITY

Empowering patients with an adequate amount of medical and drug information is one of the main recommendations of IOM to improve medication safety. Providing patients with information resources, education, and consultation regarding their medical problems and the medications they are taking is important. However, approximately 50% of Americans read at or below an eighth grade level. Understanding medical information requires a high level of health and scientific literacy. Therefore, healthcare and public health providers need to be conscientious about the information that they are delivering to the general public to ensure that the correct information is being communicated.

The following is a patient medication leaflet available at MedlinePlus, a Web site that provides medical and medication information to the general public that is maintained by the National Library of Medicine. This information resource is recommended by IOM to be used as the primary source of medical information for patients. Discuss:

- Would the general public—especially the population the information is targeting—understand the message?
- Suggest how to modify the information so the message will be better delivered.

Duloxetine (Cymbalta®). Available at: http://www.nlm.nih.gov/medlineplus/drug info/medmaster/a604030.html Accessed on March 18, 2008.

KEY TERMS

Clinical Terms

Brand name: The name provided by a pharmaceutical company when the company markets the drug. For example, Zantac® is the trade name for the generic drug, ranitidine.

Drug-Drug, Drug-Food, and Drug-Herbal Interactions: Chemical, physical, or physiologic interactions between one drug product and another drug, food, or herbal that a patient might be receiving. These interactions can result in an increase or decrease in the activity of the original drug and could therefore result in toxicity or lack of therapeutic efficacy.

Generic name: The chemical name of the drug (not the name used by the pharmaceutical company to market the agent). For example, ranitidine is the generic name of the product Zantac®.

Therapeutic drug monitoring: A process whereby healthcare professionals monitor the patients' response to medications to ensure maximum efficacy and minimum toxicity by measuring drug concentrations in patient's blood to ensure that a desired concentration has been achieved. Not all medications require therapeutic drug monitoring. This is usually only performed for those whose medications need to be dosed to a certain narrow range of blood-drug concentrations in order to achieve the maximum efficacy versus toxicity ratio.

Type A reactions: These reactions are generally an extension of the desired therapeutic effect. For example, an agent used to treat hypertension might cause dizziness in a patient as a result of excess blood pressure lowering.[22]

Type B reactions: These reactions are not an extension of the normal therapeutic effect. For example, allergic reactions associated with penicillin and other antibiotics are examples of a type B reaction.[22]

Public Health Terms

Adverse Drug Event Reporting System: (also, **MedWatch**). A system implemented by the FDA to assure the safety and efficacy of regulated, marketed medical products. The system allows reports of adverse events that are suspected to be related to a drug or medical device by healthcare professionals and patients.

Drug-Induced Disease: Defined as "an unintended effect of a drug that may result in morbidity or mortality with symptoms sufficient to prompt a patient to seek medical attention and/or require hospitalization."[3]

Adverse Drug Event (ADE): Defined as "an untoward effect or outcome associated with use of a drug."[4]

Healthy People 2010

Focus Area: Medical Product Safety

Goal: Ensure the safe and effective use of medical products.

Objectives:

17-1. Increase the proportion of healthcare organizations that are linked in an integrated system that monitors and reports adverse events.

17-2. Increase the use of linked, automated systems to share information.

17-3. Increase the proportion of primary care providers, pharmacists, and other healthcare professionals who routinely review with their patients aged 65 years and older and patients with chronic illnesses or disabilities all new prescribed and over-the-counter medicines.

17-4. Increase the proportion of patients receiving information that meets guidelines for usefulness when their new prescriptions are dispensed.

17-5. Increase the proportion of patients who receive verbal counseling from prescribers and pharmacists on the appropriate use and potential risks of medications.

Medication Reconciliation: A process that identifies, maintains, and updates the most accurate list of all medications (including non-prescription medications, herbals, and alternative medicines) that patients are taking, including dosage and route of administration.

REFERENCES

1. Institute of Medicine. In: Kohn LT, Corrigan JM, Donaldson MS, eds. *To Err Is Human: Building a Safer Health System.* Washington, DC: National Academy Press; 2000. Available at http://www.nap.edu/openbook. php?isbn=0309068371. Accessed March 18, 2008.

2. Lazarou J, Pomeranz BH, Corey PN. Incidence of adverse drug reactions in hospitalized patients: a meta-analysis of prospective studies. *JAMA* 1998;279:1200–1205.

3. Tisdale JE, Miller DA. Preface. In: Tisdale JE, Miller DA, eds. *Drug-Induced Diseases: Prevention, Detection, and Management.* Bethesda, MD: American Society of Health-System Pharmacists; 2005:xvii.

4. Cantilena LR. Adverse drug events and postmarketing surveillance. In: Flomenbaum NE, Goldfrank LR, Hoffman RS, et al. eds. *Goldfrank's Toxicologic Emergencies.* New York: McGraw Hill; 2006: 1856–1865.

5. Litaker JR, Wilson JP. Epidemiology and public health impact of drug-induced diseases. In: Tisdale JE, Miller DA, eds. *Drug-Induced Diseases: Prevention, Detection, and Management.* Bethesda, MD: American Society of Health-System Pharmacists; 2005:3–10.

6. US Food and Drug Administration. History of the FDA. The 1938 Food, Drug, and Cosmetic Act. Available at http://www.fda.gov/oc/history/historyoffda/default.htm. Accessed March 18, 2008.

7. Bernstein J. Thalidomide. *Clinical Toxicology Review.* 1999;21. Available at http://www.k-faktor.com/thalidomide/artikel5.htm. Accessed March 18, 2008.

8. National Institutes of Health, Center for the Evaluation of Risks to Human Reproduction. (n.d.). Thalidomide. Retrieved October 30, 2007, from http://cerhr.niehs.nih.gov/common/thalidomide.html.

9. U.S. Food and Drug Administration, Center for Drug Evaluation and Research. Thalidomide information. (n.d.). Retrieved September 15, 2007, from http://www.fda.gov/cder/news/thalinfo/default.htm.

10. American Association of Colleges of Pharmacy, Center for the Advancement of Pharmaceutical Education. *Educational Outcomes 2004.* (2004). Available at http://www.aacp.org/Docs/MainNavigation/Resources/6075_CAPE2004.pdf. Accessed March 18, 2008.

11. Accreditation Council for Pharmacy Education. (2006). Accreditation standards and guidelines for the professional program in pharmacy leading to the doctor of pharmacy degree. Retrieved October 30, 2007, from http://www.acpe-ccredit.org/pdf/ACPE_Revised_PharmD_Standards_Adopted_Jan15 2006.pdf

12. Bush PJ, Johnson KW. (1979). Where is the public health pharmacist? *Am J Pharmaceut Edu* 1979;43:249–253.

13. Capper SA, Sands CD. The vital relationship between public health and pharmacy. *Int J Pharmacy Edu* 2006;3(2). Available at http://www.samford.edu/schools/pharmacy/ijpe/206/206.html. Accessed March 18, 2008.

14. Einarson TR. Drug-related hospital admissions. *Ann Pharmacother* 1993;27:832–840.

15. Hallas J. Drug related hospital admissions in subspecialties of internal medicine. *Danish Med Bull* 1996;43:141–155.

16. Jhung MA, Budnitz DS, Mendelsohn AB, Weidenbach KN, Nelson TD, Pollock DA. Evaluation and overview of the national electronic injury surveillance system—cooperative adverse drug event surveillance project (NEISS-CADES). *Med Care* 2007;45:S96–S102.

17. Moore TJ, Cohen MR, Furberg CD. Serious adverse drug events reported to the food and drug administration, 1998–2005. *Arch Intern Med* 2007;167:1752–1759.

18. World Health Organization. Quality of care: patient safety (2002). Available at http://www.who.int/gb/ebwha/pdf_files/WHA55/ea5513.pdf. Accessed March 18, 2008.

19. Wysowski DK, Swartz L. Adverse drug event surveillance and drug withdrawals in the United States, 1969–2002. *Arch Intern Med* 2005;165:1363–1369.

20. Bates DW, Miller EB, Cullen DJ, Burdick L, Williams L, Laird N, et al. Patient risk factors for adverse drug events in hospitalized patients. ADE prevention study group. *Arch Intern Med* 1999;159:2553–2560.

21. Schnipper JL, Kirwin JL, Cotugno MC, Wahlstrom SA, Brown BA, Tarvin E, et al. Role of pharmacist counseling in preventing adverse drug events after hospitalization. *Arch Intern Med* 2006;166:565–571.

22. Rawlings M, Thompson W. Mechanisms of adverse drug reactions. In: Davies D, ed. *Textbook of Adverse Drug Reactions.* New York: Oxford University Press; 1991:18–45.

23. MacKichan JJ, Lee M. Factors contributing to drug-induced diseases. In: Tisdale JE, Miller DA, eds. Drug-Induced Diseases: Prevention, Detection, and Management. Bethesda, MD: American Society of Health-System Pharmacists; 2005:11–16.

24. Chase BA, Bennett NL. *Medication Safety, Systems and Communications.* (2006). Available at http://www.massmed.org/Content/NavigationMenu2/MedicationSafetySystemsandCommunication/CourseInformation/default.htm. Accessed March 18, 2008.

25. Joint Commission. Patient Safety Goals Hospital Program. (2007). Available at http://www.jointcommission.org/NR/rdonlyres/C92AAB3F-A9BD-431C-8628-11DD2D1D53CC/0/lasa.pdf. Accessed March 18, 2008.

26. Kirsch I, Jungeblut A, Jenkins L, Kolstad A. *Adult Literacy in America: A First Look at the Findings of the National Adult Literacy Survey.* Washington, DC: US Department of Education; 1993.

27. Institute of Medicine. *Health Literacy: A Prescription to End Confusion.* Washington, DC: The National Academy Press; 2004.

28. Williams MV, Baker DW, Honig EG, Lee TM, Nowlan A. Inadequate literacy is a barrier to asthma knowledge and self-care. *Chest* 1998;114:1008–1015.

29. Williams MV, Parker RM, Baker DW, Parikh NS, Pitkin K, Coates WC, et al. Inadequate functional health literacy among patients at two public hospitals. *JAMA* 1995;274:1677–1682.

30. American Medical Association. Health literacy: report of the Council on Scientific Affairs: Ad hoc committee on health literacy for the council on scientific affairs. *JAMA* 1999;281:552–557.

31. Youmans SL, Schillinger D. Functional health literacy and medication use: the pharmacist's role. *Annals Pharmacotherapy,* 2003;37:1726–1729.

32. Rudd RE, Moeykens BA, Colton TC. Health and literacy: a review of medical and public health literature. In: Comings J, Garners B, Smith C, eds. *Annual Review of Adult Learning and Literacy.* New York: Josey Bass; 1999. Available at http://www.hsph.harvard.edu/healthliteracy/litreview_final.pdf. Accessed March 18, 2008.

33. U.S. Census Bureau. Foreign-born population: 2000. (2003). Available at http://www.census.gov/prod/2003pubs/c2kbr-34.pdf. Accessed March 18, 2008.

34. Anderson DJ, Webster CS. A systems approach to the reduction of medication errors on the hospital wards. *J Adv Nurs* 2001;35:34–41.

35. Bates DW, Boyle DL, Vander Vliet MB, Schneider J, Leape L. Relationship between medication errors and adverse drug events. *J Gen Intern Med* 1995;10:199–205.

36. Institute of Medicine. *Crossing the Quality Chasm: A New Health System for the 21st Century.* Washington, DC: National Academy Press; 2001.

37. Institute of Medicine. *Preventing Medication Errors: Quality Chasm Series.* Washington, DC: National Academy Press; 2006.

38. National Patient Safety Foundation. *Ask me 3.* (n.d.). Available at http://askmethree.org/. Accessed March 18, 2008.

39. Zarcadoolas C, Pleasant A, Greer DS. Advancing Health Literacy: A Framework or Understanding and Action. San Francisco: John Wiley and Sons; 2006.

40. Bates DW, Leape LL, Cullen DJ, Laird N, Petersen LA, Teich JM, et al. Effect of computerized physician order entry and a team intervention on prevention of serious medication errors. *JAMA* 1998;280:1311–1316.

41. Poon EG, Cina JL, Churchill W, Patel N, Featherstone E, Rothschild JM, et al. Medication dispensing errors and potential adverse drug events before and after implementing bar code technology in the pharmacy. *Ann Intern Med* 2006;45:426–334.

42. Rogers G, Alper E, Brunelle D, Federico F, Fenn CA, Leape LL, et al. Reconciling medications at admission: safe practice recommendations and implementation strategies. *Joint Comm J Qual Patient Saf* 2006;32:37–50.

CROSS REFERENCE

Communicating Public Health Information

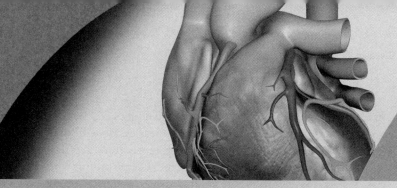

CHAPTER 7

Disease Versus Disease: How Some Diseases Ameliorate Others

E. Richard Stiehm

> Immunization, perhaps the most important therapeutic advance in medicine, resulted from a disease-versus-disease observation.[1]
>
> E. Richard Stiehm

LEARNING OBJECTIVES

By the end of this chapter, the student will be able to:

- Discuss the tangible results that have come from the discovery that one disease may prevent or modify another.
  - Clinical observations of these interactions have led to the discovery of vaccines, therapeutic antibodies, drugs, and special diets.
- Discuss the potential benefits that genetic polymorphism may have on the disease process.
  - Genetic polymorphisms, symptomatic and asymptomatic, may prevent or modify the severity of infections, including bubonic plague, tuberculosis, secretory diarrhea, malaria, *Parvovirus* B19, and HIV.
  - Genetic polymorphisms that lead to complete resistance provide unique insight into disease pathogenesis.
- Describe the ways in which viral interference may be used as a means of combating HIV.
  - Viral interference, using retroviruses similar to HIV-2 or hepatitis virus strains similar to GBV-C, should be explored as a means to combat HIV-1.
- Describe the scientific reason behind why cowpox (vaccinia) is able to prevent smallpox (variola).
  - Following vaccination with live cowpox virus, cross-reactive antibodies provide long-lasting immunity to the much more virulent smallpox virus.
- Describe the possible mechanism explaining why certain autoimmune diseases, such as inflammatory bowel disease (IBD), are modified by intestinal parasites.

- The mechanism may be immunologic diversion. The immune system is directed at the intestinal parasite and spares certain self-antigens. Worms could stimulate Th2 responses, which in turn inhibit Th1 responses both locally or centrally.
  - Alternatively, they may enroll immune cells destined for autoimmunity to the task of worm expulsion, thus diverting the immune system.
- Discuss the consequences of infection-induced immunosuppression, particularly in the case of measles.
  - Measles and other systemic viral infections cause a temporary suppression of cellular immunity. This suppression often results in remission of autoimmune diseases.
- Discuss some of the reasons why patients afflicted with trisomy-21 are usually not affected by asthma.
  - Trisomy-21 patients have subtle B- and T-cell immune defects that may favor a Th1 skewing.
  - Trisomy-21 patients also may have an increased number of bacterial infections, which favor a Th1 and a decreased Th2 response.
- Discuss the ways in which genes may prevent infection, particularly in the case of HIV.
  - HIV virus infects a blood cell by attaching to the HIV receptor CD4 and the CCR coreceptor.
  - Individuals with a homozygous hereditary mutation of the coreceptor are resistant to HIV.

INTRODUCTION

With apologies to Jane Austen, it is a truth universally acknowledged that a single person in possession of a single disease may often be afflicted with another (e.g., diabetes with arteriosclerosis, obesity with hypertension, ulcerative colitis with colon cancer, etc.). The converse of this—that one illness prevents or ameliorates another—is also surprisingly common.

In this chapter, I shall elaborate on how three such classes of disorders—infectious diseases, nutritional deficiencies, and genetic syndromes—may favorably alter the manifestations of another illness. These paradigms provide important lessons into disease prevalence and pathogenesis as well as offer preventive and therapeutic approaches.[1]

CLINICAL VIGNETTES

My interest in disease versus disease arose from my experiences during a pediatric residency at Babies Hospital in New York and medical work in Ghana and Kenya.

In New York, my toddler ward was overflowing with children with acute illnesses (e.g., diarrhea, sepsis, and pneumonia) and chronic illnesses (cystic fibrosis, heart disease, nephrosis). The admitting resident called to tell me he was admitting a child with tuberculous meningitis who needed a single isolation room. Because no such room was available, I called my attending physician. He provided the astounding recommendation, "Put him in the room with the cystic fibrosis patient. CF patients never get tuberculosis." I did, and the CF patient didn't get infected during their month together.

Shortly thereafter, an edematous boy with nephrosis (due to loss of protein in the urine) was not responding at all to albumin infusions. This time my attending said, "Put him in the same room as the patient with measles. He will surely catch measles and this may result in remission." Ten days later, measles appeared and the patient's edema promptly resolved.

Several years later in Africa, while conducting immunological studies on malnourished children in the city hospitals of Accra, Ghana, and Nairobi, Kenya, our team found extremely high levels of IgE immunoglobulin, the allergy antibody also associated with intestinal parasites. Most of these children had or were infected with intestinal parasites. Surprisingly, I never saw a child with asthma! Asthma is the leading cause of hospitalization for children in our country.

INFECTION

Cowpox and Smallpox

The best example of how one infectious disease prevents another is the use of vaccinia (cowpox) to prevent variola (smallpox). William Jenner performed this task in 1796, thus initiating the vaccine era (Figure 7-1).[2] Vaccination is probably the most significant medical advance of the last two centuries. Smallpox killed about 1 of every 10 people in Europe before vaccination, helped to conquer the American Indians, and claimed the lives of thousands of unvaccinated subjects until its complete eradication in 1978.[3]

Following vaccination with live cowpox virus, cross-reactive antibodies provide long-lasting immunity to the much more virulent smallpox virus.[3] Attenuated (weakened) virus vaccines mimic this effect and are widely used to prevent rabies, measles, mumps, varicella/zoster, and rotavirus infections.

Table 7-1 provides examples of this experience as well as other previously described disease-versus-disease events and is derived from an article on disease-versus-disease.[1]

Treating Syphilis with Malaria

Malaria was the treatment of choice for tertiary syphilis in the early 1900s prior to the discovery of penicillin.[4] Julius Wagner-Jauregg (1857–1940), a Viennese psychiatrist, noted that some of his syphilitic patients with severe weakness and paralysis (paresis) improved follow-

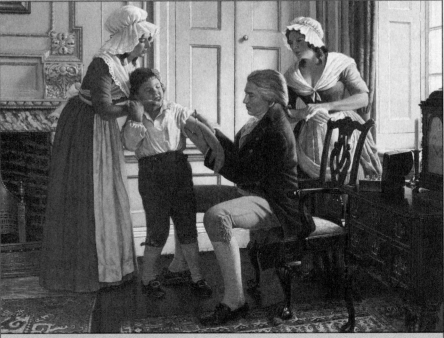

FIGURE 7-1 Painting of Dr. William Jenner Inoculating James Phipps with Pus from a Cowpox Sore on Milkmaid Sarah Nelmes' Hand. She became infected when milking her cow named Blossom. This event which occurred in 1796 in Gloucestershire, UK, ushered in the vaccine era.

Source: Robert Thom. Great Moments in Medicine.

TABLE 7-1 Disease Versus Disease and Therapeutic Implications

Protective Disorder	Protective Disorder	Therapeutic Implications
Vaccinia	Variola	Smallpox vaccine Vaccinia IG
Hemoglobin/RBC disorders* (Sickle cell disease, Thalassemia, G6PD deficiency)	Malaria	None
Male Pseudohermaphroditism	Prostatic enlargement Female hirsutism Male pattern baldness	Finasteride Finasteride Finasteride
ABO Hemolytic Disease	Rh Hemolytic disease	Rh Immune Globulin
X-lined Agammaglobulinemia	EBV infection	Rituximab (Anti-CD20)
Cystic Fibrosis*	Tuberculosis Secretory diarrhea	None CFTR inhibitors
Measles	Nephrotic syndrome	Immunosuppressives
Leprosy	Psoriasis	Immunosuppressives
Undernutrition	Celiac Disease Seizures Type 2 diabetes Renal Failure Inflammatory Bowel disease	Gluten-free diet Ketogenic diet Calorie-restricted diet Low-protein diet Elemental diet
HIV-1	Common variable immunodeficiency	HIV B-cell stimulant (?)
HIV-2	HIV-1	HIV vaccine
Hepatitis GB virus C	HIV-1	Viral Interference

Abbreviations are: IG, immunoglobulin; RBC, red blood cell; G6PD, glucose-6-phosphate dehydrogenase; ABO, a type of blood group; Rh, a type of protein on the blood cell; EBV, Epstein-Barr virus; Anti-CD20, a type of antibody; CFTR, cystic fibrosis transmembrane conductance regulator.

* Heterozygotes may have survival advantage.

Source: Used with permission from E. Richard Stiehm. Disease versus disease: how one disease may ameliorate another. *Pediatrics* 2006;117:184–191.

ing a bout of fever. Wagner-Jauregg then began treating such patients by inducing fever. He first tried injections of tuberculin but this did not reliably produce fever. In 1917, he used blood from a malarial soldier to treat nine paretic patients, all of whom got malaria. The malaria was aborted after seven to ten fever cycles with quinine. He reported that six of nine of the patients improved, one died and two were unchanged.

Within five years the "malaria fever cure" was widely used, often with dramatic benefit.[4] Wagner-Jauregg became famous and received the 1927 Nobel prized in Medicine, one of only two psychiatrists to win the award. The exact mechanism of fever therapy is not known; perhaps it alters the growth or the response of the treponema spirochete within the brain.

The Hygiene Hypothesis

A recent hypothesis suggests that early exposure to environmental endotoxins and bacterial illness prevents the later development of asthma and allergy, and, conversely, the lack of such exposure predisposes to the development of asthma and allergy.[5] The hygiene hypothesis has been offered as one explanation for the increasing prevalence of allergies in developed countries, including the United States.

Thus, improvement of water supply, less exposure to animals and soil, and prevention of childhood diseases by multiple vaccinations may focus the immune system toward allergy and autoimmunity and away from combating bacterial infections. This results in a skewing of the regulatory T cells of the immune system from a preponderance of helper T-1 (Th1) cells to a preponderance of Th2 cells.[6]

Th1 cells respond to viral and bacterial disorders by production of the cytokines interleukin (IL)-2, IL-12, and interferon-gamma, promote delayed (cellular) hypersensitivity against infections, and inhibit Th2 responses. Th2 cells respond to environmental and intestinal antigens by production of the cytokines IL-4, IL-5, and IL-13, stimulation of immunoglobulin E (IgE; allergy) antibodies causing immediate (allergic) responses and inhibit Th1 responses.

Support for this hypothesis is provided by the lessened incidence of asthma and allergic disease in developing countries, in rural areas, and in children exposed in early life to dogs and cats.[7,8] In addition, asthma is uncommon in the presence of lung disorders with chronic bacterial infection such as cystic fibrosis and tuberculosis.[9,10]

Immunologic Diversion

Certain autoimmune diseases, notably inflammatory bowel disease and multiple sclerosis, are modified by intestinal parasites. The mechanism may be immunological diversion where the immune system is directed at the intestinal parasite and spares certain self-antigens. This can be considered a corollary of the hygiene hypothesis.

The prevalence of schistosomiasis and multiple sclerosis (MS) are reciprocal; MS is less common in the tropics where schistosomiasis is endemic and more common in temperate climate where schistosomiasis is rare.[11,12] That this is not genetic is the fact that individuals formerly living in tropical climates get MS just as often as do others in the temperate zone.[11] A murine model of MS, experimental autoimmune encephalomyelitis, can be modified by deliberate infection with *S. mansoni* eggs.[13] MS is thought to result from cellular immunity to myelin basic protein of the central nervous system, which is inhibited by this organism.

Inflammatory bowel disease (IBD; e.g., regional enteritis and ulcerative colitis) is considered to be a T-cell mediated autoimmune disease directed against intestinal cells.[14,15] The presence of worms, notably *Trichuris*, may prevent or modulate these disorders; indeed, Summers et al. have proposed deliberate infection with this organism as a safe and possibly effective treatment for IBD.[16]

How intestinal parasites modulate a cellular immune autoimmune disease is not at all clear. Helminths stimulate Th2 responses, which in turn inhibit Th1 responses both locally (to intestinal epithelial cells in IBD) or centrally (to central nervous system [CNS] antigens in MS). Alternatively, they may enroll immune cells destined for autoimmunity to the task of worm expulsion thus diverting the immune system.

Infection-Induced Immunosuppression

Measles and several other systemic viral infections (particularly herpes viruses such as Epstein Barr virus) cause a temporary suppression of cellular immunity, resulting in remission of autoimmune diseases such as nephrosis.[17,18] Hansen disease (leprosy) is associated with a state of cutaneous anergy (non-reactivity to tuberculin and other antigens) and thus the common immune-mediated skin disease psoriasis is extremely rare in these patients.[19]

UNDERNUTRITION

Arteriosclerosis

The incidence of arteriosclerosis is considerably lower in underdeveloped countries where much of the population is chronically malnourished.[20] These individuals have a low calorie, low fat diet, are very thin, and expand a lot of energy in their work and their transportation (bicycling and walking). In addition, they often have nutritional anemia, as their diets are poor in vitamins and minerals, particularly iron.

Anemia *per se* is associated with fewer arteriosclerotic illnesses such as myocardial infarction and stroke, possibly by diminishing blood viscosity and thus preventing thrombosis.[21,22] The anemia can be secondary to iron deficiency, thalassemia, or hemolytic anemia. Schilling et al. showed that their patients with hereditary spherocytosis (HS) who were splenectomized and thus had a higher hemoglobin levels also had a higher incidence of arteriosclerosis than their non-splenectomized HS patients.[23] It must be noted, however, that anemia may aggravate arteriosclerosis in certain conditions such as chronic renal disease.

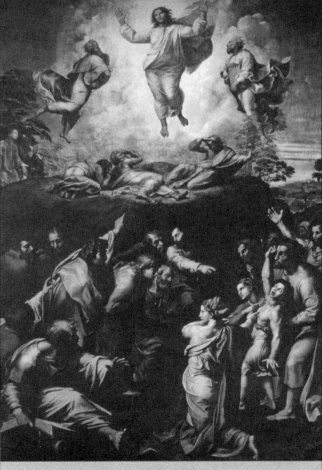

FIGURE 7-2 *Transfiguration,* an Unfinished Painting by Raphael (1483–1520).

Source: © The Print Collector/Alamey Images.

Celiac Disease

During Europe's 1944–1945 "winter of starvation," delivery of bread to the Juliana Children's Hospital in the Hague, Netherlands, was severely curtailed. PediatricianWillem-Karel Dicke observed that, unlike most of his patients, a few children gained weight and vigor on a very restricted diet that included tulip bulbs; these children had celiac disease.[24] This confirmed Dr. Dicke's long-held suspicion that wheat was the offending agent. Dicke's classic dietary studies after the war, using growth curves and stool fat excretion, firmly established that gluten was the offending agent in celiac diseases and that a gluten-free diet was the treatment of choice for celiac disease.[25]

Seizures and the Ketogenic Diet

Jesus was asked how he was able to free a possessed child of the demons (seizures). He replied, "This kind does not leave but by prayer and fasting" (Matthew 17:14–21). This event is depicted in the Italian artist Raphael's final painting, the magnificent *Transfiguration* (Figure 7-2), which depicts Christ freeing a possessed child from demons (seizures). Fasting was used for centuries in the treatment of seizures and is the precursor of the modern ketogenic diet.

The modern ketogenic diet had its origin in 1911 with the report from Guelpa and Marie, indicating that a four-day fast provided control of seizures; this was followed in 1924 by Wilder's observation that the benefit of starvation could be mimicked if ketonemia was produced by a diet rich in fat and low in carbohydrates.[26,27] A few years later, Peterman et al. reported that 69% of 57 patients treated with a ketogenic diet were seizure-free, and 35% were markedly improved. The ketogenic diet is still used today for many drug-resistant patients.[28,29]

Treatment by Caloric Restriction

Severe caloric restriction in experimental animals and probably humans can prolong life span.[30] Willi et al. used it with benefit in children with type 2 diabetes.[31] Low-protein diets are of proven benefit in chronic renal disease.[32] A calorie-restricted diet has been used successfully in the treatment of inflammatory bowel disease and childhood diabetes with obesity.[33,34]

GENETIC DISORDERS
Hemoglobinopathies and Malaria

Next to Jenner's use of cowpox to prevent smallpox, the best known example of disease-versus-disease is the modification of malaria by genetic red cell disorders such as sickle cell anemia and thalassemia. In 1948, British biologist J.B. Haldane proposed that malaria was an evolutionary force by selecting for malaria-resistance genes, thus enhancing survival of people with thalassemia major and minor (the carriers) in areas of malaria endemicity, the well-known "heterozygote advantage."[35,36] This also holds for sickle cell anemia and sickle cell trait (heterozygote carriers) and for less common hemoglobinopathies such as ovalocytosis and eliptocytosis.[37]

Subsequent studies have validated Haldane's conjecture by showing a higher frequency of these disorders in tropical regions with high malaria incidence as compared to adjacent mosquito-free highlands.[36] These patients have a reduced mortality (up to 50%) and decreased numbers of circulating parasites (by 80%).[38] The mechanism of resistance may be reduced parasite replication within the erythrocytes, or enhanced splenic clearance of parasitized erythrocytes.[39]

Asthma and Down Syndrome

Down syndrome (trisomy 21) is the most frequent chromosomal abnormality recognized at birth; it is associated with a variety of health problems, notably congenital heart disease, cancer, respiratory tract infections, sleep apnea, and autoimmune disease. Asthma, the most common cause of childhood hospitalization, is surprisingly uncommon in Down syndrome (DS).

Hilton et al. noted that only 5% of children with DS hospitalized in New South Wales for respiratory problems had asthma, as compared to 25% for other children.[40] Other studies have noted a similar finding.[41–44] When present, the asthma is often mild and of short duration. Lockitch and Ferguson noted that the serum IgE levels, a potential marker of asthma, was significantly lower in DS patients (184 µg/L) than in controls (242 µg/L).[45]

The reason for this protection may be multifactial. DS patients have subtle B- and T-cell immune defects that may favor a Th1 skewing.[46] They also may have an increased number of bacterial infection that, as noted earlier, favors a Th1 and a decreased Th 2 response. Alternatively, environmental and lifestyle factors may limit their allergen exposure.

Macular Degeneration and the Complement System

Age-related macular degeneration (AMD) is the most common cause of blindness in the elderly.[47,48] Risk factors include a positive family history, obesity, cigarette smoking, hypertension, and chronic inflammation as indicated by increased blood levels of C-reactive protein.[49] Retinal inflammation promotes progressive deposits of lipids and proteins (termed *drusin*) in the retina pigment epithelium with loss of photoreceptors, neovascularization, and progressive blindness.[47]

Chronic inflammation within the retina is associated with complement system activation This is usually held in check by the presence of complement inhibitors, notably complement factor H (CFH), in the serum and in the retina.[50] Certain gene polymorphisms that promote complement activation (e.g., of complement factor 3 [C3]) or diminish the activity of factor H increase the risk of developing AMD.[51,52] Other gene polymorphisms for C2 and factor B that decrease complement activation provide protection against AMD.[53] Thus, the very rare patients with hereditary C2 and C3 deficiencies would be expected to be protected against AMD.

It is of interest that patients with long-standing rheumatoid arthritis who have taken anti-inflammatory drugs for years have a lower incidence of AMD.[54]

Genes Prevent Infections

The most common strain of the AIDS virus (monocytotrophic HIV) infects a blood cell by attaching to the HIV receptor CD4 and the CCR coreceptor. Individuals with a homozygous hereditary mutation of the coreceptor (the CCR-Δ32 mutation) are completely resistant to HIV infection and heterozygotes have a slower rate of disease progression.[55] Drugs that interfere with coreceptors (e.g., receptor blockaders or monoclonal antibodies) are now available.

Most blacks of West African descent are resistant to malaria caused by *Plasmodium vivax*. These individuals have a red blood cell type termed *Duffy negative*, that is, *FyFy*. The Duffy red blood cell groups Fy^a and Fy^b are the receptors for *P. vivax*, and without this receptor they cannot be infected with this strain of plasmodium but are susceptible to other strains.[56]

Individuals who lack the red blood cell antigen P, that is, they are blood type pp rather than PP or Pp, cannot become infected with parvovirus B19, a common virus that causes slapped-cheek syndrome in youngsters and severe anemia in individuals with compromised immune systems.[57] The only receptor for parvovirus B19 is the P antigen on erythrocyte precursors, so that the rare individual with pp blood type is completed protected.[57]

SUMMARY

Disease-versus-disease observations have led to the discovery of vaccines, therapeutic antibodies, drugs, and special diets. Genetic polymorphisms that lead to complete resistance provide unique insight into disease pathogenesis. New associations will emerge as the database on human disease expands. So keep your eyes and minds open!

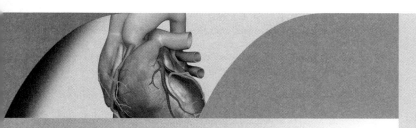

Questions for Further Research, Study, Reflection, and Discussion

For the Individual Student

It may be necessary to research the primary literature to answer these questions.

- The knowledge that one disease may prevent the onset of another is not new. For example, the discovery that cowpox vaccines can prevent smallpox dates back to 1798. What other examples of disease-versus-disease can you find outside of the text that illustrates how one illness may prevent or decrease the severity of another?
- Genetic polymorphisms can lead to complete viral resistance and provide unique insight into disease pathogenesis. How do these polymorphisms come about, and what diseases are known to be reduced in severity due to these genetic polymorphisms?

For Entire Class Discussion

- On a recent trip to a South American rainforest, three out of the four researchers came down with a bout of malaria. It was determined that the strain of malaria that infected the researchers was *Plasmodium vivax*. The first and second researchers who fell ill were Canadian, the third researcher who fell ill hailed from Portugal, and the fourth researcher who remained healthy was born in Mauritania. If all four researchers were equally exposed to the same strain, what are some possible reasons for why the fourth researcher was not affected by the malaria?
- As a prominent scientist in the field of immunology, you have been invited to speak at a conference regarding the prevalence of asthma in patients diagnosed with trisomy 21. How prevalent is asthma among patients with trisomy 21, and what are several reasons for this level of occurrence?

Acknowledgment

I thank Daniel Adam Lyons for contributing learning objectives and chapter questions.

REFERENCES

1. Stiehm ER. Disease versus disease: how one disease may ameliorate another. *Pediatrics* 2006;117:184–191.

2. Jenner E. *An Enquiry into the Causes and Effect of the Variolae Vaccinae.* London: Sampson-Low; 1778.

3. Henderson DA, Moss B. Smallpox and vaccinia. In: Plotkin SA, Orenstein WA, eds. *Vaccines,* 3rd ed. Philadelphia: WB Saunders; 1999: 74–95.

4. Raju NKR. Hot brains: manipulating body heat to save the brain. *Pediatrics* 2006;117:e320–e321.

5. Strachan DP. Family size, infection and atopy: the first decade of the "hygiene hypothesis." *Thorax* 2000;55(Suppl 1):S2–S10.

6. Sicherer SH, Sampson HA. Allergic disorders. In: Stiehm ER, Ochs HD, Winkestein JA, eds. *Immunologic Disorders in Infants and Children,* 5th ed. Philadelphia: Elsevier/Saunders; 2004:967–987.

7. Braun-Fahrlander C, Riedler J, Herz U, et al. Environmental exposure to endotoxin and its relation to asthma in school-age children. *N Engl J Med* 2002;347:869–877.

8. Ownby DR, Johnson CC, Peterson EL. Exposure to dogs and cats in the first year of life and risk of allergic sensitization at 6 to 7 years of age. *JAMA* 2002;288:963–972.

9. Shirakawa T, Enomoto T, Shimazu S, Hopkin JM. The inverse association between tuberculin responses and atopic disorders. *Science* 1997;275: 77–79.

10. Wood RE, Boat TF, Doershuk CR. Cystic fibrosis. *Am Rev Respir Dis* 1976;113:833–878.

11. Kurtzke JF. Multiple sclerosis in time and space—geographic clues to cause. *J Neurovirol* 2000;6(Suppl):S134–S140.

12. La Flamme AC, Canagasabey K, Harvie M, Backstrorm BT. Schistosomiasis protects against multiple sclerosis. *Mem Inst Oswaldo Cruz* 2004;99(Suppl 5):33–36.

13. La Flamme AC, Ruddenklau K, Backstrom BT. Schistosomiasis decreases central nervous system inflammation and alters the progression of experimental autoimmune encephalomyelitis. *Infect Immunity* 2003:71: 4996–5004.

14. Yamamoto-Farusho JK. Innovative therapeutics for inflammatory bowel disease. *World J Gastroenterol* 2007;13:1893–1896.

15. Fallon PG , Mongan NE. Suppression of Th2-type allergic reactions by helminth infection. *Nat Rev Immunol* 2007;7:220–240.

16. Summers RW, Elliott Weinstock JV. Is there a role for helminths in the therapy of inflammatory bowel disease? *Nat Clin Pract Gastroenterol Hepatol* 2005;2:62–63.

17. Blumberg RW, Cassady HA. Effect of measles on the nephrotic syndrome. *Am J Dis Child* 1947;73:151–166.

18. Lin C-Y, Hsu H-C. Histopathological and immunological studies in spontaneous remission of nephrotic syndrome after intercurrent measles infection. *Nephron* 1986;42:110–115.

19. Kumar B, Raychaudhure SP, Vossough S, Farber EM. The rare coexistence of leprosy and psoriasis. *Int J Dermatol* 1992;31:551–554.

20. Osuntokun BO. Nutritional problems in the African region. *Bull Schwiez Akad Med Wiss* 1976;31:353–376.

21. Kannel WB, Godon T, Wolf PA, McNamara P. Hemoglobin and the risk of cerebral infarction: the Framingham study. *Stroke* 1972;3:409–419.

22. Gagnon DR, Zhang TJ, Brand FN, Kannel WB. Hematocrit and the risk of cardiovascular disease—the Farmington study, a 34 year follow-up. *Am Heart J* 1994;127:674–682.

23. Schilling RF, Gangnon RE, Traver M. Arteriosclerotic events are less frequent in persons with chronic anemia: evidence from families with hereditary spherocytosis. *Am J Hemat* 2006;81:60–64.

24. Dicke WK. Coeliac disease. *Investigation of the Harmful Effects of Certain Types of Cereal on Patients with Coeliac Disease* (Thesis). University of Utrecht, The Netherlands; 1950 (in Dutch).

25. Dicke WK, Weijers HA, van de Kamer JH. Coeliac disease II. The presence in wheat of a factor having a deleterious effect in cases of coeliac disease. *Acta Paediatr Scand* 1953;42:34–42.

26. Guelpa G, Marie A: La lutte contre l'epilesie par la desintoxication et par la reeducation alimentaire. *Revue de therapie medico-chirurgicale* 1911;788–113 (in French).

27. Wilder RM. The effect of ketonemia on the course of epilepsy. *Mayo Clin Bull* 1921;2:307.

28. Peterman MG. The ketogenic diet in epilepsy. *JAMA* 1925;84:1979–1983.

29. Swink TC, Vining EPG, Freeman JM. The ketogenic diet: 1997. *Adv Pediatr* 1997;44:297–329.

30. Heilbronn LK, Ravussin E. Calorie restriction and aging: review of the literature and implications for studies in humans. *Am J Clin Nutr* 2003;78:361–369.

31. Willi SM, Martin K, Datko FM, Brant BP. Treatment of type 2 diabetes in childhood using a very-low-calorie diet. *Diabetes Care* 2004;27: 348–353.

32. Lentine K, Wrone EM. New insights into protein intake and progression of renal disease. *Curr Opin Nephrol Hypertens* 2004;13:333–336.

33. Russell RI. Dietary and nutritional management of Crohn's disease. *Aliment Pharmacol Ther* 1991;5:211–226.

34. Haarder H, Kinese B, Astrup A. The effect of a rapid weight loss on lipid profile and glycemic control in obese type 2 diabetic patients. *Int J Obes Relat Metab Disord* 2004;28:180–182.

35. Haldane JBS. The rate of mutation of human genes. *Hereditas* 1948;35(Suppl):267–273.

36. Weatherall DJ. Thalassaemia and malaria, revisited. *Ann Trop Med Parisotol* 1997;91:885–890.

37. Luzzatto L. Genetics of red cells and susceptibility to malaria. *Blood* 1997;54:961–976.

38. Nagel RL, Roth EF Jr. Malaria and red cell genetic defects. *Blood* 1989;74:1213–1221.

39. Lell B, May J, Schmidt-Ott RJ, Lehman LG, Luckner D, Greve B, Matousek P, Schmid D, Herbich K, Mockenhaupt FP, Meyer CG, Blienzle, U, Kremsner PG. The role of red blood cell polymorphisms in resistance and susceptibility to malaria. *Clin Infect Dis* 1999;28:794–799.

40. Hilton JM, Fitzgerald DA, Cooper DM. Respiratory morbidity of hospitalized children with Trisomy 21. *J Paediatr Child Health* 1999;35:383–386.

41. Coghlan MK, Evans PR. Infantile eczema, asthma and hay fever in mongolism. *Guys Hosp Rep* 1964;113:223–230.

42. Forni GL, Acutis MS, Strigini P. Incidence of bronchial asthma in Down syndrome. *J Pediatr* 1990;116:467–488.

43. Selikowitz, M. Health problems and health checks in school-aged children with Down syndrome. *J Paediatr Child Health* 1992;28:383–386.

44. Goldacre MJ, Wotton CJ, Seagroatt V, Yeates D. Cancers and immune related diseases associated with Down's syndrome: a record linkage study. *Arch Dis Child* 2004;89:1014–1017.

45. Lockitch G, Ferguson A. Reply: incidence of bronchial asthma in Down syndrome. *J Pediatr* 1990;116:487–488.

46. Ugazio AG, Maccario R, Notarangelo LD, Burgio GR. Immunology of Down syndrome: a review. *Am J Med Genet* 1990;7(Suppl):204–212.

47. De Jong PTVM. Age-related macular degeneration. *N Engl J Med* 1996;355:1474–1485.

48. Patel N, Adewoyin T, Chong NV. Age related macular degeneration: a perspective on genetic studies. *Eye* 2007;1–9.

49. Schaumberg DA, Christen WG, Buring JE, et al. High-sensitivity C-reactive protein, other markers of inflammation, and the incidence of macular degeneration in women. *Arch Ophthalmol* 2007;125:300–305.

50. Klein RJ, Zeiss C, Chew EY, et al. Complement factor H polymorphism in age-related macular degeneration. *Science* 2005;308:385–389.

51. Yates JRW, Sepp T, Matharu BK, et al. Complement C3 variant and the risk of age-related macular degeneration. *N Engl J Med* 2007;357:553–561.

52. Seddon JM, Francis PJ, George S. Association of *CFH Y402H* and *LOC 387715 A695* with progression of age-related macular degeneration. *JAMA* 2007;297:1793–1800.

53. Gold B, Merriam JE, Zernant J, et al. Variation if factor B (*BF*) and Complement component 2 (*C2*) genes is associated with age-related macular degeneration. *Nat Genet* 2006;38:458–462.

54. McGeer PL, Sibley J. Sparing of age-related macular degeneration in rheumatoid arthritis. *Neurobiol Aging* 2005;26:1199–1203.

55. Liu R, Paxton WA, Choe S, et al. Homozygous defect in HIV-1 core-ceptor accounts for resistance of some multiply-exposed individuals to HIV-1 infection. *Cell* 1966;86:367–377.

56. Spencer HC, Miller LH, Collins WE, et al. The Duffy blood group and resistance to *Plasmodium vivax* in Honduras. *J Parasitol* 1958;44:371–373.

57. Brown KE, Hibbs JR, Gallinella G, et al. Resistance to Parvovirus B199 infection due to lack of virus recepton (erythrocyte P antigen). *N Engl J Med* 2004;330:1192–1196.

CROSS REFERENCES

Achieving Asthma Control
Epidemiology of Atherosclerosis
Genetics and Public Health
Malaria

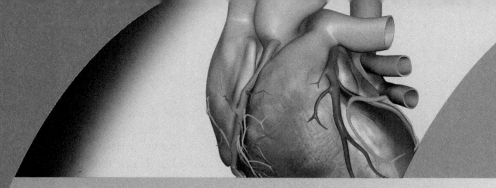

CHAPTER 8

Behavioral Determinants of Health

Frances F. Fiocchi

> One must avoid the naive view that compliance is merely a matter of enough information.[1]

LEARNING OBJECTIVES

By the end of this chapter, the student will be able to:

- Describe at least four theories of behavior change.
- Outline the process of behavior change for each of the four theories.
- List behavioral risk factors associated with the leading cause of death.
- Define specific constructs related to each of the four theories of behavior change.

BACKGROUND

Despite our best intentions, most of us engage in various degrees of unhealthy behaviors. As common examples, we may exercise too little or we may eat too much. The extent and the frequency to which we engage in these harmful behaviors will have different impacts on our health.

It is well known that the leading causes of death in the United States are chronic diseases such as heart disease, cancer, and stroke, and what cannot be overstated is the obvious fact that these mortality causes are associated with a multitude of common behavioral risk factors. In fact, about half of the U.S. deaths attributed to the 10 leading causes of death are a result of lifestyle-related behaviors such as tobacco use, poor dietary habits, inactivity, alcohol misuse, drug use, and risky sexual practices.[2] Table 8-1 shows the common behavioral risk factors

associated with the top five leading causes of death. These factors can be largely attributed to individual behavioral actions, and the totality of these risk factors accounts not only for a vast majority of deaths but also for a large portion of the medical care costs in the United States. Yet, there is hope. Despite daunting challenges that remain in intervening on these risk factors, poor health habits are potentially controllable and modifiable through direct behavior change.

Changing an individual's health practices holds a theoretical and practical potential to decrease the morbidity and mortality associated with such behaviors. This underscores the need to seriously take into account and address the issue of behavior change.

National initiatives such as ***Healthy People 2010*** have brought considerable attention to the need to target the modifiable behaviors that impact the health and well-being of Americans. Even the smallest intervention strategy addressing the behavioral risk factors most closely associated with the leading causes of death have the potential to produce significant improvements in an individual's health in addition to the broader population.

Before we attempt to modify an individual's health behavior, it is necessary to understand why people behave the way they do despite the obvious detrimental effects that are common knowledge for the individuals at risk. There are multiple factors influencing an individual's behavioral choices and actions and there is even more variability in these factors among individuals who share the same objective health behavior.[3] The more is understood about the underlying influences and determinants of an individual's behavior, the greater

TABLE 8-1 Behavioral Risk Factors Associated with the Five Leading Causes of Death in the United States

Cause of Death	Rank	Deaths	% of Total Deaths	Behavioral Risk Factors
Heart disease	1	685,089	28.0	Physical inactivity, obesity, smoking, poor dietary habits
Cancer	2	556,902	22.7	Smoking, physical inactivity, poor dietary habits, obesity, alcohol use
Stroke (cerebrovascular disease)	3	157,689	6.4	Physical inactivity, obesity, alcohol and drug use
Chronic lower respiratory disease	4	126,382	5.2	Smoking
Accidents (unintentional injuries)	5	109,277	4.5	Alcohol use, seatbelt use

Source: Data adapted from Heron MP, Smith BL. Deaths: leading causes for 2003. *Natl Vital Stat Rep* 2007;55:1–92.

the likelihood that behavior change strategies and interventions can be successful in targeting and transforming the risk factors responsible for the development and progression of disease.

The aim of this chapter is to provide students with a global but simple understanding of those determinants of health behavior and the process by which behavior change occurs.

BASIC SCIENCE FACTS/KEY CONCEPTS REVIEW

An individual's health behavior is rooted in biological, psychological, social, and environmental context factors. Addressing each of these aspects individually or the complex interplay among these factors makes the task of changing behavior far from a straightforward and clear-cut undertaking. In general, the most effective behavioral interventions are those that address each distinct undesirable factor.

Many health behavior theories and models have been developed to understand the multifaceted components of individual behavior and to explain why individuals are either successful in carrying out health-promoting practices while others fail to do so. Health behavior theories were created based on the need to explain human behavior and further comprehend an individual's personal processes of understanding, contemplating, adopting, modifying, and maintaining healthy behavior.

The theories and models of health behavior emerged from social psychology research.[4] These models and theories have been developed to create and guide practical strategies to promote healthy behaviors and facilitate effective adaptation to coping with illness.[5] Each theory or model has its own set of **constructs** and unique approaches to facilitate the process of

behavior change. Constructs can be thought of as explicit ideas that are derived for and applied to specific theories.

While several health behavior theories and models exist, it is not the intention of this chapter to provide an in-depth overview of each one of them. Instead, this chapter discusses a summary of four widely used theories: 1) Social Cognitive Theory; 2) Theory of Planned Behavior; 3) Health Belief Model; and 4) the Transtheoretical Model and Stages of Change. Put to use, each of these provides a framework for understanding how to bring about changes in knowledge, attitudes, and skills in order to produce behavior changes.

Social Cognitive Theory

The principles of social learning were first applied by Albert Bandura to explain human behavior in the Social Cognitive Theory. This theory proposes that individuals learn through observation of the behaviors of others and the rewards that others receive as an outcome of their actions.[6] It also emphasizes that cognitive processes mainly regulate an individual's behavior so that individuals do not simply respond to stimuli unconsciously, but rather they think about and interpret stimuli. Insight into how an individual processes and reflects on personal, environmental, and social factors helps predict how those factors will influence individual behavior. The concept of **reciprocal determinism** was later introduced to the Social Cognitive Theory to illustrate how individual behavior is largely determined by the reciprocal interaction of these personal, environmental, and behavioral factors.[7]

Apart from an individual's own cognitive processes, cognitive events are both stimulated and changed by an individual's experiences and, in turn, these experiences can alter the individual's expectations of **self-efficacy**.[6] The construct of self-efficacy is likely the most well-known and widely used concept to stem from the Social Cognitive Theory. Self-efficacy is the confidence that an individual has in his or her ability to successfully carry out a certain behavior in order to produce a desired outcome. This self-belief has a powerful effect on behavior. Individuals will generally choose to engage in behaviors or take on activities that they are confident that they can successfully accomplish and are inclined to steer clear of activities that they believe exceed their potential. **Outcome expectancy** is defined as an individual's belief that a certain behavior will produce certain outcomes. These constructs are key components of the Social Cognitive Theory and explain a portion of the factors that explain human behavior. Other constructs including **behavioral capability, observational learning, reinforcements**, and **emotional coping responses** account for additional determinants of behavior. Table 8-2 lists and defines the main constructs of the Social Cognitive Theory.

The Social Cognitive Theory has been applied to many behavioral risk factor interventions seeking to assess and subsequently alter an individual's level of intensity of any number of constructs in the context of a particular health problem. Interventions can focus on one specific construct, such as increasing an individual's self-efficacy related to making a targeted behavior change, or address several constructs that together influence health habits. Success of these approaches can vary depending on how effective an individual intervention is at assessing and modifying pertinent constructs.

Theory of Reasoned Action/Theory of Planned Behavior

The Theory of Reasoned Action underscores the influence of **behavioral intention** as a predictor and motivator of an individual's conduct. It focuses on variables such as attitudes and subjective norms to predict the execution of a certain behavior.[8] An individual's **attitudes** are comprised of his or her behavioral beliefs that performing certain actions will be associated with certain outcomes. **Subjective norms** are the individual's beliefs about whether other people approve or disapprove of engaging in a certain behavior. The assertion of the Theory of Reasoned Action is that an individual's decision to engage in a specific behavior is based on his or her personal attitude toward the behavior that has been indirectly influenced by the individual's own personal beliefs and subjective norms.

The Theory of Planned Behavior emerged as an extension of the Theory of Reasoned Action through the addition of a new construct: **perceived behavior control**. The construct was added to account for factors beyond an individual's immediate control that also can have an effect on the individual's intention. With the addition of an individual's self-perception of control, the Theory of Planned Behavior provides a useful blueprint for predicting the likelihood of an individual carrying out certain actions. Table 8-3 shows the direction and relationship between the key constructs influencing behavior in the Theory of Reasoned Action and Theory of Planned Behavior.

Health Belief Model

The Health Belief Model is used to describe the influence and power of perception in changing and maintaining health behavior. The principle features of the Health Belief Model emphasize an individual's desire to avoid being ill and the expectancy that a specific health behavior will ward off illness or enhance health. According to the Health Belief Model, if an individual believes that he or she is vulnerable to an illness, that individual will take necessary steps to protect against, monitor, or manage the

---

TABLE 8-2 Social Cognitive Theory

Individual Characteristics	
Self-Efficacy	A person's confidence that he or she can perform a behavior.
Behavioral Capability	A person's level of knowledge and skill in relation to a behavior.
Expectations	What a person thinks will happen if he or she makes a behavior change.
Expectancies	Whether a person thinks the expected outcome is good or likely to be rewarded.
Self-Control	How much control a person has over making a change.
Emotional Coping	A person's ability to deal with emotions involved in a behavior change.
Environmental Factors	
Vicarious Learning	A person learns by observing the behavior of others and the consequences of that behavior.
Situation	The social/physical environment in which the behavior takes place, and a person's perception of those factors.
Reinforcement	Positive or negative responses to a person's behavior.
Reciprocal Determinism	The iterative process where a person makes a change based on individual characteristics and social/environmental cues, receives a response, makes adjustments to his or her behavior, and so on.

Source: Edberg, M. (2007). *Essentials of Health Behavior.* Sudbury, Massachusetts: Jones and Bartlett Publishers, LLC.

TABLE 8-3 Components of the Theory of Reasoned Action/Theory of Planned Behavior (TRA/TPB)

Theory of Reasoned Action	Theory of Planned Behavior
Attitude • A person's beliefs about what will happen if he or she performs the behavior • A person's judgment of whether the expected outcome is good or bad	*Perceived Behavioral Control* • *Control beliefs:* A person's beliefs about factors that will make it easy or difficult to perform the behavior
Subjective Norms • A person's beliefs about what other people in his or her social group will think about the behavior • A person's motivation to conform to these perceived norms	• *Perceived power:* The amount of power a person believes he or she has over performing the behavior
Behavioral Intention • A person's intention to perform a behavior • Influenced by attitude, subjective norms, and perceived • Behavioral control, behavioral intention is most predictive of actual behavior	

Source: Edberg, M. (2007) *Essentials of Health Behavior.* Sudbury, Massachusetts: Jones and Bartlett Publishers, LLC.

disease if he or she believes that engaging in a particular behavior or action will have a positive effect on reducing their **perceived susceptibility** to the illness or the acuteness of the condition. Furthermore, provided that an individual believes that any **perceived barriers** are outweighed by the **perceived benefits** of performing a particular health-related behavior, the individual is more likely to undertake the action. Certain **cues to action** such as media publicity, a public figure's battle with an illness, or the loss of a close friend or family member due to illness also may trigger the individual to take action. Table 8-4 lists and defines the constructs of the Health Belief Model.

Transtheoretical Model: Stages of Change

The Transtheoretical Model uses stages of change to describe the distinct phases through which an individual progresses to change a behavior.[9,10] The application of this model to health behavior contends that behavior modification occurs through a series of changes: pre-contemplation, contemplation, preparation, action, and maintenance. Although listed sequentially, an individual does not necessarily experience these stages in order; rather, the individual can advance forward or backward through the stages during the behavior modification process.

TABLE 8-4 Health Belief Model Constructs

Construct	Definition
Perceived Susceptibility	An individual's perception of the probability that he or she will acquire a disease or become ill
Perceived Severity	An individual's perception of the seriousness of a disease and the consequences of having an illness
Perceived Benefits	An individual's perception of the positive aspects of the behavior being required to reduce risk
Perceived Barriers	An individual's perception of the negative aspects of the behavior being required to reduce risk
Self-Efficacy	The confidence that an individual has in his or her ability to successfully carry out a certain behavior in order to produce a desired outcome
Cues to Action	External triggers that stimulate an individual to take action

Source: Edberg, M. (2007). *Essentials of Health Behavior.* Sudbury, Massachusetts: Jones and Bartlett Publishers, LLC.

To better understand an individual's progression of behavior change according to this model, it is useful to be familiar with each stage. An individual in the pre-contemplation stage is largely unaware of his or her actions or of the consequences of his or her behavior. Individuals at this stage have not considered changing their behavior nor have any intention of altering their current behavior. In the contemplation stage, an individual has begun to become aware of the health implications associated with his or her current behavior. The individual also has started to consider what actions are required to reduce his or her possible health risks. Yet, despite these initial steps, the individual in the contemplation stage has not developed a tangible action plan for addressing his or her health risk. In the following preparation stage, an individual is set to take action soon. At this point, the individual may have decided on a particular action plan to address his or her health risk.

The first noticeable progress becomes evident during the next action stage. Although the individual has taken tangible actions to reduce his or her health risks, an individual at this stage is still at risk for relapsing and reverting back to a previous stage. In the final maintenance stage, the individual accepts the ongoing effort required to support long-term behavioral change and is working to maintain such change. The individual in this final stage must repeatedly practice and reinforce his or her newly adopted behavior and make an effort to steer clear of situations he or she associates with previous behavior that put him or her at risk. Figure 8-1 and Table 8-5 represent the stages of change that an individual must proceed through during the process of behavior change.

Strategies to modify unhealthy behaviors utilizing the Transtheoretical Model require careful consideration of an in-

dividual's readiness for change. Tailoring interventions to maximize the capacity of individuals at different stages is advisable to produce appreciable changes in behavior.

FIGURE 8-1 The Transtheoretical Model's Stages of Change.

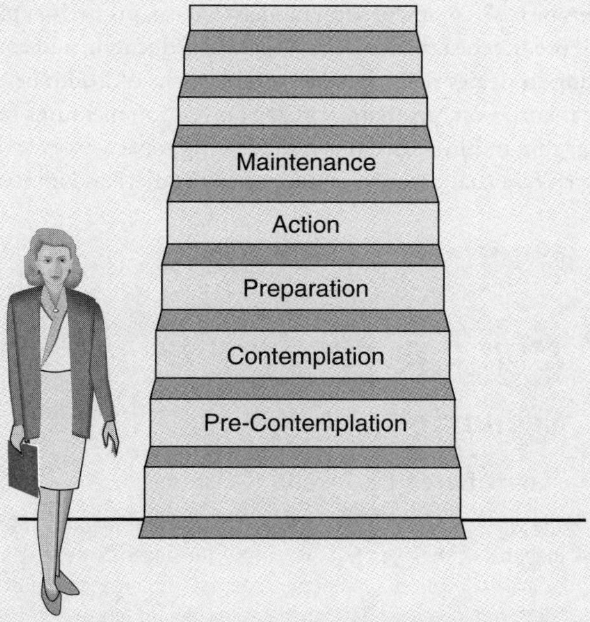

Source: Data from Bandura, A. (1977) *Social Learning Theory.* Englewood Cliffs, NJ: Prentice-Hall, Inc.
Bandura, A. The self system in reciprocal determinism. *American Psychologist.* 1978;33:344–358.

TABLE 8-5 Components of the Transtheoretical Model (TTM) and the Precaution Adoption Process Model (PAPM)

Transtheoretical Model	Precaution Adoption Process Model
Stage One: Precontemplation	Stage One: Unaware of the Issue
	Stage Two: Unengaged by the Issue
Stage Two: Contemplation	Stage Three: Deciding About Acting
Stage Three: Preparation	Stage Four: Deciding Not to Act
	Stage Five: Deciding to Act
Stage Four: Action	Stage Six: Acting
Stage Five: Maintenance	Stage Seven: Maintenance
Stage Six: Termination	

Source: Edberg, M. (2007). *Essentials of Health Behavior.* Sudbury, Massachusetts: Jones and Bartlett Publishers, LLC.

SUMMARY

In summary, in order to develop effective interventions intended to reduce health risks, it is essential that such interventions be based on theoretical models that can properly explain and predict the targeted behavior. Initial education and counseling strategies that capitalize on the tenets of health behavior theories can promote primary prevention measures (e.g., engaging in physical activity, preventing tobacco use, avoiding risky sexual practices, eating a healthy diet) and interventions aimed at secondary prevention have the potential to influence early detection of illness (e.g., compliance with breast self-examination, participation in colon cancer screening programs).[6] Public health interventions to change risky health behaviors are most effective when the knowledge of what motivates health behavior change and an understanding of the process through which it occurs are integrated into behavior change strategies.

CASE STUDY
Scenario

(Contributed by Joseph F. Pauley)

Joe P. is a 51-year-old Caucasian communications consultant. After decades of being overweight, Joe was diagnosed with Type II diabetes at the age of 45. Recently, Joe began to experience increasing blurred and distorted vision that eventually prompted him to make a medical appointment. At the recommendation of his doctor, Joe underwent a visual acuity test and retinal examinations. "Joe, you have macular degeneration in your left eye," his doctor told him. Joe's doctor continued, "Your diabetes put you at high risk for developing macular degeneration. Your diabetes can still be controlled if you are willing to do two things: lose weight and exercise two hours every day. The medicines you are taking can only do so much, but they will not cure your diabetes. However, you have a very good chance of controlling the progression of your disease if you lose one pound a week, exercise on a treadmill one hour each day, and lift weights for one hour each day. The alternative is that, in three to four years, you will be back here on dialysis because your kidneys have failed, or in a wheelchair because your feet have been amputated, and blind from your macular degeneration. Shortly after that, the heart attacks and strokes will start, if they haven't already by that point. The choice is yours."

With that, Joe's doctor left the room to see another patient, leaving him to think of the alternatives that were presented to him. The walls in his doctor's office were bare with the exception for one sign, a quote from Benjamin Franklin that read: "Those who won't be counseled can't be helped." Joe had been diagnosed with diabetes six years before and had lost 25 pounds over the past two years at the rate of one pound a month. Yet, he was still about 65 pounds overweight and had not really taken his diabetes seriously. Even though he had been losing weight, he continued to eat candy and ice cream and indulge in other sweets. Joe was confident that blindness, amputation, and kidney failure might happen to other people, but they wouldn't happen to him. This new diagnosis of macular degeneration was a wake up call. His doctor's blunt description of what lay ahead of him hopefully came just at the right time.

Defining the Issues

Several factors contributed to the progression of Joe's health condition, including:

- Resistance to change his lifestyle habits
- Denial of the risks related to the long-term effects of diabetes
- Rationalizing unhealthy behaviors

Patient's Understanding

Faced with the prospect of becoming blind as a result of his macular degeneration, Joe begins to realize that years of denial, resistance, and rationalization have led to his worsened health condition. He begins to realize that years of believing that blindness, amputation, and kidney failure only happened to other people was quickly cut short with this latest diagnosis. Only now Joe begins to understand that the decision before him is a matter of saving his life. Sitting in the doctor's office, he begins the mental exercise of acknowledging the significant lifestyle changes that he must make in order to prevent further progression of his diabetes and prolong his life.

HEALTH BEHAVIOR PERSPECTIVE FOR THE INDIVIDUAL PATIENT

The factors that contributed to Joe's diabetes and the gradual deterioration of his health are largely the result of the behavioral choices that he made in previous years. Common behavioral risk factors associated with diabetes are low physical activity level, poor diet, and obesity. These factors are causes for high blood pressure and high cholesterol, which are also risk factors for diabetes.

Level of Intervention Now

Medical treatment alone will not cure Joe's health problems. What lies ahead for Joe will be a major challenge: he must drastically alter the lifestyle to which he has grown accustomed. The changes that his doctor is urging will require considerable modifications for multiple high risk behaviors. The behavior change approach that he chooses must take into account Joe's readiness for change and should be tailored in a realistic way that encourages Joe to make healthy choices, sustains his motivation, continually assesses his progress, and provides him with feedback and support.

Potential Level Earlier

Joe could have avoided his current state of poor health had he adopted a healthier lifestyle as a young man; however, that retrospection does little for his current state.

PUBLIC HEALTH PERSPECTIVE FOR THE HEALTH OF THE GENERAL POPULATION AND OF HIGH RISK GROUPS

Joe's behavioral risk factors account for the majority of deaths and rising healthcare costs in the United States. Although these preventable risk factors place individuals like Joe at increased risk for death and disability, the encouraging news is that these factors are controllable through behavior change strategies. Local, state, and federal public health initiatives as well as an increasing interest from employers and health insurance companies has led to a greater awareness of the role of health behavior in containing healthcare costs and the need to identify sound and practical behavioral approaches for successful behavior change strategies.

By adopting and encouraging participation in wellness and prevention programs, employers and insurance companies may see a decrease in their healthcare expenditures.

For patients like Joe, their individual healthcare provider can play an important role in motivating individuals to make needed behavior changes. Primary care clinicians are valuable sources of preventive health information. Healthcare providers can assist their patients in adopting and maintaining healthful behaviors by implementing simple behavior change strategies during routine clinical care. The most common interventions that healthcare providers can deliver include counseling on smoking cessation, physical activity programs, and healthy eating.

In 1995, Congress established the Office of Behavioral and Social Sciences Research (OBSSR) as part of the Office of the Director at the National Institutes of Health (NIH), with the mission to stimulate behavioral and social sciences research and to integrate it more fully into the entire NIH research enterprise. The 2007 Strategic Plan entitled *The Contributions of Behavioral and Social Sciences Research to Improving the Health of the Nation: A Prospectus for the Future* is available at http://www.thehillgroup.com/OBSSR_Prospectus.pdf (accessed March 20, 2008). In addition to building stronger partnerships within NIH, OBSSR will address the most important research areas concerning pressing public health problems. OBSSR also will facilitate a common research language and terminology among behavioral and social scientists and with the broader scientific community. For the common research language, NIH uses the term *behavioral* to refer to overt actions; to underlying psychological processes such as cognition, emotion, temperament, and motivation; and to biobehavioral interactions.[11] The term *social* in contrast encompasses sociocultural, socioeconomic, and sociodemographic status; it refers to biosocial interactions and to the various levels of social context from small groups to complex cultural systems and societal influences.[11] Finally, it will encourage the development of new theoretical models, methodologies, and tools necessary to answer the many questions about behavioral determinants of health.

KEY TERMS

Behavioral Terms

Attitudes: Comprised of an individual's behavioral beliefs that performing certain actions will be associated with certain outcomes or attributes and an individual's personal evaluation of the importance or value of those outcomes.

Behavioral Capability: An individual's knowledge of a behavior and the skills required to perform the behavior.

Behavioral Intention: An individual's perception of their likelihood of modifying a certain behavior.

Construct: An explicit idea that is derived for and applied to a specific theory.

Cues to Action: External triggers that stimulate an individual to take action.

Emotional Coping Response: Strategies used by an individual to deal with stimuli.

Environment: Any factor that is physically external to an individual.

Observational Learning: Behavioral learning that occurs by watching the behaviors of others and the outcomes that result from others' actions.

Outcome Expectancy: An individual's belief that a certain behavior or action will produce a certain outcome.

Perceived Barriers: An individual's perception of the negative aspects of the behavior being required to reduce risk.

Perceived Behavioral Control: An individual's perception of their level of control of factors beyond their immediate control.

Perceived Benefits: An individual's perception of the positive aspects of the behavior being required to reduce risk.

Perceived Severity: An individual's perception of the seriousness of a disease and the consequences of having an illness.

Perceived Susceptibility: An individual's perception of the probability that he or she will acquire a disease or become ill.

Reciprocal Determinism: The interaction of an individual's personal factors, actions, and environmental factors that help explain the overall behavior.

Reinforcement: A response to an individual's behavior that increases or decreases the repetition of that behavior.

Self-Efficacy: The confidence that an individual has in his or her ability to successfully carry out a certain behavior in order to produce a desired outcome.

Subjective Norms: An individual's belief about whether other people approve or disapprove of engaging in a certain behavior.

Public Health Term

Healthy People 2010: A U.S. Department of Health and Human Services initiative that provides a framework for prevention of diseases in the United States. It is a statement of national health objectives designed to identify the most significant preventable threats to health and to establish national goals to reduce these threats.

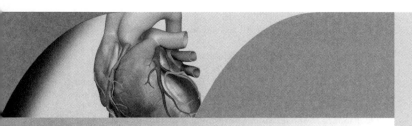

Questions for Further Research, Study, Reflection, and Discussion

For the Individual Student

In order to answer these questions, it may be necessary to research the primary literature.

- Out of the various theories discussed in this chapter, which one(s) do you think offer(s) the most convincing explanation of health-related behaviors?
- How can healthcare providers motivate patients to reduce the risks and harms associated with unhealthy behaviors?
- What are examples of brief interventions that can be integrated into routine primary care visits that can tackle some of the most common risk behaviors?

For Small Group Discussion

- What are the stages of change illustrated in Joe's case?
- How would you rate Joe's level of self-efficacy prior to his diagnosis of macular degeneration? Does his self-efficacy change after his diagnosis?
- What attitudes and social norms influence Joe's behavioral intentions?
- What interventions can Joe adopt based on the health behavior theories or models?

For Entire Class Discussion

- Look at other chapters in the book and consider the role of health behavior in the development and progression of those diseases.
- If modifying a single health behavior can improve the health risks associated with unhealthy behaviors, will intervening on multiple health behaviors have greater potential to increase the impact across different diseases?

EXERCISE/ACTIVITY

- In small groups, students should identify one health behavior that they would like to change (e.g., decreasing alcohol use or increasing daily exercise). Examples of behaviors that may be considered for this activity include, but are not limited to, physical activity, overweight and obesity, smoking, substance abuse, sexual behavior, etc. Students will design a modification plan for the selected behavior based on one of the theories of behavior change. Each group will prepare a five- to ten-page paper and an in-class presentation that includes:

1. A description of the targeted behavior
2. An overview of the selected behavior change theory or model
3. An outline of the goal of the behavior modification plan
4. A description of the application of the key constructs of the theory or model
5. A summary of the pros and cons related to the use of the selected model

Healthy People 2010

*As mentioned above, the initiatives of **Healthy People 2010** have brought considerable attention to the need to target the modifiable behaviors that impact the health and well-being of Americans. The following portions apply to Joe P.*

Indicator: Overweight and Obesity

Focus Area: Nutrition and Overweight

Goal: Promote health and reduce chronic disease associated with diet and weight.

Objectives:

19-1. Increase the proportion of adults who are at a healthy weight

19-2. Reduce the proportion of adults who are obese

REFERENCES

1. Becker MH. Theoretical models of adherence and strategies for improving adherence. In: Shumaker SA (ed). *The Handbook of Health Behavior Change*. New York: Springer Publishing Company;1990:5–43.

2. McGinnis JM, Foege WH. Actual causes of death in the United States. *JAMA* 1993;270:2207–2212.

3. Whitlock EP, Orleans CT, Pender N, Allan J. Evaluating primary care behavioral counseling interventions: an evidence-based approach. *Am J Prev Med* 2002;22:267–284.

4. Noar SM. A health educator's guide to theories of health behaviors. *Int Q Community Health Edu* 2005-2006;24:75-92.

5. Pellmar TC, Brandt EN, Baird MA. Health and behavior: the interplay of biological, behavioral, and social influences: Summary of an Institute of Medicine Report. *Am J Health Promot* 2002;16:206–219.

6. Bandura A. *Social Learning Theory*. Englewood Cliffs, NJ: Prentice-Hall, Inc.; 1977.

7. Bandura A. The self system in reciprocal determinism. *Am Psychologist* 1978;33:344–358.

8. Fishbein M, Ajzen I. *Belief, Attitude, Intention, and Behavior: An Introduction to Theory and Research*. Reading, MA: Addison-Wesley Publishing Company, Inc.; 1975.

9. DiClemente CC, Prochaska JO. Self-change and therapy change of smoking behavior: a comparison of processes of change in cessation and maintenance. *Addict Behav* 1982;7:133–142.

10. Prochaska JO, DiClemente CC. Stages and processes of self-change of smoking: toward an integrative model of change. *J Consult Clin Psychol* 1983;51:390–395.

11. Office of Behavioral and Social Sciences Research National Institutes of Health. BSSR Definition. Available at http://obssr.od.nih.gov/Content/About_OBSSR/BSSR_Definition/. Accessed March 20, 2008.

CROSS REFERENCES

Exercise

Fetal Alcohol Syndrome

Nutrition Transition

Oral Health and Diseases

Pathophysiology of Injury

Smoking

Understanding Nutrition

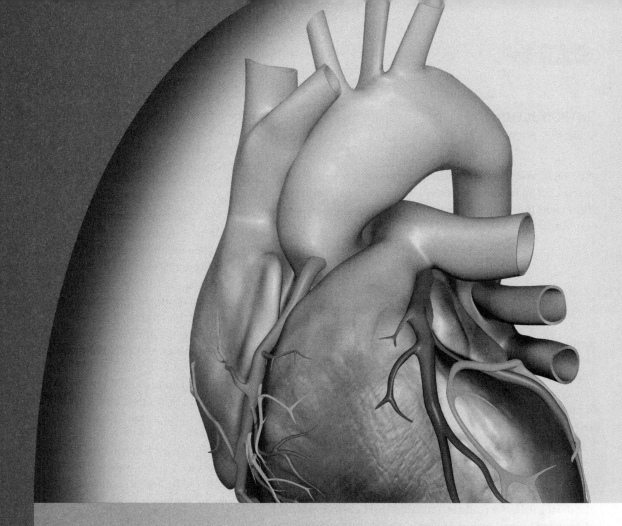

PART II

Using Public Health to Address Behavioral Change

INTRODUCTION
Constance Battle

The social sciences are intrinsically compatible with natural sciences. The two great branches of learning will benefit to the extent that their modes of causal explanation are made consistent.[1]

—EO Wilson

This Part expands upon Chapter 8, which focuses on behavioral determinants of health, by addressing new conceptualizations or models of epidemics that have behavioral and social roots rather than infectious disease causes. These new epidemics result from the consequences of tobacco use, alcohol use, seatbelt neglect, violence, physical inactivity, and poor eating patterns.

McGinnis and Foege in 1993 attempted to identify and quantify the major external (non-genetic) factors that contribute to death in the United States.[2] Their data synthesis demonstrated that the most prominent contributors to mortality in the United States in 1990 were tobacco, diet and activity patterns, alcohol, microbial agents, toxic agents, fire arms, sexual behaviors, motor vehicles, and illicit drug use. Half of the deaths that year could be attributed to these factors, which they called "**actual causes of death**" and described as **modifiable factors**. They made it clear that the public health burden these factors impose is considerable and that doing something about these contributors to death is imperative. An updated review in 2000 concluded that tobacco use, poor diet, and physical inactivity contributed to the largest number of deaths and that deaths due to the latter two factors continue to increase.[3,4] They also noted that behavior changes have led to an increased prevalence of obesity and diabetes.

Three of the chapters (9 to 11) address aspects of the steady and increasing aspects of obesity throughout the U.S. population, particularly among children and youth. The 21st century may turn out to be labeled the century of the obesity epidemic. Obesity is the second leading cause of preventable death after tobacco use. It could be the first condition to shorten the lifespan of children in comparison to that of their parents. Important aspects covered in these chapters, which lay a foundation for students to begin to consider how to develop strategies to prevent or reverse obesity, include dietary recommendations, the consequences of transition from too little to too much food, and the equal importance of exercise and activity to eating properly in order to maintain a healthy weight.

Two chapters address two addictions—Chapter 12 on alcohol and 13 on nicotine—and their long-term consequences. Cigarette smoking causes nearly one out of every five deaths each year and affects nearly every organ of the body. Cancer was among the first diseases causally linked to smoking. The varied and multiple effects of fetal alcohol syndrome last for a lifetime of limitations.

Chapter 14 outlines the importance of the relationship between injury and behavior, noting the point stressed by Henry David Thoreau, that he who receives an injury is to some extent an accomplice of the wrong-doer.

Finally, to a significant extent in some populations, behavior is an important aspect of maintaining oral health, as discussed in Chapter 15.

In summary, behavior and social factors play pivotal roles in illness and health. Behavioral sciences are thus at a crossroads in public health according to Glass and McAtee, who attempt to describe a pathway from the micro biological level to the macro sociological level for greater integration of the natural and behavioral sciences.[5] They propose a model of society-behavior-biology interactions from infancy to old age in this description of their vision of the future of behavioral science. Their envisioning follows their quotation of Wilson's exhortation.

REFERENCES

1. Wilson EO. *Consilience: The Unity of Knowledge*. New York: Alfred A. Knopf; 1998.
2. McGinnis J, Foege M, William H. Actual causes of death in the United States. *JAMA* 1993;270:2207–2212.
3. Mokdad AH, Marks JS, Stroup DF, Gerberding JL. Actual causes of death in the United States, 2000. *JAMA* 2004;291:1238–1245.
4. Mokdad AH, Marks JS, Stroup DF, Gerberding JL. Correction: actual causes of death in the United States, 2000. *JAMA* 2005;293:293.
5. Glass TA, McAtee MJ. Behavioral science at the crossroads in public health: extending horizons, envisioning the future. *Social Sci Med* 2006;62:1650–1671.

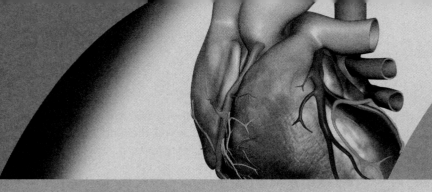

CHAPTER 9

Understanding Nutrition for the Public's Health

Elizabeth Tedrow
Jennifer A. Weber

In 1970, a link was discovered between Vitamin A deficiency and pediatric blindness and mortality, which affects close to 140 million children worldwide. Once Vitamin A supplements were introduced, overall child mortality in the developing world decreased by 34%, and Vitamin A was established as among the most cost-effective of all health interventions.[1,2]

LEARNING OBJECTIVES

By the end of this chapter, the student will be able to:

- Understand the connection between micronutrient intake and overall health status.
- Recognize the complexity and determinants of food choices (the interaction between people, environment, and food).
- Describe different types of nutrient deficiencies, their possible sources, and potential interventions.
- Describe the basic tenets of a healthy diet.
- Detail the methods of tracking the nutritional status of the U.S. population.
- Identify federal food assistance programs.

HISTORY

What we eat no doubt has been the result of our history of food production, food availability, and our cultural preferences. Food and nutrients are such an important part of our daily lives for many reasons, yet we often forget how much our diet can determine our well-being. Our diet has shaped our physical and social bodies and continues to affect our individual and collective health.

Keeping pace with medical advancements is not only relevant to the public health field, it also dictates the course of public health policies and interventions. Public health is a vehicle for practically integrating medicine into public behavior, yet this process is often challenged by the public itself. The following two examples outline how the relationship between medical science and public health efforts have both aided and hindered improvements in the public's health. With *scurvy*, public health suffered from a lack of public support, fueled by the inconsistencies of medical science. In the case of *rickets*, public health and the threat of disease were what demanded such aggressive work toward medical discovery. In both, the role of public health was both proactive and reactive to health discovery and health improvements.

Scurvy: Fruitful Cures Are Not Always Convincing

One of the most curious aspects of scurvy is how close people were to identifying its cure, and how long it took for people to accept what had proved to be true. The use of citrus fruits to cure scurvy was proclaimed as early as 1510, and ships voyaging through South America and India benefited from this "folk" advice. The Dutch East India Company went so far as to plant fruit trees at the Cape of Good Hope, where ships often stopped to reprovision. Yet citrus fruits were never considered legitimate medicine, and more powerful than the successful examples of citrus fruits was the founding medical belief that diseases were caused by the presence of something harmful, not the absence of something beneficial.

In 1617, John Woodall published *The Chirurgeon's Mate*, delineating his experiences as a ship's surgeon, and making a great case for the use of lemons or limes to cure scurvy. Woodall's book made an impact on the medical field but had little effect on public health practice, in particular because sailors were considered so expendable. It was not until 1744, when a British Commodore returned from a voyage with over 1,400 of his 2,000 sailors dead (four from battle, almost all the rest from scurvy) that the British Navy began to formally address the problem of scurvy.[3]

At this time, James Lind, a Scottish surgeon's mate for the Royal Navy, applied this concern for scurvy to the victims themselves. During his voyages, he began an in-depth investigation of scurvy's effects, and eventually experimented with scurvy's remedy. Lind himself was not convinced that scurvy could be completely cured by citrus fruits alone, and in a 1747 voyage, he developed a controlled experiment to provide what he thought would be the necessary data to prove there was more to scurvy than a lack of lemon juice. His experiment was the first controlled clinical trial in history. The results overwhelmingly demonstrated the power of citrus fruits, and Lind published his results in *A Treatise on the Scurvy*. It was Johannes Bachstrom though, who first made the assertion that scurvy's primary cause was a "want" of fresh vegetable matter, in particular citrus fruits.

Despite these valid claims, the debate over scurvy continued and featured such "promising" cures as cheese and honey or soda water. By the 20th century, the medical field still had little reliable understanding of scurvy and its cure. The 1933 *Oxford English Dictionary*, for example, defined scurvy as a disease induced by a "too-liberal diet of salted foods." Vitamin C was finally named in 1930, and shortly after classified as an ascorbic acid, as it was antiscorbutic, or anti-scurvy.[3]

The example of scurvy shows how trying a process it can be to translate medical knowledge into public health practice. Often, scientific knowledge does not fit well within a society's cultural and environmental perspectives, making it challenging for a population to accept.

Rickets: A Deficiency That Led to a Discovery

Assumptions about the cause of rickets have a long history. Despite that they were surprisingly correct, it took significant research from a variety of experiments to garner enough evidence for rickets to be understood as a Vitamin D deficiency that easily could be avoided and cured.

Populations as old as the ancient Egyptians noticed the effects of rickets. After battles, it was found that the skulls of Persians were so thin, they could be cracked when struck with a pebble, yet the skulls of Egyptians required the force of large stones to break. Egyptians attributed their thick craniums to their custom of being bareheaded in the sun, whereas Persians always covered their heads with turbans. Amazingly, the Egyptians were not far off, as rickets is the most noticeable consequence of Vitamin D deficiency, and can be avoided by sufficient exposure to sunlight.

This wisdom of the Egyptians did not survive, however, and rickets remained misunderstood and mistreated. The onset of the industrial revolution in the 19th century led to significant environmental and social changes, and a significant rise in rickets. As families left the outdoor life of farm work to work in factories, and continued to move closer into cities, rickets quickly spiraled into a plague, affecting most of Europe. Before long, rickets was so pervasive that it was nicknamed the "children's disease" in England, as it was so characteristic of children. In 1822, a Polish physician observed that children in Warsaw suffered severely from rickets, yet rickets was unheard of outside the city. He concluded that sunbathing was the cure for rickets, and, in 1882, British scientist T.A. Palm furthered this concept, finding a strong relationship between the geographic distribution of rickets and the amount of sunlight in a region. Although the specific nutrient responsible for rickets had not yet been identified, researchers continued to delve deeper into the pathophysiology of rickets.

By 1913, researchers at the University of Wisconsin had discovered that goats kept indoors without sunlight lost a great deal of skeletal calcium, and following that observation, researchers at Columbia University showed that sunlight cured rickets in children. It was finally Edward Mellanby who isolated and named Vitamin D through his work with rickets. After continued experimentation, the team at the University of Wisconsin developed and patented a process of food irradiation using ultraviolet light, supplementing the lack of Vitamin D that was common in more industrialized lifestyles. Soon after, food irradiation became standard practice for bread and milk products in the United States, effectively curbing Vitamin D deficiencies and rickets.[4]

It is important to maintain a public health perspective and notice what these discoveries can and did imply for the public's health, as well as how changes in public behavior influenced disease. This is perhaps what links nutrition so closely with public health: vitamin deficiencies are defined by their absence in individuals, and **vitamins** themselves are discovered by their deficiencies in populations.

Milestones in American Nutrition

W.O. Atwater, the first director of the U.S. Department of Agriculture's (USDA) Office of Experiment Stations, is considered the father of modern American nutrition. In the 1880s, he started publishing his calculations of the fat, protein, and carbohydrate content of various foods. The early 1900s was a time

TABLE 9-1 History of Nutrition: Efforts of Science and Public Health

Science Discoveries

1743	James Lind discovers that citrus prevents scurvy through his experiments with sailors.
1811	Iodine is discovered.
1864	Louis Pasteur invents concept of pasteurization.
1896	Christian Eijkman reproduces condition of beriberi in chickens, convincing people to stop removing the husks from rice.
1911	The term *vitamins* is coined by Casimir Frank.
1913	Elmer McCollum helps to discover Vitamins A and D, and thiamin, showing the negative effects of their deficiencies.
1918	Pellagra is found to be caused by deficiency from corn-based diet.
1920	Edward Mellanby discovers that rickets is due to a vitamin deficiency.
1930	Robert Williams discovers that it is the thiamin (Vitamin B) in rice husks that leads to the deficiency causing beriberi.
1932	Albert Szent-Gyorgvi discovers that the specific element in citrus fruits responsible for their nutritional benefits is Vitamin C.
1940	Vitamin B_{12} is discovered.
1952	Abram Hoffer starts treating schizophrenia with Vitamin C and B_3, beginning a new paradigm for thinking about vitamins and health.

Public Health Measures

1819	Iodine is used for experiments about goiters in Switzerland, yet the toxic effects of iodine overdosages cause the popularity of iodine to decline.
1826	Railroads are established, increasing the availability of foodstuffs.
1898	School lunches introduced in New York City.
1920	DHHS Children's Bureau begins first series of nutritional studies in U.S. children.
1924	Salt begins to be supplemented with iodine.
1928	The American Institute of Nutrition is formed.
1929	DHHS Children's Bureau publishes first height and weight tables for children six and under.
1939	The Food Stamp program is created.
1941	The National Nutritional Conference for Defense produces structure of dietary allowances that later become the Recommended Dietary Allowances.
1946	The National School lunch program is founded.
1946	Sir Edward Mellanby designs a post-war bread that is laced with iron compounds and B vitamins.
1966	The Child Nutrition Act is passed, expanding food programs for children.
1977	U.S. Senate publishes *Dietary Goals for the United States*.
1979	USDA defined "foods of minimal value" and set nutrition standards for foods to be considered **healthy**; restricted the sale of minimal value foods in school cafeterias.
1990	U.S. Congress passes an act requiring that **Dietary Guidelines** be revised every five years.
1990	U.S. government publishes first set of ideal height and weight tables.
1992	USDA creates first food pyramid.
1994	U.S. Congress passes the Dietary Supplement and Health Education Act, and the USDA and FDA revised regulations on food labeling, requiring all manufacturers to label the nutritional facts on their products.
2002	CDC declares obesity an epidemic in the United States.
2004	CDC declares obesity an epidemic in children as well.
2005	USDA publishes new food pyramid, focusing more intently on food content and portions.

of tremendous growth in nutrition knowledge, when many vitamins and minerals were discovered. The 1960s exposed the existence of **hunger** in America and federal feeding programs were developed in response. In 1980, the government issued the first Dietary Guidelines for Americans (Table 9-1).

Our knowledge of nutrition has greatly expanded since W.O. Atwater's time, but has the nutritional health of our population also improved? We have a country (and increasingly a world) where **overweight** and obesity are on the rise, while at the same time there are people without enough food to eat, and among those consuming enough (or too many) calories, the right proportion of foods are not being consumed, increasing risk of chronic disease.

BASIC SCIENCE FACTS/KEY CONCEPTS REVIEW

What Is Nutrition?

Nutrition is the science that studies the relationship between diet and health. Despite the straightforward definition, maintaining good nutrition is an incredibly complex and multidimensional process. Diet is often simplified to the basic pillars of protein, fat, and carbohydrates, and the necessary combination of calories, but nutrition is the value of foods beyond their caloric worth. Nutrition is the dynamic foundation of our health, requiring a delicate balance of multiple nutritional factors. Although the quantity of calories and proportion of major caloric sources are vital to our health, the nutritional quality of our diet is just as important and influential a factor in our overall well-being.

Even though there are so many processes that influence what we eat, the core purpose of eating is fundamentally to get the nutrients that allow our body to function properly. A nutrient best can be defined by its absence from the diet, so that through the lack of a nutrient, we recognize its necessity. Each nutrient has a specific effect on the body and causes specific changes in bodily processes. Nutrients are therefore very scientific in nature and must make a noticeable difference in the body's performance both when they are absent and when they are present in the diet. In general, the three main functions of nutrients are to: *help with growth and development*; *regulate cell and body processes*; and *provide fuel for metabolic functions*. Most nutrients are needed in relatively small amounts, especially when compared to calorie-based components (proteins, carbohydrates, and lipids); however, the absence of just one nutrient can result in severe health consequences.

Nutrients are classified into six classes: carbohydrates, lipids, proteins, vitamins, minerals, and water. Carbohydrates, lipids, and proteins are the pillars of *diet*, as they are the source of fuel for the body and contribute significantly to the main-

Exhibit 9-1

Six Classes of Nutrients

Macronutrients

Carbohydrates: Carbohydrates are found in grains, vegetables, legumes, and fruits; most carbohydrates are converted into glucose (a simple sugar), and their major function is to provide energy for the body.

Lipids: Lipids are various types of fats or oils, or fatlike substances such as cholesterol (also referred to as triglycerides). They are a major fuel source for the body, but they also help by providing structure to the cells, carrying fat-soluble vitamins, and providing materials to make hormones.

Proteins: Proteins are found in both animal-based and plant-based sources such as meat and beans. Proteins are comprised of amino acids, and the amino acids we get from dietary sources combine with the amino acids already in our body to make hundreds of different body proteins, which build and maintain body structure and regulate body processes.

Micronutrients

Vitamins: Vitamins are primarily responsible for regulating body processes such as energy production, blood clotting, and calcium balance. Vitamins are essential to the health of organs and tissues. There are two main types: fat-soluble (A, D, E, and K) and water-soluble (C and B), which work in very different ways. Each vitamin has a unique dietary source.

Minerals: There are 16 essential minerals in the body, including sodium, chloride, potassium, calcium, and phosphorus. Minerals play both structural and regulatory roles, and the dietary sources for minerals are incredibly diverse.

Water: The simplest and most essential nutrient, water helps with the body's temperature control, the transportation of nutrients and waste throughout the body, and hydration.

tenance of cell tissue and body structure. Vitamins and minerals are the pillars of *nutrition* and are imperative for more subtle cell and body processes. Both of these components—energy and nutrition—require equal consideration and need to be fulfilled through one's diet.

All of the various nutrients have a unique relationship, so that the *diet* is the complex and individualized pattern of how we receive *nutrients*.

Classifying Nutrients

There are several ways to classify nutrients that coincide with their significance in body functioning. Essential nutrients are those that must be present in one's diet because the body in not able to produce any or sufficient amounts of them. Nutrients also can be broken down into **macronutrients** and **micronutrients**: macronutrients are needed in large quantities, like carbohydrates, fats, and proteins; micronutrients are needed in comparatively smaller quantities. In addition, nutrients can be classified by their chemical composition, and separated into organic (containing carbon) and inorganic (carbonless) substances.

For less technical understandings of nutrients, a common way of classifying foods is according to their nutritional value, the perspective from which most people are familiar. Foods are judged by their make-up of calories, fats, protein, and basic nutritional worth, from which they can be tagged as "healthy," "low-fat," or a variety of other lay terms that help describe their appropriate place in the diet. Many foods, however, can be assessed by how functional they are beyond the nature of their macronutrition. **Functional foods** provide nutritional benefits beyond their basic caloric value, often in ways that protect against disease. For example, tomato sauce contains the compound lycopene, which has been found to reduce the risk of prostate cancer; soy protein (found in tofu, among other foods) can reduce the risk of heart disease. The characteristics and compounds attributed to functional foods are not considered nutrients, but instead **phytochemicals**, or naturally occurring plant chemicals. Phytochemicals are not essential to the body, although many are found to promote health (e.g., antioxidants). There are thousands of different kinds of phytochemicals—an orange alone has over 170 separate phytochemicals—and their main purpose is actually to protect the plants themselves from harmful things like bacteria, fungi, or ultraviolet rays. Foods also can "become" functional through fortification processes, such as fortifying salt with iodine.

Foods all have a unique nutritional profile that can be quantified by their **nutrient density**, the amount of nutrients per kilocalorie. An orange, for example, contains the same amount of sugar as a tablespoon of cane sugar or honey, yet the packaging of the orange provides many other nutritional benefits, such as Vitamin C and fiber, thus increasing the orange's nutrient density.

How Does Nutrition Affect the Body?

The elements of nutrition are crucial to the body's health and proper functioning, yet each nutrient has distinctive health properties. To ensure that an individual or a population has sound nutrition, it is important to understand the nuances of each nutrient and its relative deficiency.

Especially with the popularity of multivitamins or vitamins in pill form, it is easy to reduce vitamins themselves to simple additives that food either has or does not contain. The process of actually getting adequate vitamins through nutrition though is more complicated, as each vitamin is found in a unique form. Proteins are a very good example, because protein can be glossed over as a single nutrient in itself, yet each source of protein varies in protein quantity and quality, and proteins themselves can be composed of any combination of amino acids, some of which are and some of which are not essential to the body. Even more, once in the body, these amino acids can be recombined to serve the purposes of our body better. So when evaluating protein in a diet, it is necessary to look at not only how much protein is needed, but also what protein variety is included. Animal proteins tend to build muscle tissue quickly, yet plant proteins build tissue that tends to last longer, and a truly nutritious diet would include a combination of both.

More often than not, the "vitamins" in foods are not actually vitamins in complete form, but **precursor** forms of vitamins. These precursors combine with elements already present in the body to produce the actual vitamin. This process is effective because it allows the body to form vitamins as they are needed, avoiding the **toxicity** that high levels of certain vitamins can cause. However, these precursors are essential for vitamin production, and must be acquired from outside the body.

Understanding the unique profile of each vitamin is not only important for curing its deficiency, but also for the purpose of recognizing nutritional gaps in a diet, and analyzing effective public health solutions. Nutrients can be categorized as vitamins and **minerals**, and of those, they can be further classified as either fat-soluble vitamins and water-soluble vitamins; or major minerals and trace minerals. Although these categories help define their overarching characteristics, every individual nutrient has a distinct purpose, as the following descriptions demonstrate.

Vitamins

Fat Soluble Vitamins

Vitamins are either fat soluble or water soluble, and this determines how they are absorbed and stored within the body. Therefore, fat soluble vitamins are transported and stored with the assistance of fat molecules, allowing the body to build a vitamin reserve supply.

Vitamin A. Vitamin A is incredibly important for vision, protein synthesis within the body, and cell differentiation processes. Although its most noticeable role is in vision (and the most obvious sign of a deficiency), only one-thousandth of the body's Vitamin A supply is used in the retina. More essential to the body's functioning is Vitamin A's role in cell differentiation, where Vitamin A maintains the smooth and protective integrity of the epithelial cells that line all body surfaces both inside and out. A Vitamin A deficiency affects this process significantly, causing epithelial cells to produce a rigid protein called keratin, which is normal for the surface of hair and nails, yet dangerous for the surfaces of the mouth, bladder, reproductive organs, and eyelids.

The liver can build up a storage of enough Vitamin A to sustain bodily processes for up to two years without any outside Vitamin A replenishment, however, after that, a person would suffer fast and severe deficiency complications.

The precursor for Vitamin A is beta-carotene, which by itself is one of the most effective antioxidants, protecting against free radicals that can lead to cancer. Beta-carotene is found in orange fruits and vegetables such as carrots, sweet potatoes, and cantaloupe as well as dark green vegetables like spinach and broccoli. There are also preformed versions of Vitamin A that can be found in many animal-based foods such as liver, fish oil, milk, and eggs. Preformed Vitamin A can take one of three distinct forms, each with a different purpose within the body (while beta-carotene's utilization can be versatile).

Although there are many food sources of Vitamin A, the way that these sources are prepared greatly changes the quality of the Vitamin A within it. Vitamin A is a fat soluble vitamin, so, for example, although milk is a source of Vitamin A, the process of skimming milk and eliminating its fat also eliminates its stock of Vitamin A. Because lower-fat milks are considered healthier, it is common to fortify skim milk with Vitamin A, yet this concept developed only after Vitamin A deficiencies became apparent and were linked to the popular trend of milk skimming.

Vitamin D. Vitamin D is one of the most unique vitamins because the body does not need to consume any outside elements to make it. The liver actually makes the precursor for Vitamin D, and this precursor then travels through the body to the skin's surface, where sunlight works as its second precursor, allowing it to become an active vitamin. However, Vitamin D's second precursor also can be derived from certain foods if enough sunlight is not available (primarily liver and eggs), though it is not as effective. Once Vitamin D is active, it works like a hormone much more than a vitamin, targeting such organs as the intestine, kidneys, bones, and brain. This vitamin helps regulate organ functioning, and even the immune system.

Probably Vitamin D's most important function though is in calcium absorption; calcium cannot be properly handled and used without adequate Vitamin D. Vitamin D helps throughout the entire process of calcium absorption, stimulating calcium absorption from the gastrointestinal (GI) tract, mobilizing calcium from the bones into the bloodstream, and helping the kidneys retain calcium during blood filtering processes.

Because Vitamin D is so critical to calcium absorption, a Vitamin D deficiency inhibits the ability of bones to calcify normally. This leads to weak bones that are unable to support the body's weight and consequently bend or change shape, a disease better known as rickets. Rickets particularly affects children, as their bones are still developing, and results in bowed legs and other bone deformities. Adult rickets (osteomalacia) most often is found in women with low calcium intakes and poor sunlight exposure, who, after repeated childbirths, will deplete their body's store of calcium and begin to develop bowed legs and hunched statures. If low-to-moderate Vitamin D deficiencies persist throughout life, they will greatly increase the risk for osteoporosis in older adults.

Rickets became a major problem in the United States and Western Europe with the rise of industrialization, which brought much of the workforce indoors. Additionally, large factories polluted the skies with smoke and haze, making it even more difficult to get sunlight. Once Vitamin D was discovered, the United States began to fortify milk and bread with Vitamin D, a practice that is still common today. Although rickets is no longer a major threat, certain factors still place many populations at risk for it. For example, those groups with darker skin pigment are not able to absorb as much Vitamin D, and sunscreen also blocks Vitamin D absorption. Vitamin D **supplementation** is recommended for pregnant and breastfeeding mothers as well as infants, because this is a critical period for bone formation. Those infants who are not breastfed and are fed soy or rice milk (or unfortified milk) are at a high risk for vitamin deficiency. Lack of sunlight exposure is the greatest risk factor for Vitamin D deficiencies, yet these factors are also important to consider when addressing a population's Vitamin D levels.

Vitamin E. Vitamin E is a fat soluble vitamin known best as an antioxidant, as it protects against the oxidation of several unhealthy lipids and pollutants. It is particularly effective at reducing the harmful effects of polyunsaturated fatty acids and the harmful oxidation of pollutants inside the lungs. Unlike Vitamins A and D, Vitamin E is not stored in the liver, but instead in body fat tissue. Therefore, virtually every tissue throughout the body has some amount of Vitamin E reserve and consequently antioxidant protection. This is partly why Vitamin E is thought to be so closely associated with aging processes, yet there is no resounding evidence in support of Vitamin E as an anti-aging agent. Along the same lines, Vitamin E is also considered to be helpful at preventing or reducing the severity of chronic degenerative diseases such as heart disease, respiratory infections, and Alzheimer, although its true effectiveness is still unknown.

Because maintaining stores of Vitamin E is so dependant on fat cells, Vitamin E deficiencies often result in various fat malabsorption disorders, such as diseases of the liver, gallbladder, and pancreas. The other most significant Vitamin E deficiency consequence is erythrocyte hemolysis, a hemorrhagic condition specific to red blood cells. Additionally, Vitamin E deficiencies arise when diets are low in healthy fats, which are necessary for the storage of Vitamin E supplies throughout the body.

There are many sources for Vitamin E in various meats, dairy products, nuts, seeds, and vegetable oils. Most people only need a relatively small amount of Vitamin E and can easily acquire it from foods, assuming they do not heavily avoid fat sources (e.g., using low-fat dressings and margarines). Another key factor in Vitamin E supply is food processing. Vitamin E is easily destroyed by heat processing, so highly processed foods lose much of their Vitamin E supply. For example, almonds are considered a high source of Vitamin E, yet roasting almonds reduces their Vitamin E supply by 80 percent.[5] Even storage can cause a significant reduction of Vitamin E. Safflower oil loses half of its Vitamin E supply after three months of storage. It is therefore important to consider not only what kind of food sources people are receiving, but also the quality of these sources with respect to Vitamin E.

Vitamin K. Named after the Danish word "koagulation," Vitamin K has a clearly essential role in blood clotting.[5] Without Vitamin K, people would bleed to death from minor cuts and injuries, or develop severe hemorrhagic disorders. Vitamin K also plays a major role in bone formation, and decreased Vitamin K often leads to increased fractures. The vitamin itself though is very unique, formed from a combination of animal- and plant-based chemical compounds that are synthesized by intestinal bacteria. These compounds can be derived from non-food sources or even produced by the body if need be, and although it is not very effective in the long term, this process can prevent or delay major Vitamin K deficiencies. What more often causes Vitamin K deficiencies are antibiotics that sterilize the intestinal tract and kill those bacteria that *are* necessary to making it. Newborn babies also have sterile intestines and need to receive a dose of Vitamin K to allow their blood to properly coagulate until they start producing bacteria.

Vitamin K is stored in the liver but, unlike other vitamins, it is metabolized quickly and eliminated if not immediately needed, so Vitamin K reserves can be easily lost. The best sources for Vitamin K include cabbage, Brussels sprouts, spinach, and broccoli.

Water Soluble Vitamins

Characteristically, water soluble vitamins are easily absorbed into the bloodstream and eliminated quickly, leaving little risk of vitamin toxicity. However, this makes it necessary to consume them more frequently.

Vitamin C. Vitamin C is an ascorbic acid and functions as an antioxidant in the body. Vitamin C participates in the formation of many vital compounds, including thyroid hormones, neurotransmitters such as serotonin, and parts of DNA molecules. The most important role Vitamin C plays though is in collagen formation. Collagen is a fibrous protein that helps strengthen and support the connective tissues throughout the body, so without Vitamin C, all the structures in our body would deteriorate. Additionally, Vitamin C enhances the body's ability to absorb iron from plant foods, and works as an antihistamine.

In 1970, Linus Pauling made a worthy case of Vitamin C as a protective nutrient against infection. Since then there has been great research on Vitamin C's effectiveness against colds and flus. Although no overwhelming evidence links Vitamin C to cold prevention, it has been somewhat associated with easing symptoms and speeding recovery. Currently, there is growing evidence that Vitamin C may reduce the risk of heart disease and cancer.

The most famous consequence of Vitamin C deficiency is scurvy, a potentially fatal condition where the body loses its ability to synthesize collagen and all the connective tissues begins to break down. Scurvy can develop after only a month without Vitamin C and progresses quickly, yet can be easily reversed with the addition of Vitamin C to the diet. In fact, only 5 milligrams of Vitamin C a day is needed to prevent scurvy. The Vitamin C Recommended Dietary Allowances (RDA) for the United States is about 90 milligrams per day for men and 75 for women; those who are pregnant or regular smokers should increase that by roughly 40 milligrams. What is interesting about Vitamin C though is that the more Vitamin C one consumes, the less efficiently one's body absorbs it. For example, a person who regularly consumes 30 milligrams or less of Vitamin C will absorb and use 100 percent of it, yet a person who regularly consumes 100 milligrams or more will only absorb about 80 percent of it.[5] Excess Vitamin C is excreted daily through the urine, so Vitamin C toxicity is rare, and at worst will result in kidney problems such as kidney stones and digestive disturbances. Almost all fruits and vegetables have some Vitamin C, and many are very **good sources**; the best are citrus fruits, tomatoes, broccoli, strawberries, kiwifruit, peppers, and cabbage. Vitamin C is also very sensitive to heat and oxygen, so any type of processing dramatically reduces the Vitamin C content of foods.

Vitamin B. There are actually eight separate B vitamins, each with distinct characteristics. Overall, B vitamins help enzymes perform thousands of molecular conversions, and aid greatly in protein and DNA synthesis. B vitamins include: thiamin (B_1), riboflavin (B_2), niacin (B_3), pathothenic acid (B_5), pyroxidine (B_6), biotin (B_7), folate (B_9), and cobalamin (B_{12}).

Thiamin (B_1): Thiamin works as a coenzyme, and without it, every cell in the body would not be able to actually use energy. Among many things, thiamin helps break down glucose, make RNA and DNA, and aid in protein synthesis. Thiamin is famous for its deficiency, beriberi, which literally means "I can't, I can't," and was what patients would say to doctors when they suffered the nerve destruction and muscle weakness associated with the disease.[5] Originally discovered in Southeast Asian countries (where beriberi is still common), beriberi developed as a result of the husking and processing of rice. With rice being such a staple item of Asian diets, often because it is the most widely available foodstuff, removing the outer layers (husking) eliminated all the nutrients rice had to offer. Thiamin deficiency symptoms can arise after only ten days without thiamin and are still found in Westernized countries, mainly in those suffering from alcoholism. Developing nations also struggle with thiamin deficiencies, most often among refugee and displaced populations who must survive off basic international aid food products. Pork is one of the best thiamin sources; beans, sunflower seeds, and certain types of fish are also good sources; however, today most Americans get thiamin through enriched grain products such as breads and cereals.

Riboflavin (B_2): Riboflavin functions similarly to thiamin and was originally thought to be the same nutrient. Its primary purpose is to assist in releasing and using energy within cells. Although riboflavin deficiency is officially called ariboflavinosis, a lack of adequate riboflavin actually results in several malfunctions of bodily systems, eventually developing into anemia. Riboflavin deficiencies also disrupt the body's ability to properly metabolize other nutrients. Milk and animal liver are excellent riboflavin sources.

Niacin (B_3): Niacin is necessary for the body to metabolize energy and synthesize fatty acids, and the body can either make niacin from the amino acid tryptophan or obtain it directly from foods. Therefore, recommendations for niacin intake can

include either fully formed niacin or tryptophan sources. Niacin is well-known for its deficiency, pellagra, a disease that results in the "four D's": dermatitis, diarrhea, dementia, and death. The United States experienced a major pellagra epidemic in the early 20th century, when communities in the South relied heavily on corn for their diet. Corn does have niacin, but its niacin is bound to another protein that inhibits its absorption. It has since been discovered that soaking corn in a lime solution releases the niacin, allowing the body to absorb it. Other sources for niacin include meat, poultry, fish, and nuts. Food's niacin content is not affected during heat processing. High doses of niacin can be very toxic, inducing liver damage in just one week of a high dosage regimen.

Pyroxidine (B_6): The B_6 vitamin is involved in protein and amino acid metabolism, particularly when helping the body convert essential amino acids into the nonessential forms. This enables the body to not depend on food sources for all amino acid components. A lack of B_6 can lead to anemia, damage the nervous system, cause depression and confusion, and increase the risk of heart disease. Good sources of B_6 include meats, fish, and poultry as well as bananas and sunflower seeds.

Folate (B_9): Named for its best source, foliage, folate includes several forms, the most stable being folic acid. Folic acid is crucial in preventing birth defects such as spina bifida and neural tube defects and plays a major role in DNA synthesis, cell division, and red blood cell maturation. Folate can also reduce the risk for colon cancer by 75 percent, and breast cancer by 50 percent.[5] Surprisingly, the body absorbs 100 percent of folate from supplements or enriched sources, but only about half of folate from natural food sources. Folate deficiencies are one of the most common micronutrient deficiencies in the United States today. As a result, the U.S. FDA now recommends that folic acid be added to most enriched breads, flour, cornmeal, pastas, and rice products.

Cobalamin (B_{12}): The B_{12} vitamin is essential for the conversion of folate to an active form, so a B_{12} deficiency results in a folate deficiency. B_{12} is also unique because it is not available in any plant source and can only be acquired through manufactured sources. Vitamin B_{12} actually originates from bacteria and can be stored in the liver for years, animal liver (with B_{12} already made) and fortified cereals are the best sources for B_{12}.

Pantothenic Acid (B_5): This B vitamin is used for energy extraction from foods and for building new fatty acids. Panotothenic acid has a very universal role in the body, and therefore can be found in almost every food source, making a pantothenic acid deficiency almost impossible.

Biotin (B₇): Biotin helps with amino acid metabolism and DNA synthesis, yet little is known about biotin beyond these facts. Some sources of biotin include cauliflower, liver, and cheese. Raw eggs contain proteins that actually block biotin absorption (however, cooked eggs do not).

Antioxidants may be the key to preventing cancer. In a 2007 conference of the American Chemical Society, animals whose diets were supplemented with black raspberries showed an 80 percent reduction in colon tumors, and those fed grape seed compounds had a 65 percent reduction in tumors related to skin cancer.[6]

Minerals

Unlike vitamins, minerals are actually elemental atoms or ions rather than compounds. Therefore, minerals are needed in comparatively smaller amounts than vitamins. The body naturally absorbs minerals in small amounts, as it is very difficult to flush out extra minerals. Also, fiber and phytate (a component of whole grains) greatly increase the body's ability to absorb minerals when needed, or eliminate excess minerals when not needed. Minerals can be found in both animal and plant sources; however, mineral content in soil composition significantly affects the amount of minerals that are present in plant sources. Another important attribute of minerals is that they are not affected by heat processing (as are most vitamins).

Minerals are classified by the quantity needed by the body, falling into the category of either *major mineral* or *trace mineral*. The seven *major minerals* are: sodium, potassium, chloride, calcium, phosphorus, magnesium, and sulfur.

Major Minerals

Sodium. Perhaps the most well-known mineral, sodium regulates cellular and total body fluid and maintains blood pressure. Sodium is found in table salt and almost all processed or prepared foods, so it is rare to take in too little sodium. Too much sodium, however, leads to issues of hypertension and is a growing concern particularly in the American diet.

Potassium. Potassium, when coupled with sodium, helps the muscles contract, transmits nerve impulses, and regulates heartbeat. Moderate potassium deficiency increases the risk for hypertension, and severe deficiency levels have dangerous effects on the kidneys and heart (as can extremely high levels of potassium, too). Some good sources of potassium include bananas, lima beans, cantaloupe, apricots, clams, and halibut.

Chloride. Chloride is crucial for transmitting nerve impulses and maintaining acid-base balance throughout the body. It is also is a component of hydrochloric acid, which is needed for digestion. Chloride deficiencies usually arise quickly, for ex-

ample, after extreme or constant vomiting, and can cause potentially fatal irregularities in the heartbeat. The most common source for chloride is table salt.

Calcium. The most abundant mineral in the body, calcium is absolutely necessary for bone formation and also plays roles in muscle contraction and nerve impulse transmission. Adequate calcium intake can help with weight control and cancer risk reduction. Calcium deficiency over time will cause osteoporosis, so calcium is especially important for children, whose bones are still forming. Dairy products are the best source of calcium as well as green vegetables (except spinach, which contains, oxalate, a mineral that prevents its calcium absorption) and sesame seeds. Of all the calcium ingested through the diet, the body only absorbs about 25 percent to 75 percent of it.

Phosphorus. Phosphorus is another necessary element for bone formation and is used during processes of energy extraction from foods. Additionally, phosphorus is one of the building blocks of DNA. Phosphorus is found in many foods, so deficiencies are rare. Some conditions, like kidney disease and overuse of Vitamin D supplements, can lead to a phosphorus deficiency. Over time, prolonged high phosphorus and low calcium intake levels will negatively affect bone health. The best sources for phosphorus include yogurt, sunflower seeds, milk, oysters, and beef.

Magnesium. Magnesium participates in over 300 cellular reactions, helping with protein synthesis, DNA formation, blood clotting, muscle contractions, and adenosine-5-triphosphate (ATP) production. Therefore, a lack of magnesium would basically stop all cellular activity. Magnesium is found in many food sources, even water, yet the body only absorbs about half the magnesium it intakes. Good magnesium sources are sesame seeds, halibut, almonds, cashews, and beans.

Sulfur. Sulfur is actually a component of other vitamins, such as biotin and thiamin, and helps in protein synthesis and liver detoxification processes. Sulfur deficiencies are unheard of.

Trace Minerals

Trace minerals are just as important as major minerals, yet needed in much smaller amounts. Trace minerals include: iron, zinc, iodine, copper, selenium, fluoride, manganese, chromium, and molybdenum.

Iron. Iron's main role is helping to transport oxygen in the blood, yet it is also involved in hundreds of enzyme and metabolism reactions and in brain development. There are several factors that complicate iron absorption into the body. To begin with, the GI tract regulates iron absorption based on the body's need, and its absorption rate ranges from 1 percent to 50 percent of iron ingested. The type of iron acquired from meat sources is significantly more effective than plant-based sources, which is a particular concern for those on plant-based diets. Another difficulty in iron absorption is that calcium, iron, and zinc compete with each other during absorption, and if possible should be staggered throughout meals (e.g., taking calcium supplements apart from meals, or focusing meals on one of the three minerals). Iron is vital for newborns, as inadequate amounts impair their physical and cognitive performance. By far, the best iron sources are clams, oysters, beef liver, shrimp, steak, and lentils, although many cereals are now fortified with iron.

Zinc. Among many things, zinc helps proteins fold and shape properly, regulates gene expression and cell death, and is essential to the immune system. Zinc deficiencies are characteristic of cereal-based diets and lead to increased infections (of all kinds), abnormal growth, and low birth rates. This is why zinc supplementation in developing countries has resulted in an 18 percent reduction in diarrhea diseases and a 41 percent reduction in pneumonia incidence among children.[7] Good sources for zinc include oysters, beef, clams, and lobster.

Iodine. Iodine is essential to thyroid hormones and the thyroid itself. Because the mineral selenium also plays a role in thyroid functions, selenium deficiencies will lead to iodine deficiencies as well. The most famous aspect of iodine deficiencies is the goiter (enlarged thyroid). Iodine deficiencies also have many physiological and developmental effects to both the brain and body, and it is estimated that over two billion people have inadequate iodine intakes. Iodine's best source is the ocean, so iodine can be easily acquired from seafood. Iodine from the ocean also permeates the soil, increasing iodine content in plants. However, the more inland, the less iodine is present in soil. Other environmental factors such as heavy snowfall or glaciations (bringing more freshwater) can dilute iodine contents in soil as well, and the consumption of goitrogens (found in certain foods) can inhibit iodine's effect on the thyroid. Efforts to reduce iodine deficiencies have focused on adding iodine to salt.

Summary of Vitamins and Minerals

Lead poisoning still continues to be a major risk for children in the United States, yet many are unaware of how important good nutrition is at protecting children against lead's ill effects. In addition to their traditional health and developmental benefits, adequate iron, calcium, and Vitamin C intakes help protect against lead absorption in the body.[8]

KEY CONCEPTS FOR PUBLIC HEALTH

Although beneficial to understand how each nutrient works, there are some overarching concepts about nutrients as a whole that can help guide public health practices:

- Each nutrient is unique, can be derived from distinct sources, and is needed in varying amounts.
- The quality of nutrient sources is dramatically altered through food processing.
- Nutrient deficiencies not only have nutrient-specific consequences, but they inhibit other nutrients and affect overall health.
- Many other aspects of our diet affect how we obtain, absorb, and retain nutrients.
- The two most important factors in micronutrient nutrition are *quality* and *diversity* of nutrient sources.

The relationship between nutrition and lifelong health constantly grows tighter as more research continues to show how well nutrition can protect health, and how debilitating poor nutrition can be to the body. Nutrition affects health on multiple levels, through individual and pointed nutritional deficiencies, to hindering the body's overarching ability to recover from disease. It is established that poor nutrition can both lead to and worsen many types of cancers, but it has even been suggested that nutrition has the power to reverse early cancer growth by establishing poor conditions in which cancer cells could grow (or conversely, feeding cancer growth through dietary promoter factors). Unfortunately, there is so much scientific evidence surrounding nutrition that it often nullifies itself, and makes it extremely difficult to decipher the well-supported evidence that can be applied to nutrition practices.

PUBLIC HEALTH PERSPECTIVE FOR THE HEALTH OF THE GENERAL POPULATION AND OF HIGH RISK GROUPS

The pathophysiology of nutrients as well as the history of their discovery and incorporation into our diet demonstrates that nutrition is a complex science that cannot be treated one dimensionally. It is easy to consider nutrition as a unit, yet nutrients themselves are unique and not interchangeable. Each nutrient has a particular purpose and source, so each nutritional deficiency requires a distinct approach. Therefore, assessing and alleviating a population's nutritional issues also necessitates a tailored public health approach.

POPULATIONS AND NUTRITION

Nutritional Health of the U.S. Population

Originally focused primarily on malnutrition and deficiencies, current public health nutrition is now facing the duel,

CASE STUDIES
Nutrition and Latinos

Often one of the challenges in improving health conditions is not the condition itself, but the patient's understanding and perspective of the issue. Different cultural, social, familial, or even personal backgrounds can determine how effectively a patient or population handles its health status. The following two case studies demonstrate how what happens in the patient's environment outside the doctor's office can influence health status as much or even more than the health care they receive inside the office.

Case Study 1: Malena's Environment
Scenario

Malena emigrated from El Salvador to the United States not long before she gave birth to her second child. She moved into an urban neighborhood and worked long hours to support her two-year-old and her newborn boy. Although her neighborhood is home to many Salvadorans, she has no family or close friends from her home community.

Growing up in a farming community in rural El Salvador, Malena was used to limited but fresh foods, and the practice of making meals that her whole community enjoyed together. Now in this crowded neighborhood, Malena can only shop at local bodegas that offer little more than convenience stores, and fresh fruits and vegetables are practically unheard of. Her work schedule also prevents her from cooking the complex fresh meals she knows well, and she has been forced to find more convenient options to feed her children.

Malena continued to increase her hours in order to make her rent payments, and some weeks she could barely afford enough food for her children. She left her children with a good friend and neighbor during the day, and although they were well taken care of, they spent all their days inside, with almost no exercise or sunlight. With her work schedule, Malena could no longer breastfeed her infant, so she started providing regular milk to feed him during the day. Malena was forced to buy cheaper and cheaper foods, and she wondered how different these foods were from the fresh foods she grew up with in El Salvador.

After awhile, Malena began to worry about her youngest child, who seemed to take much longer to sit and crawl than other babies his age. Malena figured it was because she worked too much to give him the attention he needed, but a friend suggested she visit a doctor. Malena has no health insurance, yet there is a local health clinic that Malena was told offered free services for children.

Defining the Issues

During her visit with the doctor, Malena explained how she fed and cared for the baby, and he quickly pointed out that the child was not getting nearly enough nutrition. He explained that imported regular milk, in particular the least expensive brands that were not fortified (U.S. milk is required to be fortified), did not contain all the nutrients babies need, like Vitamin D. The doctor also warned that Malena's other child's weight was in close to the 90th percentile, but that she also showed signs of **malnutrition**. Malena did not really understand what this meant, but did not feel comfortable asking questions. Although Malena's English was decent, she was very unfamiliar with many of the medical terms her doctor used. The doctor ended the session by encouraging her to apply for food stamps, and start incorporating baby formula, fresh vegetables, and vitamin supplements into their diet.

Patient's Understanding

Malena left confused about her children's health. She wasn't familiar with vitamins, and did not understand the difference between breast milk and store-bought milk. She also found it impossible to cook better meals, and fresh foods were inaccessible in many ways. Malena wondered why her doctor sounded concerned about her older child being in the 90th percentile. To her, a chubby (*gordita*) child is a healthy one who will survive anything that comes its way. She was proud her child was in the 90th percentile, as such a high number clearly meant success.

Clinical Perspective

The nutritional issues for Malena and her family are extensive, primarily due to the change in her food quality. Having less fresh foods, in particular fruits and vegetables, means a dramatic reduction in effective nutrient sources of all major nutrients. Specific concerns for Malena's family include Vitamin D deficiency (darker skin pigment and lack of sun exposure), and iron deficiency for her infant (as she has replaced breastfeeding with regular milk; Figure 9-1).

FIGURE 9-1 The Traditional Healthy Latin American Diet Pyramid.

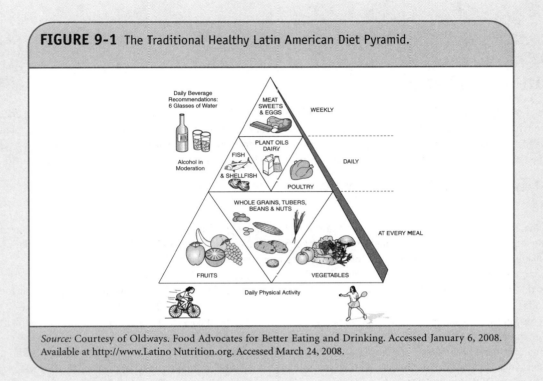

Source: Courtesy of Oldways. Food Advocates for Better Eating and Drinking. Accessed January 6, 2008. Available at http://www.Latino Nutrition.org. Accessed March 24, 2008.

Case Study 2: Cristina: Making Changes Is Hard to Do "Solo"

Scenario

Cristina is sixteen years old and diagnosed with Type 2 diabetes. Her parents emigrated from Mexico before she was born, and much of her extended family lives nearby as well. Although Cristina has not experienced many complications from her diabetes yet, the disease itself is overwhelming for her, making it hard to understand diabetes herself, let alone communicate it to those around her. Her doctor gave her good advice about nutritional changes that can help her control her diabetes, yet the examples he gave just did not fit her family's diet, and Christina does not know how to access many good food sources. Her doctor also tried to assert the importance of vitamins and minerals—macronutrient malnutrition was a culprit of the development of her diabetes—but micronutrient malnutrition will be the cause of the disease's severe morbidity. He said that micronutrients have been proven to reduce infection and absenteeism among diabetes patients; however, all Cristina can think about is how much she fears having her life crippled by this disease. She is embarrassed to be different from her peers and prefers to not think about what might come.

Defining the Issues

Her family normally determines her diet, and although they have traditional Latino foods, they now shop in more mainstream markets and use less traditional cooking methods. Cristina remembers when her grandmother would make her fresh corn tortillas made with whole corn, yet her mom only has time to buy the processed white corn tortillas at Safeway. Their meals include some vegetables, but they are often fried or cooked as part of large dishes and never fresh. Her mom has had a huge impact on her diet behaviors since she was very young. Cristina was always given the same portion sizes as the adults around her, and if she did not finish, her mother worried that she was not eating enough; her mother was very concerned about being a good mother. Being chubby was seen as healthy, and as a result, most of Cristina's family is overweight by her doctor's standards. Yet her family lives by their own standards, and in her community, their higher weight is not perceived as any cause for concern.

   Once she was diagnosed, Cristina tried to understand what a good diet would be, and read about the Food Guide Pyramid. Yet she found it difficult to put the foods she normally ate in those categories. They just did not fit. Cristina tried to share the information her doctor gave her with her family, especially because she knew her whole family was on the same unhealthy track as she, and could benefit from some nutritional changes. She did not want her little brother to get diabetes as well. Food was not just a meal. Often it was an event, and her aunts and cousins were always sharing food with her family, making it impossible for her family to change their ways. It seemed impossible for Cristina to change in this environment by herself.

Patient's Understanding

Cristina's diabetes diagnosis possibly could have been delayed by a healthier lifestyle, and although she visited the doctor at times while growing up, her mother was never able to fully understand the doctor's advice. Additionally, her mother never went to the doctor herself, for to her it seemed selfish when that time and money could be put back into her family. Cristina felt the same way, and avoided going to the doctor as much as she could, at least until she was diagnosed. Even now, she does not really feel "sick," and wonders why she needs to make all this effort.

Mostly though, for Cristina the concept of nutrition was never a part of her life, and now she finds it so difficult to make space for it. Her diet was a factor that led to this disease, but she wants to try to prevent it from getting worse by practicing good nutrition. Her doctor's messages are valid, but they just do not apply to her culture, and Cristina feels like a burden to her family when she tries to ask them to adapt to her disease. Besides, if she is sick, maybe that is just how it is supposed to be, and she should not try to interfere with her fate.

Clinical Perspective

While macronutrient malnutrition plays a bigger role in Cristina's disease, appropriate micronutrient nutrition would have made a significant difference and will be a determining factor in the severity of her disease as it progresses. Diabetes affects major systems within the body, and can impair the digestion, absorption, or storage of vitamins. For example, patients with diabetes tend to have 75 percent less thiamin in their body, leading to vascular complications.

and perhaps conflicting, concerns of overnutrition, chronic disease prevention, and health promotion. The U.S. population could be considered well fed from the perspective that we don't have widespread nutrient deficiency (excluding specific pockets of concern such as iron deficiency in pregnant women), but we also are not consuming dietary patterns associated with prevention of chronic disease. In particular, many Americans consume more calories than they need without meeting recommended intakes for a number of nutrients or food groups.

For example, in 2005 not even one quarter of the adults residing in the United States consumed five or more servings of fruits and vegetables per day.[9] Even those consuming recommended amounts of fruits and vegetables may not be consuming the appropriate types.[10]

Overconsumption is not only a concern of calories. Efforts to reduce heart disease and hypertension have focused on reducing intake of saturated and trans fats and sodium, all nutrients that are consumed in amounts exceeding recommendations by much of the population.

The mean percentage of calories from saturated fat is over 11 percent for all ages of the U.S. population (over 2 months of age). In 1999–2000, 59 percent of the population age 2 years and older reported intakes of more than 10 percent of calories from saturated fat.[11]

The estimated mean trans fatty acid intake for the U.S. population ages 3 years and older is 2.6 percent of total energy intake.[12] For individuals age 20 years and older, the estimated average daily intake of trans fat in the U.S. population is about 5.8 g per day, which represents about 2.6 percent of total energy intake.[10]

The median intakes of sodium among adult men and women age 31 to 50 are 4,300 mg and 2,900 mg of sodium per day, respectively. Approximately 95 percent of adult men and 75 percent of adult women exceed the upper level recommendation of 2,300 mg of sodium per day.[13]

Hunger–Obesity Paradox

Nutrition faces a new challenge: helping people eat more, while eating less. In public health, this dual challenge is especially daunting, often presenting **food insecurity** and obesity in the same population. The hunger–obesity paradox was first raised in the mid 1990s.[14] Numerous articles have been published since that time looking for a link between poverty or food assistance and weight. While there is not a clear consensus, the continued increase in obesity rates, coupled with increasing reports of food insecurity, contribute to a sense of urgency to address both issues. In many cases, the incidence of food insecurity and obesity appears to overlap.[15]

Nutritional Health in Developing Countries

Globally, micronutrient deficiency accounts for 7.3 percent of the total disease burden. The three most common micronutrient deficiencies are iron, Vitamin A, and iodine, together affecting one third of the global population. In terms of Disability Adjusted Life Years (or DALYs) lost, iron deficiencies account for 25 million DALYs lost, and Vitamin A deficiencies for another 18 million DALYs lost.[16] Iron deficiencies are by far the most substantial deficiency experienced, as over 2 billion people are anemic. However, all three deficiencies are pervasive: 46 percent of the African population is anemic, 69 percent of Southeast Asian preschoolers have Vitamin A deficiencies, and 54 percent of Eastern Mediterranean populations have iodine deficiencies.[16] Micronutrient malnutrition is sure to exist wherever there are issues of undernutrition from either food shortages or lack of **diet diversity**, and even diets that are energy-rich can still be micronutrient poor. Of those at risk, young children and women of reproductive age are disproportionately affected by micronutrient malnutrition.

Even moderate levels of micronutrient deficiencies can result in serious and detrimental effects, yet micronutrient malnutrition goes beyond the risk of deficiencies themselves. Micronutrient deficiencies increase the risk and burden of many other diseases, and debilitate the overall health and productivity of a population. Vitamin A deficiency, for example, not only leads to blindness but also increases the risk for severe illness and death. Among Vitamin A-deficient children who become blind, half are expected to die within a year of the onset of their blindness. Conversely, a high dose of Vitamin A supplementation can cure Vitamin A deficiency issues as well as reduce mortality from measles by 50 percent and decreases all-cause mortality by 23 percent.[16] Aside from its direct complications, Vitamin A deficiencies are considered one of the most important predictors of maternal mortality and poor pregnancy outcomes. There is a clear need to reduce the burden of micronutrient malnutrition, for both its direct effects and its influence on a population's total health.

If an individual suffers micronutrient malnutrition, they can receive personalized diet therapy from their healthcare provider, or can utilize resources and social support systems to guide them through appropriate changes. A vegetarian for example, may notice an iron deficiency, and add more iron-rich foods or an iron supplement to their diet. However, when a noticeable segment of a population, or a population as a whole, suffers micronutrient deficiencies, this may signify that they lack the knowledge or resources to reverse the deficiency's effects, and that public health measures are needed.

Exhibit 9-2

Critical Influences on Food Choices

Whether nutritional deficiencies occur on an individual or community level, treating nutritional deficiencies must begin with a thorough assessment of what factors are influencing food choices. Each person's nutrition develops through an incredibly complex and nuanced process, so that there are multiple factors that work to structure how people practice nutrition on individual, social, and global levels.

- *Environment:* What foods can a community produce, how can they produce it, what foods are convenient to a community, are able to be stored well, and are cost-effective or affordable?
  - **Bioavailability:** Bioavailability describes the quantity of vitamins provided by the food itself, and the amount of vitamins absorbed and used by the body. In general, the body is not able to process the total amount of nutrients available in a food, and may require more of a food to meet their nutritional needs, especially if they suffer concurring health issues.
- *Society:* What is accepted "cuisine," what are the traditional folk remedies and nutritional beliefs, what does a community consider appropriate nutrition, and what type of nutritional messages are advertised or target the community?
  - Many cultures have forms of cultural bias that affect their food distribution, such as allowing only men to have meat. The fact that lower classes were historically not often able to afford meat is what has led the Western diet to become so meat-focused.
- *Family/relationships:* Family has a great influence on nutrition by developing one's "system" of choosing foods. Additionally, family events and interactions with people influence what food one chooses, how one combines foods to build meals, the timing of meals, and acceptable foods.
- *Personal factors:* Time, mood, daily influences, personal preferences, etc., all play a role in food choices.

Just like most other diseases, there are epidemiological methods for detecting and monitoring nutritional deficiencies. Nutritional deficiencies have direct and noticeable health consequences, and the more severe the deficiencies are, the easier it is to record and quantify their extent within a population. Epidemiological measures such as the prevalence and incidence of a nutritional deficiency help provide insight to the scope of the problem and the appropriate level of action needed and can be used to assess improvements throughout the course of public health interventions. Some countries maintain national-level assessments of their population's nutritional status, often based on surveys of food consumption patterns. However, it can be expected that the countries that have the least **nutritional monitoring** suffer the greatest nutritional complications.

Although some nutritional deficiencies have relatively obvious markers (i.e., blindness for Vitamin A), others are not so easily distinguishable, and may often include the effects of several deficiencies simultaneously. In addition to the development of clear deficiency signs, micronutrient deficiencies also impact the overall health of a population, resulting in higher infection prevalence and greater (unnecessary) disease morbidity and mortality. Not surprisingly, when one nutrient deficiency takes a significant toll, there is a high probability others will be present as well.

Nutritional deficiencies can be detected through a variety of routes, ranging from reported food consumption surveys to blood serum level testing, all of which can provide an epidemiological representation of nutritional status. The strength of the assessment method should depend on the characteristics of the population and the state of their nutritional deficiencies. Blood serum testing, for example, is extremely important when designing a **fortification** plan, yet food consumption surveys would be instrumental in crafting food policy changes.

PUBLIC HEALTH INTERVENTIONS

Successful public health interventions must be uniquely tailored to the population and problem, yet there are several major intervention structures that nutritional deficiencies utilize. Key nutritional interventions include: **supplementation, fortification, education,** and **structural changes**.

In order to design a successful public health intervention, one must first assess the nature of the disorder; any possible social, cultural, and environmental factors that are causing it (i.e., diet traditions and patterns, farming limitations, and social hierarchy systems); and which of those can be realistically changed. Then, based on the immediacy of the problem, one can develop an intervention plan that leverages the resources of the community environment. Finally, the intervention should include both 1) direct action that alleviates the burden of the problem now and 2) long-term planning that prevents the problem's reoccurrence in the future.

Probably the most crucial aspects of intervention planning are understanding the root of the problem and communicating effectively with the population involved. A population may be experiencing micronutrient malnutrition not because they fail to consume adequate nutrients, but because they are suffering from major diseases, such as parasite infections or HIV/AIDS, that greatly inhibit their body's ability to absorb and maintain nutrient supplies. Or perhaps they are consuming sufficient sources of Vitamin A, but severely lack sources of fat or oil, which are necessary to process fat-soluble vitamins, so their Vitamin A intake is rendered almost useless. Therefore, a successful intervention would address their immediate needs through direct supplementation, yet also work to reduce their disease burden in the future. Effective communication is critical both for guaranteeing that the population participates in the intervention efforts and that they are educated to continue to recognize and prevent this nutrient deficiency after the intervention is over (Figure 9-2).

Up until the 1980s, efforts to alleviate undernutrition in developing countries were only focused on protein-energy malnutrition. Since then, the focus of nutritional remedying efforts has developed to target specific micronutrient deficiencies. In addition, the severity of micronutrient malnutrition has been brought to a global stage, allowing key industry partnerships to assist in the efforts and build resources such as the provision of salt, fortified foods, or supplementations.

Supplementation

Micronutrient supplementation is a direct dosage of a nutrient, often given in the form of a vaccine or pill, but separately from food. Much like commercial supplements such as multivitamins, supplements are designed to target a specific micronutrient deficiency quickly and effectively. The vitamin supplements we find commonly are intended to provide a day's or week's worth of a nutrient, so as not to induce toxicity. Supplementation for public health interventions, especially those in vaccine form, are designed to deliver a nutrient supply that will last months to a year. Vitamin A vaccines for example, only need to be administered two to three times a year, making it simple for a population to receive all the Vitamin A they need regardless of their diet. The body is able to store high dosages of Vitamin A because it is a fat-soluble vitamin; water-soluble vitamins, however, cannot remain in the body for long periods of time and require more frequent supplementation.

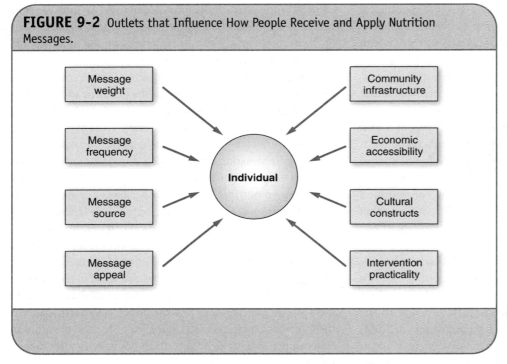

FIGURE 9-2 Outlets that Influence How People Receive and Apply Nutrition Messages.

Message weight

Message frequency

Message source

Message appeal

Individual

Community infrastructure

Economic accessibility

Cultural constructs

Intervention practicality

Supplementation interventions offer immediate and powerful results, and are especially beneficial because they can be closely controlled and monitored, ensuring that specific population segments receive appropriate nutrient levels. However, supplementation is neither cost-effective (compared to other interventions) nor sustainable, making supplementation effective for an initial reduction in deficiency burden, but not a solution to deficiency problems. Once a micronutrient deficiency is stabilized through supplementation measures, a fortification intervention can lead to more sustainable results.

Fortification

Fortification is the deliberate addition of one or more micronutrients to a particular food, so as to increase the consumption of these nutrients and correct or prevent a related deficiency. Fortification efforts can either be mass, reaching the general population, or targeted, reaching specific subgroups. The breadth of a fortification effort hinges upon what particular food is fortified. Especially with respect to cultural habits, women, men, and children may all have selective access to foodstuffs, so it is necessary to fortify the food that is regularly accessed by the targeted subgroup. The selected fortified food also must be an item that is staple to the population's diet and consumed consistently. Some nutrients are needed daily while others less often, so food fortification efforts must choose a food that a population consumes at a level that

will complement their need for that particular nutrient.

Iron is a common nutrient used in fortification interventions: in the United States, breads and cereals are often fortified with iron; in Vietnam, fish sauce is fortified with iron; in China, soy sauce is fortified with iron; and in South Africa, curry powder is fortified with iron.[16]

Education

No intervention will be effective unless the community understands and supports its purpose. Not only is education an essential part of *any* nutrition intervention, as the population must be aware of it in order to participate in it properly, education itself can be a significant aid in improving a population's nutritional perspectives and habits. The goal of any education intervention is to unify and redirect a group's efforts toward healthier behaviors and the knowledge behind them.

Education can take on many unique forms, including patient or service provider training, structured educational work-

Exhibit 9-3

Sugar Fortification in Central America

The practice of fortifying sugar with Vitamin A began in Guatemala in the 1970s and was so successful that the Guatemalan government made it mandatory by 1974. Other Central American countries soon followed suit. Now the practice has evolved to doubly fortify sugar with both Vitamin A and iron, and sometimes even zinc. Regular fortification practice, along with routine testing and responsive one-time supplementation if needed, ensures that children and communities avoid the consequences of Vitamin A deficiencies. These practices still continue in Central America and Brazil as well as parts of Africa.[17]

shops for individuals or groups, or broader educational campaigns. All education efforts, whether they are a component of a larger intervention or the intervention itself, must use the communication channels most popular among the target audience. Interpersonal communication means may be the best method for one group, whereas others may rely on technologically advanced mediums such as social networking sites and mobile devices.

Structural Changes

Although fortification interventions are relatively sustainable and certainly effective, the most desirable intervention would be to facilitate access to greater **diet diversity**, so as to eliminate the possibility of micronutrient deficiency in the future. Establishing long-term structural changes to food availability and diet diversity can take many forms, yet can often be a challenging and time-consuming endeavor. Some examples of **structural changes** include:

- Modifying farming habits to increase the diversity of crops grown
- Developing public policy to increase nutritional resources and practices (e.g., modifying school lunch options or food stamp programs)
- Increasing the availability of outside foods (building grocery stores in communities that only have small convenience stores, or improving local trade opportunities between communities)
- Working with a population to change traditional social practices (i.e., a diet that favors men, traditional cultural beliefs about nutrition for pregnant and nursing women, or the role that local doctors play in nutrition education)
- Breeding and genetic modification of plants to improve their nutrient content (**biofortification**)

There is a very broad range of possible structural changes, and they depend on the nature of the nutrient deficiency and the population's environment. Some populations may need the involvement of government policies to make sustainable changes, while others will be completely reliant on the capabilities of their small community. No matter what approach, structural approaches involve working with community stakeholders to develop the practices that will best maintain positive results for the public's health and give sustainable structure to guide the public toward long-term health outcomes. Structural changes are the key to making a lasting impression on the public's health and interweave the responsibility of maintaining nutrition practices within the community—

ideally at multiple levels—so that these practices remain a constant element of a community's lifestyle. In order to be successful, structural changes must incorporate the characteristics of the community into its foundation and design.

Micronutrient **supplementation** provides the fastest improvements; food **fortification** offers a less immediate but more sustainable impact; increasing **diet diversity** is the most desirable option, being the most natural and sustainable, but requires the most effort to implement.

PUBLIC HEALTH POLICY

Public health policy has and continues to shape nutrition standards and behaviors in the United States, forming the long-term structures needed to address nutrition issues throughout the population. Nutrition policy has developed around the population's nutritional needs, often arising from specific nutritional deficiencies, but also created to address and prevent more general nutritional concerns. Overall, public health policy has helped us better *define, assess,* and *access* nutrition information and services.

Define

Dietary Guidelines for Americans

Long before the discovery of vitamins and minerals, the U.S. Department of Agriculture (USDA) published its first dietary recommendations in 1894. In 1916, the first food guide, "Food For Young Children," was published. Its author, USDA nutritionist Caroline Hunt, divided food into five groups: milk and meat, cereals, vegetables and fruits, fats and fatty foods, and sugars and sugary foods. The current Dietary Guidelines provide science-based advice to promote health and to reduce risk for chronic diseases through diet and physical activity. The recommendations apply to the general U.S. public over two years of age.

By law, the Dietary Guidelines are reviewed and published every five years by the Department of Health and Human Services and the Department of Agriculture and form the basis of federal food, nutrition education, and information programs.[18] Development of the 2005 version included a scientific review by an external scientific Advisory Committee that served as the basis for the government's science-based key recommendations. Consumer messages were then developed for the general public. The Dietary Guidelines Advisory Committee relied on published human studies and the Dietary Reference Intake reports prepared by the Institute of Medicine.

The 2005 *Dietary Guidelines for Americans* were extensive in scope providing 41 key recommendations: 23 for the general public and 18 for special populations. These recommendations are grouped into nine general topics: Adequate Nutrients within Calorie Needs; Weight Management; Physical Activity; Food Groups to Encourage; Fats; Carbohydrates; Sodium and Potassium; Alcoholic Beverages; and Food Safety (side bar of key recommendations). These recommendations not only provide a strong scientific basis for what constitutes a healthy diet, but also highlight that most Americans need to make major changes in current intake to meet recommendations.

Current law requires the government to reissue the *Dietary Guidelines for Americans* every five years. The next issue is expected in 2010.

To help translate the extensive information in the Dietary Guidelines to the public, the federal government has numerous resources to assist consumers. The primary resource for consumers is a brochure, "Finding Your Way to a Healthier You: Based on the Dietary Guidelines for Americans,"[19] which summarizes the intent of the Dietary Guidelines into three key points:

1. Make smart choices from every food group.
2. Mix up your choices within each food group.
3. Find your balance between food and physical activity.

It also describes a healthy diet as one that:

- Emphasizes fruits, vegetables, whole grains, and fat-free or low-fat milk and milk products.
- Includes lean meats, poultry, fish, beans, eggs, and nuts.
- Is low in saturated fats, trans fats, cholesterol, salt (sodium), and added sugars.

Additional Dietary Guidelines resources available to help translate and implement the recommendations include a toolkit for health professionals, a consumer book, and Spanish materials. The resources are available on the Internet (http://www.healthierus.gov/dietaryguidelines. Accessed March 23, 2008).

Translating the Dietary Guidelines recommendations into actual practice can be daunting for even the most knowledgeable consumer. To assist, public health experts often turn to food-based dietary guidance, which essentially translates the recommendations into amounts of food to consume in a day. The U.S. Dietary Guidelines identifies two food-based systems that can help consumers meet recommendations: USDA's MyPyramid and the Department of Health and Human Services' (DHHS) **DASH diet**.

Regardless of the plan used, most Americans need to significantly change their eating style to reduce their intake of salt, fats and sugars, and increasing fruits, vegetables, whole grains, and low-fat milk. Both the reducing intake and increasing intake parts of this equation are important and concur-

rent as these foods should be replacing the low-nutrition, high-calorie foods that form the basis of many Americans diets.

MyPyramid

USDA's food guide pyramid was first unveiled in 1992. Although numerous USDA food plans preceded this program, the pyramid is considered by many to be the face of federal nutrition guidance and the 1992 version gained widespread recognition. The pyramid received a facelift—both in the underlying science and in the graphic—in 2005. This update was intended to reflect the new science presented in the Dietary Reference Intakes and *2005 Dietary Guidelines for Americans* as well as improve the effectiveness of the pyramid with consumers.

> **Dietary Reference Intakes**
>
> The Dietary Reference Intakes (DRIs) are a set of values that serve as standards for nutrient intakes for healthy persons in the United States and Canada. The DRIs, along with additional research on diet and chronic disease development, serve as the basis for the Dietary Guidelines for Americans.

The new version, called MyPyramid (Figure 9-3), is intended to offer a personalized eating plan based on age, sex, height, weight, and level of physical activity.

The messages of MyPyramid mirror those of the *Dietary Guidelines for Americans*:

- Make smart choices from every food group.
- Find your balance between food and physical activity.
- Get the most nutrition out of your calories.
- Stay within your daily calorie needs.

MyPyramid provides a plan based on food groups (grains, fruits, vegetables, milk, meat and beans, oils) and **discretionary calories**. The food intake patterns are designed to meet the Dietary Guidelines and nutrient needs, but also take into account current consumption patterns. A sample MyPyramid meal plan for a 2,000-calorie diet would include: 2 cups of fruits, 2.5 cups of vegetables, 6 ounce equivalents of grains, 5.5 ounce equivalents of meats/beans, 3 cups milk, 6 tsp oil, and a discretionary calorie allowance of about 265 calories.

Key messages align with each food group to offer additional guidance on healthy food choices. These messages include:

- Make half your grains whole
- Vary your veggies
- Focus on fruit
- Get your calcium-rich foods

FIGURE 9-3 MyPyramid.

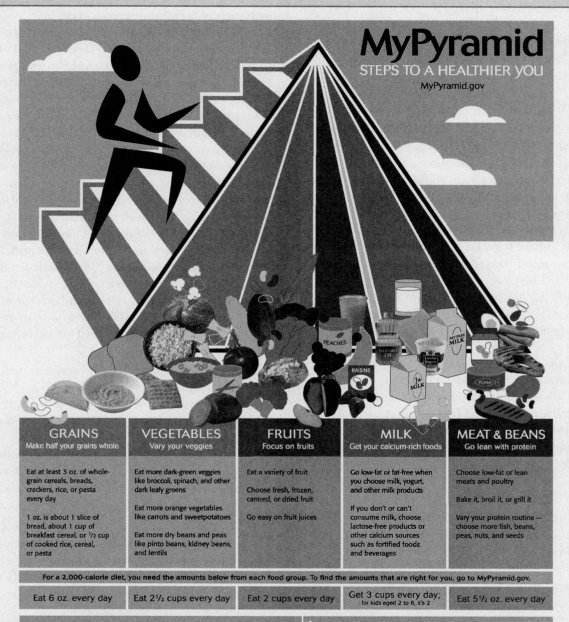

Source: Courtesy of the United States Department of Agriculture. Available at http://www.mypyramid.gov/. Accessed March 24, 2008.

- Go lean with protein
- Find your balance between food and physical activity

By entering all foods eaten and physical activity performed, consumers can get a comparison of their current eating and physical activity habits to the recommendations of the *Dietary Guidelines for Americans* (http://www.mypyramidtracker.gov. Accessed March 23, 2008).

DASH Diet

The DASH diet is based on a clinical study that tested the effects of nutrients in food on blood pressure. Study results indicated that elevated blood pressures were reduced with an eating plan that emphasizes fruits, vegetables, and low-fat dairy foods and is low in saturated fat, total fat, and cholesterol. The DASH eating plan includes whole grains, poultry, fish, and nuts and has reduced amounts of fats, red meats, sweets, added sugars, and sugared beverages compared to the typical U.S. diet. All recommendations are consistent with the *2005 Dietary Guidelines for Americans*.

A sample 2,000-calorie meal plan for a DASH diet would include six to eight servings of grains, four to five servings of vegetables, four to five servings of fruits, two to three servings of fat-free or low-fat milk and milk products, 6 ounces or less lean meats, poultry, and fish, four to five servings per week of nuts, seeds, and legumes, two to three tsp per day of fats and oils, and five or less servings per week of sweets and added sugars.

Both the MyPyramid and DASH eating plans require additional information to the amounts. For example, whole grains should be at least half of grain intake and that a variety of vegetables should be consumed.

Food Labeling

Although the USDA's dietary guidelines have helped the public frame their perspective of a good diet, it became clear that information on individual food products was needed in order for Americans to make healthy decisions. Therefore, in 1990, the U.S. Congress enacted the Nutrition Labeling and Education Act, which required all food manufacturers to provide nutrition information on their product packaging. In accordance with the Act, most packaged foods are required to carry a nutrition facts label and ingredient list. Under the label's "Nutrition Facts" panel, manufacturers are required to provide information on total calories, calories from fat, total fat, saturated fat, trans fat, cholesterol, sodium, total carbohydrate, dietary fiber, sugars, protein, Vitamins A and D, calcium, and iron. These nutrients are required because they are considered to be related to major health concerns of Americans and are both nutrients to decrease (i.e., saturated fat and cholesterol) and those to consume

(Vitamins A and D, calcium, and iron). All information in the nutrition facts label is based on one serving. To use the information accurately, it is necessary to look at the serving size and assess the number of servings consumed.

All nutrients must be declared by amount (grams or milligrams) and as percentages of the Daily Values (DV). The DV is a label reference value, and declaring nutrients as a percentage of the DV is intended to prevent misinterpretations that arise with quantitative values. For example, a food with 140 milligrams (mg) of sodium could be mistaken by a consumer as a high-sodium food because 140 is a relatively large number when it actually represents less than 6 percent of the Daily Value for sodium. On the other hand, a food with 5 g of saturated fat could be construed as being low in that nutrient when it provides one-fourth the total Daily Value for saturated fat. To help consumers use the DV, which has proven difficult to interpret, FDA is encouraging consumers to use the 5/20 rule: 5 percent DV or less is low, 20 percent DV or more is high. The Daily Value percentages are based on a 2,000-calorie diet. This is not a recommendation, but rather a reference value (Figure 9-4).

Additionally, this policy set standards for nutritional claims such as "light," "high-fiber," and "low-fat," so that each claim had valid criteria it was required to meet before products could use them. For example:

- *Low-fat* foods cannot contain more than three grams of fat per serving.
- *Good source* indicates that a food provides 10 percent to 19 percent of the Daily Value of a given nutrient per serving.
- *Healthy* implies that a food is low in fat, saturated fat, sodium, and cholesterol and contains at least 10 percent of the Daily Value for some of the following nutrients: Vitamins A and C, iron, calcium, fiber, or protein[20]

As a result of these policies, the American public has developed a reliable system for defining nutrition and understanding the nutritional value of the foods they select. Now, nutritional content is the second most influential factor affecting people's food choices. Nutritional labeling has greatly aided the availability of nutrition information and education, yet the public must still make the appropriate food choices. Requirements for making nutritional information more public have recently expanded into fast-food and restaurant markets for this purpose.

WHERE DOES PHYSICAL ACTIVITY FIT IN?

The increase in overweight and obesity has initially linked diet and physical activity, and certainly improving health and preventing disease

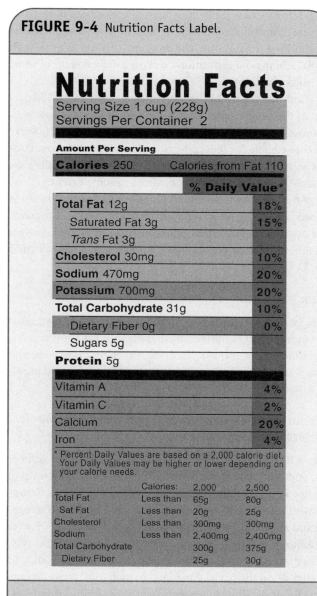

FIGURE 9-4 Nutrition Facts Label.

Nutrition Facts

Serving Size 1 cup (228g)
Servings Per Container 2

Amount Per Serving

Calories 250	Calories from Fat 110

	% Daily Value*
Total Fat 12g	18%
Saturated Fat 3g	15%
Trans Fat 3g	
Cholesterol 30mg	10%
Sodium 470mg	20%
Potassium 700mg	20%
Total Carbohydrate 31g	10%
Dietary Fiber 0g	0%
Sugars 5g	
Protein 5g	

Vitamin A	4%
Vitamin C	2%
Calcium	20%
Iron	4%

* Percent Daily Values are based on a 2,000 calorie diet. Your Daily Values may be higher or lower depending on your calorie needs.

		Calories:	2,000	2,500
Total Fat	Less than		65g	80g
Sat Fat	Less than		20g	25g
Cholesterol	Less than		300mg	300mg
Sodium	Less than		2,400mg	2,400mg
Total Carbohydrate			300g	375g
Dietary Fiber			25g	30g

Courtesy of CFSAN/Office of Nutritional Products, Labeling, and Dietary Supplements. Food and Drug Administration. Available at http://www.cfsan. fda.gov/~dms/label—dl.html. Accessed March 24, 2008.

are about both. Messages to control weight focus on finding the balance between food intake and physical activity. Additional information on health benefits of physical activity is available in Chapter 11, by Wayne Miller.

Assess

To best respond to the public's nutritional needs, there needs to be policy that helps policymakers themselves better assess and track trends in the public's nutritional health.

The **National Nutrition Monitoring and Related Research Act of 1990** is one such policy and requires that the *United States Dietary Guidelines for Americans* be reissued every five years. By taking into account the most recent scientific research and adjusting for current diet trends in the population, continuously revised guidelines can more effectively assess and respond to the public's nutritional status.

Nutritional guidelines and goals mean little if we can't measure if there is an impact on health. **Healthy People 2010** provides this framework by identifying national health objectives addressing the most significant preventable threats to health and then establishing national goals to reduce these threats.

Healthy People 2010 is utilized by federal, state, and local governments, communities, professional organizations, and others to help them develop programs to improve health and measure progress.

The Healthy People 2010 highlights the many factors that serve as markers for nutritional status, including weight status and growth, food and nutrient consumption, iron deficiency and anemia, schools, worksites and nutrition counseling, and food security in a section entitled Nutrition and Overweight.

Healthy People helps set objectives and measure progress, but we need data to actually measure progress. How do we know what people are eating and drinking? A vital resource for public health nutrition is the nation's national nutrition monitoring system. Comprised of the **National Health and Nutrition Examination Survey** (**NHANES**) and "What We Eat in America," the national nutrition monitoring system provides data on food consumption patterns and is the basis for many studies examining associations between food intake and weight. Knowing what Americans eat and how their diets affect health provides valuable information to direct health professionals as well as policymakers on food and dietary guidance, food safety, food labeling, and food assistance.

Comprised of in-person interviews and examinations, NHANES provides the best and most accurate information on what people are consuming and their health status. "What We Eat in America" (WWEIA) is the dietary intake interview component of NHANES and includes two days of 24-hour recall data.

The extent of the NHANES data collection limits the sample size. To complement NHANES, additional surveys are utilized to provide information on weight and food intake. The **Behavioral Risk Factor Surveillance System** (BRFSS) is the world's largest, ongoing telephone health survey system, tracking health conditions and risk behaviors. BRFSS is conducted by the state health departments, providing information at the state and local level.

National height and weight tables are another indicator that establishes benchmarks for the public's health and give individuals and health stakeholders a valid representation of how healthy the public really is. Height and weight tables have particular significance for nutrition's role in child development and alert health professionals to a variety of nutritional deficiencies.

Access

Raising awareness about good nutrition indeed leads the public to make more educated nutritional choices, yet in order to ensure that they can maintain good nutrition, it is necessary to ensure they have access to the healthy foods they need.

A key component of the federal government's efforts to address hunger and nutrition are food assistance programs. Nearly 1 in 6 Americans is served by 1 or more of the 15 domestic food assistance programs administered by the USDA at some point during the year. Additional Americans are served by other federal food programs.

Food Stamp Programs

The Food Stamp Program serves low-income individuals and families by providing funds to buy food. It enables low-income families to buy food with Electronic Benefits Transfer (EBT) cards in authorized retail food stores. Many states also provide nutrition education to participants. In 2005, almost 26 million people living in over 11 million households received food stamps in the United States each month. Of those, over half were children and almost 10 percent were age 60 or older. Many food stamp participants are working, with 40 percent living in a household with earnings. The average food stamp household received a monthly benefit of $209 in 2005. The minimum benefit, received by 5 percent of participants, is $10 per month.[21] To be eligible, net income must be below 100 percent of the federal poverty level and additional requirements must be met for assets and work requirements.

School Meals

The School Meals Program provides breakfast, lunch, and after-school snacks to children. The National School Lunch Program operates in over 100,000 public and non-profit private schools and residential child care institutions providing nutritionally balanced lunches to more than 29 million children each school day. Schools that participate in the lunch program get cash subsidies and donated commodities from the USDA for each meal they serve. In return, they must serve lunches that meet Federal requirements, and they must offer free or reduced-price lunches to eligible children. The School Breakfast Program (SBP) provides cash assistance to states to operate nonprofit breakfast programs in schools and residential childcare institutions. The program operates in more than 72,000 schools and institutions, serving a daily average of some 8.4 million children.

Children from families with incomes at or below 130 percent of the poverty level are eligible for free meals. Those with incomes between 130 percent and 185 percent of the poverty level are eligible for reduced-price meals. Children from families with incomes over 185 percent of poverty pay a full price, though their meals are still subsidized to some extent.

After school snacks are provided to children on the same income eligibility basis as school meals. However, programs that operate in areas where at least 50 percent of students are eligible for free or reduced-price meals may serve all their snacks for free.

Team Nutrition

This is a USDA initiative to support the meal programs through training and technical assistance for food service, nutrition education for children and their caregivers, and school and community support for healthy eating and physical activity.

Special Supplemental Nutrition Program for Women, Infants, and Children (WIC)

The WIC program serves low-income pregnant, breastfeeding, and postpartum women, and infants and children up to age five who are at nutritional risks by providing foods to supplement diets, nutrition education and counseling, and screening and referrals to healthcare and social services. In 2005, over 8 million participants were served by WIC each month. WIC services 45 percent of all infants born in the United States. To be eligible on the basis of income, participants' gross income must fall at or below 185 percent of the federal poverty level.

The WIC food package, which remained virtually unchanged over the last 30 years, is about to receive an overhaul. USDA has proposed changes to the food package that include the addition of whole grains, milk alternatives, and cash vouchers for fruits and vegetables.

Child and Adult Care Food Program (CACFP)

The CACFP provides meals to low-income children and adults who receive daycare outside of their home. Each day, 2.9 million children receive nutritious meals and snacks through CACFP. The program also provides meals and snacks to 86,000 adults who receive care in nonresidential adult day care centers. CACFP reaches even further to provide meals to children residing in emergency shelters, and snacks and suppers to youths participating in eligible after school care programs.

Elderly Nutrition Programs

Operated by the Administration on Aging, the Elderly Nutrition Program provides for congregate and home-delivered meals. These meals and other nutrition services are provided in a variety of settings, such as senior centers, schools, and in individual homes. Meals must meet nutrition standards. The Elderly Nutrition Program also provides a range of related services, by some of the aging network's estimated 4,000 nutrition service providers, including nutrition screening, assessment, education, and counseling. These services help older participants to identify their general and special nutrition needs, as they may relate to health concerns such as hypertension and diabetes.

Additional Programs

There are numerous other food programs operated at the federal, state, and local levels. While these programs may not serve the numbers of participants that those listed in this section serve, they are vital to helping many Americans obtain food for themselves and their families. Examples of these programs include: Food Distribution on Indian Reservations, The Emergency Food Assistance Program (TEFAP), the Summer Food Service Program, and Farmers Markets Nutrition Programs.

While these policies aid the population most in need, the public as a whole still suffers from poor nutritional barriers in their environment. Public health policy aimed at reducing or preventing the burden of inadequate nutrition must therefore continue to search for opportunities to affect the public arena. For example, some schools have gone "commercial-free," banning the monopolization of soda companies and processed food products on school grounds. The availability of quality foods in low-income urban areas is another major issue affecting nutrition. Low-income areas are found to have 30 percent fewer supermarkets than higher-income areas; even worse, those groceries that are available carry an average of 6 kinds of fruit, 5 kinds of vegetables, and 2 kinds of meat, compared to the 19 kinds of fruit, 29 kinds of vegetables, and 18 kinds of meat in traditional grocery stores.[22] Public health policy that increases access to nutritious foods in urban areas and promotes local farmers can consequently significantly aid at-risk communities in incorporating better nutritional behaviors, and cities such as Pittsburgh, Boston, and New York have leveraged public/private partnerships to bring supermarkets into these underserved areas.

Food marketing has a major influence on food behaviors. A 2005 report by the Institute of Medicine found that food and beverage marketing practices put children's long-term health at risk by promoting consumption of high-calorie, low-nutrient foods. The United States currently places few restrictions specifically on food advertising and marketing aimed at children, although it does have overall restrictions and guidelines for advertising during children's programming. The food and beverage industries as well as some media companies have announced voluntary efforts to shift the types of products advertised to children. Other countries have policies that limit or ban advertising to children. Australia for example, does not allow any ads during programming aimed at preschools, and Sweden and Norway prohibit any television advertising directed at children twelve years of age and under. Many other countries put strict limits on commercial sponsorships for children's products.[23]

Even proper nutritional behaviors themselves can benefit from public health policy. The CIGNA Corporation has instituted a "Working Well Moms" lactation program that offers consultation for new mothers about breastfeeding practices, and promotes breastfeeding practices in workplaces by developing more accessible and informative environments. Because breastfeeding is so beneficial for the health of newborns, policy that protects and promotes the rights of new mothers can encourage greater breastfeeding participation.

Nutrition policy has made an indelible impact on how the public defines, assesses, and accesses good nutrition. However, nutritional needs are never stagnant, and nutrition policy must continue to be reflective of the public's health.

FUTURE OF NUTRITION AND PUBLIC HEALTH

We can be certain that advancements and discoveries in nutrition science will continue. With a strong foundation of vitamin knowledge already established though, future nutrition research will begin to delve deeper into the influence of nutrients on our health and disease. The connection between nutrition science and public health will therefore grow increasingly important, as we evaluate how nutrition interplays with the major health conditions we now face, such as cancer, diabetes, cardiovascular disease, and HIV/AIDS. Public health fields in particular will need to consider how nutrition is involved in those conditions that dominate our disease burden, and how nutrition can be leveraged to improve health outcomes, both from a preventive and therapeutic perspective.

For example, nutrition services have proven to not only improve nutrition, but also overall health and compliance with other medical treatment regimens. Some medical treatments are ineffective without adequate nutritional support, while others could be avoided or minimized through proper nutrition. Diabetes is an excellent example of how nutrition affects other areas of health. Poor nutrition can be a significant risk factor for the development of diabetes as well as for debilitating outcomes of diabetes patients. For patients with HIV/AIDS, good nutrition is essential for ensuring optimal absorption of medication, and also reduces medication side effects.[24] Because outside infections are such a threat to AIDS patients (who are immunocompromised), nutrition also helps maintain their overall health and lowers their risk of contracting or developing an infection.

It is clear that nutrition can significantly reduce healthcare costs and disease burden, both directly and indirectly, and will be a very influential factor in the future course of the public's health. Whether populations struggle with securing adequate food or suffer devastating chronic disease, nutrition has a decisive role in their health outcomes, and should be regarded not only as a preventive foundation for good health, but also as a route towards improved health overall.

KEY TERMS

Clinical Terms

Bioavailability: Describes the quantity of vitamins provided by the food itself, and the amount of vitamins the body is able to absorb and use, which is often less than the total nutrients present in a food.

Biofortification: Genetically modifying agricultural products to improve their nutritional content.

Daily Values: A set of nutrient intake standards designed to inform consumers about the proper levels of nutrients to consume daily.

Discretionary Calories: After fulfilling the daily recommended values of all food categories for his or her body type, each individual will still usually need between 100 and 300 additional calories to meet the recommended daily caloric intake. Those calories are called discretionary calories because each individual can decide for himself or herself what to eat to consume the extra needed calories.

Functional Foods: Provides nutritional benefits beyond its caloric or basic nutritional value. Foods that contain antioxidants are good examples of functional foods.

Hunger: The internal, physiological drive to find and consume food, often experienced as a negative sensation; manifests as an uneasy or painful sensation. The recurrent and involuntary lack of access to food that may produce malnutrition over time.

Macronutrients: Nutrients needed in large quantities, including carbohydrates, proteins, and fats.

Micronutrients: Nutrients needed in comparatively smaller quantities, including vitamins and minerals.

Minerals: Inorganic compounds needed for growth and for regulation of body processes.

Nutrient Density: A quantitative measure of a food's nutrient value, measuring the amount of nutrients per kilocalorie.

Obese: Body mass index (BMI) above 30.

Overweight: Body mass index (BMI) between 25.9 and 29.

Phytochemicals: Naturally occurring plant chemicals that are not essential but often aid in disease protection and maintaining health. Phytochemical compounds are intended to enhance the lives of plants themselves, but have recently been found to have benefits for humans as well.

Precursor: A component of a vitamin that, when combined with other components and processes in the body, will produce a full vitamin. Precursors are most often acquired from foods and stored in the body so that the body can make whole vitamins as they needed.

Toxicity: Toxicity is the presence of too much of a single micronutrient in the body. Each nutrient has a unique threshold for toxicity and distinct harmful consequences from the ingestion of toxic amounts.

Vitamins: Organic compounds necessary for reproduction, growth, and maintenance of the body. They are required in miniscule amounts.

Public Health Terms

DASH Diet: A type of eating plan developed by the Department of Health and Human Services to minimize risks for hypertension.

Dietary Guidelines: A nutrition education measure designed to help Americans gauge the nutritional quality of their food consumption in comparison to a norm.

Diet Diversity: The nutrients available to a population based on the foods they are able to access. Populations that are sustained on two or three major crops, for example, would have a low diet diversity.

Food Insecurity: Limited or uncertain availability of nutritionally adequate and safe foods, or limited or uncertain ability to acquire acceptable foods in socially acceptable ways.

Fortification: The addition of one or more nutrients to a food source, so as to correct a micronutrient deficiency.

Good Source: If a food can be labeled a "good source" of a nutrient, it must then provide 10 percent to 19 percent of the Daily Value of that nutrient per serving.

Healthy: For a food to be labeled "healthy" implies that it is low in fat, saturated fat, sodium, and cholesterol, and contains at least 10 percent of the Daily Value of one or more of the following nutrients: Vitamins A and C, iron, calcium, fiber, or protein.

Malnutrition: Failure to achieve nutrient requirements, which can impair physical and/or mental health. It may result from consuming too little food or a shortage or imbalance of key nutrients.

National Health and Nutrition Examination Survey (NHANES): A program of studies designed to assess the health and nutritional status of adults and children in the United States. The survey is unique in that it combines interviews and physical examinations.

Nutritional Monitoring: A system of continuously measuring nutritional intake and status of a population. Nutritional monitoring is an important epidemiological tool for nutritional public health.

Structural Changes: In reference to nutritional public health interventions, structural changes involve long-term adjustments to a population's behaviors and/or environment that allow them to better meet their nutritional needs.

Supplementation: A direct dosage of a nutrient, often given as a vaccine or pill.

ADDENDUM: DIETARY GUIDELINES FOR AMERICANS: 2005 KEY RECOMMENDATIONS

[Published jointly every five years since 1980 by the Department of Health and Human Services (DHHS) and the Department of Agriculture (USDA)][10,19]

ADEQUATE NUTRIENTS WITHIN CALORIE NEEDS

Key Recommendations

- Consume a variety of nutrient-dense foods and beverages within and among the basic food groups while choosing foods that limit the intake of saturated and trans fats, cholesterol, added sugars, salt, and alcohol.
- Meet recommended intakes within energy needs by adopting a balanced eating pattern, such as the USDA Food Guide or the DASH Eating Plan.

Key Recommendations for Specific Population Groups

- *People over age 50.* Consume Vitamin B$_{12}$ in its crystalline form (i.e., fortified foods or supplements).
- *Women of childbearing age who may become pregnant.* Eat foods high in heme-iron and/or consume iron-rich plant foods or iron-fortified foods with an enhancer of iron absorption, such as Vitamin C-rich foods.
- *Women of childbearing age who may become pregnant and those in the first trimester of pregnancy.* Consume adequate synthetic folic acid daily (from fortified foods or supplements) in addition to food forms of folate from a varied diet.
- *Older adults, people with dark skin, and people exposed to insufficient ultraviolet band radiation (i.e., sunlight).* Consume extra Vitamin D from Vitamin D-fortified foods and/or supplements.

WEIGHT MANAGEMENT

Key Recommendations

- To maintain body weight in a healthy range, balance calories from foods and beverages with calories expended.
- To prevent gradual weight gain over time, make small decreases in food and beverage calories and increase physical activity.

Key Recommendations for Specific Population Groups

- *Those who need to lose weight.* Aim for a slow, steady weight loss by decreasing calorie intake while maintaining an adequate nutrient intake and increasing physical activity.
- *Overweight children.* Reduce the rate of body weight gain while allowing growth and development. Consult a healthcare provider before placing a child on a weight-reduction diet.
- *Pregnant women.* Ensure appropriate weight gain as specified by a healthcare provider.
- *Breastfeeding women.* Moderate weight reduction is safe and does not compromise weight gain of the nursing infant.
- *Overweight adults and overweight children with chronic diseases and/or on medication.* Consult a healthcare provider about weight loss strategies prior to starting a weight-reduction program to ensure appropriate management of other health conditions.

PHYSICAL ACTIVITY

Key Recommendations

- Engage in regular physical activity and reduce sedentary activities to promote health, psychological well-being, and a healthy body weight.

- To reduce the risk of chronic disease in adulthood, engage in at least 30 minutes of moderate-intensity physical activity, above usual activity, at work or home on most days of the week.
- For most people, greater health benefits can be obtained by engaging in physical activity of more vigorous intensity or longer duration.
- To help manage body weight and prevent gradual, unhealthy body weight gain in adulthood, engage in approximately 60 minutes of moderate-to-vigorous intensity activity on most days of the week while not exceeding caloric intake requirements.
- To sustain weight loss in adulthood, participate in at least 60 to 90 minutes of daily moderate-intensity physical activity while not exceeding caloric intake requirements. Some people may need to consult with a healthcare provider before participating in this level of activity.
- Achieve physical fitness by including cardiovascular conditioning, stretching exercises for flexibility, and resistance exercises or calisthenics for muscle strength and endurance.

Key Recommendations for Specific Population Groups

- *Children and adolescents.* Engage in at least 60 minutes of physical activity on most, preferably all, days of the week.
- *Pregnant women.* In the absence of medical or obstetric complications, incorporate 30 minutes or more of moderate-intensity physical activity on most, if not all, days of the week. Avoid activities with a high risk of falling or abdominal trauma.
- *Breastfeeding women.* Be aware that neither acute nor regular exercise adversely affects the mother's ability to successfully breastfeed.
- *Older adults.* Participate in regular physical activity to reduce functional declines associated with aging and to achieve the other benefits of physical activity identified for all adults.

FOOD GROUPS TO ENCOURAGE

Key Recommendations

- Consume a sufficient amount of fruits and vegetables while staying within energy needs. Two cups of fruit and 2½ cups of vegetables per day are recommended for a reference 2,000-calorie intake, with higher or lower amounts depending on the calorie level.
- Choose a variety of fruits and vegetables each day. In particular, select from all five vegetable subgroups (dark green, orange, legumes, starchy vegetables, and other vegetables) several times a week.
- Consume 3 or more ounce-equivalents of whole-grain products per day, with the rest of the recommended grains coming from enriched or whole-grain products. In general, at least half the grains should come from whole grains.
- Consume 3 cups per day of fat-free or low-fat milk or equivalent milk products.

Key Recommendations for Specific Population Groups

- *Children and adolescents.* Consume whole-grain products often; at least half the grains should be whole grains. Children 2 to 8 years should consume 2 cups per day of fat-free or low-fat milk or equivalent milk products. Children 9 years of age and older should consume 3 cups per day of fat-free or low-fat milk or equivalent milk products.

FATS

Key Recommendations

- Consume less than 10 percent of calories from saturated fatty acids and less than 300 mg/day of cholesterol, and keep trans fatty acid consumption as low as possible.
- Keep total fat intake between 20 percent and 35 percent of calories, with most fats coming from sources of polyunsaturated and monounsaturated fatty acids, such as fish, nuts, and vegetable oils.
- When selecting and preparing meat, poultry, dry beans, and milk or milk products, make choices that are lean, low-fat, or fat-free.
- Limit intake of fats and oils high in saturated and/or trans fatty acids, and choose products low in such fats and oils.

Key Recommendations for Specific Population Groups

- *Children and adolescents.* Keep total fat intake between 30 and 35 percent of calories for children 2 to 3 years of age and between 25 and 35 percent of calories for children and adolescents 4 to 18 years of age, with most fats coming from sources of polyunsaturated and monounsaturated fatty acids, such as fish, nuts, and vegetable oils.

CARBOHYDRATES
Key Recommendations

- Choose fiber-rich fruits, vegetables, and whole grains often.
- Choose and prepare foods and beverages with little added sugars or caloric sweeteners, such as amounts suggested by the USDA Food Guide and the DASH Eating Plan.
- Reduce the incidence of dental caries by practicing good oral hygiene and consuming sugar- and starch-containing foods and beverages less frequently.

SODIUM AND POTASSIUM
Key Recommendations

- Consume less than 2,300 mg (approximately 1 tsp of salt) of sodium per day.
- Choose and prepare foods with little salt. At the same time, consume potassium-rich foods, such as fruits and vegetables.

Key Recommendations for Specific Population Groups

- *Individuals with hypertension, blacks, and middle-aged and older adults.* Aim to consume no more than 1,500 mg of sodium per day, and meet the potassium recommendation (4,700 mg/day) with food.

ALCOHOLIC BEVERAGES
Key Recommendations

- Those who choose to drink alcoholic beverages should do so sensibly and in moderation, which is defined as the consumption of up to one drink per day for women and up to two drinks per day for men.
- Alcoholic beverages should not be consumed by some individuals, including those who cannot restrict their alcohol intake, women of childbearing age who may become pregnant, pregnant and lactating women, children and adolescents, individuals taking medications that can interact with alcohol, and those with specific medical conditions.

- Alcoholic beverages should be avoided by individuals engaging in activities that require attention, skill, or coordination, such as driving or operating machinery.

FOOD SAFETY
Key Recommendations

- To avoid microbial foodborne illness:
  - Clean hands, food contact surfaces, and fruits and vegetables. Meat and poultry should not be washed or rinsed.
  - Separate raw, cooked, and ready-to-eat foods while shopping, preparing, or storing foods.
  - Cook foods to a safe temperature to kill microorganisms.
  - Chill (refrigerate) perishable food promptly and defrost foods properly.
  - Avoid raw (unpasteurized) milk or any products made from unpasteurized milk, raw or partially cooked eggs or foods containing raw eggs, raw or undercooked meat and poultry, unpasteurized juices, and raw sprouts.

Key Recommendations for Specific Population Groups

- *Infants and young children, pregnant women, older adults, and those who are immunocompromised.* Do not eat or drink raw (unpasteurized) milk or any products made from unpasteurized milk, raw or partially cooked eggs, or foods containing raw eggs, raw or undercooked meat and poultry, raw or undercooked fish or shellfish, unpasteurized juices, and raw sprouts.
- *Pregnant women, older adults, and those who are immunocompromised:* Only eat certain deli meats and frankfurters that have been reheated to steaming hot.

Special nutrient recommendations are warranted for a few large subgroups of the population as follows:

- Adolescent female and women of childbearing age need extra iron and folic acid.
- Persons over age 50 benefit from taking Vitamin B_{12} in its crystalline form from foods fortified with this vitamin or from supplements that contain Vitamin B_{12}.
- The elderly, persons with dark skin, and persons exposed to little UVB radiation may need extra Vitamin D from Vitamin D-fortified foods and/or supplements that contain Vitamin D.

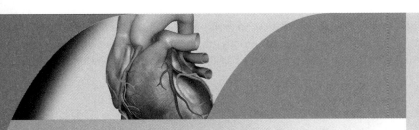

Questions for Further Research, Study, Reflection, and Discussion

For the Individual Student

In order to answer these questions, it may be necessary to research the primary literature.

- Describe the general roles that vitamins play in our body's functioning, and their typical deficiency consequences. How is this different than minerals?
- Using the history outline of nutrition, describe how public health interventions have been both proactive and reactive to nutrition science and scientific discovery, and give some examples.
- Using the categories for assessing nutritional choices, evaluate what factors influence your own nutritional habits.
- What foods would be the most efficient and effective way to increase nutritional status through diet diversity?
- Develop a timeline describing how nutrition has influenced another aspect or health condition (for example, obesity or malaria).
- Why is iron deficiency prevalent among children? What are the consequences of iron-deficiency anemia in young children?
- What are the key messages/recommendations of the *Dietary Guidelines for Americans*? How do these differ from typical intake?
- Why are most of the food assistance programs operated by the U.S. Department of Agriculture? What agencies in your state are responsible for implementing these programs?
- Why do we still have hunger in the United States?
- Why would hunger and obesity coexist?

For Small Group Discussion
Case Study 1

Assess Malena's nutritional profile, and name some major nutritional gaps in her diet. How did her diet change once she came to the United States?

What are the primary nutritional challenges Malena faces? What challenges do her children face? What clinically can be done now to help improve Malena's nutritional challenges? What could have been done before to reduce or prevent Malena's nutritional challenges? What factors in her life make it difficult for her to make nutritional changes? How does her cultural perspective aid or hinder Malena's nutritional habits? What changes to her environment or structure could help her situation? What recommendations would you make for her that would be realistic for her life? What federal food assistance programs might be available to Malena and her children?

Case Study 2

Assess Cristina's nutritional profile, and name some major nutritional gaps in her diet. How did her family's diet change from a traditional Latino diet? What are the primary nutritional challenges Cristina faces? What clinically can be done now to help improve Cristina's nutritional challenges? What could have been done before to reduce or prevent Cristina's nutritional challenges? What factors in her home life make it difficult for her to make nutritional changes? What environmental and cultural factors affect Cristina's food habits? How has her cultural perspective affected her nutritional status? What changes to her environment or structure could help her situation?

For Entire Class Discussion

- How does nutrition affect the overall health of a population?
- Explain how immigration or migration can affect the nutrition of an individual or community.
- How does culture play a role in nutrition and in nutritional public health?
- How have cultural perceptions and values shaped nutrition practices, in both beneficial and detrimental ways?
- How would you describe "good nutrition" to a population in an easy and effective way?

- If you were to conduct a nutritional public health intervention, what would be the major steps you would take to design the intervention?
- What are some environmental, structural, and social ways you can target micronutrient malnutrition issues?
- In general, how would you use a community's cultural distinctions to help them adapt more nutritionally-beneficial habits?
- How do federal dietary guidelines compare to popular diets?
- Why do people turn to diet books over the *Dietary Guidelines for Americans*?
- What is the role of public health professionals in alleviating consumer confusion about healthy diets?
- Why is it important to differentiate between obesity and good nutrition?
- Does weight imply good health?

EXERCISES/ACTIVITIES

- Pick a population outside of the United States and research characteristics about their diet and farming traditions. Identify some possible nutritional gaps and potential solutions.
- What research is currently being done about nutrients or nutrition science? Find some examples and present them to the class. What do these factors imply for public health fields?
- Consider the current public health policies that affect nutrition in the United States. How can they be improved, and what other health issues should they be taking into account, based on the U.S. health profile?
- Take a field trip to a local grocer or bodega (not a mainstream grocery store) that a neighborhood might depend on as a food source. Take a general inventory of what nutrients they do offer and those they might be lacking. Make some sample grocery lists of what would be the best used of the foodstuffs they have to offer.

Healthy People 2010

Indicator: Overweight and Obesity

Focus Area: Nutrition and Overweight

Goal: Promote health and reduce chronic disease associated with diet and weight.

Objectives:

19-5. Increase the proportion of persons aged 2 years and older who consume at least two daily servings of fruit.

19-6. Increase the proportion of persons aged 2 years and older who consume at least three daily servings of vegetables, with at least one third being dark green or orange vegetables.

19-7. Increase the proportion of persons aged 2 years and older who consume at least six daily servings of grain products, with at least three being whole grains.

19-8. Increase the proportion of persons aged 2 years and older who consume less than 10 percent of calories from saturated fat.

19-9. Increase the proportion of persons aged 2 years and older who consume no more than 30 percent of calories from total fat.

19-10. Increase the proportion of persons aged 2 years and older who consume 2,400 mg or less of sodium daily.

19-11. Increase the proportion of persons aged 2 years and older who meet dietary recommendations for calcium.

TIME LINE OF THE HISTORY OF NUTRITION: EFFORTS OF SCIENCE AND PUBLIC HEALTH

1743

James Lind, through his experiments with Scottish sailors, discovers that citrus fruits prevent scurvy.

1780s

Antoine Lavoisier, the father of nutrition, demonstrates that foodstuffs supply energy and heat for the body, introducing the term "caloric."

1811

Iodine is discovered.

1819

Iodine is used for experiments about goiters in Switzerland, yet the toxic effects of iodine overdosages cause the popularity of iodine to decline.

1826

First American railroad is built, greatly increasing the availability of foodstuffs.

1830s

François Magendie shows that proteins (amino acids) are essential for growth and health and that a deficiency in amino acids leads to widespread impairment of body and cellular functions.

1864

Louis Pasteur makes great contributions to the microbial paradigm for disease and introduces the concept of pasteurizing milk.

1895

New York City establishes milk stations to provide safe milk for infants and children, as well as educate parents about feeding.

1896

Christian Eijkman reproduces the condition of beriberi in chickens by feeding them a diet of polished (husked) rice, convincing people to stop removing the husks from rice, as they seemed to contain a preventive substance against beriberi.

1898

School lunches begin in New York City.

1906

Frederick Hopkins first delineates the concept of vitamins, such that foods contain substances beyond fats, proteins, and carbohydrates, which are essential for the health and growth of humans.

1911

Casimir Frank coins the term "vitamins."

1913

Elmer McCollum plays a significant role in the discovery of vitamins A and D, as well as thiamin, and his experiments clearly show the negative effects (such as night blindness and stunted growth) from vitamin deficiencies.

1916

David Marine uses iodine for his experiments with goiters in Ohio, achieving incredible success with his results.

1918

It is discovered that pellagra was caused by a dietary deficiency, produced from a corn-based diet.

1920

Edward Mellanby's experiments demonstrate that rickets is undoubtedly the result of a dietary deficiency, which he found to be present in butterfat, and later isolated at vitamin D.

The DHHS Children's Bureau begins first series of nutritional studies in children throughout the nation.

1924

The supplementation of salt with iodine is first introduced in Michigan, two years after Sweden introduces it.

1928

The American Institute of Nutrition is created. The addition of vitamin D to milk is initiated.

1929

The Children's Bureau publishes their first height and weight tables for children under six years old.

1930s

Robert Williams isolates the antiberiberi factor in rice husks, now known as thiamin and vitamin B.

1932

Albert Szent-Gyorgvi finds that the specific element in citrus fruits responsible for their nutritional benefit is ascorbic acid, or vitamin C.

1935

The USDA begins a nationwide food consumption survey.

1939

The Food Stamp Program is created to ensure emergency relief and food assistance to those in poverty.

1940

Vitamin B_{12} is isolated and named by scientists William Castle, William Murphy, and George Minot.

1941

The National Nutritional Conference for Defense first submits a structure of dietary allowances.

1942

The Metropolitan Life Insurance Company issues their first version of height and weight tables for all ages.

1946

The National School Lunch Program is founded.

1952

Abram Hoffer starts treating schizophrenics with Vitamins C and B_3, beginning a new paradigm of thinking about vitamins and more crucial aspects of health.

1964

The Head Start Program is created with a strong nutrition education component included.

1966

The Child Nutrition Act is passed, expanding food programs for children.

1972

WIC creates the Special Supplemental Food Program for women, infants and children.

1977

The U.S. Senate Select Committee on Nutrition and Human Needs publishes the Dietary Goals for the United States, with their recommendations on the food and nutrition practices of Americans. From this, the Nutritional Education and Training Program is established.

1990

The U.S. Congress passes an act requiring that the Dietary Guidelines be revised and republished every 5 years.

The U.S. government releases their first tables of ideal height and weight.

The Nutrition Labeling and Education Act is passed.

1992

The USDA comes out with its first Food Guide Pyramid.

1994

The U.S. Congress unanimously passes the Dietary Supplement and Health Education Act, and the USDA and FDA also revised their regulations on food labeling, requiring that all manufacturers label the nutritional facts on their products.

2002

The CDC declares obesity an epidemic in the United States.

2004

The CDC declares an obesity epidemic among children as well.

2005

The USDA publishes a new food pyramid, which focuses more intensely on food content and portions.

REFERENCES

1. Public Health News Center. The Story of Vitamin A. (2007). Johns Hopkins School of Public Health. Available at http://www.jhsph.edu/publichealthnews/press_releases/sommer_vitA.html. Accessed March 23, 2008.

2. WGBH/NOVA Science Unit. Rx for Survival—A Global Health Challenge. WGBH Education Foundation and Vulcan Productions. (2005). Available at http://www.pbs.org/wgbh/rxforsurvival. Accessed March 23, 2008.

3. Gratzer W. *Terrors of the Table: The Curious History of Nutrition.* New York: Oxford University Press; 2005.

4. National Academy of Sciences. Beyond Discovery. Unraveling the Enigma of Vitamin D. Washington, DC: NAS; 2003. Available at http://www.beyonddiscovery.org/content/view.article.asp?a=414. Accessed March 23, 2008.

5. Insel P, Turner RE, Ross D. *Discovering Nutrition,* 2nd ed. Boston: Jones and Bartlett Publications; 2006.

6. Douaud C. Conference highlights cancer-fighting foods. *AP-Food technology.* 2007:28 Mar. Available at http://ap-foodtechnology.com/news/ng.asp?id=75329. Accessed March 23, 2008.

7. Fischer WC, Black RE. Zinc and the risk for infectious disease. *Ann Rev Nutr* 2004;24:255–275.

8. Schilling J. Eliminate Childhood Lead Poisoning by 2010. *Special Primary Interest Groups Newsletters: Food and Nutrition.* American Public Health Association. 2005;Winter.

9. Centers for Disease Control and Prevention. *Behavioral Risk Factor Surveillance System.* Available at http://www.cdc.gov/brfss/. Accessed March 23, 2008.

10. Department of Health and Human Services. *Report of the Dietary Guidelines Advisory Committee on the Dietary Guidelines for Americans, 2005.* Available at http://www.health.gov/dietaryguidelines/dga2005/report/. Accessed March 23, 2008.

11. Briefel RR, Johnson CL. Secular trends in dietary intake in the United States. *Ann Rev Nutr* 2004;24:401–431.

12. Allison DB, Egan SK, Barraj LM, Caughman C, Infante M, Heimbach JT. Estimated intakes of trans fatty and other fatty acids in the U.S. population. *J Am Diet Assoc* 1999;99:166–174.

13. Institute of Medicine. *Dietary Reference Intakes for Water, Potassium, Sodium, Chloride, and Sulfate.* Washington, DC: National Academies Press; 2004.

14. Dietz WH. Does hunger cause obesity? *Pediatrics* 1995;95:766–767.

15. Weber JA. Talking about hunger in a land of plenty. *J Am Diet Assoc* 2006;106:804–807.

16. Lindsay A, de Benoist B, Dary O, Hurrel R. *Guidelines of Food Fortification with Micronutrients.* World Health Organization and Food and Agricultural Organization of the United Nations; 2006.

17. Pineda O. Fortification of sugar with vitamin A. In: *Food and Nutrition Bulletin,* 1998;19(2). Available at: http://www.unu.edu/unupress/food/V192e/begin.htm Accessed March 23, 2008.

18. Public Law 101-445; October 22, 1990. National Nutrition Monitoring and Related Research Act of 1990.

19. U.S. Department of Health and Human Services and U.S. Department of Agriculture. *Finding Your Way to a Healthier You: Based on the Dietary Guidelines for Americans.* HHS Publication number: HHS-ODPHP-2005-01-DGA-B. USDA Publication number: Home and Garden Bulletin No. 232-CP, 2005.

20. Cataldo CB, Debrunye LK, Whitney EN. *Nutrition and Diet Therapy,* 6th ed. Belmont, CA: Thompson Learning/Wadsworth; 2003.

21. Barrett A. *Characteristics of Food Stamp Households: Fiscal Year 2005.* Prepared by Mathematica Policy Research, Inc., for the Food and Nutrition Service; 2006. Available at: www.fns.usda.gov/oane. Accessed March 23, 2008.

22. Cotterill RW, Franklin AW. *The Urban Grocery Store Gap.* Storrs: Food Marketing Policy Center. University of Connecticut: Food Marketing Policy Issue Paper. No. 8; 1995.

23. Prevention Institute. *Nutrition Policy Profiles.* (2002). Available at: http://www.preventioninstitute.org/npp.html. Accessed March 23, 2008.

24. Association of Nutrition Services Agencies (ANSA). *The Power of Nutrition.* (2006). Available at: http://www.aidsnutrition.org/documents/ANSAwpFinal.pdf Accessed March 23, 2008.

ADDITIONAL RESOURCES

Hoats K. *The Cost of Being Poor in the City: A Comparison of Cost and Availability of Food in the Lehigh Valley.* Community Action Committee of the Lehigh Valley; 1993.

McDonald's Corporation. Menu Innovation and Nutrition Education Firsts. (2005). Available at http://www.mcdepk.com/passporttoplay/media/leadership_legacy_fact_sheet.pdf. Accessed March 23, 2008.

Webb P. Intrahousehold Dimensions of Micronutrient Deficiencies: A Review of the Evidence. Tufts Food Policy and Applied Nutrition Program. Discussion Paper No. 4; 2002. Available at http://nutrition.tufts.edu/docs/pdf/fpan/wp04-intrahousehold_dimensions.pdf. Accessed March 24, 2008.

HISTORY OF NUTRITION: TIME LINE RESOURCES

Boyd S. *History of Nutrition and Health.* GlycoScience and Nutrition Research and Development of Mannatech Incorporated, Texas. 2000;1(2).

Challem J. The Past, Present and Future of Vitamins. *The Nutrition Reporter. Essay 1997.* Available at http:www.thenutritionreporter.com/history_of_vitamins.html. Accessed March 24, 2008.

Department of Health and Human Services. Appendix I. History of the Dietary Guidelines for Americans. Available at http://health.gov/dietaryguidelines/dga95/12DIETAP.HTM. Accessed March 24, 2008.

Elvehjem CA. Seven decades of nutrition research. *Science.* New Series: 1949;109:354–358.

Murray RK. *Ten Major Advances in Nutrition.* GlycoScience and Nutrition. Research and Development of Mannatech Incorporated, Texas. 2000;1(28).

Center for Human Development and Disability. Nutrition. (2003). University of Washington. http://depts.washington.edu/lend/coresem/nutrition/intro.htm.

Popkin BM. Nutritional patterns and transitions. *Population Develop Rev* 1993;19:138–157.

Sherman HC. A Century of Progress in the Chemistry of Nutrition. *Scientific Monthly* 1933;37:442–447.

Thornalley PJ, Babaei-Jadidi R, Al Ali H, Rabbani N, et al. High prevalence of low plasma thiamine concentration in diabetes linked to a marker of vascular disease. *Diabetologia* 2007;50:2164–2170.

CROSS REFERENCES

Behavioral Determinants of Health
Communicating Public Health Information
Diabetes
Exercise
Information Seeking Strategies
Nutrition Transition

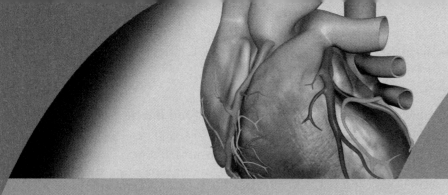

CHAPTER 10

The Nutrition Transition:
Changes in Eating Patterns and the Relationship to Chronic Illness
Mellen Duffy Tanamly

Dietary factors are associated with 4 of the 10 leading causes of death: coronary heart disease (CHD), some types of cancer, stroke, and type 2 diabetes.[1]

Since the mid-seventies, the prevalence of overweight and obesity has increased sharply for both adults and children. Data from two U.S. National Health and Nutrition Examination Survey (NHANES) surveys show that among adults aged 20 to 74 years the prevalence of obesity increased from 15.0% (in the 1976–1980 survey) to 32.9% (in the 2003–2004 survey).[2]

Projections show that chronic diseases will be the predominant global source of morbidity and death in the 21st century.[3]

LEARNING OBJECTIVES

By the end of this chapter, the student will be able to:

- Name the major nutrition-related chronic diseases causing death and disability in the United States as well as globally.

- Recognize the role of dietary patterns in the prevention and management of diabetes, cardiovascular disease (CVD), and cancer.

- Examine nutrition as a behavioral risk factor for CVD, diabetes, cancer, and obesity.

- Discover how nutritional interventions can help people living with human immunodeficiency virus/acquired immune deficiency syndrome (HIV/AIDS) to manage symptoms, reduce susceptibility to opportunistic infections, promote response to medical treatment, and improve overall quality of life.

- Describe current trends in prevention and treatment for each of the major nutrition-related chronic conditions.

- Assess the impact of the "nutrition transition" on the health of Americans and citizens of the world.

HISTORY

Historical Focus on Undernutrition

During the 1800s in the United States, the primary emphasis of public health nutrition was on improving nutrition for children and mothers to reduce mortality and morbidity. The "War on Poverty" in the 1960s focused on nutrition targeted to high risk and low income groups. Today we have the continued presence of poverty and hunger in many communities, while at the same time we have an epidemic of obesity in adults and children throughout our nation. Along with obesity trends, type 2 diabetes and other diseases for which poor eating habits are a risk factor are increasing worldwide.

The last three decades have brought important achievements in health and nutrition status in the developing world, but formidable challenges persist. The world population more than doubled in the second half of the 20th century, mostly from population growth in developing countries. High population growth poses significant challenges to national efforts to alleviate poverty and to facilitate access to basic services. Lack of adequate food and **micronutrients** in particular contributes to more than half of the deaths of young children under five in many developing countries. Malnutrition is problematic not only in poor countries (many of which have both undernutrition and obesity), but also in wealthy countries confronted with a rapidly growing prevalence of obesity.

Nutrition Transition Today

There have been steep reductions in child mortality and undernutrition in almost every country, unprecedented innovation in health technology and discoveries in medicine, and a steady decline in mortality in most regions of the world. At the same time, a significant increase has occurred in premature deaths related to chronic diseases (diabetes, pulmonary diseases, hypertension, cancer) linked to tobacco addiction and obesity. Eighty percent of chronic disease deaths take place in low and middle income countries (Figure 10-1). Many countries, including India, Egypt, and Nigeria, are facing the same pattern of "nutrition transition" that the United States and other high income nations already experienced.

Gains in identifying dietary risk factors for major noncommunicable diseases including cardiovascular diseases (CVD), diabetes, and cancer have shown that eating behaviors and other lifestyle factors play a crucial role in prevention and management of these illnesses. Throughout most of history, humans have had to exert a great deal of physical energy to obtain their food. Only over the past century has a substantial and increasing percentage of the population, especially in the United States, had access to an excess of food, with no need to exert any physical effort to obtain it. The consequence of this imbalance is that Americans are becoming fatter—an exceedingly unhealthy trend. Today, diet and physical activity patterns rank second among the factors identified as leading actual causes of U.S. deaths.

Globalization and Changing Food Habits

Furthermore, rapid changes in diets and lifestyles that have occurred with industrialization, urbanization, economic development, and market globalization have accelerated over the past decade. This is having a significant impact on the health and nutritional status of populations, particularly **vulnerable and at-risk populations** in developing countries and countries in transition. While standards of living have improved, food availability has expanded and become more diversified, and access to services has increased, there also have been significant negative consequences such as inappropriate dietary patterns and decreased physical activity, and a corresponding increase in diet-related chronic diseases, especially among poor people. Changes in the world food economy are reflected in shifting dietary patterns, for example, increased consumption of energy-dense diets high in fat, particularly saturated fat, and low in unrefined carbohydrates. Often changes in geographic location bring changes in access to fresh produce that were part of the traditional diet. These patterns are combined with a decline in energy expenditure that is associated with a sedentary lifestyle: motorized transport, labor-saving devices in the home, phasing out of physically demanding manual tasks in the workplace, and leisure time that is predominately devoted to physically undemanding pastimes.

Noncommunicable Diseases Can Be Prevented and Controlled

The experience of high-income countries clearly shows what can be achieved with sustained interventions. A "War on Cancer" was declared in 1971 and resulted in increased funding and attention to cancer. Advances in cancer biology, treatment, and prevention have led to a better understanding of the role of environment and lifestyle on cancer development and more effective education about prevention.

A tremendous achievement has been the reduction of rates of death from CVD since World War II. Death rates from

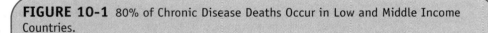

FIGURE 10-1 80% of Chronic Disease Deaths Occur in Low and Middle Income Countries.

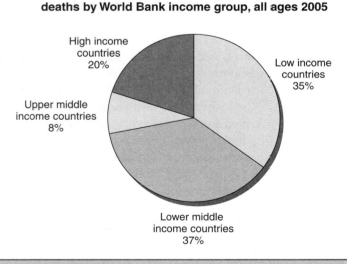

Projected global distribution chronic disease deaths by World Bank income group, all ages 2005

High income countries 20%

Low income countries 35%

Upper middle income countries 8%

Lower middle income countries 37%

Source: From Chronic Diseases and Health Promotion, World Health Organization. "Preventing Chronic Diseases: a Vital Investment." Available at http://www.who.int/chp/chronic_disease_report/presentation/en/index.html. Accessed April 2, 2008.

heart disease have fallen by up to 70 percent in the past three decades in Australia, Canada, Japan, the United Kingdom, and the United States. Between 1970 and 2000, 14 million deaths due to cardiovascular disease were averted in the United States alone. During the same period, the numbers of deaths averted in Japan and the United Kingdom were 8 million and 3 million, respectively. Nutrition interventions are important elements of prevention strategies.

Despite the tremendous progress in saving lives, CVD is still the leading cause of death in every state in the United States and the leading cause of mortality globally (Figure 10-2). It is the leading cause of death for men and for women and the leading cause of death for every ethnic and minority group.

Chronic Diseases Are a Major Global Burden

Projections show that chronic diseases will be the predominant global source of morbidity and mortality in the 21st century. Contributing factors include an increase in minority populations in the United States, especially Hispanic and South Asian, and an increase in the number and proportion of elderly in most societies due to life-saving health advancements. Cardiovascular disease is the leading cause of death for women and men in the United States today and the leading cause of mortality globally. Diabetes and cancer are affecting people and stressing health systems worldwide. By 2015, **noncommunicable diseases (NCDs)** will be the leading cause of death in low-income countries.[4] Many of those deaths occur prematurely, at an early middle age of adulthood. NCDs impose a significant economic burden, not just on patients but also on their households, communities, employers, healthcare systems, and government budgets. An increasing burden of NCDs in developing countries will put an enormous strain on their weak health systems. Many people living with AIDS (PLWA) in Sub-Saharan Africa and other nations need better nutrition care.

Policies and Health Services Should Promote Healthy Diets

These conditions cause tremendous disability before they cause death, so more effective prevention and better management are needed. Nutrition is coming to the fore as a major modifiable determinant of chronic disease, with increasing scientific evidence to support the view that alterations in diet can have strong effects, both positive and negative, on health throughout life. Most importantly, dietary adjustments may not only influence present health, but may determine whether or not an individual will develop such diseases as cancer, cardiovascular disease, and diabetes much later in life. However, these concepts have not led to changes in public policies or in health practices. Health protection, which would encompass both health promotion and prevention, is weak or nonexistent in most global health systems. In many developing countries, food policies remain focused only on undernutrition and are not addressing the prevention of chronic disease and obesity. In addition, health services are often not providing adequate quality prevention and management of these conditions.

BASIC SCIENCE FACTS/KEY CONCEPTS REVIEW

Although chronic diseases are among the most common and costly health problems, they are also among the most preventable. Adopting healthy behaviors such as eating nutritious foods and being physically active can prevent or control the devastating effects of these diseases. During the past decade, rapid expansion in a number of relevant scientific fields and,

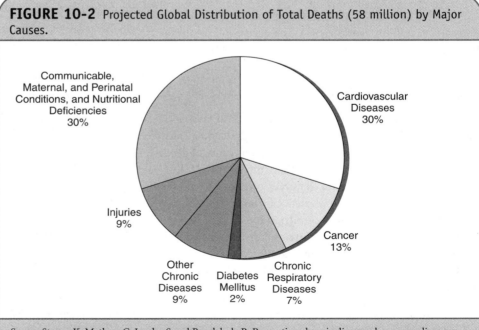

FIGURE 10-2 Projected Global Distribution of Total Deaths (58 million) by Major Causes.

Communicable, Maternal, and Perinatal Conditions, and Nutritional Deficiencies 30%

Cardiovascular Diseases 30%

Cancer 13%

Chronic Respiratory Diseases 7%

Diabetes Mellitus 2%

Other Chronic Diseases 9%

Injuries 9%

Source: Strong K, Mathers C, Leeder S and Beaglehole R. Preventing chronic diseases: how many lives can we save? *Lancet* 2005;366:1578–82.

in particular, in the amount of population-based epidemiological evidence, has helped to clarify the role of diet in preventing and controlling morbidity and premature mortality resulting from NCDs. Some of the specific dietary components that increase the probability of occurrence of these diseases in individuals, and interventions to modify their impact, have been identified also. Estimates of the joint effects of the leading chronic disease risk factors (tobacco use, raised blood pressure, and poor diet) indicate that more than 30 percent of the burden of chronic diseases and more than 50 percent of deaths from chronic disease are attributable to a relatively small number of modifiable risks.[3]

> **NUTRITION-RELATED CHRONIC ILLNESSES COVERED IN THIS CHAPTER**
>
> Cardiovascular disease
> Diabetes mellitus
> Cancer
> Overweight and obesity
> HIV/AIDS (as a chronic condition)

There are many noncommunicable diseases in which nutrition plays an important role in prevention and/or therapeutic management. This chapter addresses those that cause the largest burden of disease in the United States and globally: cardiovascular disease, diabetes mellitus, cancer, and obesity. In addition, because HIV/AIDS, an infectious disease that currently affects millions worldwide, has chronic implications for those affected, nutrition-related factors in HIV/AIDS will be included.

CARDIOVASCULAR DISEASE

Despite the tremendous progress in saving lives, CVD is still the leading cause of death in every U.S. state and the leading cause of mortality globally. Heart disease is the leading cause of death for all racial and ethnic groups in the United States, killing over 910,000 every year. More than half of persons who die each year of heart disease are women. Coronary heart disease is decreasing in some wealthy countries, but is increasing in developing and transitional countries, partly as a result of increasing longevity, urbanization, and lifestyle.

CVDs are diseases of the heart and blood vessels that include:

- Coronary heart disease (heart attack)
- Cerebrovascular diseases (stroke and transient ischemic attacks)
- High blood pressure (hypertension)

Coronary Heart Disease and Stroke

Coronary heart disease (CHD) and stroke are the most common forms of CVDs and therefore is the main focus of this chapter. CHD is the leading cause of U.S. deaths and is caused by atherosclerosis in the large- and medium-sized arteries. Stroke is a type of cardiovascular disease that affects the arteries leading to and within the brain. A stroke occurs when a blood vessel that carries oxygen and nutrients to the brain is either blocked by a clot or bursts. Deprived of oxygen, nerve cells in the affected area of the brain can't work and die within minutes. When nerve cells do not work, the part of the body they control cannot work either. The devastating effects of stroke are often permanent because dead brain cells are not replaced.

High Blood Pressure/Hypertension

The major risk factor for stroke is **hypertension**, which is high blood pressure. It usually has no specific symptoms and no early warning signs, the reasons why everyone should have their blood pressure checked regularly. **Blood pressure** is the force exerted in the arteries when the heart beats (systolic pressure) and when the heart is at rest (diastolic pressure). It is measured in millimeters of mercury (mm Hg). High blood pressure (hypertension) is defined in an adult as a blood pressure greater than or equal to 140 mm Hg systolic pressure or greater than or equal to 90 mm Hg diastolic pressure. High blood pressure directly increases the risk of coronary heart disease (which leads to heart attack) and stroke, especially when it is present with other risk factors. Often, blood pressure can be controlled just by eating a healthier diet and maintaining a healthy weight.

High blood pressure can occur in children or adults, but is more common among people over age 35. It is particularly prevalent in African Americans, middle-aged and elderly people, obese people, heavy drinkers, and women who are taking birth control pills. It may run in families, but many people with a strong family history of high blood pressure never have it. People with diabetes mellitus, gout, or kidney disease are more likely to have high blood pressure, too. According to recent estimates, nearly one in three U.S. adults has high blood pressure, but because there are no symptoms, nearly one third of these people don't know they have it. In fact, many people have high blood pressure for years without knowing it. Uncontrolled high blood pressure can lead to stroke, heart attack, heart failure, or kidney failure, which is why it is often referred to as *the silent killer*. The only way to tell if a person has high blood pressure is to have one's blood pressure checked.

African Americans have a high risk of hypertension because more than 40 percent have it. High blood pressure develops earlier in life in blacks than in whites and is usually more severe. The longer it is left untreated, the more serious its complications can become. Because high blood pressure is so serious, early detection and treatment are very important.

Women everywhere have risks for heart disease and stroke. CVD kills over 480,000 women a year—about one death per minute—in the United States. Some ethnic groups may have more or less of various risk factors, but every woman needs to know what special risks seem to fall to her racial/ethnic grouping:

- Black women have high rates of high blood pressure, high cholesterol, overweight/obesity, physical inactivity, and diabetes.
- Mexican-American women have high rates of diabetes, high cholesterol, and overweight/obesity.
- Asian or Pacific Islander women have high rates of high cholesterol levels (240 mg/dL and higher).
- American Indian/Alaska Native women have high rates of smoking, physical inactivity, and overweight and obesity.

Nutrition-Related Risk Factors

Extensive clinical and statistical studies, many sponsored by the American Heart Association, have identified several factors that increase the risk of coronary heart disease and heart attack. Some of these risks can be modified, treated, or controlled; however, the more risk factors and the greater the level of each risk factor, the greater the chance of developing coronary heart disease. For example, a person with a total blood cholesterol level of 300 mg/dL has a greater risk than someone with a total cholesterol level of 245 mg/dL, even though everyone with a total cholesterol greater than 240 is considered high risk.

The following are the major nutrition-related risk factors for CVD that can be modified, treated, or controlled by changes in lifestyle or by taking medication:

- *High blood cholesterol:* A high level ($\geq$ 240 mg/dL) of total **cholesterol** (a soft, waxy substance located within fats circulating in the bloodstream) in the blood is a major risk factor for heart disease, which raises the risk of stroke. As blood cholesterol rises, so does risk of coronary heart disease. When other risk factors (i.e., high blood pressure and tobacco smoke) are present, this risk increases even more. A person's cholesterol level also is affected by age, sex, heredity, and diet.
- *High blood pressure:* High blood pressure ($\geq$ 140/90 mm Hg) increases the heart's workload, causing it to thicken and become stiffer. It also increases the risk of stroke, heart attack, kidney failure, and congestive heart fail-

ure. When high blood pressure exists with obesity, smoking, high blood cholesterol levels, or diabetes, the risk of heart attack or stroke increases by several times.
- *Physical inactivity:* An inactive lifestyle is a risk factor for coronary heart disease. An inactive lifestyle makes it easier to become overweight and increases the chance of high blood pressure. Regular, moderate-to-vigorous physical activity helps prevent heart and blood vessel disease. The more vigorous the activity, the greater the benefits. However, even moderate-intensity activities help if done regularly and long term. Physical activity can help control blood cholesterol, diabetes, and obesity as well as help lower blood pressure in some people.
- *Obesity and overweight:* People who have excess body fat—especially if much of it is at the waist—are more likely to develop heart disease and stroke even if they have no other risk factors. Being inactive, obese, or both can increase the risk of high blood pressure, high blood cholesterol, diabetes, heart disease, and stroke. Persons with a body mass index (BMI) of 30.0 or higher are more likely to develop high blood pressure. Excess weight increases the heart's work. It also raises blood pressure and blood cholesterol and triglyceride levels and lowers HDL ("good") cholesterol levels. Diabetes is more likely to develop. Many obese and overweight people have difficulty losing weight, but losing even as few as 10 pounds can lower heart disease risk.
- *Diabetes mellitus:* Diabetes seriously increases the risk of developing cardiovascular disease. Diabetes is defined as a fasting plasma glucose (monosaccharide; blood sugar) of 126 mg/dL or more when measured on two occasions. Even when glucose (blood sugar) levels are under control, having diabetes increases the risk of heart disease and stroke, but the risks are even greater if blood sugar is not well controlled. About three-quarters of people with diabetes die of some form of heart or blood vessel disease.

Other factors that contribute to heart disease risk:

- Individual response to *stress* may be a contributing factor. Some scientists have noted a relationship between coronary heart disease risk and stress in a person's life, his or her health behaviors, and socioeconomic status. These factors may affect other established risk factors. For example, people under stress may overeat, start smoking, or smoke more than they would otherwise.
- Drinking *too much alcohol* can raise blood pressure, cause heart failure, and lead to stroke; it contributes to high triglycerides, cancer, and other diseases as well as

produces irregular heartbeats. It contributes to obesity, alcoholism, suicide, and accidents. The risk of heart disease in people who drink *moderate amounts of alcohol* (an average of one drink for women or two drinks for men per day) is lower than in nondrinkers. One drink is defined as 1½ fluid ounces (fl oz) of 80-proof spirits (such as bourbon, Scotch, vodka, gin, etc.), 1 fl oz of 100-proof spirits, 4 fl oz of wine, or 12 fl oz of beer. It is *not* recommended that nondrinkers start using alcohol or that drinkers increase the amount they drink. This is because the risks of drinking too much alcohol can outweigh the benefits and alcohol adds calories (7 kcals per gram) that most people with CVD risk can ill afford.

Mechanisms of Action

Key dietary factors for CVD and some of the evidence for their effects on heart health are as follows.

Elevated Blood Cholesterol

Too much cholesterol in the blood can lead to health problems. In the 1960s and 70s, scientists established a link between high blood cholesterol levels and heart disease. Deposits of cholesterol (called *plaque*) can build up inside arteries. Plaque can narrow arteries and reduce the flow of blood in arteries that feed the heart. This narrowing process, called **atherosclerosis**, commonly occurs in arteries that nourish the heart (the coronary arteries). An atherogenic diet (high in saturated fats and low in vegetables, fruits, and whole grains) contributes to this process. When one or more sections of heart muscle fail to get enough blood, and thus the oxygen and nutrients they need, the result may be the chest pain known as *angina*. In addition, plaque can rupture, causing blood clots that may lead to heart attack, stroke, or even sudden death. Fortunately, the buildup of cholesterol can be slowed, stopped, and even reversed. A heart attack occurs when the blood vessels supplying the heart muscle become blocked, limiting the amount of blood that can flow through the artery and thus starving it of oxygen, which leads to the heart muscle's failure or death.

A high level of total cholesterol in the blood (≥ 240 mg/dL) is a major risk factor for heart disease. *Cholesterol* is a fat-like substance made primarily in the liver. The body needs cholesterol for important biological functions. Typically, the body makes all of the cholesterol it needs from the food we eat, but adding too much cholesterol through the diet can increase the risk for heart attack and stroke. Cholesterol-carrying lipoproteins play central roles in the development of atherosclerotic plaque and cardiovascular disease. The two main types of lipoproteins—high and low lipoproteins—basically work in opposing directions.

Low-density lipoproteins (LDL) carry cholesterol from the liver to the rest of the body. When there is too much LDL cholesterol in the blood, it can be deposited on the walls of the coronary arteries. Because of this, LDL cholesterol is often referred to as the "bad" cholesterol.

High-density lipoproteins (HDL) carry cholesterol from the blood back to the liver, where it is processed for elimination from the body. HDL makes it less likely that excess cholesterol in the blood will be deposited in the coronary arteries, which is why HDL cholesterol is often referred to as the "good" cholesterol.

In general, the higher the LDL and the lower the HDL, the greater the risk for atherosclerosis and heart disease. For adults age 20 years and over, the latest guidelines from the National Cholesterol Education Program recommend the following optimal levels:

- Total cholesterol < 200 mg/dL
- HDL cholesterol levels > 40 mg/dL
- LDL cholesterol levels < 100 mg/dL

While it is well known that high blood cholesterol levels are associated with an increased risk for heart disease, scientific studies have shown that there is only a weak relationship between the amount of cholesterol a person consumes and their blood cholesterol levels or risk for heart disease. For some people with high cholesterol, reducing the amount of cholesterol in the diet has a small but helpful impact on blood cholesterol levels. For others, the amount of cholesterol eaten has little impact on the amount of cholesterol circulating in the blood.

One of the most important determinants of blood cholesterol level is fat in the diet; this is not total fat, but specific types of fat. Some types of fat are clearly good for cholesterol levels and others are clearly bad for them.

The Bad Fats

Some fats are considered "bad" because they tend to worsen blood cholesterol levels.

Saturated Fats. Saturated fats are mainly animal fats and are found in meat, seafood, whole-milk dairy products (cheese, milk, and ice cream), poultry skin, and egg yolks. Some plant foods are also high in saturated fats, including coconut and coconut oil, palm oil, and palm kernel oil. Saturated fats raise total blood cholesterol levels more than dietary cholesterol because they tend to boost both good HDL and bad LDL cholesterol. The net effect is negative, meaning it's important to limit saturated fats.

Trans Fats. *Trans fatty acids* are fats produced by heating liquid vegetable oils in the presence of hydrogen, a process is known as *hydrogenation*. The more hydrogenated an oil is, the more solid it will be at room temperature. For example, spreadable tub margarine is less hydrogenated and so has fewer trans fats than stick margarine.

Most of the trans fats in the American diet are found in commercially prepared baked goods, margarines, snack foods, and processed foods. Commercially prepared fried foods, like French fries and onion rings, also contain a good deal of trans fat.

Trans fats are even worse for cholesterol levels than saturated fats because they raise bad LDL and lower good HDL. They also fire inflammation, an overactivity of the immune system that has been implicated in heart disease, stroke, diabetes, and other chronic conditions. While intake of saturated fats should be limited, it is important to entirely eliminate trans fats from partially hydrogenated oils.

The Good Fats

Some fats are considered "good" because they can improve blood cholesterol levels.

Unsaturated Fats: Polyunsaturated and Monounsaturated. Unsaturated fats are found in products derived from plant sources, such as vegetable oils, nuts, and seeds. There are two main categories: polyunsaturated fats (which are found in high concentrations in sunflower, corn, and soybean oils) and monounsaturated fats (which are found in high concentra-

tions in canola, peanut, and olive oils). In studies in which polyunsaturated and monounsaturated fats were eaten in place of carbohydrates, these good fats decreased LDL levels and increased HDL levels.

Omega-3 fatty acids, a type of polyunsaturated fat, may decrease the risk of heart attack, protect against irregular heartbeats, and lower blood pressure. Some fish are a good natural source of omega-3s (wild salmon, halibut). However, pregnant women and women of childbearing age should avoid shark, swordfish, king mackerel, and tilefish because they contain levels of mercury high enough to pose a danger to a developing fetus. For most others, the health benefits of fish outweigh any risks associated with mercury. Omega-3s are present in smaller amounts in flaxseed oil, walnut oil, soybean oil, and canola oil; they can also be found in supplements.

Table 10-1[5] provides more information on the various types of "bad" and "good" fats.

Dietary Fiber

Dietary fiber is the term for several materials that comprise the parts of plants our bodies can't digest. Fiber is classified as soluble or insoluble. When eaten regularly as part of a diet low in saturated fat and cholesterol, *soluble fiber* has been shown to help lower blood cholesterol. Oats have the highest proportion of soluble fiber of any grain. Foods high in soluble fiber include oat bran, oatmeal, beans, peas, rice bran, barley, citrus fruits, strawberries, and apple pulp.

TABLE 10-1 Dietary Fats

Type of Fat	Main Source	State at Room Temperature	Effect on Cholesterol Levels Compared with Carbohydrates
Monounsaturated	Olives; olive oil, canola oil, peanut oil; cashews, almonds, peanuts, and most other nuts; avocados	Liquid	Lowers LDL; raises HDL
Polyunsaturated	Corn, soybean, safflower, and cottonseed oils; fish	Liquid	Lowers LDL; raises HDL
Saturated	Whole milk, butter, cheese, and ice cream; red meat; chocolate; coconuts, coconut milk, and coconut oil	Solid	Raises both LDL and HDL
Trans	Most margarines; vegetable shortening; partially hydrogenated vegetable oil; deep-fried chips; many fast foods; most commercial baked goods	Solid or semi-solid	Raises LDL*

Source: Harvard School of Public Health. Fats and Cholesterol—The Good, The Bad, and The Healthy Diet. Available at http://www.hsph.harvard.edu/ nutritionsource/fats.html. Accessed April 2, 2008.

*Trans fat increases LDL, decreases HDL, and increases triglycerides when compared to monounsaturated or polyunsaturated fat.

Insoluble fiber does not seem to help lower blood cholesterol. However, it is an important aid in normal bowel function. Foods high in insoluble fiber include whole wheat breads, wheat cereals, wheat bran, rye, rice, barley, most other whole grains, cabbage, beets, carrots, Brussels sprouts, turnips, cauliflower, and apple skin.

Sodium and Salt in the Diet

A high sodium intake increases blood pressure in some people, who are "salt sensitive." Cutting back on sodium intake will help these people the most.

The terms *salt* and *sodium* tend to be used interchangeably, but they are not really the same. Salt is a chemical made up of about 40 percent sodium and 60 percent chloride. Sodium is an essential mineral that we need to survive. Some amount of sodium is found in all foods. However, sodium that occurs naturally and salt added to foods at the dinner table are not the major sources of sodium in our diet. Most of the sodium in foods is added during food processing. In fact, up to 4,000 milligrams of sodium that the average American ingests each day comes from processed foods. While some foods have an obvious salty taste—such as pretzels, pickles, and soy sauce—many people are unaware that some favorite foods contain quite a lot of sodium, including: canned soup and dry soup mixes, barbecue sauce, cereal, catsup, luncheon meat, cheese, mustard, crackers, salad dressing, and sausage. Hidden sodium can be uncovered by reading the ingredient list on a food package. Some examples of high sodium ingredients are: monosodium glutamate (MSG), sodium benzoate, baking soda, and baking powder.

Does Folic Acid Play a Role?

There has been much enthusiasm about the possible role of folic acid supplements in preventing and treating heart disease, but multiple clinical trials involving folic acid supplements have shown no such heart benefits. Folic acid (folate) and other B vitamins help break down homocysteine, an amino acid in blood. Too much homocysteine is associated with an increased risk of heart disease. For this reason, some scientists have speculated that folic acid supplements may lower homocysteine levels, which in turn may reduce the risk of heart disease. However, this effect has not been proven. Also, it is unclear whether high homocysteine levels are a direct cause or simply the result of coronary artery disease. At this time, the American Heart Association (AHA) does not recommend use of folic acid supplements by the general public to reduce the risk of heart disease. However, if a person is at high risk of heart disease, the AHA does recommend a diet rich in folic acid (folate) and other B vitamins. Good food sources of folate include citrus fruits, tomatoes, vegetables, and grain products.

Medical science does not understand why most cases of high blood pressure occur, so it is difficult to say how to prevent it. However, we do know of several factors that may contribute to high blood pressure and raise the risk for heart attack and stroke (discussed earlier).

DIABETES MELLITUS

Diabetes affects more than 230 million people worldwide and is expected to affect 350 million by 2025. The five countries in 2003 with the largest numbers of people with diabetes were India (35.5 million), China (23.8 million), the United States (16 million), Russia (9.7 million), and Japan (6.7 million). The five countries in 2003 with the highest diabetes prevalence in the adult population were Nauru (30.2%), United Arab Emirates (20.1%), Qatar (16%), Bahrain (14.9%), and Kuwait (12.8%). By 2025, the number of people with diabetes is expected to more than double in Africa, the Eastern Mediterranean region, Middle East, and Southeast Asia, and rise by 20 percent in Europe, 50 percent in North America, 85 percent in South and Central America, and 75 percent in the Western Pacific. Each year, a further 6 million people develop diabetes.

Diabetes is the fourth leading cause of death by disease globally. Each year over 3 million deaths are tied directly to diabetes. Every 10 seconds a person dies from diabetes-related causes. At least 50 percent of all people with diabetes are unaware of their condition. In some countries this statistic may reach 80 percent. In 2003, diabetes prevalence worldwide was estimated at 5.1 percent among people aged 20 to 79 years. Although diabetes is still more common in developed countries, it is rapidly increasing in developing countries. By 2025, the worldwide prevalence is projected to be 6.3 percent, a 24-percent increase over the 2003 rate, largely due to greater food availability and increased consumption of sugar and fats. The prevalence of diabetes is higher in men than women, but the number of women with diabetes is greater than the numbers of men. The most important demographic change to diabetes prevalence across the world appears to be the increase in the proportion of people 65 years of age.

Diabetes is becoming more common in the United States. From 1980 through 2004, the number of Americans with diabetes more than doubled (from 5.8 million to 14.7 million). Diabetes affects more women than men. The prevalence of diabetes is 70 percent higher among African Americans and nearly 100 percent higher among Hispanics than among whites. The prevalence of diabetes among American Indians and Alaska Natives is more than twice that of the total population; the Pima Nation in Arizona has the highest known prevalence of diabetes in the world. People aged 65 years and older account for almost 40 percent of the population with diabetes. About one

CASE STUDIES
Cardiovascular Disease

Ahmed, an Egyptian with High Cholesterol

A 49-year-old engineer named Ahmed living in Cairo had a mild heart attack. He was admitted to a large, private hospital where tests revealed that his blood cholesterol was high and that he had numerous arteries blocked by atherosclerosis. In addition, he had uncontrolled hypertension and a family history of diabetes. Most of his siblings had developed type 2 diabetes as adults. He underwent bypass surgery and recovered sufficiently to be able to return to work.

At first he tried to eat better at the urging of his daughter, a young physician, and did a bit of strolling on a walking track at the local club, but gradually he returned to his old habits. He generally started the day with sweetened tea before leaving for work, ate a large breakfast of bread, cheese, and sometimes beans in the midmorning, and around 4 p.m. when he returned home from work, he ate a large dinner with his wife and daughters. Dinner generally consisted of meat and/or chicken, rice and/or potatoes or pasta, and cooked vegetables and salad as well as bread. Soda or fruit juice was most often the beverage consumed with the meal, followed by sweetened tea. Later in the evening, a snack consisting of cheese or yogurt and fruit were often consumed. He tried to quit smoking, but failed. Ahmed was 5'6" tall, weighed 165 pounds, and had the belly fat typical of an out-of-shape middle-aged man.

At 60 years of age, he retired and spent most of his time chatting with family and friends over endless cups of coffee and tea. His only physical activity was walking up and down the stairs in his apartment building once a day. He developed chest pains, and it was recommended that he have bypass surgery once again. Although his family pleaded with him to quit smoking, exercise regularly, and eat a healthier diet, he was content with his old behaviors. He had a massive heart attack and died at age 63.

1. What basic information have you gathered about Ahmed?
2. What information is available about Ahmed's eating habits? Are there any positive aspects to his patterns in terms of risk reduction? What harmful eating behaviors may have contributed to his risk of heart disease?
3. Are there any other lifestyle factors that played a role in his coronary vascular disease?
4. How should Ahmed's doctor have counseled him to lower his blood pressure and reduce his risk of another heart attack?

Gladys, an African-American Liscensed Practical Nurse (LPN) with Hypertension

Gladys is a widowed mother of four children aged 25, 21, 18, and 14, all of whom live with her in a low income area of Washington, D.C. She works as an LPN at a large hospital, just a few Metro stops away. Her income is barely sufficient to pay the mortgage on their home, utilities, transportation, and other expenses. Fortunately, she has medical insurance through her job for herself and her two youngest children. Her oldest son is currently unemployed and looking for work. Her second child, a daughter, is attending a local university on a scholarship. The 18-year-old boy is graduating from high school this year and thinking about joining the Marines. Her baby girl is in high school, and going through a terrible period of adolescence. Gladys loves her children, but worries about them and their futures. She sometimes feels overwhelmed by the responsibilities she carries all on her own.

Gladys has had high blood pressure since she was in her twenties. Her mother and father both had uncontrolled hypertension. They had small strokes before her mother died from a massive stroke and her father from kidney failure. She is 63 inches tall and weighs 158 pounds. Despite taking medication to control her hypertension, it still measures above 140/90 most days.

Gladys cooks breakfast and dinner at home every day. For lunch, she eats at the hospital cafeteria and the kids eat at school or in local fast food restaurants. There is a small grocery store a block from their home, and Gladys does most of her shopping there on her way home from work. Breakfast usually consists of sweetened cereal and milk during the week, but when she has weekends off, she cooks large breakfasts of ham, eggs, bacon, and toast. For dinner, she generally cooks chicken or meat with potatoes or a casserole and canned vegetables. Everyone in the family likes soda with their meals, so there is always a big container of soft drinks on the table for the family meals.

1. What information have you gathered about Gladys?
2. What nutrition-related risk factors have you identified in her eating patterns?
3. What is her BMI? What lifestyle factors are contributing to her hypertension?
4. How would you counsel Gladys to help her reduce her blood pressure?

CLINICAL PERSPECTIVE FOR THE INDIVIDUAL PATIENT

This section covers the recommendations for prevention of cardiovascular disease in individuals, and nutrition-related strategies for reducing risk factors for heart disease and stroke.

1. Nutrition-Related Prevention

For the two out of three Americans who do not smoke or drink alcohol excessively, the one choice that can influence long-term health prospects more than any other is diet (Table 10-2).

Consistently eating a diet rich in fruits, vegetables, whole grains, and low-fat dairy products can help protect the heart. Legumes, low-fat sources of protein, and certain types of fish also can reduce the risk of heart disease. Heart-healthy eating is not all about cutting back. Most people, for instance, need to add more fruits and vegetables to their diet, with a goal of five to ten servings a day. An enormous amount of data suggests that fruits and vegetables are highly effective in preventing not just cardiovascular disease, but cancer and other diseases as well. Following a heart-healthy diet means drinking alcohol only in moderation (no more than two drinks a day for men, one a day for women). At that moderate level, alcohol can have a protective effect on your heart. Above that, it becomes a health hazard.

2. Reduction of Nutrition-Related Heart Disease Risks

Although most people probably know that some of their behaviors contribute to risk of heart disease, it is often tough to change day-to-day habits. Whether one has years of unhealthy eating history or simply wants to fine-tune his or her diet, here are five heart-smart strategies to get started. Once a person knows which foods to emphasize and which foods to limit or avoid, he or she can create meal plans to stay on track.

KEY DIETARY STRATEGIES FOR HEART HEALTH

- Limit unhealthy fats and cholesterol
- Choose low-fat protein sources
- Eat more fruits and vegetables
- Select whole grains
- Practice moderation and balance

TABLE 10-2 American Heart Association (AHA) 2006 Diet and Lifestyle Recommendations for Cardiovascular Disease Risk Reduction

- Balance calorie intake and physical activity to achieve or maintain a healthy body weight.
- Consume a diet rich in vegetables and fruits.
- Choose whole-grain, high-fiber foods.
- Consume fish, especially oily fish, at least twice a week.
- Limit intake of saturated fat to 7 percent of energy, trans fat to 1 percent of energy, and cholesterol to 300 mg per day by:
  - choosing lean meats and vegetable alternatives;
  - selecting fat-free (skim), 1 percent fat, and low-fat dairy products; *and*
  - minimizing intake of partially hydrogenated fats.

Source: AHA Scientific Statement. Diet and Lifestyle Recommendations Revision 2006. *Circulation* 2006;114:82–96.

Limit Unhealthy Fats and Cholesterol. Of the possible dietary changes, limiting how much saturated and trans fats eaten is the most important step to reduce blood cholesterol and lower risk of coronary artery disease. Table 10-3 lists American Heart Association guidelines for how much fat and cholesterol to include in the diet.

The best way to reduce intake of saturated and trans fats is to limit the amount of solid fat—butter, margarine, and shortening—added to food when cooking and serving. Major sources of saturated fat include beef, cheese, whole milk, and coconut and palm oils. Sources of trans fat include deep-fried fast foods, bakery products, packaged snack foods, margarines, and crackers. Use low-fat substitutions when possible. For example, top a baked potato with salsa or low-fat yogurt rather than butter, or use sugar-free fruit spread on toast instead of margarine.

TABLE 10-3 Recommended Daily Fat and Cholesterol Intake

Type of Fat	Recommendation
Saturated fat	Less than 7 percent of total daily calories
Trans fat	Less than 1 percent of total daily calories
Cholesterol	Less than 300 milligrams a day for healthy adults; less than 200 milligrams a day for adults with high levels of LDL ("bad") cholesterol or those who are taking cholesterol-lowering medication

Source: Data are from AHA. Consumer FAQ - General Information about Fats. Available at http://www.americanheart.org/presenter.jhtml?identifier=3046391. Accessed April 2, 2008.

TABLE 10-4 Fats or Oils to Use When Cooking or Baking

Choose	Avoid
• Olive oil	• Butter
• Canola oil	• Lard
• Margarine labeled "trans fat-free"	• Bacon
• Cholesterol-lowering margarine, such as Benecol or Take Control	• Gravy
	• Cream sauce
	• Nondairy creamers
	• Hydrogenated margarine and shortening
	• Cocoa butter, found in chocolate
	• Coconut, palm, and palm-kernel oils

Source: Data are from the American Heart Association (AHA). Cooking. Available at http://www.americanheart.org/presenter.jhtml?identifier=3046053. Accessed April 2, 2008.

When using fat, choose monounsaturated fats such as olive oil or canola oil. Polyunsaturated fats, found in nuts and seeds, are a healthier choice as well. When used in place of saturated fat, monounsaturated and polyunsaturated fats may help lower total blood cholesterol. But moderation is essential. All types of fat are high in calories (9 kcal/g).

Use Table 10-4 as a guide when selecting fats or oils to use in cooking or baking.

Choose Low-Fat Protein Sources. Meat, poultry, and fish along with low-fat dairy products and eggs are some of the best sources of protein. Be careful to choose lower fat options, such as skim milk rather than whole milk and skinless chicken breasts rather than fried chicken patties.

Fish is a good alternative to high-fat meats. Some types of fish—cod, tuna, and halibut—have less total fat, saturated fat, and cholesterol than do meat and poultry. Certain types of fish are heart healthy because they are rich in omega-3 fatty acids. These fats may help lower blood fats called **triglycerides** and may reduce risk of sudden cardiac death. Omega-3 fats are most abundant in fatty, cold-water fish, such as salmon, mackerel, and herring. Lesser amounts are in flaxseeds, walnuts, soybeans, and canola oil.

Legumes—beans, peas, and lentils—also are good sources of protein and contain less fat and no cholesterol, making them good substitutes for meat. Soybeans, one type of legume, may be especially beneficial to your heart. Regularly substituting soy protein for animal protein (e.g., a soy burger instead of a beef hamburger) may help lower cholesterol and triglyceride levels.

Eat More Vegetables and Fruits. Vegetables and fruits are low in calories, a good source of vitamins and minerals, and are rich in dietary fiber. A diet high in soluble fiber (found in fruits and vegetables) can help lower blood cholesterol and reduce risk of heart disease. Vegetables and fruits also contain *phytochemicals*, substances found in plants, that may help prevent cardiovascular disease. Eating more fruits and vegetables to satisfy hunger may help a person eat less high-fat foods such as meat, cheese, and processed snack foods.

Featuring vegetables and fruits in a diet may not be as difficult as some people think. Keep raw carrots, cauliflower, and broccoli ready to eat in the refrigerator for quick snacks. Apples, bananas, grapes, or peaches in a bowl in the kitchen are a visual reminder. Choose recipes that have vegetables or fruits as the main ingredient, such as vegetable stir-fry or fresh fruit mixed into salads. Do not smother vegetables in butter, dressings, creamy sauces, or other high-fat garnishes. Avoid fruits in cream or heavy sauces.

Select Whole Grains. Whole grains have not had their bran and germ removed by milling, making them good sources of fiber (the part of plant-based foods your body cannot digest) and other nutrients. Whole grains are a source of vitamins and minerals that include: thiamin, riboflavin, niacin, vitamin E, magnesium, phosphorus, selenium, zinc, and iron. Phytochemicals also are found in whole grains. Various nutrients found in whole grains play a role in regulating blood pressure and heart health.

One can increase the amount of whole grains in the diet by making simple substitutions. For example, choose whole grain breads instead of those with refined white flour, whole wheat pasta over regular pasta, and brown rice instead of white rice. Select high fiber cereals for breakfast, such as bran flakes or shredded wheat, instead of muffins or doughnuts; select whole wheat flour rather than white flour when buying or making baked goods.

Table 10-5 lists whole grain and processed foods that may be useful when choosing what to include in a meal.

Practice Moderation and Balance. Knowing which foods to eat is the first step in creating a heart-healthy diet. However, it is also important to know how much food to consume. Overloading your plate, taking seconds, and eating until stuffed can lead to excess calorie, fat, and cholesterol intake. Portions served in restaurants are often much larger than anyone needs. Keeping track of the number of servings eaten and the use of proper serving sizes can to help control the quantity of food eaten.

A serving size is a specific amount of food, defined by common measurements such as cups, ounces, or pieces. For example, one serving of pasta is 1/2 cup, or about the size of an ice cream scoop. A serving of meat, fish, or chicken is 2 to 3 ounces, or about the size and thickness of a deck of cards. Judging serving size is a learned skill. Patients may need to use measuring cups and spoons and a scale until comfortable with their judgment.

A healthy diet is also about balance. A simple rule of thumb is to keep the portion size for meat, poultry, and fish small, about the size of a deck of cards. This helps make room for ample servings of vegetables, fruits, and whole grains.

An indulgence should be allowed every now and then, but don't let it turn into an excuse for giving up on a healthy-eating plan. If overindulgence is the exception rather than the rule, things will balance out over the long term. What is important is to eat healthy foods most of the time.

TABLE 10-5 Guide to Choosing Cereals, Breads, Rice, and Pasta

Choose	Avoid
• Whole-wheat flour	• Muffins made with white flour
• Whole-grain bread, preferably 100 percent whole wheat or 100 percent whole grain bread	• Frozen waffles
	• Corn bread
	• Doughnuts
	• Biscuits
• High-fiber cereal with 5 or more grams of fiber per serving	• Quick breads
	• Granola bars
	• Cakes
• Brown rice	• Pies
• Whole-grain pasta	• Egg noodles
• Oatmeal	• Buttered popcorn
• Other whole grains like barley, quinoa, and rye	• High-fat snack crackers
	• Chips

Source: Data are from American Heart Association. Available at http://www.americanheart.org/presenter.jhtml?identifier=1200000. Accessed April 2, 2008.

3. Additional Important Strategies to Lower Heart Disease Risk

GUIDE TO LOWERING HEART DISEASE RISK
- Maintain healthy weight
- Decrease abdominal obesity
- Choose plant stanols/sterols
- Achieve blood pressure (systolic and diastolic pressure) < 120/80 mm Hg

Maintain Healthy Weight. A desirable body mass index (BMI) to maintain is between 18.5 and 24.9 (see section on Overweight and Obesity).

Decrease Abdominal Obesity. Excess fat around the trunk of the body is often called central obesity. Waist circumference is an anthropometric measurement used to assess a person's abdominal fat. In order to lower the risk of obesity-related chronic health problems, men should measure less than 40 inches (102 centimeters) around the waist and women less than 35 inches (88 centimeters).

Choose Plant Stanols/Sterols. Plant stanols/sterols can lower LDL cholesterol levels by up to 15% and therefore are seen as a therapeutic option, in addition to diet and lifestyle modification, for individuals with elevated LDL cholesterol levels. Plant sterols work by reducing the intestinal absorption of cholesterol. Maximum effects are observed at plant stanol/sterol intakes of 2 g per day. Plant stanol/sterols are currently available in a wide variety of foods (added to some margarines, cheese, and other products), drinks, and soft gel capsules. The choice of vehicle should be determined by availability and by other considerations, including caloric content. In general, patients need to consume them daily, just as they would use lipid-lowering medication. *Note:* There is a concern that they may also reduce absorption and blood levels of carotenoids.

Achieve Blood Pressure < 120/80 mm Hg. If an adult has blood pressure of 140/90 mm Hg or above, they have hypertension and are at higher risk for heart disease, stroke, and other medical problems. They need to see a doctor and learn how to manage blood pressure and how often to have it checked. High blood pressure has no symptoms. One in three adult Americans has high blood pressure, and nearly one third of them don't know they have it.

4. Guidance to Prevent or Reduce High Blood Pressure

Choose and Prepare Foods with Little or No Salt. On average, as salt (sodium chloride) intake increases, so does blood pressure. Reduced sodium intake can prevent hypertension in nonhypertensive individuals as well as lower blood pressure in the setting of antihypertensive medication and facilitate hypertension control. Reduced sodium intake is associated with a blunted age-related rise in systolic pressure and a reduced risk of atherosclerotic cardiovascular events and congestive heart failure. In general, the effects of sodium reduction on blood pressure tend to be greater in blacks; middle-aged and older-aged persons; and individuals with hypertension, diabetes, or chronic kidney disease. Diets rich in potassium can lower blood pressure and also help blunt the blood pressure-raising effects of increased sodium intake.

> ### FOODS THAT HELP REDUCE SODIUM IN THE DIET
> - Fresh, frozen, or canned food items without added salts.
> - Unsalted nuts or seeds, dried beans, peas, and lentils.
> - Unsalted, fat-free broths, bouillons, or soups.
> - Fat-free (skim) or low-fat milk; low-sodium, low-fat cheeses; and low-fat yogurt.
> - Spices and herbs to enhance the taste of food.

Patients should be encouraged to read the labels when they buy prepared and packaged foods. They should watch for the words "soda" (soda refers to sodium bicarbonate, or baking soda) and "sodium" and the symbol "Na" on labels. These products contain sodium compounds. Most spices contain sodium in very small amounts.

Some drugs contain large amounts of sodium. Patients should make a habit of carefully reading the ingredient list on the label of all over-the-counter drugs and the warning statement to see if sodium is in the product. A statement of sodium content must appear on labels of antacids containing 5 mg or more per dosage unit (tablet, teaspoon, etc.). Some companies now make low-sodium over-the-counter products.

Healthy adults should limit their sodium intake to no more than 2,300 milligrams per day. This is about 1 teaspoon of sodium chloride (salt).

Dietary Approaches to Stop Hypertension (DASH): An Example of a Dietary Plan to Control Hypertension

The **DASH** eating plan[6] developed by the U.S. Department of Health and Human Services has been shown to prevent and reduce high blood pressure. It is rich in fruits and vegetables and low-fat dairy products, moderate in total fat, and low in saturated fat and cholesterol. The DASH diet helps to reduce blood pressure due to generous amounts of potassium. It is even more effective when salt and sodium intake are also reduced. This eating plan can help people lose weight, which also will help to lower blood pressure.

The DASH diet was developed and tested in a multi-center, randomized feeding study, designed to compare impact on blood pressure of three dietary patterns:

1. A control diet (similar to typical American diet)
2. A diet rich in fruits and vegetables
3. A combination diet emphasizing fruits and vegetables and low-fat dairy, with whole grains, and reduced fats and sweets.

The study team concluded that the dietary pattern reflected in the combination diet can substantially reduce blood pressure and, accordingly, provides an additional lifestyle approach to preventing and treating hypertension.

third of persons with diabetes in the United States are unaware they have diabetes because it has not been diagnosed.

These data indicate that the "diabetes epidemic" will continue even if levels of obesity (a major cause of diabetes) remain constant. Given the increasing prevalence of obesity, it is likely that these figures provide an underestimate of future diabetes prevalence.

Diabetes mellitus is a group of diseases characterized by high levels of **blood glucose** (sugar in blood that is the body's main source of energy) resulting from defects in insulin production, insulin action, or both. Diabetes can be associated with serious complications and premature death, but people with diabetes can take steps to control the disease and lower the risk of complications.

Types of Diabetes

Type 1 Diabetes

- Accounts for 5 to 10 percent of all cases
- Strong genetic component with possible environmental trigger
- Occurs during childhood or adolescence
- Symptoms may appear abruptly
- Classic symptoms are: frequent urination, weight loss, increased thirst, and ketoacidosis that may occur due to excessive production of ketone bodies
- Formerly called juvenile or insulin-dependent diabetes

Type 2 Diabetes

- Accounts for 90 to 95 percent of all cases
- Risk increases with age
- Principal defect is insulin resistance
- Reduced sensitivity to insulin in muscle, adipose, and liver cells
- To compensate, the **pancreas** (a digestive organ) secretes larger amounts of insulin
- Can have devastating complications
- Formerly called adult-onset or noninsulin-dependant diabetes

Gestational Diabetes

A third type of diabetes is gestational diabetes. This type is characterized by **hyperglycemia** (raised blood sugar) that is first recognized during pregnancy. With gestational diabetes, a woman may have glucose (sugar) in her blood at a higher than normal level during the second half of her pregnancy. In about 95 percent of cases, blood sugar returns to normal after the pregnancy is over. Women who develop gestational dia-

betes, however, are at risk for developing type 2 diabetes later in life.

Nutrition-Related Risk Factors

- BMI of 25 or more
- Prediabetes: impaired glucose tolerance and impaired fasting glucose
- Lack of regular exercise
- Abnormal **lipid** (fat) levels

To determine whether a patient has pre-diabetes or diabetes, healthcare providers conduct a fasting plasma glucose test (FPG) or an oral glucose tolerance test (OGTT). Either test can be used to diagnose prediabetes or diabetes. The American Diabetes Association recommends the FPG because it is easier, faster, and less expensive to perform. With the FPG test, a fasting **blood glucose level** between 100 and 125 mg/dL signals prediabetes. A person with a fasting blood glucose level of 126 mg/dL or higher has diabetes.

Link with Obesity

Type 2 diabetes is now epidemic, affecting women in greater numbers than men. It is expected to rise almost another 40% over the next 3 decades in North America and even higher in other parts of the world. In just a little more than a decade, prevalence of diabetes has nearly doubled in the American adult population, from 4.9 percent in 1990 to 8.7 percent in 2002. Adults are no longer the only victims; more and more children are developing this health-robbing disease or its precursor, prediabetes. The reason for this runaway epidemic is the increase in overweight and obesity in the population, especially the accumulation of large amounts of body fat around the abdomen.

Mechanisms of Action

Diabetes mellitus is a group of disorders characterized by elevated blood glucose concentrations and disordered insulin metabolism. In diabetes, the body is unable to secrete sufficient insulin, use insulin effectively, or both. **Glucose** is the sugar molecule that is a major source of fuel for the body. **Carbohydrates** (starches, vegetables, fruits, dairy products, and sugars) are broken down into glucose energy blocks for the cells. It is absorbed from the intestines into the blood where it travels to the liver and other organs. **Insulin** is a hormone made by specialized cells in the pancreas. Its whole job is to push glucose out of the blood into various cells of the body. Insulin secretions normally increase after ingestion of food, enabling adipose cells to take up newly absorbed glucose from the blood. This occurs between meals in smaller amounts to restrain the glucose-raising actions of **glucagon** (a pancreas-secreting hormone) and the subsequent breakdown of **glycogen** (animal polysaccharide stored in liver and muscles).

Obesity and weight gain are key risk factors for diabetes. Both are caused by a disproportionate intake of energy as food compared with the amount of energy expended through physical exercise. Each unit increase in the body mass index, a common measure of body weight, boosts the risk of diabetes by 12 percent. Central obesity, or disproportionate build-up of fat in the body's trunk region, is another leading risk factor, as is a sedentary lifestyle. Diet plays a strong role. A high intake of sugar-sweetened beverages, saturated fats, and trans fatty acids increases the risk of diabetes. In contrast, regular physical activity and diets including polyunsaturated fats, long-chain omega-3 fatty acids (found in fish oils), and rich in fiber and vegetables may reduce the risk of diabetes.

Likewise, socioeconomic status appears to influence the risk of developing diabetes, but the relationship operates differently in developed than in developing countries. In developing economies, diabetes is linked to increased affluence and Westernization, especially among indigenous populations. But in developed countries, people in lower socioeconomic groups have a higher risk of obesity and type 2 diabetes.

Weight loss helps people with diabetes in two important ways. First, it lowers insulin resistance. This allows natural insulin (in people with type 2 diabetes) to do a better job lowering blood glucose levels. If one takes a diabetes medicine, losing weight lowers blood glucose and may allow reducing the amount of medication or eliminating it altogether. Second, it improves blood fat and blood pressure levels. People with diabetes are about twice as likely to get cardiovascular disease as other people. Lowering blood fats and blood pressure is a way to reduce that risk.

CANCER

Cancer is not a single disease, but represents hundreds of diseases, each one requiring specialized approaches to treatment. Cancer is caused by a variety of identified and unidentified factors. The most important established cause of cancer is tobacco smoking. Other important determinants of cancer risk include diet, alcohol, and physical activity, infections, hormonal factors, and radiation. The relative importance of cancers as a cause of death is increasing, mostly because of the increasing proportion of people who are older but also the reduction in mortality from other causes, especially infectious diseases. The incidence of cancers of the lung, colon and rectum, breast, and prostate generally increases in parallel with economic trends.

Cancer is now a major cause of mortality throughout the world and, in the developed world, is generally exceeded only by cardiovascular diseases. An estimated 10 million new cases and over 6 million deaths from cancer occurred in 2000. As developing countries become urbanized, patterns of cancer (including those most strongly associated with diet) tend to shift toward those of economically developed countries. Between 2000 and 2020, the total number of cases of cancer in the developing world is predicted to increase by 73 percent and in the developed world by 29 percent, largely as a result of an increase in the number of older people.

Physical inactivity, obesity, and poor nutrition are major preventable causes of cancer and other diseases in the United States. The American Cancer Society estimates that in 2006, approximately one third (188,277) of the 564,830 cancer deaths expected to occur will be related to poor nutrition, physical inactivity, overweight, and obesity.

Dietary factors are estimated to account for approximately 30 percent of cancers in industrialized countries, making diet second only to tobacco as a theoretically preventable cause of cancer. This proportion is thought to be about 20 percent in developing countries, but may grow with dietary change, particularly if the importance of other causes of mortality, especially infections, declines. Cancer rates change as populations move between countries and adopt different dietary (and other) behaviors, further implicating dietary factors in the etiology of cancer. Body weight and physical inactivity together are estimated to account for approximately one-fifth to one-third of several of the most common cancers, specifically cancers of the breast (postmenopausal), colon, endometrium, kidney, and esophagus (adenocarcinoma).

Nutrition-Related Risk Factors

Research to date has uncovered few definite relationships between diet and cancer risk. Dietary factors for which there is convincing evidence for an increase in risk are overweight and obesity, high consumption of alcoholic beverages, aflatoxins, and some forms of salting and fermenting fish. There is also convincing evidence to indicate that physical activity decreases the risk of colon cancer. Factors that probably increase risk include high dietary intake of preserved meats, salt-preserved foods and salt, and very hot (thermally) drinks and food. Probable protective factors are consumption of fruits and vegetables, and physical activity (for breast cancer). After tobacco, overweight and obesity appear to be the most important known avoidable causes of cancer.

If Americans ate a healthy, balanced diet that emphasized plant foods and maintained a healthy body weight, as many as one third of all cancer deaths in the United Sates could be prevented. Factors that can affect cancer risk include types of foods, how food is prepared, portion sizes, fat content, food variety, and overall balance of the diet. For the majority of Americans who do not use tobacco, dietary choices and physical activity are the most important modifiable determinants of cancer risk. Obesity is estimated to cause 14 percent of cancer deaths in men and 20 percent of cancer deaths in women.

Over the past few decades, recommendations for healthy diets have been developed by many federal government agencies and national voluntary organizations such as the American Cancer Society. These recommendations are based on strong evidence and state-of-the-art research that demonstrate that consuming a diet of mostly plant foods (vegetables, fruits, whole grains, beans), limiting saturated fat and added sugars, and maintaining a healthy weight (BMI less than 25) are associated with a reduced risk of chronic diseases, including many types of cancer.

Numerous scientific studies have demonstrated that dietary habits affect cancers at many sites. Strong evidence has concluded that diets high in fruits and vegetables have protective effects against lung, oral, esophageal, stomach, and colon cancers. Overweight and obesity are associated with increased risk for cancers of the breast, colon and rectum, endometrium, esophagus, and kidney. Evidence is highly suggestive that obesity also increases risk for cancers of the pancreas, gallbladder, thyroid, ovary, and cervix as well as multiple myeloma, Hodgkin lymphoma, and aggressive prostate cancer. Alcohol consumption is an established cause of cancers of the mouth, pharynx, larynx, esophagus, and liver. Extensive evidence also implicates alcohol as a cause of breast cancer and probably colorectal cancer.

Limited Fruit and Vegetable Consumption Is a Cancer Risk

To help prevent cancers and other chronic diseases, experts recommend 4 to 13 servings of fruits and vegetables daily, depending on energy needs. This includes two to five servings of fruits and two to eight servings of vegetables, with special emphasis on dark-green and orange vegetables and legumes. There is no evidence that the popular white potato protects against cancer.

Fat Consumption and Cancer

Some studies have linked high-fat diets or high intake of different types of fat in the diet to several cancers, including cancers of the colon, prostate, lung, and endometrium as well as heart disease and other chronic diseases. Saturated and trans fatty acids are thought to be the most harmful fats.

More research is needed to better understand which types of fat and what amounts alter cancer risk. Although monounsaturated and polyunsaturated fatty acids have been studied for a number of years, their effects are still unclear. More recent research on the effects of trans fatty acids also has yet to reach definitive conclusions.

The *2005 Dietary Guidelines for Americans* recommend getting less than 10 percent of calories from saturated fatty acids and keeping trans fatty acid consumption as low as possible for general health and the prevention of chronic disease, including cancer and heart disease. The Guidelines also recommend keeping total fat intake between 20 and 35 percent of calories, with most fats coming from sources of polyunsaturated and monounsaturated fatty acids, such as fish, nuts, and vegetable oils.

Dietary Guidelines to Reduce Cancer Risk

DIETARY GUIDELINES TO REDUCE CANCER RISK
- Eating a variety of fruits and vegetables
- Consuming anticarcinogens
- Avoid unhealthy cooking practices
- Lose excess weight
- Specific nutrients may help

Fruits and Vegetables. Fruits and vegetables contain dietary compounds that reduce cancer risk. Consuming adequate amounts of a variety of fruits and vegetables every day is proven to reduce cancer risk. The most likely reason for the beneficial action of fruits and vegetables is their high content of anticarcinogenic nutrients and nonnutrient compounds.

Anticarcinogens. **Anticarcinogens** include polyphenols, isothiocyanates, antioxidants, phytoestrogens, folate, and fiber. Preventative anticarcinogens act by enhancing an organism's natural defenses against cancer, by deactivating **carcinogens**, or by blocking the mechanisms by which carcinogens act (such as free radical damage to DNA).

Fruits and vegetables provide a variety of anticarcinogens (polyphenols, isothiocyanates, and others) and **antioxidants** (vitamins C and E, carotenoids; adequate selenium is needed as a cofactor for free-radical scavenging enzymes) and dietary fiber (reduces fecal transit time, provides bulking, and dilutes carcinogens in the colon). Other food components likely to reduce cancer risks include phytoestrogens (in soy and other vegetables), calcium, and folate. The recent recommendations of the World Cancer Research Fund and the American Institute for Cancer Research (AICR) "to eat mostly foods of plant origin"[8] can help protect against cancers of var-

CASE STUDY
Jeff Has a Diagnosis of Prediabetes

As a 40-year-old farm manager, Jeff is a large man at 77 inches tall and weight of 270 pounds. He works seven days a week as the manager of a private New Mexico farm that raises horses, cattle, and some alfalfa. He also co-owns a small trucking enterprise and drives one of their trucks three or four days each week. Jeff is married with two young children.

Jeff sips black coffee all day and drinks an occasional diet soda. He does not drink alcohol. He eats breakfast at home, lunch on the road, and has dinner at home most evenings when he drags himself in from work. He needs a lot of fuel for his hard physical work and eats large meals three times daily. He hasn't been feeling well lately and went to see his doctor for an annual check-up. The doctor told him that he has prediabetes and must lose weight. Jeff's mother had type 2 diabetes so he knows how hard it was for her to resist sweets.

Jeff joined a local health club and works out for an hour every day when he is not on the road driving a truck. He thinks about losing weight, but denies that he is putting his health at risk by being so large. He works hard on the farm and in the trucking business and believes he should weigh a lot at 6'5"!

1. What information have you gathered about Jeff?
2. What nutrition-related habits are increasing Jeff's risk of diabetes?
3. Is his BMI putting him at risk for diabetes?
4. What should his healthcare providers do to help him reduce his risk of diabetes?

CLINICAL PERSPECTIVE FOR THE INDIVIDUAL PATIENT
Prevention of Diabetes through Good Eating Habits

FIVE STEPS TO PREVENT DIABETES
1. Lose extra weight
2. Eat plenty of fiber
3. Skip fad diets
4. Choose whole grains
5. Increase physical activity

Lose Extra Weight. For overweight people, diabetes prevention may hinge on weight loss. Every pound lost can improve health. In one study, overweight adults who lost a modest amount of weight—5 percent to 10 percent of their initial body weight—and exercised regularly, reduced the risk of developing diabetes by 58 percent over three years.

To keep weight in a healthy range, permanent changes to eating and exercise habits are important. A healthy weight depends on a person's height, so recommendations for a healthy weight are often expressed in terms of **body mass index (BMI)**, a measure of body fat based on height and weight.

Skip Fad Diets. Low-carbohydrate, high-protein, or other fad diets may help people lose weight at first, but they are not likely to help maintain a healthy weight in the long run. By excluding or strictly limiting a particular food group, one may be giving up essential nutrients. Instead, variety and portion control as part of an overall healthy-eating plan can help. The Dietary Guidelines for Americans, 2006,[7] contains solid healthy eating recommendations for the general public that can help reduce risk of diabetes and other chronic conditions.

Eat Plenty of Fiber. It's rough, it's tough, and it can reduce the risk of diabetes by improving blood sugar control. Fiber also reduces the risk of heart disease. It can even promote weight loss by helping one feel full longer. People should aim for 25 to 50 grams of fiber a day. Foods high in fiber include fruits, vegetables, beans, whole grains, nuts, and seeds.

Choose Whole Grains. Whole grains are another important piece in the diabetes prevention puzzle. Aim to make at least half of grains consumed whole grains. After eating white bread and baking with refined flour for years, switching to whole grains actually is easy. Many foods made from whole grains now come ready to eat, including various breads, pasta products, and packaged cereals. Look for the word "whole" on the package and among the first few items in the ingredients list. Choose items with at least 3 grams of fiber per serving.

Exercise. Increasing physical activity can help people lose weight. But even if it doesn't, it's still important to get off the couch. Physical activity lowers blood sugar and boosts sensitivity to insulin, which helps keep blood sugar within a normal range. A minimum of 30 minutes of moderate physical activity a day is a good goal.

When it comes to type 2 diabetes—the most common type—prevention is extremely important. Many people have no signs or symptoms to alert them to diabetes. Symptoms can be so mild that most people will not notice them. Some people have symptoms but do not suspect diabetes. Symptoms may include:

- increased thirst
- increased hunger
- fatigue
- increased urination, especially at night
- weight loss
- blurred vision
- sores that do not heal

Many people do not find out they have the disease until they have diabetes complications, such as blurry vision or heart trouble. Finding out early about diabetes is important because treatment can prevent damage to the body.

Prediabetes. Before people develop type 2 diabetes, they almost always have prediabetes symptoms that include blood glucose levels that are higher than normal but not yet high enough to be diagnosed as diabetes. About 41 million people in the United States, ages 40 to 74, have prediabetes. Recent research has shown that some long-term damage to the body, especially the heart and circulatory system, may already be occurring during prediabetes. Research also has shown that action to control blood glucose in prediabetes can delay or even prevent type 2 diabetes from ever developing.

Nutrition Management of Diabetes

Adopting and adhering to a healthy eating plan are the first steps in taking care of diabetes. The goals of **medical nutrition therapy** are:

- To keep blood glucose levels near normal by balancing food with diabetes medications and activity levels
- To reach optimal levels of fats in the blood (cholesterol and triglycerides)
- To ensure the right amount of calories for keeping or reaching reasonable weight for adults
- To prevent, delay, or treat food-related risk factors and complications
- To improve overall health through healthy living

The diabetes nutrition guidelines of the past were rigid and monotonous. Dietitians had to provide a standardized diabetic diet to all people with diabetes. The diabetic diet was a strict, artificial distribution of calories from carbohydrate, protein, and fat; the major restriction was the strict avoidance of "simple sugars." Foods with added sugar, such as desserts, were to be strictly avoided. Even the intake of fruit and milk with "natural" sugars was carefully controlled.

The American Diabetes Association and prominent researchers in the field of diabetes studied the published findings from scientific studies on nutrition and diabetes for many years. They concluded, in the *Nutrition Principles for the Management of Diabetes and Related Complications* (1994), that there was little scientific evidence to suggest that sugar is more quickly digested and absorbed into the bloodstream than starch (complex carbohydrates), or that sugar elevates blood glucose more than starch. Sugar, we have learned, has about the same effect on blood glucose as any other carbohydrate. Therefore, the use of sugar (sucrose) as part of the total carbohydrate content of the diet is okay for people with diabetes, as long as these sugar-containing foods are substituted for other carbohydrate foods as part of a balanced meal plan. Nutrition therapy is not about avoiding sugar, but rather about controlling glucose.

The current nutrition guidelines are more flexible and offer a wide variety of food choices. People with diabetes have the same nutritional needs as everyone else. Along with exercise and medications (insulin and other medication), nutrition is important for good diabetes control. By eating well-balanced meals in the correct amounts, a patient can keep blood glucose level as close to normal (non-diabetes level) as possible.

Dietitians now recommend that people with diabetes use a meal plan as a guide for healthy eating, with a balance of nutrients tailor-made for each person's food likes and dislikes, lifestyle, health risks, and diabetes medications. Instead of a diabetic diet, meal planning for people with diabetes is now called *medical nutrition therapy*.

A diabetes meal plan is a guide that tells a patient how much and what kinds of food they can choose to eat at meals and snack times. A good meal plan should fit in with one's schedule and eating habits. The right meal plan will help a patient improve blood glucose, blood pressure, and cholesterol numbers, and also help keep weight within normal limits. People with diabetes have to take extra care to make sure that their food is balanced with insulin and oral medications, and exercise to help manage their blood glucose levels. A doctor and/or dietitian or a certified diabetes educator can help create a meal plan that is appropriate for an individual and their family.

When a person with diabetes makes healthy food choices, they will improve overall health as well as prevent complications such as heart disease, some cancers, and hypertension.

ious sites. A "plant-based diet" should contain a variety of plant foods high in nutrients and include non-starchy vegetables and roots and tubers as well as fruits that are rich sources of phytonutrients.

Cooking Practices. Avoiding unfavorable cooking practices can help to reduce cancer risk. Examples of carcinogen-generating procedures are nitrite-curing, charbroiling, and smoking foods.

Overweight and Obesity. Being overweight or obese is clearly linked with an increased risk of developing several types of cancers. Some studies have shown a link between losing weight and lowering the risk of getting certain cancers such as breast cancer. While research in this area is still ongoing, people who are overweight or obese are encouraged to lose weight. The AICR recommends that we "be as lean as possible within the normal range of body weight."

Specific Nutrients. Researchers continue to investigate, for example, the possible link between lycopene (an antioxidant found in tomatoes) and reduced risk for prostate cancer; calcium and reduced risk for colon cancer; and Vitamin E and reduced risk for prostate cancer. Some studies have suggested that soy products may reduce the risk of breast and prostate cancers, although more research is needed to confirm a link.

Mechanisms of Action

Cancer develops when cells in the body begin to grow out of control. Normal cells grow, divide, and die. Instead of dying, cancer cells continue to grow and form new abnormal cells. Cancer cells often travel to other body parts where they grow and replace normal tissue. This process, called *metastasis*, occurs as the cancer cells get into the bloodstream or lymph vessels. Cancer cells develop because of damage to deoxyribonucleic acid (DNA), which is in every cell and directs all cell activities. When DNA becomes damaged the body is usually able to repair

it; however, in cancerous cells, the damage is not repaired. People can inherit damaged DNA, which accounts for inherited cancers such as some forms of breast, ovarian, and colorectal cancers. Much more often DNA becomes damaged by exposure to something in the environment, like smoke.

Diet and lifestyle often determine whether cancer develops (Table 10-6). Cancer development typically takes many years. During this time—while a tumor is still small and has not yet spread to other organs—diet and lifestyle often determine whether tumor growth continues. Many carcinogens in food promote cancer development by binding to DNA.

DNA Mutations

Most DNA mutations in cancer cells are not inherited, but rather are the result of chronic exposure to environmental or lifestyle factors such as diet and smoking. Diet-related carcinogens that cause DNA mutations include:

- polycyclic aromatic hydrocarbons (PAH; e.g., charbroiling, fat drips on hot coals);
- **aflatoxins** (in moldy foods such as peanuts);
- heterocyclic amines, nitrosamines (e.g., nitrates in the stomach form nitrosamines)

Note: Nitrite-dependent nitrosamine formation in the stomach is inhibited by ascorbic acid, which is consumed mainly with fruits and vegetables. Many of these carcinogens act by firmly binding to DNA and forming DNA adducts. This may cause a mutation due to misreading during replication of the affected DNA. PAHs and aflatoxins are examples of carcinogens that form DNA adducts.

Nutrients That May Affect Cancer

Cancer development occurs in four stages: initiation, promotion, progression, and metastasis. Some of the ways nutrients affect cancer development include:

TABLE 10-6 Summary of Strength of Evidence on Lifestyle Factors and the Risk of Developing Cancer

Evidence	Decreased Risk	Increased Risk
Convincing[a]	Physical activity (colon)	Overweight and obesity (esophagus, colorectum, breast in post-menopausal women, endometrium, kidney)
		Alcohol (oral cavity, pharynx, larynx, esophagus, liver, breast)
		Aflatoxin (liver)
		Chinese-style salted fish (nasopharnyx)
Probable[b]	Fruits and vegetables (oral cavity, esophagus, stomach, colorectum[b])	Preserved meat (colorectum)
		Salt-preserved foods and salt (stomach)
	Physical activity (breast)	Very hot (thermally) drinks and food (oral cavity, pharynx, esophagus)
Possible (insufficient)	Fiber	Animal fats
	Soy	Heterocyclic amines
	Fish	Polycyclic aromatic hydrocarbons
	omega-3 fatty acids	Nitrosamines
	Carotenoids	
	Vitamins B_2, B_6, folate, B_{12}, C, D, and E	
	Calcium, zinc, and selenium	
	Non-nutrient plant constituents (e.g., allium compounds, flavonoids, isoflavones, lignans)	

Source: World Health Organisation. Diet, nutrition and the prevention of chronic diseases. Report of a Joint WHO/FAO Expert Consultation. WHO Technical Report Series 916. Section 5.5.4 Strength of evidence.
[a] The "convincing" and "probable" categories in this report correspond to the "sufficient category of the IAPC report on weight control and physical activity in terms of the public health and policy implications.
[b] For colorectal cancer, a protective effect of fruit and vegetable intake has been suggested by many case-control studies but this has not been supported by results of several large prospective studies, suggesting that if a benefit does exist it is likely to be modest.

- *Phase II enzymes:* Phase II enzymes in the liver conjugate or otherwise may inactivate carcinogens. The detoxification and elimination of carcinogens are enhanced by phase II enzymes. This varied group of enzymes includes those that conjugate carcinogens (glucuronide, glutathione, etc.) and others that make them less reactive. Inducers of phase II enzymes decrease the cancer-causing potential of carcinogens. Phase II inducers are consumed with several groups of vegetables, particularly with cabbages, radishes, and broccoli (because they contain isothiocyanates) and with onions, garlic, and leeks.
- *Free radicals:* Oxidative metabolism produces free radicals which chemically alter lipids, proteins, and DNA. Free radicals are normal byproducts of oxidative metabolism; the most important ones are hydroxyl radicals, superoxide anions, and hydrogen peroxide. Free radicals may react with lipids, proteins, or DNA and oxidize them; reaction with unsaturated fatty acids (e.g., those in membrane phospholipids) generates more free radicals and starts a chain reaction.
- *Free radical defense:* Enzymes and antioxidants (water- and fat-soluble) defend against free radicals. Defense against free radicals in the body includes a number of mechanisms that require specific nutrients with antioxidant potential: intracellular enzymes (some require selenium), water-soluble antioxidants (e.g., ascorbate) and fat-soluble antioxidants (e.g., vitamin E, carotenoids including beta-carotene). Vitamin E must be regenerated by ascorbate after each reaction with a free radical; without this regeneration, it is a free-radical-generating oxidant itself.

Role of the Environment

The environments in which Americans, and increasingly people in other Western and urban areas of industrialized cities, live, work, play, and go to school are barriers to healthy lifestyles and contribute powerfully to the obesity epidemic. Attempts to change individual behavior without addressing environmental barriers will have limited long-term impact on health outcomes. Research is currently under way to determine the impact of and strategies for addressing a variety of environmental issues. These may include the widespread availability, marketing, and advertising of inexpensive, energy-dense processed foods and beverages (especially targeting children and youth) and increasing portion sizes (especially of restaurant and fast-food meals).

Clinical Perspective for the Individual Patient

Prevention of Nutrition-Related Risks

The Food and Agriculture Organization and the World Health Organization have developed the following recommendations for reducing the risk of developing cancer globally:

- Maintain weight (among adults) such that BMI is in the range of 18.5 to 24.9 kg/m² and avoid weight gain (> 5 kg) during adult life.
- Maintain regular physical activity. The primary goal should be to perform physical activity on most days of the week; 60 minutes per day of moderate-intensity activity, such as walking, may be needed to maintain healthy body weight in otherwise sedentary people. More vigorous activity, such as fast walking, may give some additional benefits for cancer prevention.
- Consumption of alcoholic beverages is not recommended. If consumed, then do not exceed two drinks per day (American Cancer Society recommendations: Drink no more than 2 per day for men and 1 drink per day for women).
- Chinese-style fermented salted fish should only be consumed in moderation, especially during childhood. Overall consumption of salt-preserved foods and salt should be moderate.
- Minimize exposure to aflatoxins in foods.
- Have a diet that includes at least 400 g per day of total fruits and vegetables.
- Those who are not vegetarian are advised to moderate consumption of preserved meat (e.g., sausages, salami, bacon, ham).
- Do not consume foods or drinks when they are at a very hot (scalding hot) temperature.

Nutrition in the Management of Cancer

Cancer patients have special nutrition needs and special issues related to eating. Information to help maintain a patient's health and cope with treatment strategies is an important part of treatment.

Diet and lifestyle factors have limited (if any) effect on continued growth of established cancers. While diet and lifestyle can lower cancer risk effectively, the same dietary and lifestyle factors have limited if any effect on established cancer tissue. However, the guidelines for cancer prevention still apply to people whose cancer has been treated successfully, because they are at risk for developing new unrelated cancers, just like everyone else. Cancer patients often lose weight because of poor appetite, nausea, or difficulties eating. An important concern with people who already have cancer is to prevent undesirable weight loss.

The effectiveness of diets or supplements in reducing the size or aggressiveness of an established cancer has not been shown, yet.

OVERWEIGHT AND OBESITY

Obesity involves having an abnormally high proportion of body fat. Obesity is defined as having a BMI of 30 or higher and overweight as having a BMI of 25 or higher.

Two thirds of American adults are overweight. About one in three American adults is considered to be obese and childhood obesity is at an all-time high. Obesity is more than a cosmetic concern. Being seriously overweight puts you at greater risk of developing high blood pressure and many other serious health risks. Ultimately, obesity can even be life-threatening. Annually in the United States, more than 300,000 deaths are linked to obesity.

BMI is also recommended to identify children who are overweight or at risk of becoming overweight. Cutoff criteria are based on the 2000 BMI-for-age-growth charts for the United States developed by the CDC. Based on current recommendations of expert committees, children with BMI values at or above the 95th percentile of the sex-specific BMI growth charts are categorized as overweight.

Obesity prevalence in the United States has been increasing for at least 100 years, with an apparent acceleration in the past three decades. Since the mid-seventies, the prevalence of overweight and obesity has increased sharply for both adults and children. Data from two U.S. National Health and Nutrition Examination Survey (NHANES) surveys show that among adults aged 20 to 74 years the prevalence of obesity increased from 15.0 percent (in the 1976–1980 survey) to 32.9 percent (in the 2003–2004 survey). The distribution of BMI has increased modestly in median and moderately in mean. What has increased far more dramatically is the positive (right-tailed) skewness of the distribution, such that the most obese segments of the distribution are far more obese than in years past. Obesity has increased in every age, sex, race, and smoking-status stratum of the population, which has correctly been taken to indicate that changes in the distribution of age, race, sex, and smoking status cannot completely account for the epidemic.[9]

In the United States, we have an epidemic in diabetes that parallels (it actually follows in time) the epidemic in obesity.

We used to characterize people with diabetes as overweight, over 40, and underexercised. This epidemic is growing faster in the younger generation; there is a 70 to 80 percent increase in people in their 20s and 30s. In the past, pediatricians rarely saw a case of type II diabetes in kids. Now, about a third to half of the cases of diabetes found in our leading centers in the country is in children.

Globally, for overweight and obesity, not only has the current prevalence already reached unprecedented levels, but the rate at which it is annually increasing in most developing regions is substantial. The public health implications of this phenomenon are staggering and already becoming apparent. The rapidity of the changes in developing countries is such that a double burden of disease may often exist. India, for example, at present faces a combination of communicable diseases and chronic diseases, with the burden of chronic diseases just exceeding that of communicable diseases. Another eloquent example is that of obesity, which is becoming a serious problem throughout Asia, Latin America, and parts of Africa, despite the widespread presence of undernutrition. In some countries, the prevalence of obesity has doubled or tripled over the past decade.

Generally, although men may have higher rates of overweight, women have higher rates of obesity. For both, obesity poses a major risk for serious diet-related noncommunicable diseases, including diabetes mellitus, cardiovascular disease, hypertension, stroke, and certain forms of cancer. Its health consequences range from increased risk of premature death to serious chronic conditions that reduce the overall quality of life.

Currently, more than 1 billion adults are overweight and at least 300 million of these are clinically obese. Obesity levels range from below 5 percent in China, Japan, and certain African nations, to over 75 percent in urban Samoa. Even in relatively low prevalence countries like China, rates are almost 20 percent in some cities. Childhood obesity is already epidemic in some areas and on the rise in others. An estimated 17.6 million children under five are estimated to be overweight worldwide.

According to the U.S. Surgeon General, in our country the number of overweight children has doubled and the number of overweight adolescents has tripled since 1980. The prevalence of obese children aged 6 to 11 years has more than doubled since the 1960s. Obesity prevalence in youths aged 12 to 17 has increased from 5 percent to 13 percent in boys and from 5 percent to 9 percent in girls between 1966 and 1970 and 1988 to 1991.

The problem is global and increasingly extends into the developing world; for example, in Thailand the prevalence of obesity in 5- to 12-year-olds children rose from 12.2 percent to 15.6 percent in just two years. Obesity accounts for 2 percent to 6 percent of total healthcare costs in several developed countries; some estimates put the figure as high as 7 percent. The true costs are undoubtedly much greater as not all obesity-related conditions are included in the calculations.

Nutrition-Related Risk Factors

Factors that increase the risk of being obese include:

Diet. Regular consumption of high-calorie foods, such as fast foods, contributes to weight gain. High-fat foods are dense in calories. Loading up on soft drinks, candy, and desserts also promotes weight gain. Foods and beverages like these are high in sugar and calories.

Inactivity. Sedentary people are more likely to gain weight because they don't burn calories through physical activities.

Psychological Factors. Some people overeat to cope with problems or deal with emotions, such as stress or boredom.

Genetics. If one or both parents are obese, the chances of being overweight are greater. Genes may affect the amount of body fat stored and where that fat is distributed, but this does not guarantee obesity.

Age. As people get older, they tend to be less active. In addition, the amount of muscle in the body tends to decrease with age. This lower muscle mass leads to a decrease in metabolism. These changes also reduce calorie needs. If people do not decrease their caloric intake as they age, they will likely gain weight.

Pregnancy. During pregnancy, a woman's weight necessarily increases. Some women find this weight difficult to lose after the baby is born. This weight gain may contribute to the development of obesity in women.

Medical Problems. Uncommonly, obesity can be traced to a medical cause, such as low thyroid function, excess production of hormones by the adrenal glands (Cushing syndrome), or other hormonal imbalances, such as polycystic ovary syndrome. A low metabolic rate is rarely the cause of obesity. A medical problem, such as arthritis, also may lead to decreased activity, which can result in weight gain.

Alcohol. Drinking alcohol adds calories to your diet; just one regular beer is about 150 calories. If you don't cut back somewhere else, adding a single beer daily could cause a weight gain of more than one pound a month. Additionally, excessive drinking can stimulate your appetite and make you less likely to control portion sizes.

Mechanisms of Action

Weight is largely determined by the balance calorie intake from food in relation to the energy used in everyday activities. Consumption of more calories than those expended in exercise results in weight gain. The body stores surplus calories as fat, which is important for storing energy and insulating your body, among other functions. The human body can handle carrying some extra fat, but beyond a certain point body fat can begin to interfere with health. Eating too many calories and not getting enough physical activity are the main causes of obesity, especially in combination. Many other factors can contribute to obesity as well including genetics.

The **metabolic syndrome** is characterized by a group of metabolic risk factors in one person. These traits and medical conditions include:

- Abdominal obesity (excessive fat tissue in and around the abdomen)
- Atherogenic dyslipidemia (blood fat disorders—high triglycerides, low HDL cholesterol and high LDL cholesterol—that foster plaque buildups in artery walls)
- Elevated blood pressure ($>$ 130/85 mm Hg)
- Insulin resistance or glucose intolerance (the body can't properly use insulin or blood sugar)

Those who have metabolic syndrome are at increased risk of coronary heart disease and other diseases related to plaque buildups in artery walls (e.g., stroke and peripheral vascular disease) and type 2 diabetes. Metabolic syndrome has become increasingly common in the United States—an estimated 50 million Americans have it—and the world.

The dominant underlying risk factors for this syndrome appear to be abdominal obesity as measured by elevated waist circumference (40 inches or more in men and 35 inches or more in women) and insulin resistance. **Insulin resistance** is a generalized metabolic disorder in which the body cannot use insulin efficiently, which is why the metabolic syndrome is called the *insulin resistance syndrome.*

Other conditions associated with the syndrome include physical inactivity, aging, hormonal imbalance, and genetic predisposition. Recent research has shown that high levels of magnesium in the diet may reduce risk of developing metabolic syndrome and, thus, lower risk of heart disease and diabetes. More studies are needed to confirm this finding and to determine the needed levels of magnesium in the diet.

Clinical Perspective for the Individual
Obesity Prevention

The goal of obesity prevention is to maintain a stable, healthy weight over time. Staying at a healthy body weight increases the chances of living a long and healthy life by avoiding many of the chronic health problems addressed in this chapter. The key to maintaining a healthy weight is "energy balance," in which energy intake from food and beverages equals the energy expended through basal metabolism and physical activity. When energy consumed is greater than energy used, excess calories (the unit that measures the energy content of food) are stored in the body, which results in weight gain. When energy intake is less than energy expended, the negative energy balance results in weight loss. Adults often gain weight gradually over time as a result of excess food intake, limited physical activity, and slower metabolism. The prevention objective should be to remain at a healthy weight or lose weight and maintain the weight loss. To accomplish this, calorie intake must match energy use. This basically means eating less and/or moving more.

Defining a Healthy Body Weight. The body mass index (BMI) describes relative weight for height. A BMI of 18.5 to 24.9 is considered healthy. A person with a BMI of 25 to 29.9 is considered overweight, and a person with a BMI of 30 or more is considered obese and should talk with a health provider about losing weight for his or her health. Weight classification based on BMI is the best assessment tool for adults and children 2–20.

Body Mass Index (BMI) = wt/ht

BMI measures your weight in relation to your height, and is closely associated with measures of body fat. You can calculate your BMI using this formula:

$$BMI = \frac{weight\ pounds \times 703}{height\ squared\ (inches^2)}$$

For example, for someone who is 5 feet, 7 inches tall and weighs 220 pounds, the calculation is:

$$BMI = \frac{220\ pounds \times 703}{67\ inches \times 67\ inches} = \frac{154,660}{4,489} = 34.45$$

For children and adolescents, BMI is calculated based on age and gender and should be graphed on a gender-specific BMI chart to determine the percentile. In 1997, a consensus panel recommended that BMI for age be used routinely to screen children for overweight.[10] They also recommended cut points of between the 85th and 95th percentiles to identify children and adolescents as at risk of overweight and at or above the 95th percentile to identify children and adolescents as overweight.

BMI reflects height and weight measure, but not *body composition*, which refers to the proportion of muscle, bone, fat and other tissue that make up a person's total weight. An athlete may have a BMI above normal but have little adipose tissue and considerable muscle mass. That is why determining how much of the body is fat and where it is located are two additional steps that should be taken to help assess health risks associated with body weight and body fat. If you carry fat mainly around your waist, you are more likely to develop health problems than if you carry fat mainly in your hips and thighs. This is true even if your BMI falls within the normal range. A person's waist circumference is the most practical indicator of the fat distribution and abdominal fat.

> **Waist circumference:** An anthropometric measurement used to assess a person's abdominal fat. Abdominal fat increases the risk of many of the serious conditions associated with obesity. Women's waist measurements should be less than 35 inches. Men's should be less than 40 inches.

Prevention Starts in Childhood. Childhood is the optimum time to begin overweight and obesity prevention efforts. Childhood obesity prevention involves maintaining energy balance at a healthy weight while protecting overall health, growth and development, and nutritional status. To balance energy intake and energy expenditure is extraordinarily complex when considering the multitude of genetic, biological, psychological, sociocultural, and environmental factors that affect both sides of the equation and the interrelationships between these factors. American children live in a society that has changed dramatically in the three decades over which the obesity epidemic has developed. The same factors are changing in many third world cities as well.

A preventive approach is urgently needed so that all children may grow up physically and emotionally healthy. Preventing obesity involves promoting healthful eating behaviors and regular physical activity with the goal of achieving and maintaining energy balance at a healthy weight. Health providers, families, schools, and other community groups must be involved to encourage and support children and adolescents to adopt behaviors that promote better health. Some promising approaches for preventing obesity as noted by the Centers for Disease Control and Prevention[11]:

- Breastfeeding is associated with a reduced risk of overweight in children.
- Regular physical activity is a key part of any weight control effort. Community strategies that increase physical activity levels include community-wide campaigns, "point-of-decision" prompts (such as signs placed by elevators and escalators that encourage people to use nearby stairs), and physical education in schools. Enhancing access to places for physical activity combined with informational outreach is successful as are non-family social supports and individually adapted health behavior changes.
- Reducing the time children spend watching television appears to be effective for controlling their weight.
- For children and adolescents who are overweight, increasing physical activity helps them to: reduce many of the risks for illnesses associated with obesity; maintain their weight loss; and prevent weight gain.

Nutrition in Management of Obesity

Although the ideal is to maintain desirable BMI between 18.5 and 24.9, the good news is that losing even modest amounts of weight can lower blood pressure, reduce risk of cardiovascular disease and stroke, improve glucose control in diabetes, improve signs and symptoms of osteoarthritis and sleep apnea, and lower the risk of cancer.

This usually requires reducing weight by approximately 5 percent to 10 percent. That means that a person weighing 200 pounds who is obese by BMI standards would need to lose at least 10 to 20 pounds to start. Slow and steady weight loss of one or two pounds a week is considered the safest way to lose weight and the best way to keep it off.

In many cases, losing weight can be accomplished by committing to eating a healthier diet, exercising, and changing behaviors. Other treatments for obesity include prescription medications and surgery.

Dietary Changes. Consuming fewer calories is an important factor for successful weight loss. The number of calories needed to maintain weight each day depends on several factors, including age and activity level. A doctor can help determine daily calorie goals to lose weight and may recommend working with a dietitian or a reputable weight-loss program.

Crash diets to reduce calories aren't recommended because they can cut so many calories and nutrients that they lead to other health problems, such as vitamin deficiencies. Fasting isn't the answer, either. Most of the weight initially lost is from water, and it's not good for the body to go without food for extended periods.

Very low calorie liquid diets are sometimes prescribed as an intervention for seriously obese people. These mainly liquid diets, such as Medifast® or Optifast®, provide about 800 calories a day; most adults consume roughly 2,000 to 2,500 calories a day. While people are usually able to lose weight on these very low calorie diets, most people regain the weight just as quickly when they stop following these diets.

Over-the-counter liquid meal replacements, such as Slim-Fast®, also cut calories. These plans suggest that you replace one or two meals with their product—a low-calorie shake—then eat snacks of vegetables and fruits and a healthy, balanced third meal that is low in fat and calories. This can be as effective as a traditional calorie-controlled diet.

To lose weight and keep it off, one should eat moderate amounts of nutrient-rich, low-fat, low-calorie foods. The following factors are the fundamentals of healthy eating.

Energy Density. *Energy density* is the number of calories in a given volume of food. Eat a food that's energy dense, such as fat, and you can't eat much of it without consuming a lot of calories. On the other hand, eat a food with low energy density, including most vegetables and some fruits, and you can consume a huge amount for few calories. For example: A tablespoon of butter has the same number of calories as 20 cups of leaf lettuce. Which would leave one feeling fuller?

Nutrient-Rich Foods. Healthy foods include vegetables, fruits, grains, and lean sources of protein, including beans, fish, low-fat dairy products, and lean meats. These foods optimize nutrition and taste and promote a healthy weight. Eat a variety of healthy foods in lieu of junk foods.

The Right Carbohydrates. Nutrition experts generally agree that 45 percent to 65 percent of one's total daily calories should come from carbohydrates. Steer away from simple carbohydrates, such as table sugar and other sweeteners, and limit fruit juice, which is a type of carbohydrate concentrated in calories. Instead, try to eat plenty of complex, high-fiber carbohydrates, such as whole-grain bread and pasta, brown rice, and other grains, such as oatmeal.

Limit Sweets. Limit candies, cakes, cookies, muffins, pies, doughnuts, and frozen desserts because they are a large source of calories. Better dessert choices include angel food cake, vanilla wafers, fig-bar cookies, low-fat frozen yogurt, and sorbet or sherbet.

Reduce Fat. Because fat has more than twice the calories of carbohydrate and protein ounce for ounce, reducing fat content is an important way to cut calories. Foods high in fat include most fast foods, pastries, red meats, full-fat dairy products, oils, margarine, butter, salad dressings, and mayonnaise. Current dietary guidelines recommend that healthy Americans get between 20 percent and 35 percent of total calories from fat, with less than 10 percent of total calories coming from saturated fat sources.

Portion Sizes. A single 2-ounce serving of fish or poultry is about the size of a deck of cards. A 2-ounce serving of cheese or 1 teaspoon of butter is about the size of four dice. A small apple or a medium orange is comparable in size to a tennis ball. A hockey puck is about the size of one-half a bagel or a slice of whole-grain bread. It's especially important to watch serving sizes when eating out because many restaurants serve oversized portions.

Count Calories. It is important to read food labels. Foods that are low in fat can sometimes be very high in calories. Processed foods—most products other than fresh foods—often have hidden fat and sugar. Sugary soft drinks are high in calories and do not add any nutritional value to the diet.

Increase Physical Activity. Recommendations for diet and nutrition in the prevention of chronic diseases should emphasize the need for sufficient physical activity. This is consistent with the trend to consider physical activity alongside the complex of diet, nutrition, and health. Energy expenditure through physical activity is an important part of the energy balance equation that determines body weight. A decrease in energy expenditure through decreased physical activity is one of the major factors contributing to the global epidemic of overweight and obesity.

Simple ways to increase activity are:

- Taking the stairs (not the elevator).
- Parking in the farthest spot in the parking lot.
- Walking or biking to work or to the store.
- Walking during the lunch hour.
- Playing with children instead of watching them play.
- Walking with the family after dinner.
- Doing weekend chores the physical way (e.g., use a push mower to mow the lawn or wash the car manually).
- Buying an exercise bike and pedaling during TV shows or while talking on the phone.
- Using a pedometer and trying to increase the number of steps walked each day.

HIV/AIDS

Human immunodeficiency virus (HIV) infection has become increasingly prevalent globally, with more than 40 million infected individuals worldwide, the majority of whom live in the resource-limited world, especially sub-Saharan Africa and Asia. There are nutritional and metabolic issues that significantly impact morbidity and mortality in HIV-infected populations, and those whose disease has progressed to the **acquired immune deficiency syndrome (AIDS)**. In addition, malnutrition has been associated with an increased risk of transmission of HIV from infected mothers to infants, and malnutrition may further compromise HIV-infected individuals who have tuberculosis or persistent diarrheal disease. The introduction of highly active antiretroviral therapy will have a significant impact on the mortality of HIV but will not completely alleviate the malnutrition associated with HIV infection in the global setting.

More alarmingly, nutritional status is deteriorating in 26 countries, many of them in Africa, where the nexus between HIV and undernutrition is strong and mutually reinforcing. Once a person is infected with HIV, the body's immune system generally keeps the virus in check for quite a few years, depending on the overall health of the person. Today, when tests of the immune system indicate that the virus is beginning to win, anti-retroviral therapy is started. The drugs, as powerful as the chemotherapeutic agents used to fight cancer, slow the virus' ability to replicate. Other drug cocktails boost the immune system. However, the drugs have serious side effects, including diarrhea and nausea, which, along with the disease itself, affect the nutritional well-being of HIV patients. But the drugs do save lives.

Now, many people in the United States and elsewhere with HIV are surviving indefinitely. For them, HIV is nearly a chronic disease, but a disease with a new set of health problems. Wasting (dramatic weight loss) threatens about one third of those with HIV. The pressing needs are to develop guidelines for promoting optimum nutrition for **persons living with HIV/AIDS (PLWHA)**. Counseling HIV-infected mothers concerning breastfeeding their infants is an important subject about which considerable evidence-based data are becoming available to guide health workers and women in making the best choice for their baby.

Nutrition-Related Risk Factors

Good nutrition is essential for people living with HIV. HIV affects nutrition in three overlapping ways:

1. Nutritional status affects HIV disease progression and mortality; improving nutritional status may improve some HIV-related outcomes.
2. Counseling and other interventions to prevent weight loss probably have their greatest impact early in the course of HIV infection.
3. Nutritional supplements, particularly antioxidant vitamins and minerals, may improve HIV-related outcomes, particularly in nutritionally vulnerable populations.

In addition, all mothers should increase their food intake and eat nutrient-rich food during lactation. Breastfeeding uses energy and other nutrients that need to be replaced to keep a mother healthy. Nutritional support is particularly important for the HIV-infected mother because HIV puts an additional strain on her energy and nutrient stores, which may affect her appetite.

Mechanisms of Action

Effects of HIV/AIDS on nutrition:

- Decrease in the amount of food consumed
- Impaired nutrient absorption
- Changes in metabolism
- Good nutrition helps keep the immune system strong, enabling a person living with HIV/AIDS to better fight disease. A healthy diet improves quality of life.
- Weight loss, wasting, and malnutrition continue to be common problems in HIV, despite more effective antiretroviral medications, and can contribute to HIV disease progression.
- Good nutrition helps the body process the many medications taken by people with HIV.
- Diet (and exercise) may help with symptoms such as diarrhea, nausea, and fatigue, and with fat redistribution and metabolic abnormalities such as high blood sugar, cholesterol, and triglycerides.

Clinical Perspective for the Individual Patient
Nutrition in the Management of HIV/AIDS

Nutrition counseling, care, and support are integral to comprehensive HIV care, including care given to HIV-positive individuals (Figure 10-3). There are several nutrition and food-related interventions to consider. Appropriate actions depend on the local conditions, the HIV-positive individual's lifecycle state (e.g., child, pregnant or lactating, other adult), degree of disease progression (e.g., asymptomatic, symptomatic, AIDS), and whether they have initiated anti-retroviral (ARV) therapy. Integrating nutritional care and support interventions strengthens home-, clinic-, and community-based care and ARV services. Nutrition interventions may improve the quality and reach of care and promote successful treatment. Nutrition counseling may improve adherence to lifesaving ARV drugs and medications for treating HIV-related infections.

The main nutritional interventions are:

- *Counseling* to manage nutrition-related symptoms of common HIV related illness/opportunistic infections (e.g., loss of appetite, oral sores, fat malabsorption),
- *Prescribed/targeted nutrition supplements.* Three different types of nutrition supplements should be considered:

1. *Food rations* to manage mild weight loss and nutrition-related side effects of ARV therapy and to address nutritional needs in food insecure areas.
2. *Micronutrient supplements* for specific HIV-positive risk groups.

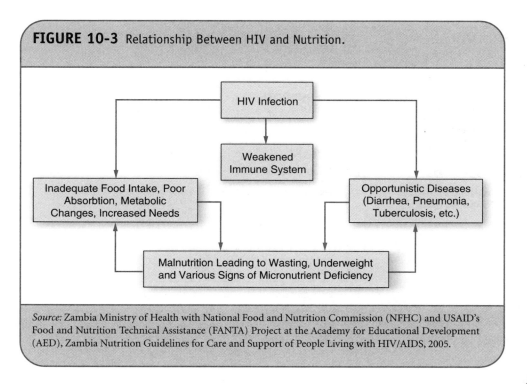

FIGURE 10-3 Relationship Between HIV and Nutrition.

HIV Infection

Weakened Immune System

Inadequate Food Intake, Poor Absorbtion, Metabolic Changes, Increased Needs

Opportunistic Diseases (Diarrhea, Pneumonia, Tuberculosis, etc.)

Malnutrition Leading to Wasting, Underweight and Various Signs of Micronutrient Deficiency

Source: Zambia Ministry of Health with National Food and Nutrition Commission (NFHC) and USAID's Food and Nutrition Technical Assistance (FANTA) Project at the Academy for Educational Development (AED), Zambia Nutrition Guidelines for Care and Support of People Living with HIV/AIDS, 2005.

3. *Therapeutic foods* for rehabilitation of moderate and severe malnutrition in HIV-positive adults and children.

PUBLIC HEALTH PERSPECTIVE FOR THE HEALTH OF THE GENERAL POPULATION AND OF HIGH RISK GROUPS

Chronic diseases—such as heart disease, cancer, and diabetes—are the leading causes of death and disability in the United States. These diseases account for 7 of every 10 deaths and affect the quality of life of 90 million Americans. By the last decade of the 20th century, chronic diseases had superseded communicable diseases as the leading cause of death in all areas of the world except sub-Saharan Africa and the Middle East, and within the next 15 years, chronic diseases are projected to account for nearly three quarters of all deaths in low-income regions of the world. Although chronic diseases are among the most common and costly health problems, they are also among the most preventable (Figure 10-4). Adopting healthy behaviors such as eating nutritious foods, being physically active, and avoiding tobacco use can prevent or control the devastating effects of these diseases.

Diet and nutrition are important factors in the promotion and maintenance of good health throughout the entire life course. Their roles as determinants of chronic conditions are well established and therefore occupy a prominent position in prevention activities.

Role of Public Health Systems

If we are not working on heart disease, stroke, and cancer as a society, we are not working on the things that are the real killers. In all likelihood, chronic diseases will be the predominant global source of morbidity, death, and disease during the 21st century. Poor diet and lack of exercise are major **risk factors**. If we are not working on the top set of conditions, which are the risks and actual causes, we are only working on the margin of the problems of our society.

How might the goal to reduce mortality and morbidity from nutrition-related chronic diseases be achieved? There are four basic components in a comprehensive chronic disease control program:

1. Chronic disease surveillance
2. Primary prevention
3. Secondary prevention
4. Diagnosis, treatment, and management

All four components are needed to achieve the global goal of chronic disease prevention and control. However, in countries with weak health systems, reaching the people needing these interventions through health service delivery mechanisms and improved basic nutrition is challenging. Health system strengthening is vital to address the growing burden of NCDs because their management and prevention require long-term, sustained interaction with multiple levels of the health system. Significant advances have been made on understanding the determinants of the major chronic conditions; however, HIV/AIDS, obesity, and new pandemics will continue to challenge countries in the future. Country public health surveillance systems must be ready to detect and respond to promote behavioral changes and effective policies to reduce the growing burden of NCDs.

Chronic Disease Surveillance

Surveillance systems that track noncommunicable diseases of public health significance are essential to track the current and future burden of disease, provide evidence for planning

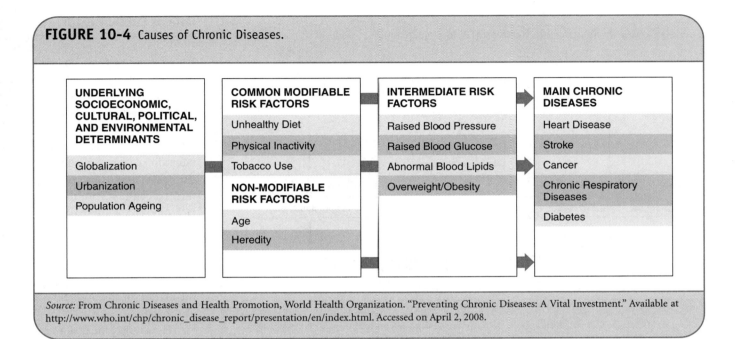

FIGURE 10-4 Causes of Chronic Diseases.

Source: From Chronic Diseases and Health Promotion, World Health Organization. "Preventing Chronic Diseases: A Vital Investment." Available at http://www.who.int/chp/chronic_disease_report/presentation/en/index.html. Accessed on April 2, 2008.

research priorities, and monitor the outcomes of prevention and treatment programs. In the case of NCDs, behavioral risk surveillance, which involves collecting data to better understand the extent of risk behaviors for various health conditions (i.e., alcohol use, obesity, cancer screening, nutrition, physical activity, tobacco use, and more), is an integral part of surveillance that enables public health agencies to monitor the progress of prevention efforts, and helps public health professionals and legislators to make more timely and effective decisions.

Primary Prevention

The goal of primary prevention is to prevent premature deaths and avoid unnecessary disability due to chronic diseases. The solutions exist now, and many are simple, cheap, and cost effective. Primary prevention involves the elimination or reduction of exposure to recognized risk factors in susceptible populations. **Health promotion**, education, and raising awareness are key strategies. In the case of nutrition-related chronic diseases, the focus is on promoting consumption of healthy foods and controlling overweight and sedentary behaviors. The key risk factors for CVD and diabetes (obesity, physical inactivity, and unhealthy diets) require interventions to change unhealthy lifestyles.

Health Promotion Is Fundamental. The health promotion infrastructure of a country is fundamental to health protection of the population. Health promotion as defined by the World Health Organization is "the process of enabling people to increase control over, and to improve, their health." Health pro-

motion works to help people change their lifestyle to move toward better health by developing personal skills, embracing community action, and fostering appropriate public policies, health services, and supportive environments. Lifestyle change can be facilitated through a combination of efforts to enhance awareness, change behavior, and create environments that support good health practices. The role of the health sector must move increasingly in a health promotion direction, beyond its responsibility for providing clinical and curative services. Health services need to embrace an expanded mandate that is sensitive and respects cultural needs. This mandate should support the needs of individuals and communities for a healthier life and open channels between the health sector and broader social, political, economic, and physical environmental components.

The ability to make healthy choices is often affected by factors in the environments in which people live, work, learn, and play. Public, private, and community organizations should work to create social and physical environments that support the adoption and maintenance of healthful nutrition and physical activity behaviors.

- Increase access to healthful foods in schools, worksites, and communities.
- Provide safe, enjoyable, and accessible environments for physical activity in schools and for transportation and recreation in communities.
- Promote policies to increase access to healthy food products in resource-poor neighborhoods.

Summary of Global Health Promotion Messages on Food and Nutrition

GLOBAL HEALTH PROMOTION MESSAGES ON FOOD AND NUTRITION

Maintain a healthy weight throughout life	Be physically active
Increase intake of fruits and vegetables	Control high blood pressure
Maintain healthy cholesterol levels	Moderate alcohol consumption
Control or delay onset of diabetes	

Maintain a Healthy Weight Throughout Life

- Balance caloric intake with physical activity.
- Avoid excessive weight gain throughout life.
- Achieve and maintain a healthy weight if currently overweight or obese.

Increase Intake of Fruits and Vegetables

New dietary guidance recommending increased intake of fruits and vegetables is based on evolving evidence of the benefit of eating a diet rich in fruits and vegetables. The average combined recommendation for fruits and vegetables of 10 servings (5 cups) in the United States is twice the level targeted by **Healthy People 2010** and about twice the current average intake. Additional servings of fruits and vegetables should replace sources of "empty calories" in the diet, such as added sugars (honey, syrup, soft drinks) and solid fats (butter, sour cream), to avoid taking in too many calories. Individuals should be especially encouraged to consume dark green/orange varieties of vegetables such as broccoli or carrots, and legumes or dried beans, such as pinto beans or lentils.

- Control high blood pressure.
- Maintain healthy cholesterol levels.
- Be physically active.
- Control or delay the onset of diabetes.
- Alcohol (in moderation): Scores of studies suggest that having an alcoholic drink a day lowers the risk of heart disease. Moderation is clearly important, since alcohol has risks as well as benefits. For men, a good balance point is one to two drinks a day. For women, it is at most one drink a day.

Controlling the Global Obesity Epidemic

Increasing levels of overweight and obesity among children and adults are now a major threat to America's health. Overweight children often become obese as adults. Obesity in-

creases the risk of developing and dying from a number of cancers as well as heart disease, diabetes, and other health problems. The proportion of children aged 6 to 19 who are overweight has tripled over the past three decades and it appears that this trend is continuing. The percentage of adults who are obese rose from 15 percent in 1976 to 31 percent in 1999 to 2002. Recommendations have been developed to counteract the rising rates of obesity and overweight among children and adults. Approaches can be taken at the national, state, and local levels to promote physical activity and healthy nutritional choices, thereby restoring caloric balance.

The health of young people and the adults they will become is linked to the starting of healthy behaviors in childhood. Risk factors such as unhealthy dietary patterns and physical inactivity during childhood and adolescence can result in life-threatening cancers, CVDs, and other major illnesses later in life. It is far easier to establish healthy practices early in life than to change behaviors later.

"Obesity is one of today's most blatantly visible—yet most neglected—public health problems. Paradoxically coexisting with undernutrition, an escalating global epidemic of overweight and obesity ("globesity") is taking over many parts of the world. If immediate action is not taken, millions will suffer from an array of serious health disorders." Preventing obesity from occurring or worsening is an important part of achieving a healthier population. Prevention includes maintenance of healthy weight, maintenance of weight loss, and prevention of weight gain. Identifying risk factors that can lead to obesity or cause related health problems, and learning strategies toward achieving a healthy weight are the keys to successful prevention.

Obesity prevention programs encourage children, adolescents and adults to adopt behaviors that promote better health. There are prevention programs for individuals and groups, in the workplace, in schools, and communities. Prevention of obesity in children and youth should be a national public health priority. It will require federal, state, and local governments to commit adequate and sustained resources for surveillance, research, public health programs, evaluation, and dissemination. Source: http://www.who.int/nutrition/topics/obesity/en/index.

Cardiovascular fitness and physical activity have been shown to reduce significantly the effects of overweight and obesity on health. Physical activity and food intake are both specific and mutually interacting behaviors that are and can be influenced partly by the same measures and policies. Lack of physical activity is already a global health hazard and is a prevalent and rapidly increasing problem in both developed and developing countries, particularly among poor people in large cities. In order to achieve the best results in preventing chronic diseases, the strategies and policies that are applied must fully recognize the essential role of diet, nutrition, and physical activity.

A shift in priorities is needed for developing strategies for action, placing nutrition—together with the other principal risk factors for chronic disease, namely, tobacco use and alcohol consumption—at the forefront of public health policies and programs.

Beware of the Metabolic Syndrome

Experts estimate that as many as 25 percent of Americans have metabolic syndrome, presenting a massive public health problem. Metabolic syndrome is the tendency of several conditions to occur together, including obesity, insulin resistance, diabetes or prediabetes, hypertension, and high lipids. Identifying factors that could lower the risk of metabolic syndrome—particularly in young people—could help individuals improve their health while boosting the health of the nation as a whole. Because heart disease and diabetes are costly both in human terms and in dollars, it is important to find ways to lower the risk of millions of people around the world.

Addressing the Global Epidemic of Diabetes

Diabetes is the fourth leading cause of death by disease globally. At least 50 percent of all people with diabetes are unaware of their condition; however, in some countries this statistic may reach 80 percent. The devastating complications of diabetes, such as blindness, kidney failure, and heart disease, are imposing a huge burden on healthcare services. It is estimated that diabetes accounts for between 5 percent and 10 percent of a nation's health budget. Better prevention and treatment strategies are needed to help patients and health systems cope with this tremendous burden of morbidity.

Efforts to prevent type 2 diabetes involve lifestyle interventions—changes in diet and increased physical activity—among people at high risk. Lifestyle interventions have been shown to reduce the incidence of type 2 diabetes dramatically. There is not enough evidence to show that type 1 diabetes can be prevented.

Reducing the Burden of Cardiovascular Disease

An estimated 17 million people die of CVDs, particularly heart attacks and strokes, every year. Following tobacco use, physical inactivity and unhealthy diet are the main risk factors that increase individual risks to cardiovascular diseases. One of the strategies to respond to the challenges to population health and well-being due to the global epidemic of heart attack and stroke is to provide actionable information for development and implementation of appropriate policies. Although CVD is emerging in developing countries with the increase in risk factors such as physical inactivity and unhealthy diets, little is known outside of Western countries about comprehensive preventive measures for controlling its expansion.

One emerging area of focus is on reducing trans fats found in processed foods, including crackers, cookies, and fried and baked goods. They cannot be eliminated from the diet completely, because small amounts appear in the meat and milk of cows and other ruminant animals. A healthy goal is to trim trans fat intake to less than 1 percent of total calories. Manufacturers must now list trans fats on the food label, right beneath saturated fats. New York and Philadelphia have passed measures eliminating its use in restaurants, and other cities are considering similar bans. Trans fat intake in the United States is still high. Reducing trans fat intake should remain an important public health priority.

Cancer Is Complex

Choosing the right health behaviors and preventing exposure to certain environmental risk factors can help prevent the development of cancer. For this reason, it is important to follow national trends data to monitor the reduction of these risk factors. In the United States, the four most common cancers are prostate, female breast, colorectal, and lung cancers. The higher incidence of stomach, liver, and cervical cancers in developing countries is mainly due to public health systems' failure to control contaminants, bacterial and viral infections, and the lack of effective prevention and treatment for these cancers. High incidence of esophageal cancer may reflect in part the consumption of traditional beverages at extremely high temperatures. Cancers that are becoming increasingly common in developing countries—lung, breast, and colorectal cancers—reflect longer life spans, the adoption of Western diets, and the globalization of tobacco markets.

Comprehensive cancer control programs are needed to deliver understandable and actionable cancer prevention and treatment information that increases patients' health literacy. Increasing trends in weight gain and obesity raise concern over future cancer rates. Trends in children are especially alarming. Research on effective environmental and policy changes to impact overweight and obesity trends is currently under way.

Healthy eating habits and other factors could reduce cancer mortality in the United States by as much as 30 percent. Cancer risk can be reduced by adopting an overall dietary pattern that emphasizes plant foods (vegetables, fruits, whole grains, beans) and helps to maintain a healthy weight, being physically active on a regular basis, and limiting alcohol consumption.

Secondary Prevention

Secondary prevention includes risk appraisal and screening to emphasize early detection and diagnosis of disease. Secondary prevention begins at the point where pathology of a disease may occur. It encompasses diagnostic services that include screening, surveillance, and clinical examinations. Screening strategies should include follow-up education, counseling, and health referral.

Examples of secondary prevention include cholesterol screening for early detection of cardiovascular problems. Lifestyle interventions that target extremely obese individuals and women with previous gestational diabetes are examples of secondary prevention of type 2 diabetes. Other interventions include blood glucose screening to detect diabetes in its early stages, and managing the disease to reduce its complications. A high-risk approach would include testing for impaired glucose tolerance and impaired fasting glucose in those with high risk of diabetes to determine if they have prediabetes. Those who are in the preclinical phase of type 2 diabetes should be provided with dietary and physical activity education and support to prevent or at least delay development of the disease.

Diagnosis, Treatment, Management

The disease burdens from CVD, diabetes, and related conditions of high blood pressure, high cholesterol, and excessive body weight are increasing worldwide. Primary healthcare systems need to develop guidelines and training for staff to enable them to manage chronic diseases effectively, using latest available knowledge. It is essential for all countries to make treatment available to all, especially those in the poorest settings. Reorienting health services to provide good quality NCD management also requires stronger attention to health research as well as changes in professional education and training. Now that the human genome has been mapped, attention is focusing on exploring genetic and environmental influences on common diseases. In the case of many chronic conditions, "Genes load the gun, and environment pulls the trigger."[12,13] Research that attempts to systematically examine the gene-environment-disease relationship has the potential to improve health providers' knowledge leading to more effective targeted prevention, diagnosis, and treatment.

For example, the quality of diabetes care generally remains poor worldwide, regardless of a country's level of development, healthcare system, or population size. Yet, the growing diabetes pandemic warrants greater attention and rapid ac-

tion. An array of effective interventions to prevent diabetes and its complications is available, with varying degrees of implementation feasibility. It is important for health planners and policy makers to realize that glycemic control costs less than managing the complications that arise in its absence. Diabetes education and organized care delivery are perhaps the most essential interventions today. Together, they reap substantial benefits at a low cost. Two interventions have proven especially cost-effective and feasible in low-resource settings.

The first involves glycemic control through diet and physical activity, oral medications to reduce glucose, and insulin injections, combined with patient education to foster compliance with medication and diet and exercise regimens. Glucose is usually poorly controlled among people with diabetes in developing countries because of lack of access to insulin and other diabetes treatment supplies. Hence, an important aspect of these interventions in developing countries is to guarantee these supplies.

Secondly, diabetes education is an integral part of diabetes care because it helps people with diabetes learn about and understand their disease, recognize emergency health problems, and adhere to self-care practices and lifestyle changes. A review of literature suggests that self-managed diabetes education may reduce medical costs in developing countries. A study in Latin America showed that a low-cost education program reduced the cost of drugs by 62 percent. In the United States, diabetes self-management education in community sites such as churches is a promising strategy, especially for those who do not have access to comprehensive health insurance.

Food and Nutrition Support for People Living with HIV/AIDS

The HIV/AIDS epidemic poses an inescapable challenge to the world at large and to Africa in particular. A massive effort is needed to cushion the impact of the epidemic, and nutritional care and support should be integral elements of any action taken. An evidence-based response is required to alleviate the overall burden of malnutrition and to reduce the severity and complexity of the impact that HIV/AIDS and malnutrition have on each other. Clear and culturally acceptable messages are required for patients and communities. Innovative partnerships are needed to ensure the optimal diet that local conditions permit is achieved.

Preventing Mother-to-Child Transmission. HIV passes via breastfeeding to about one of seven infants born to HIV-infected women. However, in many situations where there is a high prevalence of HIV, not breastfeeding dramatically increases the risk of infant mortality. Infants can die from either the failure to appropriately breastfeed or from the transmission of HIV through breastfeeding. In many programs to prevent mother-to-child transmission of HIV, the emphasis to date has been on the provision of antiretroviral drugs to prevent transmission around the time of delivery. Programs need to expand coverage and provide mothers with information, guidance, and support that allow them to choose and adhere to the safest infant feeding strategy for their situation.

CONCLUSION

If a country wants to reduce the burden of chronic disease within its population, it is essential to pay attention to diet. Healthy eating habits are fundamental to good health and help prevent morbidity and premature mortality from the most common global chronic conditions. Health protection should include promotion of healthy eating patterns and steering populations away from adopting diets based on cheap, high-energy, low-nutrient foods.

Ensuring good nutrition for all, starting in childhood and extending throughout the life cycle, is an integral part of public health.

KEY TERMS

Biology Terms

Acquired Immune Deficiency Syndrome (AIDS) (also, HIV disease): Advanced infection with the human immunodeficiency virus (HIV), which is a retrovirus that kills helper T cells, the primary defense in the body against infection and illness.

Aflatoxins: Highly toxic compounds produced by mold fungus in agricultural crops, especially peanuts, and in animal feeds that have not been carefully stored. High-level aflatoxin exposure can cause liver cancer.

Anticarcinogen: Any chemical that reduces the occurrence of cancers, reduces the severity of cancers that do occur, or acts against cancers that do occur, based on scientific evidence.

Antioxidants: Compounds that protect others from oxidation by being oxidized themselves; this action prevents the breakdown of substances in food or the body, particularly lipids.

Atherosclerosis: Often called "hardening of the arteries." Process by which artery walls become progressively thickened due to accumulation of fatty deposits, smooth muscle cells, and fibrous connective tissue (plaque). Narrowing of the lumen of an artery occurs that restricts blood flow. Too much cholesterol in the blood increases the risk that fatty deposits (plaque) will form in arteries.

Blood Glucose (also, blood sugar): The main sugar found in the blood and the body's main source of energy.

Blood Glucose Level: The amount of glucose in a given amount of blood and is noted in milligrams per deciliter (mg/dL).

Blood Pressure: The force of blood exerted on the inside walls of blood vessels. Blood pressure is expressed as a ratio (example: 120/80, read as "120 over 80"). The first number is the systolic pressure or the pressure when the heart pushes blood out into the arteries; the second number is the diastolic pressure or the pressure when the heart rests.

Body Mass Index (BMI): A measure of underweight and overweight calculated as weight (kg) divided by height squared (m^2); also a formula that uses weight and height to estimate body fat and health risks. A BMI between 19 and 24 is considered to be a healthy weight range for height. A BMI between 25 and 29 is considered overweight. A BMI of 30 or greater is considered obese. Anyone with a BMI of 30 or greater should talk to a health provider about losing weight for their health.

Cancer: Over 100 diseases characterized by growth and invasiveness of abnormal cells. Normal cells grow, divide, and die. Cancer cells do not die but continue to grow uncontrollably, replacing normal tissue cells with cancer cells. Cancer cells either multiply in a specific place (benign tumor) or cells can break away from the primary tumor, migrate via the bloodstream or lymph vessels, and subsequently invade other tissues of the body (metastasis). Those who inherit damaged DNA have inherited cancers. More often, DNA in cells is damaged by exposure to environment carcinogens (e.g., cigarette smoke).

Carcinogen: A substance or agent known or believed to cause cancer.

Cardiovascular Disease (CVD): A disease of the heart and blood vessels (arteries, veins, and capillaries).

Cerebrovascular Disease: Damage to blood vessels in the brain. Vessels burst and bleed or become clogged with fatty deposits; after the blood flow is interrupted, brain cells die or are damaged, resulting in a stroke.

Carbohydrate: One of the three main nutrients in food that include starches, vegetables, fruits, dairy products, and sugars.

Cholesterol: A naturally occurring, soft, waxy substance found among fats (lipids) circulating in the bloodstream and in all cells in the body and essential for functioning. The body makes some cholesterol and the rest comes from ingested animal products (e.g., meat, poultry, fish, eggs, butter, cheese, and whole and 2% milk). Not found in foods from plants.

Dietary Approaches to Stop Hypertension (DASH) Diet: Developed by the U.S. Department of Health and Human

Services, this diet plan reduces blood pressure due to generous amounts of potassium.

Diabetes Mellitus: A condition characterized by hyperglycemia resulting from the body's inability to use blood glucose for energy. In type 1 diabetes, the pancreas no longer makes insulin and therefore blood glucose cannot enter the cells to be used for energy. In type 2 diabetes, either the pancreas does not make enough insulin or the body is unable to use insulin correctly.

Dietary Fiber: Undigestable nonstarch polysaccharides from plants and their components including cell walls, pectins, gums, and brans, which help absorb water and move food through the digestive system, making defecation easier. Fiber is classified as soluble or insoluble.

Glucagon: A hormone secreted by special cells in the pancreas in response to low blood glucose concentration that elicits the release of glucose from liver glycogen stores.

Glucose: A monosaccharide; sometimes known as blood sugar.

Glycogen: An animal polysaccharide composed of glucose; manufactured and stored in the liver and muscles as a storage form of glucose.

High-Density Lipoprotein (HDL) (also, "good" cholesterol): A type of fat found in the blood that takes extra cholesterol from the blood to the liver for removal.

Human Immunodeficiency Virus (HIV): A retrovirus that causes AIDS (see Acquired Immunodeficiency Syndrome) by infecting helper T cells of the immune system thereby rendering the HIV patient vulnerable to infections and illnesses. Transmitted via direct contact with blood or blood products (needle stick), genital secretions (semen, vaginal fluid), or breast milk. This virus mutates rapidly but has an insidiously long gestation period that may be a decade or longer. While new therapies are being developed that can prolong life, currently there is no cure for this debilitating and fatal disease.

Hyperglycemia: Excessive blood glucose. Fasting hyperglycemia is defined as a blood glucose level above normal after a person has fasted for at least eight hours. Postprandial hyperglycemia is defined as a blood glucose level above normal one to two hours after a person has eaten.

Hypertension (also, high blood pressure): A condition present when blood flows through the blood vessels with a force greater than normal; results in heart strain, damage to blood vessels, and increased risk of heart attack, stroke, kidney problems, and death.

Insulin: A hormone that helps the body use glucose for energy. The beta cells of the pancreas make insulin. When the body cannot make enough insulin, it can be needle injected or by using an insulin pump.

Insulin Resistance: The body's inability to respond to and use the insulin it produces; may be linked to obesity, hypertension, and high levels of fat in the blood.

Low-Density Lipoprotein (LDL) (also, "bad" cholesterol): A type of fat found in the blood that transports cholesterol through the body to where it is needed for cell repair; also deposits on the inside of arterial walls (see Hypertension).

Lipid: A naturally occurring, fat-soluble molecule (e.g., triglycerides, oils, waxes, cholesterol, sterols, etc.) used as energy storage, components of cell membranes, and cell signaling.

Metabolic Syndrome: Characterized by a group of metabolic risk factors in one person; these may include: obesity, insulin resistance or intolerance, hypertension, and altherogenic dyslipidemia.

Noncommunicable Diseases (NCDs): A lifestyle or opportunistic infection or disease not typically spread person-to-person. Includes cancers, heart disease and stroke, chronic respiratory diseases, and type 2 diabetes.

Obesity: A condition where the body has a greater than normal amount of fat; more severe than overweight, having a body mass index of $\geq$ 30.

Overweight: An above-normal body weight with a body mass index of 25 to 29.9.

Pancreas: An digestive organ that makes insulin and enzymes; located behind the lower part of the stomach and is about the size of a hand.

Plant Stanols/Sterols: Naturally occurring substances found in plants, present in small quantities in many fruits, vegetables, vegetable oils, nuts, seeds, cereals, and legumes. Important because they block the absorption of cholesterol in the small intestine, thus safely reducing LDL cholesterol by 6 percent to 15 percent without lowering HDL cholesterol (see Low-Density Lipoprotein; High-Density Lipoprotein; Cholesterol).

Persons Living with HIV and AIDS (PLWHA): A biopsychosocial way to define humans infected with HIV and those whose disease has progressed to AIDS.

Risk Factor: An attribute or exposure that is causally associated with an increased probability of a disease, injury, and/or death.

Triglycerides: The chief form of fat in the diet and the major storage form of fat in the body. High levels of triglycerides often mean a low level of HDL ("good") cholesterol and a high level of LDL ("bad") cholesterol; levels $\geq$ 150 mg/dL may increase the risk for heart disease and diabetes. (See High-Density Lipoprotein; Low-Density Lipoprotein.)

Waist Circumference: Anthropometric measurement used to assess a person's abdominal fat; excess abdominal fat increases the risk of many of the serious conditions associated with obesity. Women's waist measurements should be < 35 inches and men's < 40 inches.

Public Health Terms

Dietary Guidelines for Americans: A report published by the U.S. Department of Agriculture and U.S. Department of Health and Human Services that explains how to eat to maintain health; form the basis of U.S. nutritional policies and are revised every five years. This chapter refers mostly to the 2000 guidelines.

Healthy People 2010: A national public health initiative under the jurisdiction of the U.S. Department of Health and Human Services (DHHS) that identifies the most significant preventable threats to health and focuses efforts toward eliminating them.

Medical Nutrition Therapy: Use of specific nutrition counseling and interventions, based on an assessment of nutritional status, to manage a condition or treat an illness or injury.

Micronutrients: Vitamins and minerals required in small amounts daily (e.g., vitamin A and iron).

Vulnerable and At-Risk Populations: High-risk groups of people who have multiple health and social needs. Examples include pregnant women, people with HIV infection, substance abusers, migrant farm workers, homeless people, poor people, infants and children, elderly people, people with disabilities, people with mental illness or mental health problems or disorders, and people from certain ethnic or racial groups who do not have the same access to quality health care services as other populations.

Primary Prevention: Healthcare services, medical tests, counseling, health education, and other actions designed to prevent the onset of a targeted condition. Routine immunization of healthy individuals is an example of primary prevention.[5]

Secondary Prevention: Measures such as healthcare services designed to identify or treat individuals who have a disease or risk factors for a disease but who are not yet experiencing symptoms of the disease. Papanicolaou (Pap) tests and high blood pressure screening are examples of secondary prevention.[5]

Health Promotion: Any planned combination of educational, political, regulatory, and organizational supports for actions and conditions of living conducive to the health of individuals, groups, or communities.

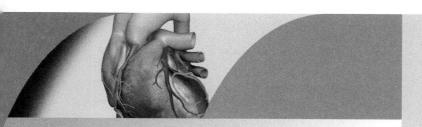

Questions for Further Research, Study, Reflection, and Discussion

For the Individual Student

In order to answer these questions, it may be necessary to research the primary literature.

1. What is the metabolic syndrome, and how can it be avoided?

2. A new field of study in the cancer arena is called *Nutrogenomics*. What are scientists discovering about the role of genes and interaction with food consumption and prevention of cancer?

3. Can poor nutrition raise a person's risk of contracting HIV/AIDS? Are any micronutrients protective against the virus?

4. The second edition of the seminal study *Disease Control Priorities in Developing Countries* estimates the cost effectiveness of several lifestyle interventions that target risk factors associated with NCDs. For example, cost-effective interventions to prevent high risk drinking or to mitigate its effects include population-based interventions, such as legislation and taxes, improved law enforcement, restricting sales, breath-testing, bans on advertising, and mass media campaigns. Consult the DCPP publications at their Web site (http:// www.dcp2.org/pubs/DCP. Accessed March 27, 2008) to find what evidence-based cost-effective interventions are recommended for the nutrition-related chronic diseases covered in this chapter.

For Small Group Discussion

1. *Case Study: Ahmed.* How could the social support from the family have been helpful to Ahmed in re-ducing his risk of future heart attacks? What elements of his lifestyle were harmful? Could his family have played a more effective role in helping him manage his CVD?

2. *Case Study: Gladys.* What assistance could Gladys' family provide to help her manage her hypertension? What role does stress play in her situation?

3. *Case Study: Jeff.* What is the impact of diabetes on Jeff's ability to work and maintain his current lifestyle? What could his wife do to help Jeff lose weight?

For Entire Class Discussion

1. In most countries, priority in health funding is given to curative care in hospitals and clinics. How does this impact the ability of the health system to prevent and manage nutrition-related chronic illnesses?

2. What are the likely trends in diabetes and obesity and how might they affect future health system costs?

3. What steps should a developing country with limited resources for health sector spending take to lower mortality from cardiovascular disease?

4. What environmental changes are needed in the United States to lower the risk of cardiovascular disease for African Americans?

5. How can a country with few resources and food insecurity best assure that people living with HIV/AIDS receive the nutritional care and support they need to manage their condition and maximize the benefits of treatment?

6. If you were the Minister of Health or Secretary of Health of a country, what priority actions would you select to reduce the burden of disease caused by nutrition-related chronic diseases?

EXERCISE/ACTIVITY

Identify a person with a chronic illness such as diabetes, hypertension, coronary heart disease, or HIV/AIDS who would be willing to talk with you about his or her challenges in managing his or her disease through dietary changes.

Healthy People 2010: An Addendum

The emerging threat of obesity receives significant and widespread attention in Healthy People 2010, as illustrated by what follows below:

Of the **Focus Areas**, 10 are directly relevant to this chapter. Many others are linked.

1. **Access to Quality Health Services**
2. Arthritis, Osteoporosis, and Chronic Back Conditions
3. **Cancer**
4. Chronic Kidney Disease
5. **Diabetes**
6. Disability and Secondary Conditions
7. **Educational and Community-Based Programs**
8. Environmental Health
9. Family Planning
10. Food Safety
11. **Health Communication**
12. **Heart Disease and Stroke**
13. **HIV**
14. Immunization and Infectious Disease
15. Injury and Violence Prevention
16. Maternal, Infant, and Child Health
17. Medical Product Safety
18. Mental Health and Mental Disorders
19. **Nutrition and Overweight**
20. Occupational Safety and Health
21. Oral Health
22. **Physical Activity and Fitness**
23. **Public Health Infrastructure**
24. Respiratory Diseases
25. Sexually Transmitted Diseases
26. Substance Abuse
27. Tobacco Use
28. Vision and Hearing

Similarly, of the Leading Health Indicators, the top two are directly related to this nutrition and chronic illness, while the last is important for prevention, treatment, and management.

- **Physical Activity**
- **Overweight and Obesity**
- Tobacco Use
- Substance Abuse
- Responsible Sexual Behavior
- Mental Health
- Injury and Violence
- Environmental Quality
- Immunization
- **Access to Health Care**

Several Chapters in HP 2010 are relevant:

5. Goal

   Through prevention programs, reduce the disease and economic burden of diabetes, and improve the quality of life for all persons who have or are at risk for diabetes.

12. Goal

    Improve cardiovascular health and quality of life through the prevention, detection, and treatment of risk factors; early identification and treatment of heart attacks and strokes; and prevention of recurrent cardiovascular events.

19. Goal

    Promote health and reduce chronic disease associated with diet and weight.

    Many of the HP 2010 Objectives are focused on nutrition-related chronic diseases.

1-3. Increase the proportion of persons appropriately counseled about health behaviors.

3-10. Increase the proportion of physicians and dentists who counsel their at-risk patients about tobacco use cessation, physical activity, and cancer screening.

5-1. Increase the proportion of persons with diabetes who receive formal diabetes education.

5-2. Prevent diabetes.

5-7. Reduce deaths from cardiovascular disease in persons with diabetes.

5-8. (Developmental) Decrease the proportion of pregnant women with gestational diabetes.

5-17. Increase the proportion of adults with diabetes who perform self-blood-glucose monitoring at least once daily.

7-11. Increase the proportion of local health departments that have established culturally appropriate and linguistically competent community health promotion and disease prevention programs.

12-11. Increase the proportion of adults with high blood pressure who are taking action (for example, losing weight, increasing physical activity, and reducing sodium intake) to help control their blood pressure.

12-13. Reduce the mean total blood cholesterol levels among adults.

12-14. Reduce the proportion of adults with high total blood cholesterol levels.

12-15. Increase the proportion of adults who have had their blood cholesterol checked within the preceding 5 years.

12-16. (Developmental) Increase the proportions of persons with coronary heart disease who have their LDL-cholesterol level treated to a goal of less than or equal to 100 mg/dL.

19-1. Increase the proportion of adults who are at a healthy weight.

19-2. Reduce the proportion of adults who are obese.

19-3. Reduce the proportion of children and adolescents who are overweight or obese.

19-5. Increase the proportion of persons aged 2 years and older who consume at least two daily servings of fruit.

19-6. Increase the proportion of persons aged 2 years and older who consume at least three daily servings of vegetables, with at least one third being dark green or orange vegetables.

19-7. Increase the proportion of persons aged 2 years and older who consume at least six daily servings of grain products, with at least three being whole grains.

19-8. Increase the proportion of persons aged 2 years and older who consume less than 10 percent of calories from saturated fat.

19-9. Increase the proportion of persons aged 2 years and older who consume no more than 30 percent of calories from total fat.

19-10. Increase the proportion of persons aged 2 years and older who consume 2,400 mg or less of sodium daily.

19-11. Increase the proportion of persons aged 2 years and older who meet dietary recommendations for calcium.

19-15. (Developmental) Increase the proportion of children and adolescents aged 6 to 19 years whose intake of meals and snacks at schools contributes to good overall dietary quality.

19-17. Increase the proportion of physician office visits made by patients with a diagnosis of cardiovascular disease, diabetes, or hyperlipidemia that include counseling or education related to diet and nutrition.

22-1. Reduce the proportion of adults who engage in no leisure-time physical activity.

22-6. Increase the proportion of adolescents who engage in moderate physical activity for at least 30 minutes on 5 or more of the previous 7 days.

22-8. Increase the proportion of the Nation's public and private schools that require daily physical education for all students.

REFERENCES

1. Office of Disease Prevention and Health Promotion, U.S. Department of Health and Human Services. *Healthy People 2010.* Bethesda: USDHHS; November 2000.

2. Centers for Disease Control and Prevention, National Center for Health Statistics. *National Health and Examination Survey 2003-2004.* Atlanta: CDC; June 2005.

3. *Joint WHO/FAO Expert Consultation on Diet, Nutrition and the Prevention of Chronic Diseases.* Geneva, Switzerland: World Health Organization; 2002.

4. Lopez AD, Mathers CD, Ezzati M, Jamison DT, Murray CJL, eds. *Global Burden of Disease and Risk Factors.* New York: Oxford University Press; Washington, DC: World Bank; 2006.

5. Harvard School of Public Health. Fats and Cholesterol: The Good, the Bad, and the Healthy Diet. 2007. Available at http://www.hsph.harvard.edu/nutritionsource/fats.html. Accessed March 28, 2008.

6. U.S. Department of Health and Human Services, National Institutes of Health. *Your Guide to Lowering Blood Pressure with DASH. DASH Eating Plan.* 2006. Available at http://www.nhlbi.nih.gov/health/public/heart/hbp/dash/new_dash.pdf. Accessed March 28, 2008.

7. U.S. Department of Health and Human Services, Office of Disease Prevention and Health Promotion. Dietary Guidelines for Americans. Updated 2006. Available at http://www.health.gov/DietaryGuidelines/. Accessed March 28, 2008.

8. Second Expert Report. Food, Nutrition, Physical Activity, and the Prevention of Cancer: a Global Perspective. Washington, DC: American Institute of Cancer Research (AICR); 2007. Available at http://www.aicr.org/site/PageServer?pagename=res_report_second. Accessed March 28, 2008.

9. Centers for Disease Control and Prevention, National Center for Health Statistics. National Health and Nutrition Examination Survey (NHANES). Homepage; 2007. Available at http://www.cdc.gov/nchs/nhanes.htm. Accessed March 28, 2008.

10. Barlow SE, Dietz WH. Obesity evaluation and treatment: expert committee recommendations. *J Pediatr* 1998;102(3):e29. Available at http://pediatrics.aappublications.org/cgi/content/full/102/3/e29. Accessed March 28, 2008.

11. U.S. Department of Health and Human Services, Centers for Disease Control and Prevention. *Preventing Obesity and Chronic Diseases Through Good Nutrition and Physical Activity.* 2005. Available at http://www.cdc.gov/nccdphp/publications/factsheets/Prevention/obesity.htm. Accessed March 28, 2008.

12. Bulik, Cynthia. 2007. Weight Management Center, Department of Psychiatry and Behavioral Sciences. Available at http://www.aedweb.org/media/shapeup.cfm. Accessed March 28, 2008.

13. Institute of Medicine. Crossing the Quality Chasm: The IOM Health Care Quality Initiative. 2006. Available at: http://www.iom.edu/CMS/8089.aspx. Accessed March 28, 2008.

RESOURCES

Sun Q, Ma J, Campos H, Hankinson SE, Manson JE, Stampfer MJ, Rexrode KM, Willett WC, Hu FB. A prospective study of *trans* fatty acids in erythrocytes and risk of coronary heart disease. *Circulation* 2007;115:1858–1865.

American Cancer Society. *Cancer Facts and Figures 2006.* Atlanta. Available at http://www.tcsg.org/tobacco/Cancer Stats2006.pdf. Accessed March 28, 2008.

American Cancer Society. Cancer Prevention and Early Detection Facts and Figures 2006. Available at http://www.cancer.org/downloads/STT/CPED2006PWSecured.pdf. Accessed March 28, 2008.

National Cancer Institute, National Institutes of Health, Department of Health and Human Services. Cancer Trends Progress Report—2007 Update. Bethesda; 2005. Available at http://progressreport.cancer.gov. Accessed March 28, 2008.

Wild S, Green A, Sicree R. Global prevalence of diabetes. Estimates for year 2000 and projections for 2030. *Diabetes Care* 2004;27:1047–1053.

He K, Liu K, Daviglus ML, Morris SJ, Loria CM, Van Horn L, Jacobs DR Jr, Savage PJ. Magnesium intake and incidence of metabolic syndrome among young adults. *Circulation* 2006;113:1675–1682.

Mokdad AH, Ford ES, Bowman BA, Nelson DE, Engelgau MM, Vinicor F, Marks JS. Diabetes trends in the U.S. 1990-1998. *Diabetes Care* 2000;23:1278–1283.

Mokdad H, Bowman BA, Ford ES, Vinicor F, Marks JS, Koplan JP. The continuing epidemics of obesity and diabetes in the United States. *JAMA* 2001;286:1195–2000.

Ezzati M, Lopez AD, Rodgers A, Vander Hoon S, Murray CJL, Comparative Risk Assessment Collaborating Group 2002. Selected major risk factors and global and regional burdens of disease. *Lancet* 2004;360:1347–1360.

Joint WHO/FAO Expert Consultation on Diet, Nutrition and the Prevention of Chronic Diseases. *Diet, nutrition and the prevention of chronic diseases: report of a joint WHO/FAO expert consultation.* WHO Technical Series 916. Geneva, Switzerland: WHO; 2002. Available at http://www.fao.org/WAIRDOCS/WHO/AC911E/AC911E00.HTM. Accessed March 28, 2008.

Lopez AD, Mathers CD, Ezzati M, Jamison DT, Murray CJL, eds. *Global Burden of Disease and Risk Factors.* New York: Oxford University Press; 2006.

Venkat Narayan KM, Zhang P, Kanaya AM, Williams DE, Englegau MM, Imperatore G, Ramachandran A. Diabetes: The Pandemic and Potential Solutions (chapt 30). In: *Disease Control Priorities in Development Countries,* 2nd ed. New York: Oxford University Press; 2006:591–603. *Note:* The Disease Control Priorities Project (DCPP) is an ongoing effort to assess disease control priorities and produce evidence-based analysis and resource materials to inform health policymaking in developing countries. DCPP has produced three volumes providing technical resources that can assist developing countries in improving their health systems and ultimately, the health of their people. The Disease Control Priorities Project is a joint enterprise of the Fogarty International Center of the National Institutes of Health, the World Health Organization, the World Bank, and the Population Reference Bureau.

Doll R, Peto R. *The Causes of Cancer.* New York: Oxford Press; 1981.

McGinnis JM, Foege WH. Actual cause of death in the United States. *JAMA* 1993;270:2207–2212.

Strong K, Mathers CD, Leeder S, Beaglehole R. Preventing chronic diseases: how many lives can we save? *Lancet* 2005; 366:1578–1582.

The Linkages Project. *Breastfeeding and HIV/AIDS Frequently Asked Questions (FAQ).* FAQ Sheet 1. (Updated 2004.) Available at http://www.pronutrition.org/files/Frequently AskedQuestions_HIV_eng.pdf. Accessed March 28, 2008.

National Food and Nutrition Commission. *Zambia Nutrition Guidelines for Care and Support for People Living with AIDS.* Lusaka, Zambia: Fanta Publications; 2004. Available at http://www.fantaproject.org/publications/zambia_guide2005.shtml. Accessed March 28, 2008.

McQueen DV. Continuing efforts in global chronic disease prevention. *Prev Chronic Dis* [serial online] 2007:4. Available at http://www.cdc.pcd/issues/2007/apr/07_0024.htm. Accessed March 28, 2008.

Barlow SE, Dietz WH. Obesity evaluation and treatment: expert committee recommendations. *Pediatrics* 1998;102:e29.

World Cancer Research Fund/American Institute for Cancer Research (AICR). *Food, Nutrition, Physical Activity, and the Prevention of Cancer: a Global Perspective.* Washington, DC: AICR; 2007.

CROSS REFERENCES

Cancer Prevention

Colon Cancer

Diabetes

Epidemiology of Atherosclerosis

Exercise

History of Nutrition

HIV/AIDS

Hypertension

Stroke

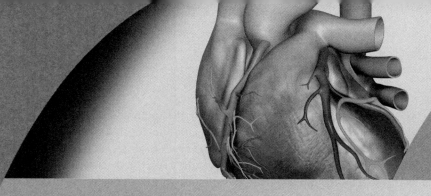

CHAPTER 11

Exercise: The Vaccine and Antidote for Obesity

Wayne C. Miller

Walking an extra 400 meters a day can reduce Americans' premature mortality risk by almost 10%.[1]

LEARNING OBJECTIVES

By the end of this chapter, the student will be able to:

- Describe how Americans' perception of health and beauty has changed over the past century.
- Recognize how the medical profession and fashion industry have contributed to the fat phobia seen in America.
- Discuss the concept of energy balance in the body, and how exercise affects the different components of energy balance.
- Evaluate exercise use at all levels of prevention for obesity.
- Interpret the paradox that exists between cultural, social, and environmental factors that promote obesity and the behavioral factors that prevent obesity.
- Observe the complexity of public health issues related to obesity prevention.

HISTORY

What comes to mind when you hear the words *voluptuous woman*? Your image is most likely much different from the image that comes to your parents' minds or grandparents' minds. During the 20th century, our vision of attractiveness and health changed dramatically. In fact, you might say our vision of desirable body size has taken a one-eighty (180°) degree turn. A voluptuous woman of the early 1900s was full-figured, robust, and had large hips, whereas a voluptuous woman of today is petite, thin, and has small hips. Why has our vision of health and physical attractiveness changed so much in 100 years? Has our modern definition of health defined our perception of attractiveness? Or, is it the other way around: has our modern perception of attractiveness dictated our definition of health? The answer is both. Events that occurred in the health insurance industry paralleled events occurring in the fashion industry to pre-program us into faulty thinking that health, thinness, fitness, and attractiveness are inseparably connected.

The Healthy Body Myth:
HEALTH = THINNESS = FITNESS = ATTRACTIVENESS

How Overweight Got Such a Bad Name

Let's look at how things changed. Life insurance companies of the early 1900s wanted to define variables that predicted premature mortality. Therefore, they began collecting and analyzing data on policy holders that could be used as screening factors for disease risk and mortality. Body weight was an easy measure to obtain on all applicants, so it was obviously thrown in the mix of potential predictive variables. The first outcome of the statistical analyses on body weight was the height-weight tables, published around the turn of the 20th century and updated several times until their latest version of 1983.[2] The first tables were sex- and age-specific and contained normative values for current policy holders. However, later versions of the tables reported what was originally called "normal" as now "desirable" and then as being "ideal." "Ideal" body weights in the newer tables no longer varied by age, and "ideal" was defined by weights at the lowest mortality rates for 20- to 29-year-olds.

In what was probably an unrelated coincidence, the fashion industry concurrently promoted thinness with styles that departed dramatically from the "voluptuous" styles of earlier years. The "flapper" style of the 1920s and 1930s promoted a new sleek boyish look. In 1947, fashion designer Christian Dior introduced the "wasp" look for women that accentuated the 17-inch waist, which only could be obtained by use of a corset. The fleshy look of Marilyn Monroe in the 1950s was soon replaced by the emaciated look of the British model, "Twiggy," in the 1960s, and this has continued through to models like today's Kate Moss. Thus, two totally unrelated industries—life insurance and fashion—pounded Americans with a new message: body fat is unfashionable as well as unhealthy.

But that was not all. During the early 1940s when the world was at war, loyal Americans submitted themselves to food rationing in an effort to provide more resources for our fighting men. Because obesity was viewed as a result of overeating (and not as a result of less physical activity), self-indulgence and overweight were seen as borderline treason, because consuming less would provide more food for our armed forces. No longer was overweight just seen as unfashionable and unhealthy, but now it was seen as immoral. This immorality of overeating has persisted today, when food is defined as "good" and "bad." As for good tasting food, isn't it *sinfully* delicious?

Commercialism of Weight Control and Exercise

One factor overlooked through more than half of the last century was the contribution of inactivity to overweight. However, this came to the forefront as an issue during the 1950s when European children were performing better than American children on physical fitness tests. President Eisenhower sought to remedy the situation by creating the President's Council on Youth Fitness (currently called the President's Council on Physical Fitness and Sports). President John F. Kennedy, who followed Eisenhower in office, was young and athletic, and further promoted children's fitness into the 1960s. The 1960s also brought us Kenneth Cooper, M.D., M.P.H., the man who defined **aerobics** (continuous exercise endurance) when he published his landmark book entitled, *The Aerobics Way*. About the same time, Jean Nidetch began holding weekly meetings in her home with friends who wanted to discuss the best ways to lose weight. These weekly meetings in Queens, New York were the start of the commercial enterprise Weight Watchers, Inc.®, one of the largest weight-loss companies in the world. Such early beginnings of the 1960s spawned two large weight-related industries: the weight loss industry and the fitness industry.

Coupled with the weight loss industry was the pharmaceutical industry's commercialization of weight loss. This industry has been frantically researching for decades to find an effective weight loss drug. During the 1950s and 1960s, **amphetamines** were used for weight loss, thinking that they would stimulate the metabolism. Other types of drugs to suppress appetite also have been tried over the years. Then what seemed to be the miracle drug was discovered to be effective in the early 1990s. The combination of two drugs, fenfluramine hydrochloride and phentermine resin (fen-phen) showed moderate success with sustained weight loss. The number of prescriptions written for fen-phen increased from 60,000 in 1992 to 1.1 million in 1995.[2] This explosion of use led to the establishment of clinics devoted just to the prescription of weight loss medications. Unfortunately, the success of this drug combination did not last long. The Food and Drug Administration (FDA) withdrew fen-phen from the market because of reports of **valvular heart disease** and **pulmonary hypertension** in women taking the drug combination. One report showed that 30 percent of women taking fen-phen demonstrated abnormal echocardiograms, even without symptoms. To date, there have not been any other drugs marketed with as much fervor and acceptance as fen-phen. Regardless, a review of the weight loss research using prescription drugs never has been promising. The data show that the difference in weight loss between treatment groups and control groups, for any weight loss drug tested, is only 2 to 3 kg after several months of treatment.

The commercialism around diet, exercise, and weight control has been further supported by claims, statements, and position stands coming from the healthcare industry, health agencies, and the national government. The American Heart Association declared physical inactivity as an independent risk factor for cardiovascular disease in 1992,[4] proposing that it has equal magnitude of risk with smoking, hyperlipidemia, and hypertension. Because these diseases are associated with obesity, obesity itself was soon added to the list of primary risk factors for cardiovascular disease. Shortly afterwards (1995), the Surgeon General for the United States produced the first report on physical activity and health.[5] The recommendation was that adults get 30 minutes of moderate-intensity physical activity on most, if not all, days of the week. However, the newest *Dietary Guidelines for Americans* (2005)[6] recommends 60 minutes of moderate intensity physical activity a day to help manage body weight and prevent weight gain; and recommends 60 to 90 minutes of daily moderate physical activity to sustain weight loss.

As the 20th century closed, the war on obesity became more ferocious than ever. The first Federal guidelines on the identification, evaluation, and treatment of overweight and obesity in adults were finally released in 1998 by the National Heart, Lung, and Blood Institute in cooperation with the

National Institute of Diabetes and Digestive and Kidney Diseases.[7] Then in 1999 an article published in the *Journal of the Americal Medical Association* reported that obesity kills approximately 300,000 Americans a year.[8] Obesity mortality rates of 300,000 to 400,000 have been batted around for the past several years, with arguments about their validity on both sides of the spectrum. Nonetheless, the only message the public has heard is that obesity kills. Furthermore, the Surgeon General, Richard H. Carmona, M.D., M.P.H., F.A.C.S., has stated on several occasions that obesity is the terror within and is a greater threat to Americans than weapons of mass destruction or terrorist attacks.

BACKGROUND: THE PUBLIC REACTION TO THE WAR ON WEIGHT

So how have Americans adapted to the bombardment of messages that we are too fat? We have not adapted well. The prevalence of obesity and overweight continues to rise in all segments of the population. The percentage of Americans who are physically active remains at the same level as it has been for years. However, the prevalence of eating disorders has doubled since the 1960s, while the mortality rate for eating disorders has been estimated to be as high as 20 percent. Moreover, a disorder that is so new that it does not have a set of diagnostic criteria has emerged. Among other things, this new disorder has been called compulsive exercise disorder, excessive exercise disorder, and anorexia athletica. A person with this disorder uses exercise to control body weight, body composition, or level of fitness to the extent that the exercise becomes compulsive and detrimental to emotional and/or physical health, rather than beneficial. Excessive exercise disorder is somewhat prevalent in overweight individuals, but more prevalent in athletes, highly fit individuals, and fitness professionals.

Thus, we see a dichotomy in the population that is paradoxical. We have become fat phobic, but are becoming fatter. In an effort to lose weight and become healthy, we are participating in unhealthy weight loss behaviors. This dichotomy even becomes comical at times. For example, we spend time running on the treadmill, but drive the car half a mile to the store because we are in a hurry. We drive our children to the park so they can get exercise during baseball practice. We sit on the sideline of a football field reading a book while our children practice soccer. We insist that bicycle paths be constructed in our neighborhoods, but we don't own a bicycle. We eat fast food (which is generally unhealthy and concentrated in calories), but order a diet drink with our meal. We institute Standards of Learning in our schools, because we want our children to have healthy and alert minds; but then we ignore their physical health by eliminating physical education from the curricula. We e-mail a message to our coworker and hope he will see it and reply quickly, rather than walk 30 feet down the hall to his office to talk to him. We finally get out and burn 300 kilocalories (kcal) in exercise, but then re-hydrate with a sport drink that contains 200 kcal.

Unlike many other **epidemics** that have come upon us in the past, the obesity epidemic does not have one cause and will not have one solution. A myriad of psychological, physiological, economic, social, cultural, moral, and behavioral factors and more affect the fragile energy balance that is at the root of this epidemic. Curbing the obesity epidemic is probably the greatest public health challenge the world has seen to date.

BASIC SCIENCE FACTS/KEY CONCEPTS REVIEW
Components of Energy Expenditure

The 24-hour energy expenditure can be broken down into three components: the thermal effect of food (TEF), the resting metabolic rate (RMR), and the energy cost of physical activity (Figure 11-1). The TEF is defined as the amount of energy required to digest, absorb, and further process the energy-yielding nutrients in food (i.e., fat, protein, carbohydrate). These energy-expending processes for preparing food prior to its use in intermediary metabolism generate heat, and are therefore collectively called the *thermal* effect of food, or alternatively, dietary-induced *thermogenesis*.

The contribution of the TEF to the total 24-h energy expenditure is minimal and averages about 8 percent. Given a daily energy expenditure of 2,000 kcal (8.37 MJ) the TEF would be approximately 160 kcal (670 kJ). Because the metabolic pathways for storing excess dietary fat in the body are more efficient than converting excess carbohydrate and protein into their storage forms—glycogen and fat—the TEF for a high-protein or high-carbohydrate meal is greater than that for a high-fat meal. However, the TEF varies at most by around 40 kcal (167 kJ) per day when altering the macronutrient composition of the diet to the extreme, and therefore would not contribute much to reducing body weight in the short term. For example, it would take over seven years for an individual to lose 30 pounds (13.6 kg) by only changing diet macronutrient composition. Furthermore, research shows that variance in the TEF does not seem to make a difference in body fat stores within or among individuals.

Resting Energy Expenditure

Because the RMR constitutes the largest portion of the 24-hour energy expenditure, anything that affects the RMR has the potential to substantially impact body fat stores. Restrictive dieting and exercise exert opposing forces on the RMR. However, the effects of exercise and restrictive dieting on

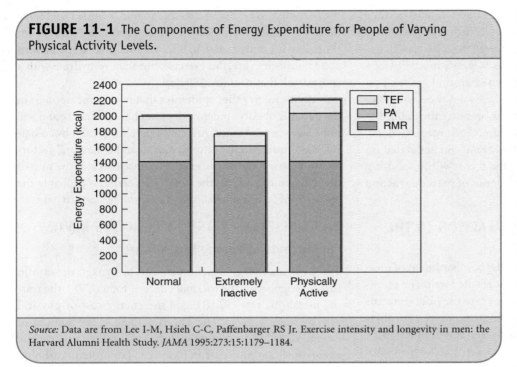

FIGURE 11-1 The Components of Energy Expenditure for People of Varying Physical Activity Levels.

Source: Data are from Lee I-M, Hsieh C-C, Paffenbarger RS Jr. Exercise intensity and longevity in men: the Harvard Alumni Health Study. *JAMA* 1995:273:15:1179–1184.

requirement of exercising muscles. Exercise physiologists have contended for years that aerobic exercise training causes a small, but significant increase in RMR. More recent investigations, however, infer that aerobic exercise training does not automatically increase RMR appreciably.

Because it is well accepted that strength training can increase muscle mass and that muscle mass is very active metabolically, Byrne and Wilmore (2001) examined how strength training may differentially affect RMR in comparison to aerobic exercise training.[10] This cross-sectional study found that there was no significant difference in RMR among strength-trained, aerobically trained, and untrained women. In another randomized controlled clinical trial, moderately obese men and women were assigned to one of three groups; diet plus strength training, diet plus aerobic training, or diet only.[11] The exercise protocols were designed to be **isoenergetic**. The mean weight loss among groups did not differ significantly after eight weeks, but the strength-trained group lost less lean tissue mass than the other two groups. The RMR declined significantly in each group, with no difference among groups. These studies indicate that neither strength training nor aerobic exercise training prevents the decline in RMR caused by restrictive dieting, and that exercise per se does not raise the RMR significantly.

The benchmark review of the effect of exercise on RMR during weight loss is a meta-analysis by Ballor and Poehlman.[12] When diet-induced reductions in RMR were corrected for changes in body weight, RMR was reduced by less than 2 percent. These meta-analytical data indicate that exercise training does not differentially affect RMR during weight loss nor enhance RMR during weight loss, and that reductions in RMR normally seen during weight loss are proportional to the loss of the metabolically active tissue.

Thus far, we have seen that the TEF and RMR are not subject to perturbations that would cause increases in the 24-hour energy expenditure substantial enough to affect body fat stores appreciably. It is also impossible to voluntarily change the metabolic rate of the TEF and RMR. Therefore, it must be concluded that these two components metabolism are relatively fixed, and that we cannot do anything voluntarily to change

RMR are almost exclusively related to their affects on lean body mass. When an overweight or obese person loses weight, his/her RMR decreases in proportion to the amount of lean body mass (LBM) lost. If an individual gains muscle mass through exercise training, his/her RMR increases in proportion to the muscle mass gained. Although RMR drops while a person is on a very-low-calorie diet, most authors agree that when energy intake is restored to pre-dieting levels, the RMR also returns to pre-dieting levels, unless there is a net decrease in lean body mass. In that case, the post-diet RMR per lean body mass ratio (RMR:LBM) would be equivalent to pre-dieting levels. However, an early research paper contests that severe energy restriction lowers RMR:LBM significantly.[9] During this study, obese women were placed on a very-low-calorie diet for three weeks. RMR:LBM declined to 94 percent, 91 percent, and 82 percent of the original value on days 3, 5, and 21, respectively. Unfortunately, no follow-up was done in this study to see if the RMR:LBM would have returned to normal after energy intake was resumed to pre-diet levels. More research needs to be conducted in order to determine the long-term effects of energy-restricted diets on RMR, both for the chronic dieter as well as the person with anorexia.

Even though less than 20 percent of the RMR is attributed to skeletal muscle, the most dramatic effect on metabolic rate is strenuous exercise. During strenuous exercise, the total energy expenditure of the body may increase 15 to 25 times above resting levels. This enormous elevation in the body's metabolic rate is the result of a 200-fold increase in the energy

them. On the other hand, the energy expenditure associated with physical activity, whether structured exercise or not, is under voluntary control.

Exercise Energy Expenditure

Because heavy exercise can increase metabolic rate 20 times above resting levels, even short bouts of daily exercise may have a profound effect on body fat stores. In terms of comparison, the RMR of a 70-kg human is approximately 1.2 kcal per minute (5.0 kJ), whereas the energy cost during strenuous exercise can be 18 to 30 kcal per minute (75–125 kJ). At first glance, these numbers look promising for weight loss in that the energy cost of a 60-minute exercise bout would be from 1,080 to 1,800 kcal (4,518–7,531 kJ). This translates into an exercise-induced weight loss of about one-third to one-half pound a day. However, theoretical estimates of energy expenditure during exercise, such as those previously described, are not realistic for the overweight or obese individual for several reasons. First, an intense exercise bout lasting 60 minutes is beyond the reach of most overweight people, because the functional capacity of the overweight person is generally much less than the normal weight individual. Overweight people, who have a history of inactivity, generally can only increase their total energy expenditure by about eight-fold during maximal exercise exertion, and most of these people find it very difficult to sustain an exercise intensity of 75 percent maximal effort for 20 minutes. Therefore, the best initial expectation for the overweight person would be to exercise for 20 minutes at an intensity that is six times the RMR (6 metabolic equivalents [**METS**]). Under these conditions (20 minutes at 6 METS), the predicted energy expenditure of the exercise session would only be about 150 kcal (628 kJ). If one were to obtain 30 minutes of moderate intensity exercise per day, as the Surgeon General suggests, the total energy expenditure would be approximately 225 kcal (941 kJ).

Figure 11-1 illustrates how the three components of metabolism contribute to the 24-hour energy expenditure under normal conditions, conditions where a person is extremely sedentary, and where a person obtains 30 minutes of moderate intensity exercise. Although it may seem that the absolute contribution of the energy cost of exercise to offset the daily energy balance during weight loss treatment is small, the relative contribution of exercise to the 24-hour energy expenditure is important. The 30-minute exercise bout described above may account for 10 percent or more of the daily energy expenditure for an obese person. Furthermore, exercise may have a metabolic effect beyond that which is accounted for during the actual exercise session itself.

It is well established that metabolic rate remains elevated for some period of time following exercise. This phenomenon has been termed *excess post-exercise oxygen consumption*

(EPOC). Studies have shown that the magnitude of EPOC is linearly related to the duration and intensity of exercise, and that EPOC following a moderate intensity exercise bout accounts for about 15 percent of the total energy cost of the exercise. The time for metabolism to return to baseline following an acute exercise session can vary from as little as 20 minutes to more than 10 hours, depending on the duration and intensity of exercise. Increments of EPOC may play a significant role in the energy balance of the body. Unfortunately, the EPOC is not sufficiently predictable as a measurable variable in exercise prescription for weight control.

Exercise and Reduced Weight Maintenance

Several reviews have been written on exercise and weight control, and each concludes that exercise is a key factor in reduced weight maintenance. A consistent finding is that the more exercise, the better the maintenance of weight loss. Patients who expend at least 1,500 to 2,500 kcal (6.3–10.5 MJ) a week are more likely to maintain their full end-of-treatment weight loss.[13–15] Similar findings have been reported from the National Weight Control Registry, which includes a total of 784 males and females who have maintained an average weight loss of 30 kg for an average of 5.6 years.[16] Participants in the National Registry reported expending approximately 2,830 kcal per week (11.8 MJ), or the equivalent of walking about 28 miles per week. However, it must be remembered that these individuals only consumed about 1,400 kcal or 5,860 kJ a day during the study.

More exact estimates of exercise energy expenditure required for maintaining reduced weight come from Schoeller and colleagues, who used **doubly labeled water** to estimate the metabolic cost of an exercise program needed to maintain weight loss in previously obese women.[17] Metabolic measurements revealed that the women were exercising 700 kcal per day (2,930 kJ) to maintain their reduced body weight. This translates into 80 minutes a day of moderate physical activity, 35 minutes a day of vigorous activity, or walking about 7 miles per day. Several years later, a similar study was conducted and the results were identical to the first.[18] However, in this later study, a comparison group of those who gained weight during a one-year follow-up period was included. The weight gainers expended 491 kcal (2,054 kJ) a day in physical activity. Thus, the difference between the maintainers and gainers was 211 kcal (883 kJ). This amount of additional physical activity is obtainable by exercising for 30 minutes a day at a moderate intensity (Figure 11-1).

Health Benefits of Exercise

It was previously mentioned that obesity is a comorbidity and major risk factor for many diseases such as cardiovascular disease, diabetes, and hypertension. It is also well established that physical activity is great preventive medicine; whether instituted at the primary, secondary, or tertiary level. The most prominent public health message of this century is to *be physically active.* The benefits of physical activity can integrate into all aspects of our health. Among other things, physical activity (or physical fitness) has been associated with decreased blood pressure, decreased risk of cardiovascular disease, improved glucose control, decreased cancer risk, improved mental health, and lower rates of premature mortality. It is even more interesting to note that most of the unhealthy conditions that are ameliorated with exercise are also comorbid to obesity. Moreover, the health benefits of exercise can be obtained without weight loss.

The past decade has produced several studies to show that physical activity or physical fitness can improve health status of the overweight/obese person in the absence of weight loss. One of the first, and most notable, studies was published by Barlow et al. in 1995.[19] This early study revealed that mortality rates of overweight and obese individuals are the same as their lean counterparts, when groups are stratified according to level of fitness. In other words, fitness, not fatness, is the determinant of mortality. Several studies since then have shown that improvements in health can occur in as few as seven days in obese people who exercise and still do not lose weight.

If weight loss is not the issue, then the question becomes: how much exercise is necessary to improve health in a population that is predominantly overweight? The answer to this question was answered over 40 years ago, but has since been forgotten in the midst of the search for a cure to the obesity epidemic. One of the earliest epidemiological studies in public health focused on physical activity and cardiovascular disease. The study compared the incidence of ischemic heart disease in bus drivers to conductors in the London public bus transportation system. The five-year study showed that the bus drivers had an incidence of heart disease that was 83 percent higher than that of the conductors. It became clear that the preventive health factor for the conductors was physical activity, in that they were walking much of the day and climbing up and down stairs to reach passengers on the upper deck of the bus.

The results of a subsequent study, which also seem to have been lost in the midst of the "more is better" mindset of the fitness promoters, show that it only takes a small amount of physical activity to reduce premature mortality significantly (Figure 11-2).[20] The data come from the Harvard Alumni study. Mortality risks were calculated for men who reported their physical activity levels in 1962 or 1966, and then were followed until 1988. Men who participated in vigorous physical activity (> 6 **METS**) in their earlier years reduced their mortality risk significantly. In fact, the mortality rates of those who expended between 150 and 400 kcal per week (628–1,674 kJ) in vigorous physical activity were no worse than those who expended more than 1,500 kcal per week (6,276 kJ; Figure 11-2). Translating this into lay terms, you can reduce your risk for mortality by about 10 percent simply by briskly walking or jogging as little as a quarter of a mile a day (400 meters). This amount of exercise is less than the Surgeon General suggests, and within the limits of exercise capacity for overweight individuals that was discussed earlier in this chapter. Walking or jogging 400 meters a day is a goal that most of the 66 percent of American adults who are overweight can achieve. Imagine the public health messages that could be built around that simple goal: *join the quarter miler club – do the daily 400 – sneak your 400 in during coffee break – 400 first – quarter miler, not quarter pounder.*

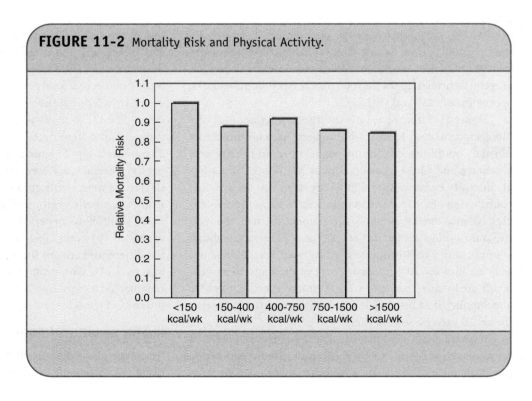

FIGURE 11-2 Mortality Risk and Physical Activity.

CASE STUDY

Scenario

John, a 58-year-old African-American truck driver with a high school education, was recently diagnosed with hypertension. His resting blood pressure at time of diagnosis was 144/92 mm Hg. John's physician has prescribed an angiotensin II receptor blocker (80 mg QD) and suggested that John lose weight to help manage his blood pressure. (Angiotensin II is a hormone that causes the blood vessels to constrict. As angiotensin II receptor blockers inhibit the action of angiotensin II, the blood vessels are able to relax and blood pressure is reduced.)

John has come to you, a health promotion specialist, to help him lose weight. John is 5'10" tall (178 cm) and weighs 231 pounds (105 kg). John's body mass index (BMI) is currently 33.1. John understands the importance of taking his medication and has not missed a dose in the past four weeks, since his diagnosis. His blood pressure is currently stable at 128/84. John does not have any other medical conditions and his physician has cleared him for exercise.

John lives in Atlanta, Georgia, with his wife of 35 years. They have four children who are all grown and living in the Atlanta area. John's wife is obese, and he describes her as the best Southern cook in Georgia. John travels a lot for his job and is usually on the road for eight to ten days a month. When he is home, John loves getting together with his extended family. John has not exercised regularly since he was an athlete in high school.

Defining the Issues

1. John is not physically active and has an occupation that does not encourage physical activity. Barriers to becoming more physically active need to be addressed and diminished.
2. John's wife is a great Southern cook, which means he probably consumes a high-fat diet when at home. Although he does not yet present other comorbidities, John is at risk for cardiovascular disease. He and his wife need to be educated and given skills for healthy eating within their cultural context.
3. John is on the road a lot. This presents another barrier for healthy eating and exercise. When and how will John be able to exercise when on the road? How can John make healthy food choices while traveling?
4. John likes to get together with his extended family when he is home. Most likely these gatherings involve large meals and overeating. An assessment of these family gatherings needs to be made, with intervention where necessary.
5. John has been living this lifestyle for many years. Lifestyle change will probably be difficult. Possible emotional, social, cultural, and religious barriers to habit change need to be evaluated.

Patient's Understanding

John understands the importance of medication for controlling his blood pressure, in that he has consistently taken his medication since the time of his diagnosis. However, John does not understand well the role lifestyle and habitual behavior play in reducing disease symptomatology. Like many people, John thinks in terms of "all or nothing" or "black and white." His perception of exercise is training three hours a day for athletic competition, like he did in high school. His perception of a healthy diet is eating only green salad. John still needs to learn that moderate changes in lifestyle, without becoming obsessive, can cause dramatic changes in health status. The long-term prevention program for John is one that ensures successful lifestyle change that is realistic for him.

Unfortunately, John is like many Americans. He was very physically active in high school and enjoyed athletic competition. However, after becoming an adult, family responsibilities and a hectic work schedule pushed physical activity out of the forefront of John's life, while fast food and quick meals took the place of healthier planned meals. John would be in a healthier condition now if throughout his young adulthood he had practiced health-promoting behaviors. However, John did not gain the lifestyle skills necessary to promote healthy living and therefore is suffering the consequences of years of sedentary living and a poor diet. Furthermore, John is now faced with the burden of developing health promotion behaviors and changing deep-rooted habits.

CLINICAL PERSPECTIVE FOR THE INDIVIDUAL PATIENT

Treatment for the obese person who has an underlying medical condition consists of intervening to reduce body weight (fatness) as well as to ameliorate symptoms of the related comorbidity. Treatment of the presenting medical condition will almost always receive priority over obesity treatment. Sometimes successful treatment of the underlying medical condition will cure the obesity problem. However, oftentimes obesity persists following treatment for the comorbidity. In these cases, extended treatment for the obesity will be necessary.

Aerobic exercise training causes a decrease in both systolic and diastolic blood pressures, even for individuals with normal blood pressure. Aerobic exercise is also the type of exercise that has the most significant effect on body weight. Because John is obese, he is also at risk for other comorbidities of obesity, particularly cardiovascular disease and diabetes. Aerobic exercise is also a great prevention strategy for these conditions.

PUBLIC HEALTH PERSPECTIVE FOR THE HEALTH OF THE GENERAL POPULATION AND OF HIGH RISK GROUPS

It is very unlikely that the cure for the obesity epidemic will be a vaccine, a weight loss pill, or a single behavioral intervention because the etiology of obesity is multifaceted and the determinants of obesity are interrelated and multitiered. Furthermore, because obesity afflicts all segments of the population, any treatment for obesity—whether primary, secondary, or tertiary prevention—will need to be targeted at specific subsets of the population. It almost seems that there will need to be as many treatments for obesity as there are overweight individuals.

Financial Issues

This overwhelming challenge to public health brings with it several issues to be addressed. First and probably foremost is the question of who will pay the cost for obesity treatment and prevention? The costs are going to be astronomical. Just think of how much a treatment plan for two-thirds of the population will be, especially when the intervention needs to be individualized. Few insurance companies currently pay for wellness programs and all refuse to pay for obesity treatment; even if they decided to pay the costs, insurance premiums would skyrocket. What about those without health insurance? Health disparities in this country would increase rather than decrease. In addition to a staggering rise in individual health insurance premiums, taxes would need to increase dramatically just to cover increasing Medicaid and Medicare expenses.

On the other side of the cost issue is the multi-billion dollar business of obesity treatment. Obesity treatment is already lucrative, so think of the trillions of dollars in potential revenue to those providing obesity treatment services. Would commercial programs like Weight Watchers® and Jenny Craig® be able to collect insurance reimbursement for their programs? Will dietitians, personal trainers, and lifestyle counselors be able to cash in on the need for obesity prevention? What about government agencies themselves, like the USDA extension services? Will they become healthcare providers? The legal battles alone to be fought over this big pot of money will themselves be lucrative. Last but not least is the issue of the Internet. Would products and services sold over Internet Web sites be covered by insurance? What about weight loss books? Could an individual be reimbursed for the cost of a weight loss book? Who would decide whether a person can receive a treatment plan or not? The personal physician? The cost for office visits alone to receive physician approval would increase a physician's income substantially.

Service Delivery

The second issue to be addressed, which is closely tied to the financial issue, is dissemination. Even after it is decided who will deliver the services, how will these services be disseminated to such diverse subsets of the population? For example, how will we reach the elderly? How will we reach low-income elderly? How will we reach low-income elderly African-Americans? How will we reach urban versus rural low-income elderly African-Americans? How will we reach urban low-income African-Americans living in subsidized housing? How will we reach urban low-income African-Americans living in subsidized housing who are illiterate? How will we reach male urban low-income African-Americans living in subsidized housing who are illiterate? How will we reach male urban low-income African-Americans living in subsidized housing who are illiterate and English is their second language? This line of questioning can go on for different climates, different regions of the country, varying religious affiliations, etc. Then it can start all over for other ages, racial groups, ethnicities, children, and more.

Environmental Change

Another issue to be addressed is the environment. How can we change our environment so that it is more conducive to eating healthy and being physically active? The same line of questioning used above can be used when we address the issue of environment. How can we change the environment of male urban low-income African-Americans living in subsidized housing who are illiterate and English is their second language? What must be done to make their environment more conducive to physical activity? Financial issues will come up again when we look at changing the environment. Who will pay for building sidewalks, constructing parks, and other types of community planning?

Political, Social, and Moral Challenges

The last major public health issue to be addressed is the one that involves political, social, and moral challenges. This can be illustrated by use of an example. It is generally accepted that foods high in refined sugar, fat, salt, and calories are unhealthy and lead to obesity if not consumed sparingly. These are commonly called *junk food*. The political issue used in this example is a proposal to levy a federal tax on all junk food. The positive aspect would be that this tax could help subsidize the obesity treatment costs already discussed in this chapter. Look now at the political, social, and moral issues that will be debated in this type of legislation. First of all, who will be the key players? In the legal battle, it will be the food producers, advertisers, stores and businesses, restaurants, food distributors, parents, human rights activists, the public, the media, food scientists, educators, and more. Next, what will their individual positions be? How will a consensus be achieved? Who will be the winners and who the losers? It is easy to see that this issue will become quite volatile.

Individual Behavior Change

Behavior change is the last public health issue to be considered. Resolution of all of the issues discussed thus far will only serve to encourage, support, facilitate, and provide the environment for successful behavior change. The obesity epidemic will only be halted if people change their behaviors to fall in line with what primary, secondary, or tertiary prevention strategies dictate. The process of behavior change itself needs to be understood and behavior change skills need to be taught to each individual who is overweight or at risk of being overweight. The challenge is, how can this be done on a large scale? How can we teach behavior change skills to masses of adults? How can we teach masses of children primary prevention skills? Not until we resolve this and all of the heretofore mentioned issues will we be in a position to reverse the obesity epidemic.

Public Health Challenges to Address the Obesity Epidemic

- Designing population interventions that also meet individual needs
- Financing obesity treatment and prevention
- Delivering services to widely diverse subsets of the population
- Restructuring the physical and social environments that currently discourage physical activity and healthy eating
- Overcoming political, social, and moral issues
- Facilitating individual behavior change

KEY TERMS

Clinical Terms

Aerobics: Refers to exercise where the predominant energy source is dependent upon the utilization of oxygen to liberate energy for muscle contraction. In lay terms, aerobics refers to continuous endurance exercise such as jogging, swimming, walking, and rowing.

Amphetamine: A type of drug that stimulates the central nervous system; prolonged use may cause drug dependence.

Doubly Labeled Water: A chemically altered molecule of water where nonradioactive isotopes of hydrogen and oxygen are used to track their utilization rates in the body. The difference between the loss of hydrogen and oxygen in the body constitutes carbon dioxide production, which is directly related to metabolic rate.

Isoenergetic: Equal in energy value, whether it be energy intake or energy expenditure.

Metabolic Equivalent (MET): The resting metabolic rate or amount of energy expended at rest, which is approximately 35 mL oxygen per kg body weight per minute.

Pulmonary Hypertension: An increase in blood pressure in the arteries of the lungs that can lead to shortness of breath, dizziness, fainting, and decreased exercise tolerance. If severe, pulmonary hypertension can cause right heart failure.

Valvular Heart Disease: Disease affecting any one of four valves in the heart. The affect may be stenosis (narrowing of the valve so blood cannot pass freely) or regurgitation (failure of the valve to close, allowing blood to go back through the valve in the wrong direction).

Public Health Term

Epidemic: A classification of a disease or condition (in this context obesity) in which new cases in the human population, during a given time period, occur at a rate that substantially exceeds what is expected, based on past experience. The widespread prevalence of obesity across whole continents and the world make obesity a pandemic.

Healthy People 2010

Indicator: Physical Activity

Focus Area: Physical Activity and Fitness

Goal: Improve health, fitness, and quality of life through daily physical activity.

Objectives:

22-2. Increase the proportion of adults who engage regularly, preferably daily, in moderate physical activity for at least 30 minutes per day.

22-1. Reduce the proportion of adults who engage in no leisure-time physical activity.

22-6. Increase the proportion of adolescents who engage in moderate physical activity for at least 30 minutes on 5 or more of the previous 7 days.

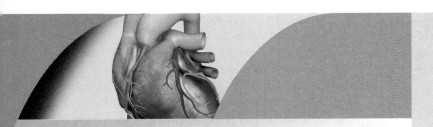

Questions for Further Research, Study, Reflection, and Discussion

For the Individual Student

In order to answer these questions, it may be necessary to research the primary literature.

- Overweight in adults is defined as having a BMI above 25, where obesity is defined as having a BMI above 30. What is the relationship between BMI and adiposity? Is BMI the best indicator of adiposity and associated disease risk?
- Health at Every Size (HAES) is a new paradigm that believes obsessions with dieting and weight have caused more harm than good. HAES promotes healthy eating and physical activity without focusing on body weight or size. The underlying assumption of HAES is that, regardless of size, all people can become healthier by eating well and being physically active. Do you think the HAES approach has a place in the fight against obesity? What are the strengths and weaknesses of such an approach?
- The bulk of the daily energy expenditure is accounted for by the resting metabolic rate (RMR). We have seen that it is unlikely that a person's RMR will increase through exercise, diet, or pharmaceuticals. On the other hand, do you think that obesity is caused by a defective RMR?
- What are the benefits of regular exercise for the normal weight person versus those for the overweight person?

For Small Group Discussion

- What things in John's family environment could possibly be used to help motivate and support his lifestyle change? What things in his family environment are obstacles to his necessary lifestyle change, and how can these be overcome?
- How might John overcome the tangible barriers to regular exercise, such as time and place to exercise? What about obstacles to eating healthily?
- How might John's wife be used as a support system for behavior change?
- Unhealthy behaviors are often controlled by one's emotions. For example, it is common for people to consume chocolate or ice cream when feeling depressed. What might be some emotions that control John's behaviors? What can be done to help John manage these emotions in a healthier way?

For Entire Class Discussion

- The prevalence of overweight and obesity is increasing in children. What effect will this have on the adult workforce, especially during the next 20 years as the "baby boomers" retire?
- It has been estimated that, because of the obesity epidemic, the current generation of children will be the first who will not outlive their parents (i.e., have a shorter life expectancy than their parents). What effects will this have on society and the healthcare system?
- Should benefits be given to people who are normal weight? In other words, should insurance companies give reduced premiums for those who are low risk? Should normal weight individuals be given health insurance premium reductions?
- Should the government regulate the production and sale of obesity-promoting foods? What would be the ramifications if this happened?

EXERCISE/ACTIVITY

Go to the library or Internet and read about some of the community and public health promotion programs that have been developed for weight control in adults and children. Prepare a written report on one of the notable programs such as: Minnesota Heart Health, SPARK (Sports, Play, & Active Recreation for Kids), Agita São Paulo, and WIN (Weight-control Information Network).

REFERENCES

1. Lee I-M, Hsieh C-C, Paffenbarger RS Jr. Exercise intensity and longevity in men: the Harvard alumni health study. *JAMA* 1995;273:1179–1184.

2. Metropolitan Life Insurance Company. 1983 Height and weight tables. *Statistical Bulletin Metropolitan Insurance Company* 1984;64:2–9.

3. National Task Force on Obesity. Long-term pharmacotherapy in the management of obesity. *JAMA* 1996;276:1907–1915.

4. Fletcher GF, Blair SN, Blumenthal J, Caspersen C, Chaitman B, Epstein S, Falls H, Froelicher ES, Froelicher VF, Pina IL. Statement on exercise. Benefits and recommendations for physical activity programs for all Americans. A statement for health professionals by the Committee on Exercise and Cardiac Rehabilitation of the Council on Clinical Cardiology, American Heart Association. *Circulation* 1992;86:340–344.

5. U.S. Department of Health and Human Services. Physical activity and health. A report of the surgeon general. Executive summary. Accessed from: http://www.cdc.gov/nccdphp/sgr/pdf/execsumm.pdf.

6. U.S. Department of Health and Human Services. Dietary guidelines for Americans. Accessed from: http://www.health.gov/dietaryguidelines/.

7. National Institutes of Health National Heart, Lung, and Blood Institute. Clinical guidelines on the identification, evaluation, and treatment of overweight and obesity in adults: the evidence report. *Obesity Res* 1998;6:S51–S210.

8. Allison DB, Fontaine KR, Manson JE, Stevens J, VanItallie TB. Annual deaths attributable to obesity in the United States. *JAMA* 1999;282:1530–1538.

9. Fricker J, Rozen R, Melchior J-C, Apfelbaum M. Energy-metabolism adaptation in obese adults on a very-low-calorie diet. *Am J Clin Nutr* 1991;53:826–830.

10. Byrne HK, Wilmore JH. The relationship of mode and intensity of training on resting metabolic rate in women. *Int J Sport Nutr Exerc Metab* 2001;11:1–14.

11. Geliebter A, Maher MM, Gerace L, Bernard G, Heymsfield SB, Hashim SA. Effects of strength or aerobic training on body composition, resting metabolic rate, and peak oxygen consumption in obese dieting subjects. *Am J Clin Nutr* 1997;66:557–563.

12. Ballor DL, Poehlman ET. A meta-analysis of the effects of exercise and/or dietary restriction on resting metabolic rate. *Eur J Appl Physiol* 1995;71:535–542.

13. Hartmann WM, Stroud M, Sweet DM, Saxton J. Long-term maintenance of weight loss following supplemented fasting. *Int J Eating Disorders* 1993;14:87–93.

14. Jakicic J, Wing R, Winters C. Effects of intermittent exercise and use of home exercise equipment on adherence, weight loss, and fitness in overweight women. *JAMA* 1999;282:1554–1560.

15. Jeffrey RW, Wing RR, Thorson C, Burton LR. Use of personal trainers and financial incentives to increase exercise in a behavioral weight loss program. *J Consult Clin Psychol* 1998;66:777–783.

16. Klem ML, Wing RR, McGuire MT, Seagle HM, Hill JO. A descriptive study of individuals successful at long-term maintenance of substantial weight loss. *Am J Clin Nutr* 1997;66:239–246.

17. Schoeller DA, Shay K, Kushner RF. How much physical activity is needed to minimize weight gain in previously obese women? *Am J Clin Nutr* 1997;66:551–556.

18. Weinsier RL, Hunter GR, Desmond RA, Byrne NM, Zuckerman PA, Darnell BE. Free-living activity energy expenditure in women successful and unsuccessful at maintaining a normal body weight. *Am J Clin Nutr* 2002;75:499–504.

19. Barlow CE, Kohl HW III, Gibbons LW, et al. Physical fitness, mortality and obesity. *Int J Obesity* 1995;19(Suppl 4):S41–S44.

20. Lee I-M, Hsieh C-C, Paffenbarger RS Jr. Exercise intensity and longevity in men: the Harvard alumni health study. *JAMA* 1995;273:1179–1184.

RESOURCE

Morris JN, Kagan A, Pattison DC, Gardner MJ, Raffle PAB. Prediction of ischemic heart disease in London businessmen. *Lancet* 1966;2:553–559.

CROSS REFERENCES

Communicating Public Health Information
Hypertension
Nutrition Transition
Understanding Nutrition

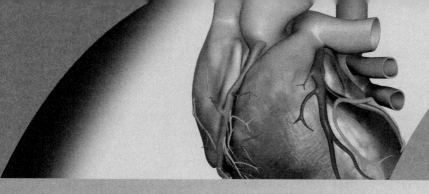

CHAPTER 12

Fetal Alcohol Syndrome: A Lifespan Perspective

Harolyn M. E. Belcher
Sabrina J. Roundtree

Fetal alcohol syndrome (FAS) is the most common preventable cause of **mental retardation** in the United States![1] In addition, FAS is reported to be the most common preventable cause of birth defects and developmental disabilities in the United States.[2]

LEARNING OBJECTIVES

By the end of this chapter, the student will be able to:

- Identify three facial features of FAS.
- Describe the spectrum of alcohol-related disorders.
- Enumerate the adverse outcomes associated with FAS and fetal alcohol effects.

HISTORY

Based on cumulative research findings, the U.S. Surgeon General has stated that, "no amount of alcohol consumption can be considered safe during pregnancy."[3,4] In fact, since biblical times, public health advocates have warned, "Behold, thou shalt conceive and bear a son. Now therefore, be careful not to drink wine or strong drink," Judges 13:3-4, 7. Ancient cultures in Carthage, Sparta, and East Asia forbade the use of alcohol for newlyweds. As early as 1876, the effects of fetal alcohol exposure on the newborn were documented in the medical literature.[5] However, our current understanding and continuous study of the effects of alcohol stem from the late 1960s, at which time in Nantes, France, Dr. Lemoine published a report about a series of 127 children of mothers with alcoholism who exhibited similar physical and growth features born to mothers who were alcoholics. During the same period in the United States, a pediatric resident, Dr. Christy Ulleland, was studying children with failure to thrive. She noted that all of the children in her study had a common history of maternal alcoholism.[6] By 1973, these clinical findings led to the term fetal alcohol syndrome (FAS) by Dr. Jones.[6]

BASIC SCIENCE FACTS/KEY CONCEPTS REVIEW

Proving Causality of Teratogens

A **teratogen** is a substance or exposure that is capable of disrupting fetal growth and producing malformations. As outlined in James Wilson's *Teratology: Principles and Techniques*,[7] manifestations of teratogens may include death, malformations, growth deficiency, and functional impairment. For a potential teratogen to be identified as a causal agent, it should meet causation criteria outlined by Sir Bradford Hill in 1965.[8] Namely, there must be a: 1) strength of association (e.g., the odds or relative risk of the adverse outcome given the teratogen exposure should be greater than one); 2) consistency (e.g., multiple studies demonstrating similar findings); 3) specificity of the association (e.g., findings are specific to exposure); 4) **temporality** (teratogen exposure must precede the disorder); 5) demonstration of a **dose response** relationship (e.g., heavier exposure produces more severe outcomes); 6) **biological plausibility** (e.g., research demonstrating the teratogen's effects in animals or at the cellular level); 7) coherence (conclusions drawn from data should be consistent with generally known facts; alternative explanations of the adverse outcome should be explored); 8) experiment (e.g., exposure produces adverse effects and lack of exposure produces no adverse outcome); and 9) analogy (given evidence of the effects of other infectious and chemical agents, similar evidence supports similar causal conclusions for teratogen agent under investigation) (Table 12-1).

Over the last 30 years, studies of the effects of alcohol on the developing fetus have satisfied each of these criteria for demonstrating causal relationships between alcohol exposure and adverse fetal outcome. In addition, fetal alcohol exposure is associated with all possible adverse outcomes of teratogen exposure, namely death, malformation, growth deficiencies, and functional impairments.[6,9–12]

Alcohol's Effects on the Developing Fetus

Animal Studies

Animal models demonstrate varying effects of alcohol on neurotransmitter receptors and nerve cells in the developing fetal brain. Organized nerve cell migration is of paramount importance for functional brain development. Gamma-aminobutyric acid (GABA) is the brain's major inhibitory neurotransmitter. $GABA_B$ receptors are involved in nerve cell motility. Alcohol decreases $GABA_{B1}$ receptor expression during specific developmental periods, especially in the cerebral cortex, which may effect nerve cell migration and lead to the development of distorted nerve cell networks.[13] In a study of rats exposed to alcohol during pregnancy, offspring were found to have a smaller diameter of nerve cells in the hippocampal, dorsal, and ventral blades of the dentate gyrus.[14] Alcohol was found to reduce the role of mitogen-activated/extracellular signal regulated protein kinases in immature neurons (nerve cells), which is hypothesized to lead to impaired granule cell migration.[15] The

aforementioned animal studies demonstrate alcohol's adverse effects on nerve cell migration and brain development.

Human Studies

Similar to the findings in animal studies, children with alcohol exposure may have abnormalities of brain development and poor weight gain, despite adequate caloric intake.[16] While neurological deficits are largely understood based on animal and magnetic resonance imaging (MRI) studies, the cause of growth retardation and poor weight gain in children with FAS is not fully understood.[17,18]

Scope of Human Neurological Effects Associated with Alcohol Exposure. Multiple central nervous system abnormalities in humans are attributed to alcohol exposure, including agenesis and malformations of the corpus callosum (the nerve fiber tract connecting the left and right cerebral hemispheres that is associated with attention, reading, verbal memory, and psychosocial functions), reduced volume of the basal ganglia (brain region involved in motor coordination, inhibition of inappropriate behavior, spatial memory, and other cognitive functions), and volume asymmetries in the hippocampus (the area of the brain responsible for consolidation of memories).[19–23]

Alcohol exposure is associated with an increased risk of developing attention deficit hyperactivity disorder, depression, suicidal ideation, mental retardation, and learning disabilities.[9,19,24,25] These factors may lead to poor school and life performance, in addition to increased risk of alcohol and drug disorders.[9,25,26]

Facial Features of FAS. Most importantly, alcohol exposure causes recognizable facial features (Figure 12-1 and Table 12-2). The facial features associated with alcohol exposure include microcephaly (head size smaller than the second percentile), small palpebral fissures (eye slits), flat philtrum, and thin upper lip.[17,18]

Other Alcohol-Related Birth Defects. The Institute of Medicine proposed using the terms *alcohol-related neurodevelopmental disorder (ARND)* and **alcohol-related birth defects (ARBD)** to describe the spectrum of clinical findings associated with alcohol exposure.[27] Birth defects associated with alcohol exposure effect multiple organ systems. Common alcohol-related malformations include: 1) cardiac **anomalies**, (e.g., atrial septal defects, ventricular septal defects, and tetralogy of Fallot); 2) skeletal anomalies (e.g., hypoplastic nails, shortened fifth digits, scoliosis, hemivertebrae, Klippel-Feil syndrome, radioulnar synostosis); 3) renal anomalies that may include aplastic or dysplastic kidneys, or horseshoe kidneys; 4) ocular anomalies (e.g., strabismus, retinal vascular anomalies); and 5) auditory impairments (hearing loss).[4]

TABLE 12-1 Causation Criteria

Sir Bradford Hill's Causation Criteria

1. Strength of Association
2. Consistency
3. Specificity of Association
4. Temporality
5. Dose Response Relationship
6. Biological Plausibility
7. Coherence
8. Experimental Proof
9. Analogy

Source: Data from Hill AB. The environment and disease: association or causation? *Proceedings of the Royal Society of Medicine* 1965;58:293–300.

FIGURE 12-1 Child with Fetal Alcohol Syndrome.

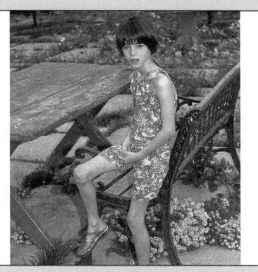

Source: © David Young Wolff/Photo Edit, Inc.

TABLE 12-3 Characteristic Findings in Children Exposed to Alcohol In Utero

- Characteristic facial anomalies
  ○ Short palpebral fissures
  ○ Ptosis
  ○ Flat midface
  ○ Upturned nose
  ○ Smooth philtrum
  ○ Thin upper lip
- Growth retardation
  ○ Low relative birth weight
  ○ Growth retardation despite adequate nutrition
  ○ Low weight relative to height
- CNS neurodevelopmental findings
  ○ Microcephaly
  ○ Structural brain abnormalities, including agenesis of the corpus callosum and cerebellar hypoplasia
  ○ Other neurological signs, such as fine motor difficulties, sensorineural hearing loss, poor gait coordination, and poor eye-hand coordination
- Unexplained behavioral abnormalities
  ○ Learning disabilities
  ○ Poor school performance
  ○ Poor impulse control
  ○ Problems with social perception
  ○ Poor language abilities
  ○ Poor abstract reasoning
  ○ Poor math skills
  ○ Impaired memory and judgment
- Birth defects (including but not limited to):
  ○ Congenital heart defects
  ○ Skeletal and limb deformities
  ○ Anatomical renal abnormalities
  ○ Ophthalmologic abnormalities
  ○ Hearing loss
  ○ Cleft lip or palate

Adapted from Institute of Medicine diagnostic criteria, 1996.

Source: Tifft C, Thackray H. Fetal alcohol syndrome. *Pediatr Rev* 2001; 22:47–55.

The term **fetal alcohol effects** (FAE) is used to describe children who do not meet the full criteria for FAS but have fetal alcohol exposure and evidence of central nervous system involvement (Table 12-3).[28] Children with fetal alcohol exposure have significantly poorer motor coordination, social functioning, and judgment.

Behavioral Phenotype. In addition to the facial structure and **body system** abnormalities associated with alcohol exposure, alcohol is associated with a behavioral phenotype (Table 12-4).

TABLE 12-2 Alcohol-Related Signs

FAS Facial Features
- Small palpebral fissures
- Flat philtrum
- Thin upper lip

Alcohol-Related Birth Defects
- Cardiac anomalies
- Skeletal anomalies
- Renal anomalies
- Ocular anomalies
- Auditory impairment

In a study of secondary disabilities in 415 individuals with FAS or FAE (mean age 14.2 years, range 6–51 years), 94 percent of the subjects with alcohol exposure had mental health disorders.[9,25] The mean intelligence quotient (IQ) range for this study cohort was found to be in the low average range; however, **adaptive skills** (skills of daily living) were in the moderate deficit range (median = 62). Of the mental health problems noted for children, attention deficit hyperactivity disorder was most common, occurring in 61 percent of the individuals, followed by

TABLE 12-4 Definitions of Alcohol-Related Effects

- Fetal alcohol syndrome (FAS; all categories must be present for diagnosis)
  - Confirmed maternal alcohol exposure (excessive drinking characterized by regular intake or heavy episodic drinking)
  - Characteristic facial anomalies
  - Growth retardation
  - Central nervous system (CNS) neurodevelopmental findings
- Partial FAS with confirmed maternal alcohol exposure
  - Confirmed maternal alcohol exposure
  - Characteristic facial anomalies
  - Either growth retardation, CNS neurodevelopmental findings, or other unexplained behavioral abnormalities
- Alcohol-related birth defects
  - Confirmed maternal alcohol exposure
  - Birth defects
- Alcohol-related neurodevelopmental disorder
  - Confirmed maternal alcohol exposure
  - Either CNS neurodevelopmental abnormalities or other unexplained behavioral abnormalities

Adapted from Institute of Medicine diagnostic criteria, 1996.
Source: Tifft C, Thackray H. Fetal alcohol syndrome. *Pediatr Rev* 2001; 22:47–55.

TABLE 12-5 Signs and Symptoms of Fetal Alcohol Syndrome by Age Group

Age Group	Signs and Symptoms
Newborn	Characteristic facial features*
	Low birth weight
	Poor growth
	Microcephaly, hypotonia
	Irritability, poor bonding with caregivers
Toddler	Characteristic facial features*
	CNS neurodevelopmental abnormalities
	Poor growth
School-age child	Characteristic facial features*
	CNS neurodevelopmental abnormalities*
	Other unexplained behavioral abnormalities
	Poor growth
Adolescent	CNS neurodevelopmental abnormalities
	Other unexplained behavioral abnormalities
Adult	CNS neurodevelopmental abnormalities
	Other unexplained behavioral abnormalities

*Most useful features for diagnosis.
Source: Tifft C, Thackray H. Fetal alcohol syndrome. *Pediatr Rev* 2001;22:47–55.

depression (22%) and suicide threats (19%). Depression was most common in adults with alcohol exposure, occurring in over one half of the adult subjects, followed by suicide threat (43%) and suicide attempts (23%) (Table 12-5).[9,25]

Poor adaptive skills (or skills of daily living; i.e., personal hygiene, communication, socialization skills) in combination with mental health disorders cause individuals with FAS and FAE to be at high risk for poor judgment, work-related difficulties, social and relationship problems, and independent living. Inappropriate sexual behaviors were documented in 42 percent of individuals over 12 years of age with FAS and 52 percent of individuals with FAE.[9,25] Individuals with alcohol exposure who were victims of violence were four times more likely to demonstrate sexually inappropriate behaviors.[9,25] Interaction with police or the judicial system was reported in 14 percent of the 6- to 11-year-olds and 61 percent of adolescents with alcohol exposure.[9,25]

PUBLIC HEALTH PERSPECTIVE FOR THE HEALTH OF THE GENERAL POPULATION AND OF HIGH RISK GROUPS

One of the primary focus areas of Healthy People 2010 is Maternal, Infant, and Child Health. The overarching goal of this focus area is to "improve the health and well-being of women, infants, children, and families."[31] Specifically focusing on reduction of alcohol use, Goal 16–17 harkens to the biblical recommendation to "Increase abstinence from alcohol, cigarettes, and illicit drugs among pregnant women," and Goal 16–18 follows with the logical outcome once Goal 16–17 has been accomplished, namely, "Reduce the occurrence of fetal alcohol syndrome (FAS)."[31] For Goal 16–17, 17 percent of the target goal had been achieved for reduction of cigarette use during pregnancy by 2005.[32] No data are available yet for alcohol abstinence and reduction of FAS (Table 12-6).

Alcohol use is highly prevalent in American families; according to the 2005 National Household Survey on Drug Abuse, over half of the United States' population, 126 million individuals, are current alcohol users.[33] Current users are defined as those individuals who had at least one drink of alcohol in the 30 days prior to interview.[33] One drink is defined as a can or bottle of beer (12 ounces), a 4-ounce glass of wine or wine cooler, or one ounce of hard liquor or mixed drink with liquor. More than one fifth (22.7%) of the persons 12 years and older admitted to binge drinking (defined as 5 or more drinks at one sitting or within a couple of hours on at least one day within the past 30 days) and heavy alcohol use (5 or more drinks on the same occasion on each of five days within the past 30 days) was reported in 6.6 percent of the population.[33]

TABLE 12-6 Maternal Complications of Alcohol Abuse

Central Nervous System	Respiratory	Cardiovascular	Cancer	Gastrointestinal	Injury and Violence Unintentional	Gynecological	Hematology	
Arcus senilis	Respiratory irregularity	Alcoholic cardiomyopathy	Breast cancer	Alcoholic hepatitis	Falls	Amenorrhea	Thrombocytopenia	**D**
Alcohol withdrawal		Alcohol-induced hypertension		Cirrhosis	Fires	Anovulation	Anemia	**E**
Anxiety				Gastritis	Motor vehicle accidents	Luteal phase dysfunction		**A**
Cerebellar degeneration, anterior lobe				Liver dysfunction	At-risk behaviors			**T**
Depression				Nutrional/ vitamin deficits				**H**
Delirium tremens				Pancreatitis				
Hallucinations				Vomiting				
Loss of consciousness								
Memory loss								
Peripheral neuropathy								
Retrobulbar neuropathy leading to amblyopia								
Seizures								
Sleep disturbance								
Tremors								
Wernicke–Korsakoff syndrome (nystagmus, sixth nerve palsy, ataxia, confusion, Korsakoff psychosis)								

Sources: (1) Goodwin DW. Alcohol: Clinical Aspects. In: Lowinson JH, Ruiz P, Millman RB, Langrod JG, eds. *Substance Abuse: A Comprehensive Textbook*, 2nd ed. Baltimore: Williams and Wilkins; 1992:144–151.

(2) Bobo JK. Tobacco use, problem drinking, and alcoholism. *Clin Obstet Gynecol* 2002;45:1169–1180.

(3) Ponnappa BC, Rubin E. Modeling alcohol's effects on organs in animal models. *Alcohol Res Health* 2000;24:93–104.

CASE STUDY
Scenario

A lifespan perspective for an individual with FAS is captured in SA's story derived from his medical and psychosocial history and physical examination.

History of Present Illness

SA is a 37-year-old man with diagnosis of fetal alcohol syndrome who comes in for a physical examination, accompanied by his adult foster brother. Foster brother, Mr. B, is petitioning the court for transfer of guardianship of SA from Mr. B's biological mother to Mr. B. Mr. B's mother, who has been SA's foster mother from the time SA was 5 weeks to 15 years and then from 18 years to adulthood, is now in her late 70s and thus Mr. B would like to take over the responsibility of guardianship.

Perinatal History

SA was a term birth infant. There was heavy alcohol use by his mother during her pregnancy. No information was available on the father. Birth weight was unknown, and SA was given up by his biological mother shortly after birth. He came to live with his foster family, the B family, at five weeks of age.

Past Medical History

SA had a history of heart murmur and possible atrial septal defect, which resolved spontaneously. SA also had a history of repeated episodes of otitis media. Audiology evaluation results were normal. There were no known allergies or medications.

Developmental and Behavioral History

SA had slow early development in gross motor, fine motor, language, and adaptive skills. There was no history of regression of developmental skills. At 15 years of age, SA was transitioned to a group home. Increasing difficulties with judgment, inattention, and impulse control caused SA to have difficulty with self-care. Behavioral difficulties noted in the group home setting included increased distractibility, verbal aggression, and inappropriate sexual behavior. When SA was 18 years old, Mrs. B reapplied for and received guardianship of SA.

SA has had legal difficulties including a two year conviction for rape. With regard to the rape conviction, his foster brother reports that SA was romantically involved with the young lady; apparently, however, in the "passion of the moment," SA didn't understand that the young lady did not want to have sex.

Occupational History. SA has worked in a sheltered work environment for seven years without difficulty. He rides a bike to work.

Previous Evaluations. Adaptive functioning was measured on the Vineland Adaptive Behavior Scale. Communication domain standard score was 44, Daily Living was 59, Socialization was 50, and Adaptive Composite was 47. On the Wechsler IQ test, Verbal IQ was 63, Performance was 65, and Full Scale was 61.

Social History. SA currently lives with his foster brother and foster brother's wife.

Physical Exam

Alert, cooperative, young man with facial features consistent with fetal alcohol syndrome. Head was 54 cm, tenth percentile. Height 5'2". Forehead was hirsute, small palpebral fissures, hypotelorism, smooth philtrum, thin upper lip, posteriorly rotated ears. Full affect, oriented to person, place, and time. Eyes: right esotropia (inward eye deviation), full eye movement and retinal reflexes. Tympanic membranes scarred. Oropharynx: tongue midline, palate intact, no tonsillar exudates or hypertrophy. Nares clear and neck supple, without adenopathy. Chest: no boney deformities. Lungs: clear. Cardiovascular: regular rate and rhythm, quiet precordium, full and symmetric pulses. Abdomen: soft nontender, positive bowel sounds, no hepatosplenomegaly. Genito-urinary: deferred. Extremities: full range of motion; strength symmetric 5/5. Skin: clear. Back: straight.

Neurological Exam

Right esotropia, as previously noted. Facial sensation and movement were normal. Symmetric palate elevation. Strong bilateral shoulder shrug, and tongue protrusion was normal. Normal bulk and strength on motor evaluation. Mildly increased lower extremity tone and diminished axial tone. No tics, tremors, or ataxia. Normal gait. Deep tendon reflexes were 3+. Response to sensory stimulation was normal.

Developmental Testing. Gesell drawings were scored at the 9-year level. Durrell paragraph comprehension was at the 6th grade level. On the Wide Range Achievement test, the Reading standard score was 79 (6th grade level) and Arithmetic standard score was 60 (3rd grade level).

Defining the Issues

In considering the lifespan perspective for individuals with FAS, SA provides an excellent case study. At each stage of his life, there were identified challenges that were met. From birth to the present time, identification of a concerned caregiver was (is) of paramount importance. Whether the caregiver is a sober biological family member, foster or adoptive parent, sibling, group home, it is important that the caregivers understand the scope of physical and mental health disabilities that may accompany FAS. Patience and understanding of the spectrum of alcohol-related effects allow the development of appropriate guidance and interventions by caregivers, teachers, supervisors, caseworkers, and physicians throughout the lifespan of individuals with FAS. Supervised and safe environments keep the individual safe and productive; allowing healthy relationships to develop. Because adaptive skills and judgment may be impaired in individuals with FAS, confusion and frustration may result as the individual reaches maturity, especially with regard to intimate relationships and independence. Continued support, advocacy, structured living environments, and supervision may be necessary to identify and address challenging life circumstances, including early identification and treatment of mental health disorders and prevention of substance abuse (that are found more commonly in individuals with FAS than in their non–alcohol-exposed peers).

Patient's Understanding

This case demonstrates the significant lifelong challenges associated with providing care for a child and adult with FAS. SA entered the child welfare system early, when his biological mother was unable to care for him. He received special education throughout his school career due to his mild mental retardation and challenging behaviors. By age 15 he was transferred to a group home; however, his behaviors worsened and he became uncontrollable, prompting his foster mother to resume his care. As an adult, he was incarcerated for two years for a rape conviction that was possibly the result of his poor social judgment and impulse control during a romantic encounter. The foster mother's biological son now has guardianship of SA, as his mother is now an infirmed senior citizen. SA lives in an in-law apartment in the same house with Mr. B and his wife. Mr. B states that because of SA's previous conviction, SA is listed on the sex offense registry and therefore the family is moving out of the state because it is no longer comfortable for them to live in the neighborhood. Mr. B has enrolled SA in a structured supervised work environment and provides supervision in the home environment, while allowing SA some independence. SA is fortunate to have a caring and committed family.

CLINICAL PERSPECTIVE FOR THE INDIVIDUAL PATIENT

In considering the clinical perspective of SA an integrated multilevel public health prevention approach is best. **Universal prevention** begins with communication to the public about the adverse consequences of alcohol during pregnancy. Prevention may take place at the individual, family, and community levels (Figure 12-1). Secondary school health courses and medical school curricula contain information about the effects of alcohol. Counseling all women during health monitoring visits, prior to pregnancy, is a key window of opportunity to prevent FAS. Alcohol containers that have warning labels describing the consequences of alcohol ingestion during pregnancy increase the knowledge of alcohol-related effects for the public who consume alcohol.

Level of Intervention Now

SA currently volunteers daily in an indicated (tertiary) prevention program, which is a structured supervised work environment for individuals with cognitive limitations. He independently bikes to work and lives within close proximity (an in-law apartment) to his foster brother. SA's foster brother manages SA's finances and bills. SA understands his need for assistance with his business concerns and agrees to have his foster brother act as a guardian and advocate on his behalf. SA's understanding of his disability increases his ability to access services and maintain employment and may reduce the likelihood of SA being involved in future inappropriate sexual behaviors and, consequently, decrease involvement with the criminal justice system. Thus, SA's emotional well-being and life satisfaction are enhanced.

For individuals with FAS, **targeted prevention** and **indicated prevention** interventions may overlap. Prevention interventions have two targets, the first are pregnant women who are drinking heavily and the second are the children of those mothers.

Systematic obstetric screening for alcohol and drug use for all pregnant women (targeted) and referral of identified patients (indicated) to drug and alcohol treatment programs may reduce alcohol use and promote abstinence. For SA's mother, early identification and alcohol treatment may have reduced SA's exposure to alcohol. Studies have demonstrated the effectiveness of brief interventions to reduce high risk alcohol behaviors.[27,29]

Potential Level Earlier

Evaluation of all infants (universal) after birth for physical and development effects of alcohol exposure may result in early identification (targeted) and intervention (indicated). SA was diagnosed with FAS during the neonatal period. He was placed in foster care with the B family before he was two months old. For preschoolers, Dr. Patricia Halverson, a clinical psychologist who has worked for many years with Native American parents with alcohol dependence on the Indian Oasis School District in Arizona, recommends reducing overstimulation in the environment by limiting the number of toys out at one time, giving clear and brief directions, making sure the child's attention is on your face when giving directions, and teaching the differences between strangers and familiar people.[30] SA did receive special education early in life and continued in special education throughout his school years. Success with educating children with FAS may be facilitated by structure, consistency, brevity, variety, and persistence. For older children, encouraging independence and self-esteem are paramount; offer support, not criticism; foster self-help; set and consistently maintain limits; be brief and clear with directions; get the child ready for school before going to bed (organizing homework, clothes for the next day, etc.); and find a child advocate at the child's school. SA's foster mother tried, unsuccessfully, to transition SA to group home where he could mature with individuals his own age in a more independent environment.

In summary, FAS and alcohol-related disorders result in lifelong physical, emotional, social, and developmental challenges in infancy, childhood, and adulthood. The disorder is costly in personal and monetary terms. FAS is 100 percent preventable—no alcohol, no FAS—yet almost 500,000 children continue to be exposed each year to alcohol during their fetal growth.

Among adults, ages 18 to 25 years, 55.4 percent of women and 66.3 percent of men reported current alcohol use. An estimated 12.1 percent of pregnant women reported current alcohol use and 3.9 percent reported binge drinking.[33] These data suggest that almost 500,000 infants are exposed to alcohol and 159,900 exposed to binge drinking during their gestation. Heavy alcohol use was rare (0.7%) among pregnant women.[33] In 1991, the Substance Abuse and Mental Health Services Administration (SAMHSA) estimated that 26.8 million children of alcohol abusers live in the United States.[34] The National Association for Children of Alcoholics reports that almost one in five adult Americans (18%) lived with an alcoholic parent while growing up.[35–38]

Based on the latest population-based FAS Surveillance Network data from 1995 to 1997, the prevalence rate of FAS is estimated to be between 0.2 and 2.0 per 1,000 live births in the United States.[39–41] Other prenatal alcohol-related conditions, including ARND and alcohol-related birth defects (ARBD), are estimated to occur approximately three times as frequently as FAS.[42] From the data from the FAS Surveillance Network, the rate of FAS per 1,000 children by race was 0.2 for white and Hispanic children, 1.1 for African American children, and 3.2 for American Indian/Alaska Native.[43] The rate of FAS is almost five times higher for African Americans and 16 times higher for Native Americans than their white and Hispanic peers, despite similar rates of binge alcohol use during pregnancy among white (1.2/1,000), black (1.4/1,000), and Hispanic women (1.0/1,000) during the same time period.[44,45] This led to the hypothesis that alcohol in combination with other maternal factors, for example, genetic vulnerability, may play a role in the higher rate of FAS in the African American population. Specific alleles of genes regulating alcohol metabolism, alcohol dehydrogenase (ADH2-1/3) have been found in higher proportions in African-American women. Research has found that this maternal genotype was associated with high alcohol consumption (70% vs. 44%) and an increased odds (2.49) of having an infant with alcohol-related physical findings.[45]

Various medical economists have estimated the costs associated with FAS.[46–49] Based on the prevalence rates used and the costs (e.g., medical care, special education, etc.) that are included, the United States spends $2.3 billion to $11.1 billion per year on individuals with FAS. Total lifetime costs for an individual with FAS including medical care, special education, residential care, and loss of productivity are estimated to be 2.0 million fiscal year 2002 dollars.[50]

CONCLUSION

FAS is a preventable cause of mental retardation and birth defects. Along with the characteristic facial findings, individuals with FAS have a behavioral phenotype. An individual with FAS has differing needs across the lifespan, the most important being a nurturing, structured, supervised caregiving environment. Individuals with FAS are at increased risk for cognitive, behavioral, and emotional disorders. Continued education and prevention efforts are mandatory to reduce this preventable cause of neurodevelopmental disabilities. Public health prevention and intervention programs are necessary across the lifespan for individuals with FAS and their parents.

KEY TERMS
Biology and Behavioral Terms

Adaptive Skills: Skills of daily living including knowledge of basic self care, maintenance of personal hygiene, dressing, social, social judgment, and communication skills.

Alcohol-Related Birth Defects: Fetal or infant body system disorders of structure or function associated with alcohol exposure during gestation (see Table 12-2).

Anomaly: Abnormal development of a body system.

Body System: Group of organs that function together for example, cardiovascular system, gastrointestinal system, neurological system, respiratory system, etc.

Fetal Alcohol Effects (FAE): (Sometimes called *partial FAS* or, less commonly, *possible fetal alcohol effects.*) Includes individuals with intrauterine alcohol exposure who meet some of the facial features and at least one of the other criteria of fetal alcohol syndrome, including growth retardation, neurodevelopmental abnormalities, or behavioral or cognitive disorders.

Fetal Alcohol Syndrome (FAS): Includes individuals with a history intrauterine alcohol exposure who have the identifiable facial features, growth retardation, and neurobehavioral dysfunction.

Mental Retardation: Intellectual deficit measured by IQ and adaptive tests. An individual must have both IQ and adaptive skills test scores less than two standard deviations below the mean (≤ 70) to meet diagnostic criteria for mental retardation. Mental retardation is divided into mild (70–55), moderate (54–40), severe (39–25), and profound (< 25). Approximately 2.5 percent of the population has mental retardation; 85 percent of individuals with mental retardation are in the mild category.

Teratogen: Agent that causes birth defects, death, growth deficiency, and/or functional impairment.

Public Health Terms

Biological Plausibility: Epidemiological findings of association between the proposed causal agent and the biological disorder supported by existing knowledge of biological systems; also termed *coherence.* If biological knowledge is absent, replication studies in other populations may be necessary to prove *biological plausibility.*

Dose Response: As the exposure to the proposed causal agent increases, the response (risk) of the biological disorder increases.

Indicated Prevention: (Also called *tertiary prevention.*) A type of strategy applied to populations who demonstrate the disease (disorder or behavior) to prevent further morbidity or illness.

Targeted Prevention: (Also called *selective* or *secondary prevention.*) A strategy that focuses on individuals who are at-risk for a disease or disorder to help deter or avoid it altogether.

Temporality: Timing of exposure to the proposed causal agent must occur before the disease process.

Universal Prevention: (Also called *primary prevention.*) A strategy that targets the entire population (no-risk to high-risk individuals) to help deter or avoid a disease, disorder, or behavior.

Healthy People 2010

Indicator: Substance Abuse

Focus Area: Maternal, Infant, and Child Health

Goal: Improve the health and well-being of women, infants, children, and families.

Objectives:

16-17. Increase abstinence from alcohol, cigarettes, and illicit drugs among pregnant women.

16-18. Reduce the occurrence of fetal alcohol syndrome (FAS).

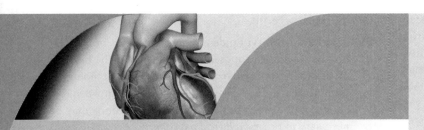

Questions for Further Research, Study, Reflection, and Discussion

For the Individual Student

In order to answer these questions, it may be necessary to research the primary literature.

- What is a possible reason for impairment of prenatal and postnatal growth observed in fetal alcohol syndrome?
- What factors may lead to higher risk of behavioral disorders in children with fetal alcohol syndrome?

For Small Group Discussion

- What strategies would you use to improve the outcome of children with FAS?
- Pretend one class member has FAS, another is the caregiver, another is the physician, another a case worker, and another is a teacher. How might these individuals work together to develop an intervention plan for the individual with FAS at different ages in the individual's life: infancy, school age, emerging adult?

For Entire Class Discussion

- How would you improve surveillance to determine a true incidence rate for fetal alcohol syndrome?

EXERCISE/ACTIVITY

- Study and develop a universal prevention for fetal alcohol syndrome.

REFERENCES

1. Substance Abuse and Mental Health Services Administration. Fetal Alcohol Spectrum Disorders by the Numbers. Rockville: U.S. Department of Health and Human Services; 2007.

2. Floyd RL, Sobell M, Velasquez MM, et al. Preventing alcohol-exposed pregnancies: a randomized controlled trial. *Am J Prev Med* 2007;32:1–10.

3. Carmona RH. U.S. Surgeon General Releases Advisory on Alcohol Use in Pregnancy. 2005. Available at http://www.come-over.to/FAS/SurGen Advisory.htm. Accessed April 3, 2008.

4. Committee on Substance Abuse, Committee on Children with Disabilities. Fetal alcohol syndrome and alcohol-related neurodevelopmental disabilities. *Pediatrics* 2000;106:358–361.

5. Haddon J. On intemperance in women, with special reference to its effects on the reproductive system. *BMJ* 1876;1:748–750.

6. Jones KL, Smith DW, Ulleland CN, Streissguth AP. Pattern of malformation in offspring of chronic alcoholic mothers. *Lancet* 1973;1:1267–1271.

7. Wilson JG, Warknay J. *Teratology: Principles and Techniques.* Chicago: University of Chicago; 1965.

8. Hill AB. The environment and disease: association or causation? *Proc Royal Soc Med* 1965;58:293–300.

9. Streissguth AP, Barr HM, Kogan J, Bookstein FL. Understanding the Occurence of Secondary Disabilities in Clients with Fetal Alcohol Syndrome (FAS) and Fetal Alcohol Effects (FAE). Centers for Disease Control and Prevention Grant No. R04/CCR008515 ed. Seattle: University of Washington School of Medicine; 1996.

10. Streissguth AP, Aase JM, Clarren SK, Randels SP, LaDue RA, Smith DF. Fetal alcohol syndrome in adolescents and adults. *JAMA* 1991;265:1961–1967.

11. Clarren SK, Smith DW. The fetal alcohol syndrome. *N Engl J Med* 1978;298:1063–1067.

12. Riley EP, Mattson SN, Li TK, et al. Neurobehavioral consequences of prenatal alcohol exposure: an international perspective. *Alcohol Clin Exp Res* 2003;27:362–373.

13. Li SP, Kim JH, Park MS, Bahk JY, Chung BC, Kim MO. Ethanol modulates the expression of GABA(B) receptor mRNAs in the prenatal rat brain in an age and area dependent manner. *Neuroscience* 2005;134:857–866.

14. Milotová M, Riljak V, Bortelová J, Marešová D, Pokorný J, Langmeier M. Changes of hippocampal neurons after perinatal exposure to ethanol (perinatal ethanol abuse and hippocampal neurons). *Physiol Res* 2007 (Epub ahead of print).

15. Kumada T, Jiang Y, Cameron DB, Komuro H. How does alcohol impair neuronal migration? *J Neurosci Res* 2007;85:465–470.

16. Centers for Disease Control and Prevention. *Guidelines for Identifying and Referring Persons with Fetal Alcohol Syndrome,* 54 ed. Atlanta: Centers for Disease Control and Prevention (CDC), U.S. Department of Health and Human Services; 2005.

17. Astley SJ, Clarren SK. A case definition and photographic screening tool for the facial phenotype of fetal alcohol syndrome. *J Pediatr* 1996;129:33–41.

18. Hoyme HE, May PA, Kalberg WO, et al. A practical clinical approach to diagnosis of fetal alcohol spectrum disorders: clarification of the 1996 institute of medicine criteria. *Pediatrics* 2005;115:39–47.

19. Mattson SN, Schoenfeld AM, Riley EP. Teratogenic effects of alcohol on brain and behavior. *Alcohol Res Health* 2001;25:185–191.

20. Mattson SN, Riley EP, Sowell ER, Jernigan TL, Sobel DF, Jones KL. A decrease in the size of the basal ganglia in children with fetal alcohol syndrome. *Alcohol Clin Exp Res* 1996;20:1088–1093.

21. Riley EP, Mattson SN, Sowell ER, Jernigan TL, Sobel DF, Jones KL. Abnormalities of the corpus callosum in chldren prenatally exposed to alcohol. *Alcohol Clin Exp Res* 1995;19:1198–1202.

22. Autti-Ramo I, Autti T, Korkman M, Kettunen S, Salonen O, Valanne L. MRI findings in children with school problems who had been exposed prenatally to alcohol. *Dev Med Child Neurol* 2002;44:98–106.

23. Guerri C. Mechanisms involved in central nervous system dysfunctions induced by prenatal ethanol exposure. *Neurotox Res* 2002;4:327–335.

24. Streissguth AP, Bookstein FL, Sampson PD, Barr HM. Attention: prenatal alcohol and continuities of vigilance and attentional problems from 4 through 14 years. *Dev Psychopathol* 1995;7:419–446.

25. Streissguth AP, Bookstein FL, Barr HM, Sampson PD, O'Malley K, Young JK. Risk factors for adverse life outcomes in fetal alcohol syndrome and fetal alcohol effects. *J Dev Behav Pediatr* 2004;25:228–238.

26. Baer JS, Sampson PD, Barr HM, Connor PD, Streissguth AP. A 21-year longitudinal analysis of the effects of prenatal alcohol exposure on young adult drinking. *Arch Gen Psychiatry* 2003;60:377–385.

27. National Academy of Sciences Committee of Fetal Alcohol Syndrome. *Fetal Alcohol Syndrome: Diagnosis, Epidemiology, Prevention and Treatment.* Washington, DC: National Academy Press; 1996.

28. Streissguth AP. *Fetal Alcohol Syndrome: A Guide for Families and Communities.* Baltimore: Paul H. Brookes Publishing Company; 1997.

29. Bertrand J, Floyd RL, Weber MK. Guidelines for Identifying and Referring Persons with Fetal Alcohol Syndrome. *Morbid Mortal Wkly Rep* 2005;54:1–15.

30. Personal communication with Dr. Halverson. June 19, 2006.

31. U.S. Department of Health and Human Services. *Healthy People 2010,* 2nd ed. With Understanding and Improving Health and Objectives for Improving Health. 2 vols. Washington, DC: Government Printing Office; 2000.

32. U.S. Department of Health and Human Services. *Maternal Infant and Child Health. Healthy People 2010. Midcourse Review.* Washington, DC: Government Printing Office; 2005:16-3–16-41.

33. Substance Abuse and Mental Health Services Administration. *Results from the 2005 National Survey on Drug Use and Health: National Findings.* DHHS Publication No. SMA 06-4194 ed. Rockville: Office of Applied Studies; 2006.

34. Substance Abuse and Mental Health Services Administration. *The Fact Is Alcoholism Tends to Run in Families.* Rockville, MD: National Clearinghouse for Drug and Alcohol Information; 1992.

35. Eigen L, Rowden D. *A Methodology and Curent Estimate of the Number of Children of Alcoholics in the United States.* Children of Alcoholics Selected Readings. Rockville: National Association of Children of Alcoholics; 1995.

36. Cotton NS. The familiar incidence of alcoholism: A review. *J Studies Alcohol* 1979;40:89–116.

37. National Association for Children of Alcoholics. *Facts About COAs.* National Association for Children of Alcoholics; 1995.

38. National Center for Health Statistics. *Exposure to Alcoholism in the Family: United States, 1998.* Rockville, MD: National Institute on Alcohol Abuse and Alcoholism; 1991.

39. Centers for Disease Control and Prevention. *Surveillance for fetal alcohol syndrome using multiple sources.* Atlanta, Georgia, 1981–1989, 46 ed. Atlanta: Centers for Disease Control and Prevention; 1997.

40. Centers for Disease Control and Prevention. *Update: trends in fetal alcohol syndrome. United States, 1979-1993,* 44 ed. Atlanta: Centers for Disease Control and Prevention; 1995.

41. Egeland GM, Perham-Heser KA, Ingle D, Berner JE, Middaugh JP. Fetal alcohol syndrome in Alaska, 1977 through 1992: an administrative prevalence derived from multiple data sources. *Am J Public Health* 1998;88:781–786.

42. Centers for Disease Control and Prevention. *Fetal Alcohol Spectrum Disorders.* Atlanta: CDC; 2006.

43. Centers for Disease Control and Prevention. *Fetal Alcohol Syndrome. Alaska, Arizona, Colorado, and New York, 1995-1997,* 51 ed. Atlanta: Centers for Disease Control and Prevention; 2002.

44. Office of Applied Studies. *1997 National Household Survey on Drug Abuse: Discussion 119.* Rockville: Substance Abuse and Mental Health Services Administration; 1997.

45. Stoler JM, Ryan LM, Holmes LB. Alcohol dehydrogenase 2 genotypes, maternal alcohol use, and infant outcome. *J Pediatr* 2002;141:780–785.

46. Abel EL, Sokol RJ. A revised estimate of the economic impact of fetal alcohol syndrome. *Recent Dev Alcohol* 1991;9:117–125.

47. Abel EL, Sokol RJ. A revised conservative estimate of the incidence of FAS and its economic impact. *Alcohol Clin Exp Res* 1991;15:514–524.

48. Abel EL, Sokol RJ. Incidence of fetal alcohol syndrome and economic impact of FAS-related anomalies. *Drug Alcohol Depend* 1987;19:51–70.

49. Harwood HJ, Napolitano DM. Economic implications of the fetal alcohol syndrome. *Alcohol Health Res World* 1985;10:38–43.

50. Lupton C. *The Financial Impact of Fetal Alcohol Syndrome.* Rockville: Substance Abuse and Mental Health Services Administration; 2003.

CROSS REFERENCES

Behavioral Determinants of Health

Smoking

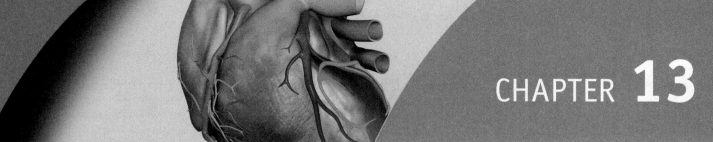

CHAPTER 13

Smoking, Nicotine, and Addiction: Tobacco or Health?

Vincent A. Chiappinelli

"Smoking remains the leading cause of preventable death and has negative health impacts on people at all stages of life. It harms unborn babies, infants, children, adolescents, adults, and seniors."[1]

LEARNING OBJECTIVES

By the end of this chapter, the student will be able to:

- Describe the major adverse effects of tobacco use on human health.
- Describe addiction, and define tolerance, dependence, and withdrawal.
- Describe how nicotine produces changes in the brain that lead to addiction.
- Describe factors that contribute to or discourage smoking initiation.
- Identify smoking cessation therapies.

HISTORY

Tobacco has played an important role in the cultural life of the Americas since Mayan times. The expression "smoking the peace pipe" comes to us from Native American ceremonies during which ritual smoking of tobacco leaves was one of many sacred and honored traditions that solidified bonds between individuals and tribal groups. The tobacco plant is indigenous only to the Americas, so the arrival of Europeans in the late 15th and early 16th centuries created a new market for this product.

Tobacco use grew rapidly in Europe, and a number of European colonies in America depended for their survival on growing tobacco as a trade item and cash crop. The downside of tobacco use was soon recognized, with smokers experiencing hacking coughs, respiratory distress, and compulsive use. But it was not until the early 20th century that true havoc was wreaked on the human population by the purveyors of this deadly plant, with the development of the manufactured cigarette.

Cigarettes provide a much milder smoke so they are preferred by smokers over cigars or pipes. Cigarette smoke is usually inhaled deeply into the lungs, resulting in a very rapid (similar to an intravenous injection) and efficient uptake of organic compounds in the smoke, some of which then enter the bloodstream and gain access to the brain in seconds.[2] Soon after their introduction by the tobacco industry, cigarettes became the preferred method of smoking tobacco. This resulted in a large increase in tobacco usage especially among men between and after the two World Wars, as tobacco companies sent millions of free cigarettes to soldiers overseas. A dramatic and parallel increase in the number of lung cancers in males was observed twenty years later, caused by cigarette smoking. In the 1960s, advertising for the brand "Virginia Slims" and a changing cultural image of women resulted in marked increases in cigarette smoking among women, and a similarly delayed increase in lung cancers has been observed. The result is that lung cancers are now the deadliest of all cancers among both men and women in the United States.[3]

INTRODUCTION

The Centers for Disease Control and Prevention (CDC) estimates that 438,000 Americans die prematurely each year from cigarette smoking (Figure 13-1). This is more annual deaths

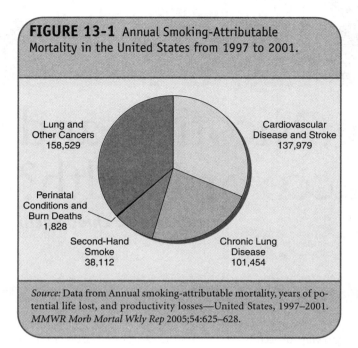

FIGURE 13-1 Annual Smoking-Attributable Mortality in the United States from 1997 to 2001.

Source: Data from Annual smoking-attributable mortality, years of potential life lost, and productivity losses—United States, 1997–2001. *MMWR Morb Mortal Wkly Rep* 2005;54:625–628.

than the combined total from AIDS, motor vehicle accidents, heroin, cocaine, suicide, and homicide. Yet 20 percent to 25 percent of the U.S. population still smokes cigarettes, even though surveys indicate that nearly everyone is fully aware of the risks of smoking. Why do people continue to smoke cigarettes and use other tobacco products (i.e., smokeless tobacco) when numerous scientific studies and the Surgeon General have linked tobacco use to serious health problems, including death from respiratory and cardiovascular disease and cancer? The reason is that tobacco contains substantial amounts of an organic compound called nicotine. Nicotine is the most **addictive** substance that can be purchased legally in the United States without a prescription.

Cigarette smoking is harmful to many organs in the body. Major causes of death due to smoking include damage to the lungs, heart, brain, and circulatory system. Non-smokers die as a result of the toxic effects of second-hand smoke, and 918 people die each year in fires caused by burning cigarettes (Figure 13-1).

BASIC SCIENCE FACTS/KEY CONCEPTS REVIEW

Nicotinic Receptors in the Brain

After nicotine enters the brain, it selectively activates a class of membrane-spanning neurotransmitter receptors that are located either presynaptically (on nerve terminals) or postsynaptically (on the dendrites or cell bodies of neurons) in many areas of the brain.[4] These receptors, called *nicotinic receptors*, are normally activated by the endogenous neurotransmitter acetylcholine.[5] When nicotine (or acetylcholine) binds to a nicotinic receptor, a central pore in the pentameric (5-subunit-containing) receptor widens for just a few milliseconds, allowing positively charged ions (especially Na+ and Ca^{2+}) to flow from the extracellular fluid into the neuron. This flow of positively charged ions into the neuron briefly depolarizes the neuron and excites it, leading to generation of an action potential and/or enhanced release of a neurotransmitter.

The Midbrain Reward Pathway

Nicotine has a lot in common with other addictive drugs such as morphine, heroin, and cocaine. All of these drugs bind to specific neurotransmitter receptors or transporters in the brain to activate what is termed the **midbrain reward pathway**. Morphine and heroin bind to opioid receptors, cocaine binds to dopamine transporters, and nicotine binds to nicotinic receptors. The normal role of these receptors and transporters in the reward pathway is to reinforce certain beneficial behaviors, such as eating and sex. But the addictive drugs artificially enhance activity in the reward pathway by increasing the release of a neurotransmitter called *dopamine*, especially within the brain nucleus called the nucleus accumbens.[6] The overall

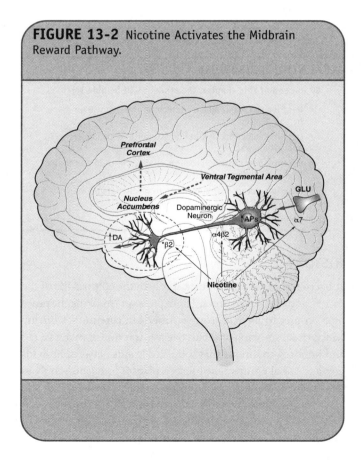

FIGURE 13-2 Nicotine Activates the Midbrain Reward Pathway.

effect of nicotine in the nucleus accumbens is to enhance the release of dopamine (Figure 13-2), but the minute-to-minute effects of nicotine in this and other brain regions are complex because prolonged nicotine can actually desensitize (inactivate) some nicotinic receptors and due to the presence of multiple subtypes of nicotinic receptors with differing properties.[7] The two most prominent nicotinic receptor subtypes in the brain are the α_7 and the $\alpha_4\beta_2$. There is evidence from knockout mice studies indicating that β_2-subunit-containing nicotinic receptors are essential for addiction to occur.[8]

Dopaminergic neuronal cell bodies located in the ventral tegmental area (VTA) send their axons into the nucleus accumbens, where their release of dopamine (DA) leads to a sensation of pleasure in the prefrontal cortex. Nicotine acts at several locations to increase this dopamine release. In the VTA, nicotine activates postsynaptic $\alpha_4\beta_2$ nicotinic receptors to directly excite the dopaminergic neurons and also activates presynaptic α_7 receptors located on nerve terminals containing the excitatory transmitter glutamate (GLU). The released glutamate further excites the dopaminergic neurons so that there is a marked increase in action potentials (APs) in the dopaminergic cell bodies. The action potentials travel down the axons and cause the release of DA in the nucleus accumbens. This release is further enhanced in the nucleus accumbens by nicotine acting on several subtypes of presynaptic nicotinic receptors containing one or more β_2 subunits ($^*\beta_2$).

Nicotine and Addiction

The excessive dopamine release in the reward pathway following nicotine may lead to a variety of emotional responses in the individual, ranging from dysphoria and anxiety (commonly seen in first-time users) to a feeling of well-being, mild euphoria, relaxation, or excitation in more experienced users. Some of the emotional effects of nicotine appear to be mediated by nicotinic receptors in other brain regions, including the amygdala and the insula.[9,10] In contrast, nicotinic receptors located in the visual system and thalamus are likely to be particularly important for the attention-enhancing properties of nicotine.[11,12] In many brain regions, nicotine activates presynaptic nicotinic receptors to enhance the release of neurotransmitters other than dopamine, including the major inhibitory transmitter GABA and the major excitatory transmitter glutamate.[13]

A hallmark of addictive drugs is that once they are consumed for several weeks or months, abruptly quitting (termed **withdrawal**) leads to a spectrum of unpleasant adverse effects that can only be prevented by taking more of the addictive substance. The mechanism behind the withdrawal effect is that neurons change in response to prolonged exposure to an addictive substance so that they become adjusted to the presence of the drug, a state called **tolerance**. For example, prolonged cigarette smoking more than doubles the number of $\alpha_4\beta_2$ nicotinic receptors in the human brain[14] and these receptors remain elevated in number even one week after smoking cessation has begun, making quit attempts more difficult.[15] After tolerance develops, an individual needs to continuously take the addictive substance in order to feel "normal" and avoid the adverse withdrawal symptoms, a condition termed **dependence**. In the case of cigarette smoking, adverse effects commonly observed upon cessation of smoking include headache, irritability, inability to concentrate, weight gain, and craving for cigarettes. According to surveys, most cigarette smokers want to quit smoking and have tried to quit, but found these adverse effects overwhelming and went back to smoking to prevent them.

CASE STUDY
Scenario

Judy Smith was born underweight and one month premature in 1970, the second child in her Caucasian family. Her father left the family when she was six months old. Her mother was the sole wage-earner for the family and earned a modest income as a waitress. Her mother smoked 1.5 packs of cigarettes per day throughout the pregnancy and continued smoking until she died of lung cancer when Judy was 32 years old.

Judy had frequent respiratory infections as an infant and child, and was diagnosed with asthma at age 8 years. She was easily distracted from her studies and was not athletic, and became overweight as she entered middle school. Judy began experimenting with cigarettes when she was 13 years old, taking them initially from her mother's packs. Within a few months, she was smoking at least 10 cigarettes per day and found that her appetite for food was reduced. She lost 10 pounds and this made her feel more attractive. She also felt that smoking helped her concentrate on her schoolwork. By age 15 she was smoking openly at home and averaging one pack per day. The cost of her cigarettes was supported by babysitting. After graduating from high school, she began full-time work as a clerk at a department store.

Judy became pregnant at age 22. She stopped smoking for the first month of pregnancy because cigarettes made her nauseous, but despite encouragement from her doctor and her boyfriend, she began smoking again and continued throughout the pregnancy. At age 32, the combination of her mother's death from lung cancer and her daughter's pleas for her to stop smoking led her to a serious quit attempt. She stopped smoking for five months, but began again because she was gaining too much weight and because of stress in her relationship with her boyfriend. Over the next three years, she made ten unsuccessful attempts to quit smoking, each lasting between two days to three months. After her workplace became smoke-free, Judy made frequent trips outside to smoke and was disciplined numerous times for being away from her station. In order to keep her job, she cut her smoking during the day by half, but often made up for this at home in the morning and evening.

At age 35, Judy was having repeated asthma attacks, shortness of breath, and a chronic cough. Her blood pressure was elevated. When her boyfriend left her, Judy decided to turn over a new leaf and stop smoking for good. With the help of a telephone quit line and nicotine skin patch therapy, she succeeded in stopping smoking and also began walking 30 minutes a day with her daughter for exercise. She gained eight pounds over the next six months, but felt physically healthier because of the walking. Her cough subsided and her bouts of asthma became less frequent. Her blood pressure was reduced to the high normal range.

Judy's daughter began smoking at age 13, and despite her mother's emphatic attempts to convince her not to smoke, her daughter became a one pack a day smoker at age 15 years.

Defining the Issues

Judy's mother smoked heavily at a time when the true health consequences of cigarettes were not understood by most Americans, 50 percent of whom smoked. When Judy began smoking in 1983, the dangers of cigarettes were just beginning to become widely known. She was unaware that many risk factors increased the likelihood that she would begin smoking, including adolescence, in utero and childhood exposure to maternal smoking, and lower socioeconomic status. Smoking initially empowered her by making her feel more attractive. She smoked during her pregnancy, and probably was unaware how much risk this created for her daughter. Her mother's death from lung cancer prompted her to try quitting, but multiple "cold turkey" quit attempts were unsuccessful. She persisted, and eventually quit with the help of combined behavioral and pharmacological smoking cessation treatment.

Patient's Understanding

Judy's daughter began smoking in 2006 and was very aware of the dangers of smoking from her own family experience and from public awareness campaigns directed at teenagers and the general population. Nonetheless, she began smoking at an early age, having a set of risk factors for smoking initiation and addiction very similar to those of her mother.

CLINICAL PERSPECTIVE FOR THE INDIVIDUAL PATIENT

Adolescents and Smoking Initiation

Smoking initiation for most people occurs between 12 and 19 years of age, and the adolescent brain (which is still developing) may be particularly vulnerable to addictive drugs such as nicotine (Figure 13-3). Some teens become dependent on cigarettes within weeks of smoking initiation, whereas other teens take months to develop signs of dependence on tobacco. Genetic factors may contribute to this variation, as do environmental factors.[16] In one large study, young teens whose mothers smoked while pregnant were two to three times more likely to initiate and maintain smoking than teens born to non-smoking mothers.[17] In the same study, teens whose mothers smoked only after delivery had initiation rates similar to those whose mothers never smoked, indicating that there is a critical prenatal period during which exposure to nicotine (and/or other chemicals in tobacco) is particularly harmful.

The reasons adolescents first try cigarettes vary, but included among them are age-related risk-taking, wanting to appear grown-up, being "cool" with their friends, and doing something "counter-culture." They are greatly influenced by mass media culture, and studies show that teens who frequently watch movies in which actors smoke cigarettes are more likely to initiate smoking.[18] Compelling evidence that culture can influence smoking behavior comes from studies comparing smoking rates among different

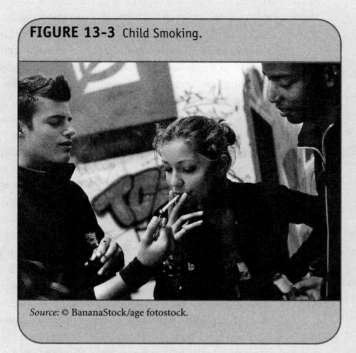

FIGURE 13-3 Child Smoking.

Source: © BananaStock/age fotostock.

racial and ethnic groups within the United States. Native American teenagers have the highest smoking rates (over 23%), while blacks (6.5%) and Asians (4.3%) have much lower rates of smoking.[19]

In the Case Study, Judy and her daughter were both at high risk for initiating smoking due to exposure to maternal smoking and socioeconomic status. Genetic factors also could have predisposed them to smoking because three generations smoked; however, no genetic tests were done and in any case the genetic criteria that make smoking more likely are not currently understood.

Treatment Options

Once dependent on cigarettes, it is typically very difficult to quit. Most quit attempts end in failure, and most successful quitters try more than once before they succeed. "Cold turkey" attempts (abrupt cessation) are successful less than 10 percent of the time. This success rate is significantly improved when the smoker receives assistance from a professional trained in **smoking cessation** methods. Various cessation techniques are successful, from telephone-based "quit lines" that smokers can call if they feel the urge to smoke, to meditation techniques and palmtop computer-delivered approaches. The idea is to provide a support mechanism at those times when the individual is most susceptible to succumbing to the urge to smoke.

Pharmacological Treatments

The most successful smoking cessation programs combine behavioral methods with one of several Food and Drug Administration (FDA)-approved smoking cessation drugs. The most widely used smoking cessation drug is nicotine itself, which is available without a prescription in the United States in a variety of forms including skin patch, gum, nasal spray, and lozenge. At first, it may seem counterproductive to use these nicotine-containing products when the goal is to eliminate the individual's dependence on the nicotine in tobacco. However, the amounts of nicotine recommended during the quit attempt are less than those delivered by smoking cigarettes, and the dose of nicotine is slowly decreased during the quit attempt, reducing withdrawal symptoms when compared with abrupt cessation. Even with a quit program that combines behavioral methods with nicotine, quit success rates are generally no better than 20 percent to 25 percent, which is 1.5- to twofold higher than the success rate for doing it cold turkey.[20]

Two prescription drugs that are FDA-approved for smoking cessation are buproprion and varenicline. Buproprion, which is also FDA-approved as an antidepressant, appears to assist smoking cessation by altering dopamine levels in several brain regions. Quit success rates with buproprion are generally comparable to those seen with nicotine. Varenicline is a partial agonist at $\alpha_4\beta_2$ nicotinic receptors in the brain, meaning that it is much less effective at activating these receptors than nicotine, and likely prevents nicotine from fully activating these receptors.[21] Varenicline became available for general use only in 2006, but preliminary studies are encouraging and suggest quit rates up to 45 percent may be possible with this drug.[22]

In the Case Study, Judy made a number of quit attempts on her own, a pattern that is commonly seen. While many people do succeed in quitting for good this way, many others require a much more organized program that includes at least one smoking cessation intervention. Had Judy stopped smoking for good before she became pregnant, her daughter's risk factors for smoking initiation would have been substantially reduced, illustrating the importance of early intervention.

Current Recommended Level of Intervention

Healthcare workers should always encourage smokers to quit and try to assess their readiness to make a quit attempt. When the patient is ready, the best chance of success is with a well-planned smoking cessation program that includes both a behavioral and a pharmacological component.

PUBLIC HEALTH PERSPECTIVE FOR THE HEALTH OF THE GENERAL POPULATION AND OF HIGH RISK GROUPS

Role of the Tobacco Industry in Perpetuating Smoking Behavior

Cigarettes are one of the very few legal products for sale in the United States that *when used as directed* are very likely to cause serious harm or death to the user. A multibillion-dollar industry profits from the sale of cigarettes and other tobacco products and spends substantial amounts of money encouraging smoking through various forms of advertising. In 2003, cigarette companies spent over $15 billion on advertising and promotions in the United States, or $53 for every person in the country.[23] Some experts say that the tobacco industry is the most irresponsible U.S. corporate presence because no other industry's product is responsible for anything approaching the 438,000 deaths per year attributable to smoking tobacco. The industry counters that it now spends millions of dollars to discourage smoking initiation among teenagers, and that most of its advertising merely reinforces brand loyalty among existing smokers. However, a recent study demonstrates that tobacco industry advertising campaigns directed against teenage smoking are ineffective because their main message is that the choice to smoke should wait until adulthood, but little is said about the serious adverse effects of smoking. Teenagers confronted with this message may actually be encouraged to initiate smoking, because cigarettes are being associated with being an adult.[24] Bearing in mind both that the tobacco industry must recruit new smokers to maintain profit levels and that nearly all smokers initiate smoking before the age of 20, the industry clearly is financially motivated to make their deadly product appealing to teenagers.

Health Policies That Reduce Smoking Behaviors

Smoking rates in the United States have declined from 50 percent to 25 percent over the past 30 years, although recently this decline has leveled off. There are several reasons for this decrease in smoking rate, including increased awareness of the serious health hazards of smoking, increased taxes on cigarettes (cost is particularly important to teenagers), elimination of television and radio advertising of tobacco products, and the smoke-free movement. As airports, restaurants, bars, hospitals, office buildings, and government buildings become smoke-free, it is more difficult for smokers to frequently smoke cigarettes, and a social stigma becomes attached to smoking that can discourage lighting up. In 2006, the Surgeon General reported that **second-hand smoke** (also called **environmental tobacco smoke**) is a killer, causing lung cancer and heart disease in non-smoking adults and asthma and respiratory infections in children.[25] This means that there is no safe exposure level to cigarette smoke in the environment and provides further justification to employers and governments to go smoke-free to protect non-smokers from unhealthy air and to protect themselves from liability claims.

A major goal of Healthy People 2010 is to "Reduce illness, disability, and death related to tobacco use and exposure to secondhand smoke."[26] Recognizing that making **non-smoking the norm** is crucial for further reductions in smoking rates and exposures, the report emphasizes the need for population-based interventions including the prevention of smoking initiation, reduced exposure to second-hand smoke, and policy changes in healthcare systems. For example, the costs of smoking cessation medications and behavioral therapy are currently not covered expenses on many healthcare plans, which is a major deterrent to smokers who are otherwise ready for a quit attempt. The report also emphasizes disparities in the adverse consequences of smoking, with lower socioeconomic status, lower educational level, and in some cases minority status associated with significantly higher health risks. While a few metrics have shown some progress toward meeting the Healthy People 2010 goals (e.g., recent reductions in lung cancer death rates and reduced exposure of children to second-hand smoke), most metrics have not shown the progress needed to meet the stated goals.[26]

CONCLUSION

Tobacco use is by far the greatest preventable cause of serious illness and death in many countries of the world, including the United States. Americans continue to smoke and to initiate smoking as teenagers even though they are fully aware of the serious adverse health effects of this habit. Cigarette smokers quickly become addicted to the nicotine in tobacco and find it difficult to quit because of unpleasant withdrawal symptoms during quit attempts.

The good news is that U.S. smoking rates have been cut in half due to both a decrease in initiation and to smoking cessation. Behavioral methods such as quit lines and drugs that assist smoking cessation have helped millions to quit. Individual smokers should always be encouraged to quit by healthcare professionals regardless of their age and number of years they have smoked and be provided with information on available smoking cessation programs and referrals.[27,28] The smoke-free movement is a powerful public health force that seeks to make non-smoking the norm and to protect non-smokers as well as smokers from the harmful effects of tobacco smoke. About 50 percent of the population of the United States now lives in localities where there are bans on indoor smoking in at least some buildings. Several public health policies can improve the situation even more. These include a total ban on smoking in all public spaces and buildings, prohibition of all forms of tobacco product advertising and promotion, and significant increases in the cost of cigarettes through taxation, with proceeds of taxes going towards smoking cessation efforts and to the excessive health care costs of smokers.

KEY TERMS

Biology Terms

Addiction (also **Dependence**): Compulsive use of a drug, even in the face of significant adverse effects and consequences.

Tolerance: A state resulting from changes in the brain that occur in response to chronic exposure to an addictive drug. An individual exhibiting tolerance to a drug requires repeated and possibly increasing amounts of that drug to feel "normal."

Withdrawal: Unpleasant adverse effects caused by abrupt cessation of a drug in an individual addicted to that drug.

Midbrain Reward Pathway: A dopaminergic pathway in the brain that is activated by certain beneficial behaviors such as eating and sex as well as by addictive drugs, to produce a sensation of pleasure.

Public Health Terms

Environmental Tobacco Smoke (or **Secondhand Smoke**): Cigarette smoke blown into the environment by active smokers; proven to cause cancer, death, and respiratory illnesses in non-smokers.

Non-Smoking as the Norm: Movement that seeks to isolate smokers, discourage initiation, and eliminate the proven hazards of environmental smoke by emphasizing everyone's right to breathe air free of toxic tobacco smoke.

Smoking Cessation: An attempt to quit smoking, either unaided ("cold turkey") or assisted by behavioral and/or pharmacological treatments.

SMOKING, PREGNANCY, AND ASTHMA

Over 11% of pregnant women in the United States continue to smoke during their pregnancy, putting their fetuses at markedly increased risk for low birth weight, birth defects, and sudden infant death syndrome.[29] Cigarette smokers must have strong motivation to successfully quit, and pregnancy is a key time because it creates increased incentive and urgency to quit. Most mothers are aware they are harming their own health, but may underestimate the adverse health effects to their fetus if they continue to smoke. They may be aware that young children of smoking mothers are at increased risk for asthma and respiratory infections. But they probably do not know that in utero exposure to maternal smoking increases the likelihood of wheezing and asthma in the first years of life.[30] Furthermore, in utero exposure to maternal smoking increases the likelihood that an adolescent will initiate smoking and doubles the likelihood that smoking initiation will lead to asthma.[31] Smoking is the leading cause of adult-onset asthma, but is also a major environmental factor in the development of asthma in infants and children. The health professional must encourage all pregnant women to stop smoking, at least during their pregnancy, for the sake of their unborn children. The early months of pregnancy are a time when cigarette smoke and taste are more likely to produce nausea and aversion, and this may also assist a quit attempt.

Healthy People 2010

Indicator: Tobacco Use

Focus Area: Tobacco Use

Goal: Reduce illness, disability, and death related to tobacco use and exposure to secondhand smoke.

Objectives

27-1. Reduce tobacco use by adolescents and adults.

27-3. Reduce the initiation of tobacco use among children and adolescents.

27-5. Increase smoking cessation attempts by adult smokers.

27-6. Increase smoking cessation during

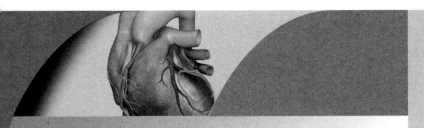

Questions for Further Research, Study, Reflection, and Discussion

For the Individual Student

In order to answer these questions, it may be necessary to research the primary literature.

- Are teenagers who smoke cigarettes more likely than non-smokers to experiment with other addictive drugs?
- Nicotine has many effects on behavior and mood. In certain psychiatric conditions, including schizophrenia, could nicotine be helpful?
- Are there genetic variants that are associated with an increased risk of nicotine addiction? Which neurotransmitter systems would be likely targets for such a study?

For Small Group Discussion

- There are cycles of addiction that impact a single individual as well as multiple generations and communities. Use the Case Study to explore these cycles.
- What types of interventions might have worked for Judy to help her stop smoking?

For Entire Class Discussion

- State governments have become "addicted" to the tax revenue they receive from cigarette sales. What percentage of this revenue is spent on healthcare or smoking cessation?
- Tobacco companies have agreed to pay billions of dollars to the states over a number of years in order to reduce their liability in court. What percentage of these payments is spent on healthcare or smoking cessation?
- Advertising and movie placements have a major impact on smoking initiation. Is there any problem with making such commercial activities illegal in the case of marketing cigarettes?
- Research several nationwide campaigns that have tried to reduce tobacco use among adolescents. What strategies did these campaigns use to affect behavior? How effective have these campaigns been? How do you measure their success?

EXERCISES/ACTIVITIES

- Become a volunteer at a telephone-based smoking quit line.
- Create a video or Powerpoint presentation directed towards adolescents who are thinking about smoking initiation.
- Compare tobacco product regulations including those covering advertising, purchasing, and smoke-free buildings in several industrial countries and several third world countries.

pregnancy.

27-7. Increase smoking cessation attempts by adolescent smokers.

27-8. Increase insurance coverage of evidence-based treatment for nicotine dependency.

27-9. Reduce the proportion of children who are regularly exposed to tobacco smoke at home.

27-11. Increase smoke-free environments in schools.

27-13. Increase smoke-free environments in worksites.

27-14. Reduce illegal sales to minors.

27-16. Eliminate tobacco advertising and promotions that influence adolescents.

27-21. Increase the average Federal and State tax on tobacco products.

More Americans die each year due to cigarette smoking than were killed in combat in all five years of World War II (438,000 deaths vs. 405,399 deaths).[32,33]

REFERENCES

1. Office of Disease Prevention and Health Promotion, U.S. Department of Surgeon General's Report, Factsheet, 28. *Surgeon General's Reports on Smoking and Health, 1964-2004.* (2004). Available at http://www.cdc.gov/tobacco/data_statistics/sgr/sgr_2004/00_pdfs/28reports.pdf. Accessed April 3, 2008.

2. Dani JA, Harris RA. Nicotine addiction and comorbidity with alcohol abuse and mental illness. *Nat Neurosci* 2005;8:1465–1470.

3. American Cancer Society. Cancer Facts & Figures 2007. Atlanta: American Cancer Society; 2007.

4. Nong Y, Sorenson EM, Chiappinelli VA. Fast excitatory nicotinic transmission in the chick lateral spiriform nucleus. *J Neurosci* 1999;19:7804–7811.

5. Gotti C, Clementi F. Neuronal nicotinic receptors: from structure to pathology. *Prog Neurobiol* 2004;74:363–396.

6. Balfour DJ. The neurobiology of tobacco dependence: a preclinical perspective on the role of the dopamine projections to the nucleus accumbens [corrected]. *Nicotine Tob Res* 2004;6:899–912.

7. Rice ME, Cragg SJ. Nicotine amplifies reward-related dopamine signals in striatum. *Nat Neurosci* 2004;7:583–584.

8. Picciotto MR, Zoli M, Rimondini R, Lena C, Marubio LM, Pich EM, et al. Acetylcholine receptors containing the beta2 subunit are involved in the reinforcing properties of nicotine. *Nature* 1998;391:173–177.

9. Franklin TR, Wang Z, Wang J, Sciortino N, Harper D, Li Y, et al. Limbic activation to cigarette smoking cues independent of nicotine withdrawal: a perfusion fMRI study. *Neuropsychopharmacology* 2007;32:2301–2309.

10. Naqvi NH, Rudrauf D, Damasio H, Bechara A. Damage to the insula disrupts addiction to cigarette smoking. *Science* 2007;315:531–534.

11. Lawrence NS, Ross TJ, Stein EA. Cognitive mechanisms of nicotine on visual attention. *Neuron* 2002;36:539–548.

12. Guo JZ, Liu Y, Sorenson EM, Chiappinelli VA. Synaptically released and exogenous ACh activates different nicotinic receptors to enhance evoked glutamatergic transmission in the lateral geniculate nucleus. *J Neurophysiol* 2005;94:2549–2560.

13. Guo JZ, Tredway TL, Chiappinelli VA. Glutamate and GABA release are enhanced by different subtypes of presynaptic nicotinic receptors in the lateral geniculate nucleus. *J Neurosci* 1998;18:1963–1969.

14. Perry DC, vila-Garcia MI, Stockmeier CA, Kellar KJ. Increased nicotinic receptors in brains from smokers: membrane binding and autoradiography studies. *J Pharmacol Exp Ther* 1999;289:1545–1552.

15. Staley JK, Krishnan-Sarin S, Cosgrove KP, Krantzler E, Frohlich E, Perry E, et al. Human tobacco smokers in early abstinence have higher levels of beta2* nicotinic acetylcholine receptors than nonsmokers. *J Neurosci* 2006;26:8707–8714.

16. Swan GE, Hudmon KS, Jack LM, Hemberger K, Carmelli D, Khroyan TV, et al. Environmental and genetic determinants of tobacco use: methodology for a multidisciplinary, longitudinal family-based investigation. *Cancer Epidemiol Biomarkers Prev* 2003;12:994–1005.

17. Al Mamun A, O'Callaghan FV, Alati R, O'Callaghan M, Najman JM, Williams GM, et al. Does maternal smoking during pregnancy predict the smoking patterns of young adult offspring? A birth cohort study. *Tob Control* 2006;15:452–457.

18. Wellman RJ, Sugarman DB, DiFranza JR, Winickoff JP. The extent to which tobacco marketing and tobacco use in films contribute to children's use of tobacco: a meta-analysis. *Arch Pediatr Adolesc Med* 2006;160:1285–1296.

19. Racial/ethnic differences among youths in cigarette smoking and susceptibility to start smoking—United States, 2002–2004. *MMWR Morbid Mortal Wkly Rep* 2006;55:1275–1277.

20. Silagy C, Lancaster T, Stead L, Mant D, Fowler G. Nicotine replacement therapy for smoking cessation. *Cochrane Database Syst Rev* 2004;CD000146.

21. Mihalak KB, Carroll FI, Luetje CW. Varenicline is a partial agonist at alpha4beta2 and a full agonist at alpha7 neuronal nicotinic receptors. *Mol Pharmacol* 2006;70:801–805.

22. Nides M, Oncken C, Gonzales D, Rennard S, Watsky EJ, Anziano R, et al. Smoking cessation with varenicline, a selective alpha4beta2 nicotinic receptor partial agonist: results from a 7-week, randomized, placebo- and bupropion-controlled trial with 1-year follow-up. *Arch Intern Med* 2006;166:1561–1568.

23. Federal Trade Commission. Cigarette Report for 2003. (Issued 2005.) Washington, DC: Federal Trade Commission Available at http://www.ftc.gov/reports/cigarette05/050809cigrpt.pdf. Accessed April 3, 2008.

24. Wakefield M, Terry-McElrath Y, Emery S, Saffer H, Chaloupka FJ, Szczypka G, et al. Effect of televised, tobacco company-funded smoking prevention advertising on youth smoking-related beliefs, intentions, and behavior. *Am J Public Health* 2006;96:2154–2160.

25. United States Public Health Service, Office of the Surgeon General. The health consequences of involuntary exposure to tobacco smoke: a report of the Surgeon General. Rockville, MD: DHHS, Public Health Service, Office of the Surgeon General; 2006.

26. United States Department of Health and Human Services. *Healthy People 2010: Understanding and Improving Health*, rvsd ed. Boston: Jones and Bartlett Publishers; 2001.

27. Pederson LL, Blumenthal DS, Dever A, McGrady G. A web-based smoking cessation and prevention curriculum for medical students: why, how, what, and what next. *Drug Alcohol Rev* 2006;25:39–47.

28. Association of American Medical Colleges. *Physician Behavior and Practice Patterns Related to Smoking Cessation.* Washington: AAMC; 2007.

29. Centers for Disease Control and Prevention. *Tobacco Use, Multistate Exhibits, 2002 Pregnancy Risk Assessment Monitoring System Surveillance Report.* Available at http://www.cdc.gov/prams/2002PRAMSSurvReport/MultiState Exhibits/Multistates13.htm. Accessed April 3, 2008.

30. Agency for Toxic Substances and Disease Registry. *Environmental Triggers of Asthma*. Publication No. ATSDR-HE-CS-2002-0001. Washington DC: U.S. Department of Health and Human Services; 2002.

31. Gilliland FD, Islam T, Berhane K, Gauderman WJ, McConnell R, Avol E, et al. Regular smoking and asthma incidence in adolescents. *Am J Respir Crit Care Med* 2006;174:1094–1100.

32. Annual smoking-attributable mortality, years of potential life lost, and productivity losses—United States, 1997–2001. *MMWR Morb Mortal Wkly Rep* 2005;54:625–628.

33. Fischer H. *American War and Military Operations Casualties: Lists and Statistics*. Washington, DC: Library of Congress, CRS Report for Congress, Congressional Research Service; 2005.

RESOURCE

Roberts KH, Munafo MR, Rodriguez D, Drury M, Murphy MF, Neale RE, et al. Longitudinal analysis of the effect of prenatal nicotine exposure on subsequent smoking behavior of offspring. *Nicotine Tob Res* 2005;7:801–808.

CROSS REFERENCES

Asthma

Behavioral Determinants of Health

Fetal Alcohol Syndrome: A Lifespan Perspective

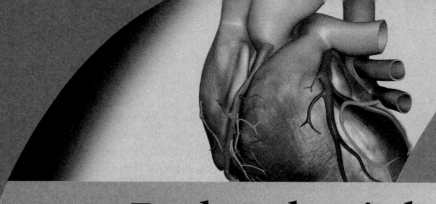

CHAPTER 14

Pathophysiology of Injury: Why Gravity Is Your Enemy

Mary Pat McKay

Worldwide, injuries are the NUMBER ONE killer of young people ages 4 to 34.[1]

LEARNING OBJECTIVES

By the end of this chapter, the student will be able to:

- Identify energy as the main cause of injury.
- Describe how anatomy and physics combine to create injury patterns.
- Recognize injury risk factors.
- Illustrate how the "five E's" of injury control (education, engineering solutions, economic incentives, enforcement, and empowerment) are used to prevent injuries.

HISTORY

On August 31, 1869, Mary Ward, an accomplished scientist and author, became the first recorded fatality from a motorized vehicle when she slipped from her seat and fell under the wheels while her steam carriage was rounding a corner in the city of Birr, County Offaly, Ireland.[2]

Thirty years later, on September 14, 1899, at the corner of 74th and Central Park West in New York City, Henry Bliss stepped in front of an electric vehicle and became the first U.S. fatality in the ongoing conflict between pedestrians and vehicles.[3]

Injury is the leading cause of death for Americans age 1 to 44 and the primary cause of lost years of productive life.[4] For those aged 1 to 34, injury claims more lives than all other causes

combined. The majority—68 percent—of the 160,000 fatalities per year are unintentional. Of these, more than 42,000 fatalities are from motor vehicles crashes alone. Of course, most injured people survive, but many need medical care. There are nearly 35 million emergency department (ED) visits for injuries annually, accounting for about one third of all ED visits in the United States.

The total cost of injuries including acute and rehabilitative medical care, lost wages, and lost productivity tops $406 billion/year (2000 dollars).[5] This represents about 4 percent of the U.S. gross national product (GNP).

INJURIES ARE NOT ACCIDENTS!

BASIC SCIENCE FACTS/KEY CONCEPTS REVIEW

The first point in studying the pathophysiology of injury is to firmly understand that injuries are not accidents. They are not mishaps that "happen unexpectedly, without a deliberate plan or cause."[6] In fact, most injuries are predictable and preventable, just like other health problems. Like other types of illness, injuries have specific causes and risk factors and are amenable to routine public health interventions for prevention as well as medical treatment to optimize recovery.

The idea that injuries are preventable may be easiest to understand for those injuries that are intentionally caused by another human such as those due to assault, domestic violence, attempted murder, war, or self-harm (suicide). Preventing one person's conscious behavior is not necessarily easy but it is generally accepted as possible to accomplish. For instance, conflict resolution, limiting access to weapons, diplomacy, and successful treatments for substance abuse and/or mental illness can all prevent many intentional injuries.

Unintentional injuries are also preventable, but the interventions may be different. Thus, non-slip surfaces help prevent slipping and falling, the plastic guard on the power tool helps prevent fingers from being amputated, and enforced speed limits help prevent serious injuries from motor vehicle crashes. Just like other public health issues, both intentional and unintentional injuries have risk and protective factors and can be prevented or limited in severity by public health interventions.

Underlying Concepts

Injuries come in different shapes and sizes, from those that are very minor and don't leave any persistent physical scar, to others that are life-threatening or cause permanent disability. They are among the most common health problems on earth; nearly every person eventually has an injury of some kind. The final common pathway for the pathophysiology of all injuries is the same: *injuries occur when the tissues of the human body absorb energy that is above the tissue threshold.*

The four types of energy that can be involved in an injury are: kinetic energy (i.e., falls, motor vehicle crashes), electrical energy (lightning strikes, downed wires), chemical energy (poisonings), and thermal/radiant energy (steam or flame burns). Injuries also can occur when a critical requirement for life is unavailable (i.e., oxygen), such as drownings and suffocations.

The Body's Response to Injury

Each body tissue has a unique ability to absorb and dissipate energy without injury until a critical threshold is reached. Thus, a minor bump to the arm may cause a noticeable feeling but leaves no mark and causes no pain. A more forceful strike may cause pain and some bleeding under the skin (a bruise) but no permanent scar. A strike with even more force may cause a bruise and a laceration of the skin deep enough to require repair, and this will leave a permanent scar. If even greater force is applied, the bones may break or dislocate.

Pain initially occurs just as the tissue's critical threshold is reached and can give the person an opportunity to act to limit the degree of damage. Each type of tissue in the body responds differently to specific types of energy, and so different tissues have different types of pain and pressure sensors. In the skin, sensors relay pain in response to significant compression, stretch, and temperature changes. These are specifically designed to allow the person to move away from the source of the problem. Internal pain sensors are more designed to signal a serious problem to the person. Some major internal organs, such as the spleen and kidney, have a capsule with sensors that measure stretch, and pain is only felt when the organ is swollen. This can occur from infection, but may occur also when there is bruising or laceration to internal organs. The periosteum, a tissue full of sensors that overlies each of the bones of the body, is particularly sensitive to stretch; this occurs when the bone breaks, telling the person to stop moving that body part, if possible. Thus, the degree and location of pain can help identify injuries requiring treatment, even if they lie below the skin's surface.

Tissue Fragility and Injury Thresholds

The type of tissue involved in an injury event determines to a large extent the severity of the injury itself. Each type of tissue in the body has different **viscoelastic** properties and responds differently to applied energy. Thus, the **cornea** (the thin clear part of the eye that we see through) suffers thermal burns more quickly than intact skin. Skin is relatively resistant to compression but tears when stretched. The brain responds particularly poorly to being compressed; it has very little elasticity. Bone is very resistant to compression along the longitudinal (long) axis (or else we could never walk upright), but less resistant to compression in cross section; it breaks when struck laterally. **Ligaments** do fine in compression but fail when overstretched.

In addition to properties inherent in the type of tissue, **comorbid factors** play a role in the development of an injury. In fact, a tissue's ability to absorb energy without injury is related to the *quality* of the tissue. Age plays a major role in this; as we age, most of the body's tissue becomes less elastic and less viscous or stiffer. The thin skin of a 90-year-old is much less elastic than that of a 20-year-old and thus less able to cope with even minor stretch. It may tear or bruise when minimal pressure is applied. The overall effect of age is to increase the mortality risk when the person is injured. In fact, the **case fatality rate** (number of deaths/number of injuries $\times$ 100) is less than 1 for those under 45 but increases by more than 3 times (to 3.34) for people 85 and older.[7]

Because they are growing, children's bodies are different than adults' and they respond differently to energy than adults. For instance, the bones of infants and toddlers bend noticeably before they break (called *plastic deformation*) and may require physicians to break them in order to straighten them out. Adult bones no longer deform in this way; they simply break.

Certain diseases decrease the injury threshold for a given tissue. **Osteoporosis** causes bones to thin, leading to an increased risk of fracture. Certain vascular syndromes (*collagen vascular diseases*) increase the risk of bleeding from minimal trauma to blood vessels. People taking blood thinners or who have alcoholic liver disease are more likely to bleed profusely from small blood vessels. If these vessels are in the brain, the effect can be catastrophic.

Tissue Healing

Each injury heals in a set series of phases. The easiest type of injury to consider is a simple laceration. The primary damage is done at the time of the injury with trauma to the skin, subcutaneous fat, and perhaps underlying musculature. Immediately, the wound bleeds. As the blood clots, the bleeding stops. Inflammation is the next step, causing swelling in the area of the wound. Naturally, lacerations caused by sharp objects have less surrounding swelling than lacerations caused by blunt trauma because more tissue is involved in the latter. This inflammatory response is critical to the process of healing. The inflammation can be painful, but the types of cells that are called in and cause inflammation are the ones that will do the repair work. During this initial phase the wound itself is weak and it may reopen fairly easily. Stitches are used (when necessary) to hold the area closed in order to allow faster healing with a more cosmetic scar. By about day three, special cells (*fibroblasts*) are organizing in the wound and begin to lay down collagen, which acts as a tissue connector. As collagen content increases, the wound site strengthens. Much of the strength of the area is repaired in the first two weeks, and the scab falls off by the end of that time. However, the wound continues to heal for many months, the scar matures and the area is remodeled. As collagen is replaced, the thick stiff scar gradually becomes softer, less raised, and less red. This phase of healing and recovery is prolonged and even minor wounds may take a year or two to reach their final appearance. Healing of other injuries, such as fractures or brain injuries, occurs in much the same way. There is an initial period of swelling, followed by slow healing and prolonged recovery.

This healing process also can be complicated by local infection, serious health issues such as heart failure or kidney failure, or even a serious infection in some other body part. Other diseases increase the risk of complications after an injury, during the second stage. Diabetes increases the risk of tissue infection as a result of even minor trauma. Peripheral vascular disease, a problem with narrowing of the blood vessels to the limbs, leads to slow wound healing. Obesity may offer some protection from internal injury due to kinetic energy but significantly increases the risk of complications during healing, and the likelihood of future arthritis if a weight-bearing joint is injured.

Finally, late complications can affect healing. Late complications include persistent infection, failure of healing with chronic wounds, or fractures that fail to unite. These may require a number of procedures to attempt to remove tissue that has failed to repair itself and move "better" tissue into the area to try and stimulate healing. These complications significantly prolong the period of disability for the person who suffers them.

Injury Mechanics

Injuries can be defined by the type of energy applied. Kinetic energy (i.e. falls, assaults, motor vehicle crashes) causes the majority of injuries, so the rest of this chapter will focus on injuries due to kinetic energy.

Penetrating Injury

Penetrating injuries indicate something sharp or edged entered the body and can be subclassified in a number of ways. Perhaps the easiest to understand is to separate firearm injuries from non-firearm injuries. This leaves knife wounds, cuts from glass shards, and impalement on sharp objects in one category.

Cutting, Slashing, Piercing. Penetrating injuries from sharp objects such as knives or glass slice tissue open in a defined track. It is easy to see what was cut or injured. They don't traumatize surrounding tissue or affect distant areas. If a person has a laceration to their index finger from cutting a bagel, there is no concern that their knee is damaged.

The mortality from cutting/piercing injury is quite different based on the intent of the injury. The case fatality rate is higher for all intentional injury than for unintentional injury, meaning that when injury is intended it is more likely to kill. For a cutting/piercing injury, the case fatality rate for unintentional injury is essentially zero, while that for intentional injury (stabbing) is 7.6.[7]

Firearms. Penetrating injury from firearms is considerably more complicated than cutting/piercing injury. Bullets have greater speed and therefore greater force is applied to the body. They directly crush tissue with a "splash" effect related to **yaw**, causing a temporary cavity around the bullet itself, and thus affecting several centimeters of tissue surrounding the bullet track. Often they bounce off body structures (most often the bones) and rebound to take a circuitous path, striking distant organs. Finally, bullet fragmentation increases the volume of tissue affected. The net result is an injury that is far more likely to be fatal than other mechanisms. The case fatality rate for unintentional firearm injuries is 8.4 (fatal 8% of the time), but when a firearm injury is intentional (assault, attempted homicide), the case fatality rate is 24.74, or fatal nearly a quarter of the time.[7] When the intention is self-harm (suicide) the case fatality rate rises to 85.

Blunt Injury

The pathophysiology of blunt injury is much more complicated than penetrating injuries. Gravity, the constant pull earthward, is the major problem. If this pull were less intense, the effect of falling onto the outstretched arm might not be a wrist fracture and it wouldn't matter as much that the person catapulted from his bicycle struck his head on hard concrete (because it would not hit as hard). Sadly, gravity is not something we can control so we must learn to live with it.

In blunt injuries, there are often internal events that are not obvious from external inspection. In fact, in *deceleration injury*—where the body comes to a sudden, unanticipated stop—there is a second, internal collision inside each body cavity that can lead to serious injury within the head, thorax, or abdomen. Thus, injury can occur because of a direct blow or indirectly through the movement of the body. For example, a motorcyclist hits a large pothole and is ejected from his vehicle. His head and body come to a stop when he hits the pavement. His brain continues forward and strikes the interior of the skull nanoseconds later. Because the brain has elastic properties, it rebounds and strikes the interior of the opposite side of the skull. (This is known as a *contrecoup* injury.) While there will be an obvious bruise for the first injury, there will likely be no external sign of trauma for the contrecoup injury.

Basic Rules of Physics (with Apologies to Isaac Newton)

There are clues to understand exactly how blunt injuries occur. In fact, all blunt injury follows three basic rules of physics. When the understanding of simple physics is combined with understanding basic human anatomy, it becomes possible to predict what injuries will occur in a given situation.

Rule 1: Objects in Motion Remain in Motion Until an External Force Is Applied

This is **Newton's First Law**, somewhat paraphrased: an object at rest tends to stay at rest until acted upon. The converse is also true. In terms of injuries, this is best illustrated by considering the following two events:

Example 1. A young man jumps off a one foot high stone wall. His feet strike the ground first, coming to a near-instantaneous stop. The force is transmitted up the bones of his legs into the pelvis. As yet unchecked, his torso continues downward, being caught and held upright by the action of the muscles in his thighs competing against gravity. His **hamstrings** and **quadriceps** grip to keep his knees from buckling, and the **gluteal** and hip muscles contract to allow him to bend rather than fall over. His back and neck muscles then contract to keep him upright.

This is an everyday event that most often will not result in an injury. But the body's ability to compensate for the forces applied could be quite different if the stone wall is 20 feet high.

Example 2. A car slides out of control on a wet road and strikes a tree; inside, the driver is wearing her lap and shoulder safety belt. The frame of the vehicle engages the tree and is forced to come to a sudden halt; however, the driver continues to move forward at the same rate of speed until her torso is caught by her safety belt and brought to a stop. Her head (which is not restrained) continues forward until the limit of motion by her neck musculature. Because of the elastic properties of the skeletal and muscular tissues of her neck, her head then rebounds back against the headrest. Her brain, which sits in a hard, bone casing cushioned by a small amount of fluid, comes to a stop and rebounds just milliseconds behind the head, taking slightly longer to come to a stop. Internally, when her chest motion is stopped by the safety belt, the rear portions of her chest continue forward until reaching the limit of compression of the ribcage, and her chest rebounds. During this phase, the internal organs—the heart and lungs—are compressed and then released. In her abdomen, the same thing occurs, compressing her **liver**, **spleen** and intestines against the lap portion of the safety belt.

If this entire event occurs with low force (meaning low speed), there may be little or no injury to the driver. If it occurs at high speed, the forces experienced by the internal and external tissues of the body are likely to be above the injury threshold.

Rule 2: The Amount of Energy Involved in a Collision Equals the Mass Times the Acceleration

This is **Newton's Second Law**, where the acceleration of an object as produced by a net force is directly proportional to the magnitude of the net force, in the same direction as the net force, and inversely proportional to the mass of the object. More succinctly, Force = mass × acceleration (F = ma).

In terms of injuries, there are two key points about this law. The first is that we are mostly talking about deceleration (or negative acceleration) causing injury: it is not going fast that creates the problem, it is the stopping that leads to the injury. Acceleration is the distance traveled divided by the time (d/t), but for most injuries, this time period is extremely short. Most car crashes occur in less than 100 milliseconds. Thus, a reasonable approximation is to consider the velocity at the time the impact begins as the acceleration.

The second point is to highlight the importance of mass. A 350-pound person jumping off a stone wall exerts a lot more force on his feet and ankles than a 150-pound person jumping off the same wall. This is the effect of earth's gravitational acceleration, 9.8 m/sec^2 (32 ft/sec^2) multiplied by the mass of the person (F = ma).

This particular rule is the one that has driven much public education, legislation, and enforcement about child safety seats over the last thirty years. Put simply, a 20 pound 11-month-old infant traveling in a vehicle going 25 mph per hour would exert more than 500 pounds of force on the encircling arms of her mother during a collision. Clearly, in this case no human parent could successfully prevent an unrestrained infant from flying forward and striking the dashboard. In addition, the unrestrained mother would then crush the baby against the dashboard as her body moved forward as a result of Newton's first law. An understanding of injury pathophysiology has motivated all U.S. states and territories to require child safety seats be used for every child under age four. These seats use a five point harness system (top of both shoulders, each side of the pelvis and between the legs) to distribute the force across the torso in order to limit the infant's motion and prevent injury.

Rule 3: Total Energy Is Preserved

The total amount of energy in the universe is static. Thus, the potential energy available in a collision has to go somewhere. Some of it may be dissipated in heat (friction on the brakes and tires) or noise, but the majority is spent on or in some physical object. Injury-producing collisions are **inelastic collisions**, meaning that at least some of the kinetic energy is absorbed or dissipated by one or more of the colliding partners. In practice, this typically means that the weaker or softer item absorbs energy from the stiffer, more unyielding one. You can readily understand the importance of this concept by imagining the effects of a human punching a pillow, a panel of drywall, or a brick wall.

At some point, the amount, type, and location of the injury overwhelm the body's defenses and the human dies. This is a relatively rare event when the injury is unintentional and the mechanism is blunt trauma. For every fatality from blunt trauma, there are 10 to 20 people injured enough to be hospitalized and 150 to 500 who eventually seek some type of medical care. This makes up the *injury pyramid* (Figure 14-1). Importantly, this pyramid is very wide at the bottom when the injury is unintentional but much narrower if the injury is intentional, and reversed if the intent is self-harm (suicide) and the mechanism is a firearm.

Injury Patterns

Injuries and injury patterns can be predicted if you understand basic physics and human anatomy.

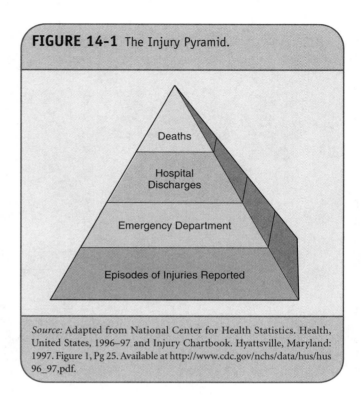

FIGURE 14-1 The Injury Pyramid.

Deaths

Hospital Discharges

Emergency Department

Episodes of Injuries Reported

Source: Adapted from National Center for Health Statistics. Health, United States, 1996–97 and Injury Chartbook. Hyattsville, Maryland: 1997. Figure 1, Pg 25. Available at http://www.cdc.gov/nchs/data/hus/hus 96_97,pdf.

Example

The abdomen has a soft casing of skin, subcutaneous tissue, and muscles. It contains solid organs (liver, spleen, and **pancreas**) and hollow organs (stomach, small intestine, large intestine, and bladder) and is bounded on the back by the **retroperitoneum** containing the kidneys, major blood vessels such as the **aorta** and **inferior vena cava**, and the thoracolumbar portion of the spinal column. Thus, the back portions are more protected than the organs lying in front of the spinal column (Figure 14-2).

Blunt injuries to the abdomen can occur by several mechanisms, and both the mechanism and the amount of force applied matter when considering the type of injury that will result. A direct blow with a booted foot (e.g., during an assault) will result initially in a contusion of the abdominal wall. If a great deal of force is applied to the center of the abdomen, the hollow organs will be compressed against the boney surface of the anterior vertebral bodies. The result may cause a contusion (*bruise*) or laceration of the intestine. Either of these can be catastrophic. A contusion may cause enough swelling to directly obstruct the flow of food through the gastrointestinal system and in the worst cases may cause the affected area of intestine to die completely (*necrosis*). A laceration causes the bacteria residing in partially digested food to spread throughout the abdomen, leading to a potentially life-threatening infection (*peritonitis*). At its worst, a direct blow to the upper

FIGURE 14-2 Abdominal Organs.

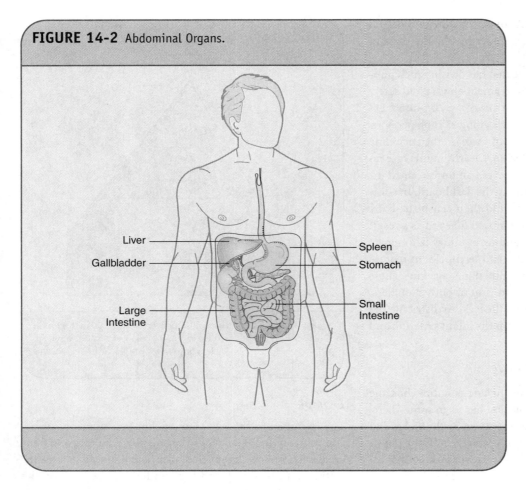

Liver
Gallbladder
Large Intestine
Spleen
Stomach
Small Intestine

abdomen may lead to **transection** of the pancreas, which resides just in front of the bones of the spine and produces potent digestive juices. Laceration or transection of this organ is a surgical emergency, as those juices will quickly begin to digest the unprotected tissues of the human body. This is what happens to a young child in a crash who is riding without a booster seat and wearing the lap portion of the safety belt across the upper abdomen.

If the force is applied linearly across the abdomen, such as in the case of an unrestrained driver who slides forward on the seat and impacts the lower rim of the steering wheel, simultaneous lacerations of the solid organs (liver and spleen) often result. As recently as 20 years ago, all of these injuries required emergent surgery to attempt to stop the bleeding that results. More recently, some patients with serious liver or spleen lacerations may be observed without surgery.

Injury Outcomes and Disability

Interestingly, those torso injuries that are most likely to be life-threatening, such as lacerations to the spleen, liver, heart, or lungs, are less likely to be associated with permanent disability. If the patient survives a liver laceration, future liver function is very likely to be normal. If the lung laceration heals, the patient's respiratory function is normal. Although patients who have undergone a splenectomy may need antibiotics to prevent certain infections such as those from dental work, their life expectancy is essentially normal.

The same is not true of patients with serious traumatic brain injuries. These injuries are both life-threatening in the acute phase and often require an extensive period of recovery with no expectation of return to pre-injury functioning. Patients with significant spinal cord injury are almost always permanently disabled (quadriplegic or paraplegic). There are few medical interventions that significantly change the long-term effects of these injuries.

Boney injuries, particularly extremity fractures, are also (perhaps surprisingly) associated with significant long-term disability. The degree of impairment is often related to the patient's pre-injury occupation. For instance, a day laborer with an ankle fracture that does not require surgery will be placed into a cast and put on crutches. He will be unable to work for 6 to 12 weeks while the injury heals, but the ankle may be stiff or weather-sensitive for years afterward, which may seriously impair his return to his previous type of work. The same injury to a stockbroker may impair his golf game, but is less likely to impair his earning capacity.

Finally, the long-term psychosocial effects of injury are worth mentioning. As many as 25 percent of young men with minimal facial injuries (mostly lacerations) suffer from posttraumatic stress disorder (PTSD) as much as a year later.[8] Even for those who do not meet criteria for the diagnosis of PTSD may make significant alterations in their lifestyles, such as refusing to drive on the highway after a motor vehicle crash. These effects are as yet poorly understood, and the interventions to minimize the long term psychological effects of trauma have not been well studied. In addition, for each person with an injury, there may be serious psychological effects on friends and family members who experience the "second trauma" of learning of the event and watching their loved one go through the recovery phase.

Injury Risk Factors

Although basic physics and anatomy can predict the event and type of an injury, there are risk factors for this event that mimic many other disease risk factors, such as the risk factors for contracting the common cold or flu or a sexually transmitted disease (STD). The type and severity of injury vary by age, race, gender, socioeconomic level, education, substance use, and personality traits. Each of these characteristics is associated with behaviors that put individuals at risk of injury.

> **INJURY RISK FACTORS**
> Age
> Gender
> Personality
> Alcohol

Age

For infants under age 1, the biggest cause of death is suffocation (either intentional or unintentional), while the most common cause of injury is falling. The most severe falling injuries are the result of an older person putting the infant on a surface high above the floor and providing insufficient protection to prevent the infant from rolling/falling off. Baby walkers with wheels turn barely mobile infants into poorly controlled racecars that readily careen down stairs and are therefore no longer recommended for use. Newly walking toddlers are at risk of falling from standing (not very far) and from running into the proverbial coffee table.

For Americans from ages 1 to 44, the greatest risk for severe or fatal injury comes from motor vehicle crashes. This cause alone accounts for 31.7 percent of the unintentional injury deaths for those aged 1 to 4 but 69.6 percent of the deaths between ages 15 and 34. Only in one subgroup, 15- to 44-year-old African-American men, does intentional injury (homicide) cause more fatalities than all types of unintentional injuries, moving motor vehicle crashes to second place.[9]

Gender

Gender plays an important role in injury epidemiology. From an early age, males are more likely to die from injuries than females, but this becomes nearly exponential in adolescence and the effect persists throughout the lifespan.[6] This is thought to be due to an increased interest in risky behaviors by men, but there may be more to it than that. The rate per population of non-fatal injuries is higher among boys and young men than among women, but the trend reverses over 65 when women have a higher rate of non-fatal injury. At older ages, men die from injuries more frequently than women, but women have more injuries.

Personality

Risk-taking behavior is a common theme among injury risk factors. Those who engage in more risky behaviors are more likely to become injured, just as those who engage in risky sexual behaviors are more likely to become infected with an STD. Individuals with sensation-seeking personality styles are more likely to be willing to place themselves at risk. For injuries, risk-taking behaviors include aggressively participating in sports without appropriate protective equipment, driving without safety belts, speeding, and physically acting out from anger.

Alcohol

No discussion of injury risk factors would be complete without mentioning the huge increase in both the risk of an injury of any severity and the risk of severe or fatal injury from using alcohol. Alcohol is a neurotoxin and neurodepressant that causes measurable slowing of physical response times, and cognitive ability declines after drinking a level as low as 0.05 blood alcohol concentration (BAC). Its initial effect on the brain is mild euphoria that is quickly followed by disinhibition. If the person continues to imbibe, the result is obvious dis-coordination and finally coma and death. Alcohol's effects include an increase in willingness to take risks and a decreased ability to respond in hazardous situations. It is implicated in nearly half of all drowning deaths and 38 percent of motor vehicle fatalities (down from 70% in 1966). Fifty to sixty percent of trauma patients who survive to hospital admission were not sober at the time of the injury. Alcohol is associated with becoming the victim of and acting as the perpetrator of an intentional assault. Between 30 and 40 percent of patients who present to the emergency department with an injury had been drinking within the two hours before the trauma occurred.

Summary

Injuries are among the most common health problems for humans. All injuries are the result of energy being applied to the tissues of the body above their tolerance thresholds. There are specific risk factors for specific types of injuries, and the type of injury can be predicted if the type, amount, and location of force applied are well understood. Injuries can be predicted, prevented, and controlled using the same public health concepts as for any other disease.

CASE STUDIES

Scenario 1

Dorothy was 79 and in generally good health when she fell and broke her hip. At the time, she was living alone in the house where she and her late husband had raised four kids. She had tripped while bringing a load a laundry up the basement stairs. Unable to walk and nowhere near a telephone, she lay on the basement floor for 36 hours until her daughter stopped by. When the paramedics brought her into the Emergency Department, she was embarrassed about the state of her clothing, which was soaked in urine. X-rays showed a fracture of her right hip (Figure 14-2). She was admitted to the hospital and underwent surgery the next day to replace the hip. After the operation, Dorothy was placed on blood thinning medicine and went to spend three weeks in a rehabilitation hospital. She did well and was able to be released, but continued to need to walk with a cane. Neither she nor her family was comfortable with the idea of her living alone and she moved into an assisted living facility.

After simply tripping, Dorothy was forced to give up her home of 50 years and move into a one bedroom apartment. Because it is farther from her children's homes, she sees a lot less of them and the grandchildren, and there is no room for the sleep-overs with the kids that she enjoyed before.

Defining the Issues

Better lighting, handrails, and non-skid coverings on the stairs might have prevented the fall. Use of an automated button necklace to call for help might have ensured that Dorothy was found earlier. The best falls prevention method for older adults seems to be regular exercise, particularly walking and balance training. A class at the senior center might have helped keep Dorothy from falling. In this case, preventing the osteoporosis or better treatment of this comorbid condition could have decreased the risk of the injury even if she did fall.

Patient's Understanding

"This was just an accident. Something that was going to happen sometime. It's just too bad now I can't live alone," said Dorothy.

Scenario 2

Jim graduated from college only two years ago and was working at his first job in advertising. He worked hard and played hard, working out at the gym five days a week and mountain biking on the weekends to stay in shape. Every other Friday evening there was a happy hour for the people in his company at a pub about two blocks from the office and he occasionally attended. One week, after a particularly good day—his rather stern boss had even congratulated him on a job well done—he decided to attend. A group of people from work decided follow the happy hour event up by going to a new restaurant across town. Jim had had five drinks but felt "OK" and offered to drive two of his coworkers to dinner.

On the way there, his car was T-boned by a dumptruck driver who ran a red light. Jim clearly had the right of way. Jim got away with a broken arm, a stiff neck, and some bruises, but the coworker sitting in the front passenger seat was killed and the rear seat passenger suffered a permanent brain injury. Jim's blood alcohol content was 0.120. He was charged with drunk driving, his license was immediately suspended, and he had to quit his job because he couldn't cope with the reactions of the rest of the people at work. He's still waiting to hear what punishment the judge is going to give him.

Defining the Issues

Alcohol use impairs judgment and likely impaired Jim's ability to recognize how drunk he was. More than two drinks in one hour will put most medium weight people into risky driving range of blood alcohol (over 0.05% blood alcohol concentration). More than three drinks in an hour will put most medium weight people over the legal limit (now 0.08 in most states). However, no one stopped him (not his coworkers, bartender, or parking attendant), and the others were willing to get into the car with him. In fact, the crash was not his "fault" because the dumptruck driver ran a red light. However, the alcohol likely made Jim take longer to recognize the risk and prolonged his reaction time. Without it, he might have been able to stop or accelerate out of the way.

Red light running is happening more frequently over the last two decades as drivers have become more aggressive. The large mass of the truck striking the less protected passenger side of Jim's vehicle meant his passengers bore the brunt of the energy transfer during the crash.

Red light cameras significantly decrease drivers' willingness to run the red light but are politically contentious in many areas.

Patient's Understanding

Jim says, "It wasn't my fault. That guy shouldn't have run the light; I had the right of way. My drinks had nothing to do with the crash and I hope the judge knows it!"

CLINICAL PERSPECTIVE FOR THE INDIVDUAL PATIENT

It should be apparent by this point in the chapter that human behaviors and choices play a crucial role in the pathophysiology of injuries. In the 21st century, many methods for reducing injuries have become part of everyday life. We "babyproof" the house to prevent toddlers from sticking their fingers into electrical sockets, drinking cleaning products, or falling down the stairs. We expect our homes and workplaces to have smoke detectors. Almost everyone I know is appalled to see small children riding loose in a passing vehicle; small children should be strapped into car seats. But for an individual to change behaviors takes an effort, and the process is not instantaneous.

Instead, individuals go through a process of change that includes considering the new behavior, planning on/for it, performing it, and finally automating or maintaining it. The Transtheoretical (Stages-of-Change) Model contains the following stages: precontemplation (benefits of lifestyle change are not being considered); contemplation (starting to consider change but not yet begun to act on this intention); preparation (ready to change the behavior and preparing to act); action (making the initial steps toward behavior change); and maintenance (maintaining behavior change while often experiencing relapses).[10]

Education appears to be critical to starting the process; the individual must know about the behavior and begin to understand that it is "good" or desirable in some way. ("Seat belts save lives.") The person has to internalize both the risk of the event ("I could be in a car crash") and personalize the potential benefit ("Wearing my seat belt could save my life"). At some point, the person makes a conscious decision ("I will wear my seat belt") and then acts upon it. While there may be backsliding and "forgetting," if the person continues to intend and use the behavior, it gradually becomes habitual and begins to feel odd not to engage in it ("I can't imagine not wearing my seat belt, I feel naked without it"). Of note, social norms also play a large role in choosing and maintaining safety behaviors. If the behavior is "normal" or "acceptable" behavior in the individual's social group, they are much more likely to perform it ("Everyone is wearing theirs, so I should wear mine").

PUBLIC HEALTH PERSPECTIVE FOR THE HEALTH OF THE GENERAL POPULATION AND OF HIGH RISK GROUPS
Injury Control

Injury control is the broad label applied to the concept of both preventing injury and optimally caring for those who develop injuries. This is a broad term that encompasses primary prevention (preventing the injury from occurring in the first place), secondary prevention (preventing the complications of the injury), and tertiary prevention (preventing re-injury by addressing risk factors). This is a complex issue and there are opportunities at every turn, but it wasn't until a landmark paper in 1968 that a usable framework was created to organize the opportunities for intervention. William Haddon, Jr. proposed the following concept: time is divided into pre-, during, and post-event phases, and human, vector, and environmental factors are considered.[11] Table 14-1 illustrates the matrix of his basic concepts, updated for today's environment.

In each cell of Table 14-1, there is an opportunity for intervention. The types of intervention include education (why seat belts save lives), engineering solutions (better guardrails, air bags), economic incentives (fines for speeding, failure to use seat belts, safety inspections), enforcement (jail for driving while intoxicated), and empowerment (changing social expec-

tations that people will not drive after drinking and will buckle up). These are known as the "Five Es" of injury control.

THE FIVE Es OF INJURY CONTROL
Education
Engineering Solutions
Economic Incentives
Enforcement
Empowerment

Some injury risks can be changed dramatically through engineering. A perfect example is the kind of glass in your vehicle's windshield. The use of safety glass, which splinters into little cubes after impact, has ended the era of people being scalped (literally) when they struck a windshield made of plate glass (which breaks into long, sharp shards). The creation and installation of **Jersey barriers** to prevent head-on crashes have greatly diminished these high energy events simply by preventing one out-of-control vehicle from crossing over the highway.

Much of the work of injury control is aimed at changing human behavior, however, either to limit the risk of having a crash (speeding, running red lights) or to limit the risk of an injury in the event of a crash (safety belts). It turns out that a

TABLE 14-1 Haddon Matrix for Motor Vehicle Crashes

	Human	Vector/Vehicle	Physical/Social Environment
Pre-Event	Intoxication Safety belt use Speed Alertness/sleepiness Experience	Tire pressure Brake functioning I beams Crumple zones	Speed cameras Weather Social culture Willingness to allow others to drive drunk
During Event	Frailty Age Size	Speed of impact Air bags Size Stiffness of surfaces Stability control	Flammability Guardrails Stiffness of fixed objects Barriers Embankments
Post-Event	Body mass index Age Comorbid conditions	Degree of crush Fuel system integrity	EMS response Trauma center availability Rehab programs

Source: Data from Haddon W Jr. The changing approach to the epidemiology, prevention, and amelioration of trauma: the transition to approaches etiologically rather than descriptively based. Am J Public Health Nations Health. 1968 August; 58(8):1431–1438.

combination of the Five Es is most effective in motivating behavior to change. Education alone (at a cost of millions during the 1970s and early 1980s) only got 14 percent of the American public to buckle up their seat belts by 1984. When states began to pass seat belt legislation (that made failure to use the belt a moving violation with a fine of $10–$25), belt use began to creep upward. States that have strengthened their belt use laws have seen further increases in belt use, and the U.S. national average is now over 80 percent.

Finally, all public health efforts cost money, first to do research to identify successful interventions, and second to implement and maintain those efforts. Federal funding in the United States for injury research and programming has lagged behind other diseases. The total number of years of productive life lost from injuries is greater than cancer and heart disease combined. The 2006 U.S. federal budget funded the National Cancer Institute at $4.8 *billion* and the National Heart, Lung, and Blood Institute at $2.9 *billion*. The National Center for Injury Prevention and Control received only $139 *million* and about $694 *million* of the National Highway Traffic Safety Administration's budget is spent on related topics, which total about $833 million or less than 1/10th of the spending on cancer and heart disease.

KEY TERMS

Physiology Terms

Aorta: The main arterial pipeline of the body. It originates at the top of the heart, curves up into the neck supplying the arteries to the head, face, and arms, and then dives down following the spinal column to finally divide at the level of the umbilicus into the main arteries to the lower extremities.

Comorbid Factors: The coexistence of two or more disease processes; usually used to indicate medical conditions already existing at the time of the injury.

Cornea: The thin clear part of the eye that allows images to enter the eye and reach the retina so vision can occur.

Hamstrings: Muscles in the back of the leg that extend or straighten the hip.

Inferior Vena Cava: Large vein that collects the blood flow from the legs and abdominal organs and carries it back to the heart.

Gluteal Muscles: Muscle group in the buttock that rotates and extends (straightens) the hip.

Ligament: Fibrous tissue that connects one bone to another.

Liver: Organ of the gastrointestinal system that resides in the right upper quadrant of the abdomen.

Osteoporosis: Abnormal loss of bony tissue resulting in fragile porous bones attributable to a lack of calcium; most common in postmenopausal women.

Pancreas: An organ in the gastrointestinal system that resides in the middle of the upper abdomen and supplies digestive juices to the intestines and insulin into the blood.

Quadriceps: Muscle in the front of the thigh that flexes (bends) the hip and extends (straightens) the knee.

Retroperitoneum: Area behind (posterior to) the abdominal cavity. It contains the spinal column, kidneys, aorta, and inferior vena cava.

Spleen: An organ of the immune system that resides in the left upper quadrant of the abdomen.

Transection: Cut in half.

Physics Terms

Inelastic Collision: Is a collision in which some or all of the kinetic energy of the colliding bodies is absorbed by at least one of the partners.

Jersey Barrier: Large, prism shaped concrete blocks that separate lanes of traffic (often opposing lanes of traffic) with a goal of minimizing vehicle crossover in the case of accidents. The shape is designed to use the vehicle's momentum to send it back into the flow of traffic in the same direction rather than into oncoming traffic lanes or across lanes.

Newton's First Law: Objects in motion remain in motion until an external force is applied. The converse is also true: an object at rest tends to stay at rest until acted upon.

Newton's Second Law: The acceleration of an object as produced by a net force is directly proportional to the magnitude of the net force, in the same direction as the net force, and inversely proportional to the mass of the object. More succinctly, Force = mass $\times$ acceleration ($F = ma$).

Viscoelastic: Having both a relatively high resistance to flow and being capable of resuming original shape after stretching or compression.

Yaw: To lean suddenly, unsteadily, and erratically from the vertical axis. When used in relationship to bullets, recall that bullets spin rapidly around their long axis. When they impact human tissue, this spinning is often partially disrupted.

Public Health Term

Case Fatality Rate: Number of deaths/total number of injuries $\times$ 100. Essentially the percentage of people with that type of injury who die.

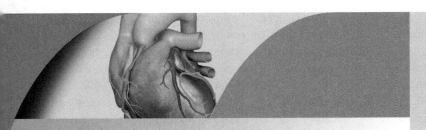

Questions for Further Research, Study, Reflection, and Discussion

For the Individual Student

In order to answer these questions, it may be necessary to research the primary literature.

- Name five things you and/or your family could do to improve your personal safety and prevent injuries in your home, at work, at the park, or at school.
- Why is alcohol such a big risk factor for injuries? Why is it legal? Why is the legal drinking age 21 when people can vote at 18? What community level interventions might help prevent alcohol-related injury?
- Use WISQARS™ (the CDC's Web-based Injury Statistics Query and Reporting System) to evaluate the effects of age, race, and gender on unintentional injury.
- Use the HCUPnet (Health Care Utilization Partnership Web-based query system) to evaluate the costs of acute hospital care for injuries. A hint: Injuries are ICD-9 codes 8000-9999.
- Besides both intentional and unintentional injuries, what other public health concerns are likely to arise in individuals with a sensation-seeking personality? Are there any interventions that can successfully limit risk-taking behaviors?

For Small Group Discussion

- A 28-year-old man, the breadwinner for a family of 4 (wife and two kids, ages 6 months and 8 years), falls down on the job and breaks his leg. He is placed in a cast and must use crutches for the next eight weeks.
- What are the effects on him and his family if he is a stockbroker? What if he is an illegal alien and works as a day laborer? What if he drives a cab?
- How will this injury affect the rest of the family relationships? Finances?
- A 25-year-old man goes to a baseball game and has four beers over the course of the game. He gets stopped by police on the way home and has a blood alcohol level of 0.120. What should the legal response be? What if he runs over and kills a 3-year-old pedestrian instead of just being stopped by police? What if the 3-year-old is his child who was riding in his car when he ran a red light and was struck by another vehicle?
- A young couple is having marital problems. During an argument, he picks her up and throws her against a wall. He is immediately sorry and repentant, and she is bruised but otherwise uninjured. What is the likelihood of a repeat offense? What should she do? What are her options? Many women stay in the relationship after this type of event. Why? What effects of witnessing domestic violence do the children in the family experience?
- Handguns in the home are more likely to be used by family members against themselves or other family members or friends than as self-protection against a burglar or other criminal. What is likely to be going on in the home when the gun is used against a family member or friend? Who might be using it in such a situation? What environmental or engineering solutions exist to prevent this type of event?
- A 75-year-old man begins to have trouble with short-term memory and his family believes that he should no longer drive a car. He disagrees. Who should decide when he legally MUST stop driving? What are the effects on his social life and mental and emotional states? What are the effects of the argument itself on other members of the family, and how are they affected when he does stop driving? How are the answers different if he lives in an area with great public transportation? How do they differ if his ability to walk more than two blocks is limited by his emphysema?
- One argument against legislation aimed at preventing injuries through the use of safety devices (such as primary safety belt laws, motorcycle helmets, gun locks) is the concept that the government should

not legislate adult behavior to prevent injury solely to that adult. In other words, if I'm an adult and I'm the only one who will be injured if I don't use this device, the govern.ment shouldn't require me to use it. What are three rebuttals to this attitude?

For Entire Class Discussion

- In 2000, the cost of just medical care for U.S. traffic victims was estimated at over $150 billion per year. Motor vehicle crashes are the number one cause of lost years of productive life in the United States, but receive much less federal research dollars than other causes. What reasons are there for this disparity?

- The majorit y of the world's 1.7 million fatalities from traffic crashes occur in the developing world, where public health efforts to curtail their impact must compete for scarce resources with AIDS, malaria, malnutrition, and other infectious diseases. All told, there are more fatalities from injuries (~6 million total) than from any of these competing issues. What would it take to get injuries onto the global public health radar and generate effective outreach programs?

- Even on the morning news traffic report, collisions are reported as "accidents" and the majority of the public continues to view them as "not MY fault." Somehow, injuries are considered to be an "acceptable risk." How might the view of the problem be reoriented in public debate?

- In areas of the world with few privately owned vehicles, the majority of drivers are young men being paid to drive trucks, buses, and taxis. The majority of the risk of injury is to pedestrians (and in an interaction between a vehicle and a pedestrian, the pedestrian ALWAYS loses). In many of these areas there is limited police effectiveness. How might companies and other community-based organizations effectively influence the behavior of both the drivers and the pedestrians?

- All states require doctors, nurses, police officers, teachers, and others in authority to report any concern about child abuse and let the local social work system investigate to find out if there is really a problem. Some legislators believe there should be a similar requirement for reporting intimate partner violence (domestic violence). What are some potential consequences of this legislation?

EXERCISE/ACTIVITY

Divide the class into groups of four to eight. Assign each group a topic below (or think of your own) and ask the group to suggest a method for intervening with a concrete end result. Give the class a time line and budget (such as 3 years with $200,000/year available), and allow about 30 minutes for group planning and discussion. Ask each group to present their plan to the rest of the class for consideration. During each presentation, assign other students to be the mayor, chief of police, town treasurer, medical director of the local hospital, or other relevant players.

A. The pedestrian struck rate at our urban university has reached epidemic proportions with 30 students struck within the last year.

B. The suicide rate for older men living in our rural county has doubled over the last 10 years. Most of these are accomplished with guns.

C. At the quarry outside town is there is a "NO swimming" sign but there have been two deaths and eight serious spinal cord injuries there in the last three years.

D. An elderly housing community is on the opposite side of the road from a strip mall containing a popular restaurant and a supermarket. The road has three lanes in either direction, an "either way turn lane" in the middle, and there is no stop sign or traffic signal. Three elderly people have been struck crossing in that area this year.

E. There have been 5 fatalities and 34 serious injuries from motor vehicle crashes among teenagers in this suburban county in the last year. Thirty-four percent of the teenage drivers had been drinking.

Healthy People 2010

Indicator: Injury and Violence

Focus Area: Injury and Violence Prevention

Goal: Reduce injuries, disabilities, and deaths due to unintentional injuries and violence.

Objectives:

15-1. Reduce hospitalization for nonfatal head injuries to 45 hospitalizations per 100,000 population from a baseline 60.6/100,000 in 1998.

15-13. Reduce deaths caused by unintentional injuries to 20.8 deaths per 100,000 population from 35.0 in 1998.

15-15. Reduce deaths caused by motor vehicle crashes to 9.0 deaths per 100,000 population and 0.8 death per 100 million vehicle miles traveled (VMT) (baseline 1.6, down to 1.47 in 2006).

15-19. Increase use of safety belts to 92 percent of the total population (69% in 1998, 84% in 2006).

15-27. Reduce deaths from falls to 2.3 deaths per 100,000 population from 4.7 in 1998.

15-37. Reduce physical assaults to 25.5 physical assaults per 1,000 persons aged 12 years and older from 31.1 in 1998.

REFERENCES

1. National Center for Health Statistics. *Ten leading causes of death by age group, United States—2003*. Available at: ftp://ftp.cdc.gov/pub/ncipc/10LC-2003/JPEG/10lc-2003.jpg Accessed April 4, 2008.

2. Fallon I, O'Neill D. The world's first automobile fatality. *Accid Anal Prev* 2005;37:601–603.

3. "Fatally hurt by automobile." *New York Times* September 14, 1899: 1.

4 Centers for Disease Control and Prevention. *Ten Leading Causes of Death, United States, 2005*. Available at http://www.cdc.gov/nchs/pressroom/data/state_mortality_rank_05.htm Accessed April 4, 2008.

5. Finkelstein EA, Corso PS, Miller TR. *Incidence and Economic Burden of Injuries in the United States*. New York: Oxford University Press; 2006.

6. Dictionary.com; "accident." http://dictionary.reference.com/browse/accident. Accessed 4/28/08

7. Vyrostek SB, Annest JL, Ryan GW. Surveillance for fatal and nonfatal injuries—United States, 2001. *MMWR Morbid Mortal Wkly Rep Surveill Summ* 2004;53:1–57.

8. Glynn SM, Asarnow JR, Asarnow R, Shetty V, Elliot-Brown K, Black E, Belin TR. The development of acute post-traumatic stress disorder after orofacial injury: a prospective study in a large urban hospital. *J Oral Maxillofac Surg* 2003;61:785–792.

9. Centers for Disease Control, National Center for Injury Prevention and Control. *WISQARS Leading Causes of Death Reports, 1999–2005*. Available at http://webappa.cdc.gov/sasweb/ncipc/leadcaus10.html Accessed April 4, 2008.

10. Prochaska JO, DiClemente CC. Stages and processes of self-change of smoking: toward an integrative model of change. *J Consult Clin Psychol* 1983;51:390–395.

11. Haddon W Jr. The changing approach to the epidemiology, prevention, and amelioration of trauma: the transition to approaches etiologically rather than descriptively based. *Am J Public Health Nations Health* 1968;58:1431–1438.

CROSS REFERENCES

Aging in America

Behavioral Determinants of Health

Epidemiological and Public Health Perspectives on Aging in America

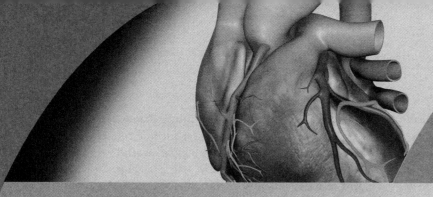

CHAPTER 15

Oral Health: The Neglected Epidemic in Public Health

Michael A. Tabacco
Tareq A. Yousef

> Oral health is integral to general health. You cannot be healthy without oral health. Oral health and general health should not be interpreted as separate entities. Oral health is a critical component of health and must be included in the provision of health care and the design of community programs.[1]
>
> Donna E. Shalala
> Former Secretary of Health and Human Services
>
> "We must seize this unprecedented opportunity to ensure that the mouth becomes reconnected to the rest of the body in health policies and programs."[2]
>
> Myron Allukian Jr., DDS, MPH
> Former president of the American Public Health Association

LEARNING OBJECTIVES

By the end of this chapter, the student will be able to:

- Understand the history of oral health and past public health initiatives to improve oral health.
- Describe the most common threats to oral health.
- Describe the current state of oral health from a public health perspective.
- Identify current issues in the field of oral health and be able to discuss potential public health interventions to address them.

A BRIEF "ORAL" HISTORY OF PUBLIC HEALTH

An awareness of the importance of **oral health** has existed for thousands of years. Ranging from the practice of oral hygiene, technological improvements in dental practice, and the incep-

tion of dentistry as a distinct profession, a vast amount of knowledge has been discovered to allow individuals to live with good oral hygiene. The following time line highlights some milestones in the history of oral health from a public health standpoint:

- Several ancient civilizations, including those in India, China, Mesopotamia, Greece, and Rome, practiced oral health care.[3]
- The history of governmental regulations on dentistry can be traced back as far as 2500 BC.[3]
- The world's first dental school, the Baltimore College of Dental Surgery, was established in 1840. As a result, dentistry became a distinct profession and was separated from the field of medicine.[3]
- The American Dental Association was established in 1859.[4]
- In one of the earliest major public health interventions aimed at oral health, Grand Rapids, Michigan, was the first city in the world to fluoridate its community water supply in 1945. By 2002, 67 percent of Americans who live in communities with public water supply systems consume fluoridated water.[3]
- Advances in restorative materials, bleaching, veneers, and implants during the 1990s created a new emphasis on esthetic dentistry.[5]

CURRENT STATE OF ORAL HEALTH

Oral health is sometimes regarded as the "neglected epidemic" in public health.[6–9] It is a common misconception that oral medicine, oral health, and dental hygiene are elective health-care specialties and that they can therefore conveniently be marginalized. This tendency towards marginalization includes: the lack of recognition that the stomatognathic (literally: *oral-jaws*) organ system is indispensable and integral to human survival, the lack of awareness that oral diseases affect the entire organism, and the failure to invest resources towards ensuring the oral health of the most vulnerable members of the population, the young and the elderly.

Both academics and practitioners in the field of public health should be aware of the following issues concerning oral health:

- Oral and dental health are intrinsically important.
- Oral and dental health are good indicators of overall health; and if dental visits are recommended every six months, they provide a good, if properly utilized, opportunity to assess overall health.
- Oral health is being neglected compared to other health domains. For example:
  - Only about half of the United States population has some form of dental insurance. So, if a diabetic person visits a doctor's office with a leg ulcer, the patient would be covered under medical insurance. However, if that same individual needs dental attention because of a mouth ulcer, their care would not be covered unless they have dental insurance.[3]
  - Only 20 percent of children who have health insurance through Medicaid receive dental care, even though dental services, aimed specifically at children, are included in Medicaid (according to a Government Accounting Office study in 2000). In response to deficits, many states have removed dental care from adult Medicaid.[3]
  - Ninety-three percent of people in the United States over the age of 40 have not had their mouths and necks checked for oral cancers in the past year. "Oral cancers are more prevalent than cervical cancer, yet most women receive pap smears routinely."[3]
  - Eighty-one percent of nursing home residents have not had an annual oral exam. The 19 percent who did were screened only after the resident was rushed by ambulance for emergency care.[3]
  - "As a percentage of total health expenditures, dental service expenditures have decreased 28 percent, from 6.4 percent in 1970 to about 4.6 percent today."[3]

Oral diseases are a *neglected epidemic* in our country, and the oral health disparities of the underserved and under-insured are becoming the norm rather than exception. This effect may be exacerbated in lower-income countries where the dentist-to-population ratio may be much lower than in higher-income countries (as low as 1:150,000 in Africa compared to 1:2,000 in most industrialized countries).[10]

BASIC SCIENCE FACTS/KEY CONCEPTS REVIEW

Although it has frequently been considered synonymous with healthy teeth, the construct of **oral health** has taken on a broader meaning in recent times. The term *oral* refers to the mouth, which is comprised of the teeth and gums (including connective tissues, ligaments, and bone), the tongue, the lips, the salivary glands, the masticatory (chewing) muscles, the jaws, the temporomandibular joints, the hard and soft palate, skeletal nerves, and the mucosal lining of the mouth and throat. Oral health is freedom from diseases and disorders that affect the craniofacial complex (oral, dental, and craniofacial tissues). Beyond the simple absence of infirmity, oral health also encompasses the notion of well-being that contributes to an individual's overall physical and mental health.

Several factors can affect oral health. The most common oral diseases are dental caries, gum disease, and oral cancer. **Dental caries** (tooth decay) is the most common childhood disease in the United States and is characterized as the breakdown of tooth structure caused by a build-up of acid waste product produced by the bacteria in **dental plaque**, a sticky substance containing diverse microorganisms that compose the oral flora of the mouth and adhere on the surface of teeth. The main species in plaque involved in dental caries is the highly cariogenic *Streptococcus mutans*, which begins the process of decay by colonizing on the hard surface of teeth. These organisms may also adhere to smooth surface teeth by synthesizing sucrose into insoluble polysaccharides. Finally, *S. mutans* ferments sucrose to produce lactic acid, leading to the chemical dissolution of hydroxyapatite crystals, the main substance in the tooth enamel that consists primarily of positively charged calcium ions and negatively charged phosphate ions. In its most aggressive form, rampant or acute dental caries, lactic acid overwhelms the normal remineralization of the tooth by saliva and production of secondary dentin by the tooth pulp, thus leading to tooth abscesses. Its effects are exacerbated by a high sucrose diet where sugars can be fermented to produce high levels of lactic acid, acidic beverage consumption that aids in dissolving tooth substance (mainly calcium phosphate), and poor oral hygiene that may increase the concentration of *S. mutans* in dental plaque. **Protective factors** that decrease the likelihood of developing dental caries include the presence and normal flow of saliva, which is critical in replacing calcium phosphate ions dissolved by the lactic acid, as well as sufficient exposure to optimal levels of fluoride that promote remineralization and hardening of the tooth enamel.

Periodontal disease involves bacterial infections and inflammation of the oral soft and hard tissues surrounding and supporting the teeth. It includes two stages: **gingivitis**, which affects the soft tissues alone, and **periodontitis**, which also targets the supporting alveolar bone surrounding the teeth. Gingivitis is considered the early stage of gum disease in which inflammation and redness occurs in the gums. The oral soft tissues may also bleed easily and become irritated, revealing signs that the gums are unhealthy. This stage of gum disease only affects the soft tissues and does not progress to the underlying bones surrounding the teeth (Figure 15-1).

A more serious form of gum disease, periodontitis, occurs when the bacterial infection and inflammation caused during gingivitis spread to the underlying hard tissue that consists of the ligaments and bone. Later stages of periodontitis cause the teeth to become loose, increasing the likelihood for the spread of craniofacial infections to occur in the spaces, or pockets, between the loose teeth. An immunological response is initiated by the body to fight the bacterial infection in the pockets from spreading. However, enzymes (specifically collagenase) produced by the body in response to toxins excreted by the bacteria break down the bones and ligaments supporting the teeth. A sufficient amount of destruction of the bones and connective tissue will eventually lead to tooth loss if the disease is not treated at its early stages. Routine flossing, brushing, and dental examinations of the teeth to maintain good oral hygiene reduce the likelihood of developing periodontal disease.

Oral cancer, another major public health issue dealing with the oral cavity, affects over 30,000 Americans and causes nearly 7,800 deaths per year.[3] This form of cancer, which may develop in the mouth or neck, is caused by mutagenic effects in the DNA of cells. Excessive consumption of alcohol, tobacco smoking, and chewing tobacco increases its likelihood by damaging these cells. Although it is painless and difficult to detect at its early stages, signs of oral cancer include: sores that do not heal and unusual red and white patches in the mouth as well as lumps in the mouth or neck. Routine dental check-ups are effective in the detection of oral cancer, but clinical detection may only spot the cancer at its late stages (stages 3 and 4). Fortunately, new devices are critical in detecting it in earlier stages (stages 1 and 2). However, frequent dental check-ups may help the dentist to detect local spread of an oral cancer as early as possible and to institute proper treatments for the already diagnosed patient.

The implementation of community water fluoridation has been a positive outcome in the reduction of dental caries, especially among children and the elderly who are most vulnerable to tooth decay. It is considered the most well-known public health intervention designed to improve oral health and has been included as one of the ten most significant public health interventions of the 20th century. A study conducted by the U.S. Public Health Service in 1945 on four communities in which fluoride was added to the drinking water showed a 48 percent reduction of decay among children between the ages of twelve and fourteen.[3] Further studies that were conducted were just as accurate in proving fluoride's effectiveness in preventing dental caries. Fluoride is an ion that comes from one of the most abundant elements on earth, fluorine. Negatively charged, it can only exist in combination with other elements. For example, fluoride was combined with sodium ions as sodium fluoride in June 1945 when the community of Newburgh, New York, added the compound to its drinking water as a result of the positive outcomes it gave to the community in Grand Rapids, Michigan, the first city to fluoridate its drinking water.

Fluoridation of teeth may be administered in two forms: topical and systemic. Topical fluoride is applied to the surface of the teeth while systemic fluoride is ingested. If given in moderation, systemic fluoride can help reduce dental caries in children whose teeth are developing by increasing the presence of fluoroapatite in the tooth enamel. When the tooth's main substance, **hydroxyapatite**, is dissolved by the acid produced by bacteria in plaque, topical fluoride is effective in remineralizing the teeth by forming **fluoroapatite**, a substance containing

FIGURE 15-1 Picture of Periodontitis (Gum Disease).

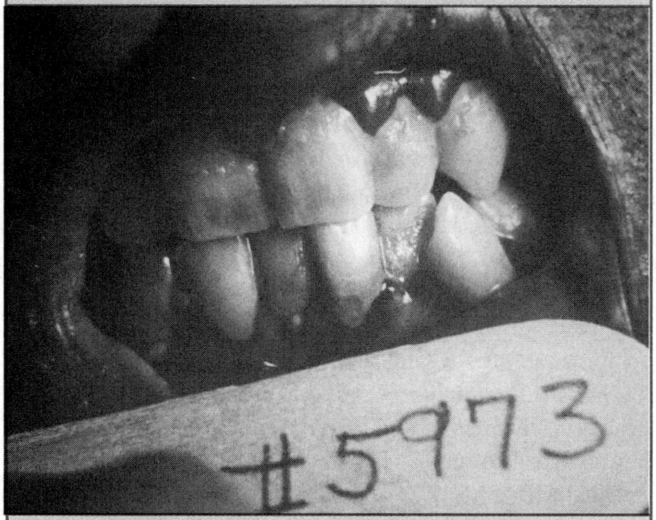

Source: Courtesy of CDC.

calcium, phosphate, and fluoride ions that provides the surface of teeth with a harder, less penetrable barrier to acid dissolution compared to hydroxyapatite.

However, excessive ingestion of fluoride can lead to dental fluorosis, a condition that causes tooth discoloration if too much fluoride is ingested during the time period when the tooth enamel is developing in children. A mild form of fluorosis, characterized by chalky-white patches on the tooth enamel, is the most prevalent form observed in children in the United States. A more severe form also exists in which yellow or brown discolorations occur in the affected areas of the tooth's surface. Fluorosis is a condition that mainly affects the appearance of the tooth and does not require medical attention.

In 1908, a young dentist by the name of Frederick S. McKay of Colorado Springs, Colorado, led many experiments to figure out why some individuals of the community had discolorations of the teeth (Figure 15-2). Children living in communities with naturally occurring fluoridated water at high levels had these discolorations while children in communities without fluoride in their drinking water did not have these stains. Known as the *Colorado Brown Stain phenomenon*, Dr.

FIGURE 15-2 Picture of Dr. Frederick S. McKay.

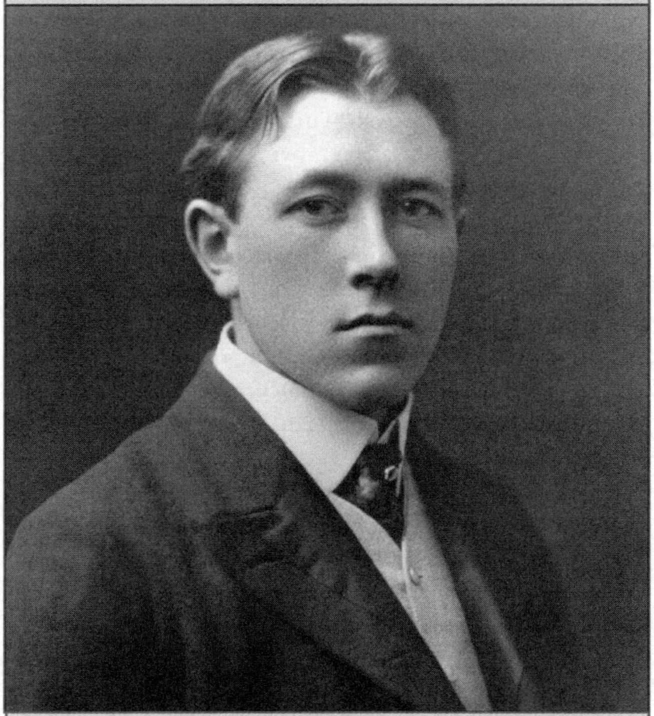

Source: Courtesy of CDC.

McKay was able to conclude in 1931 that the ingestion of high levels of fluoride was responsible for the discoloration, yet the use of this ion was critical in inhibiting dental caries. Further experiments showed that the use of optimal levels of fluoride, measured at 1 ppm (parts per million), in drinking water would reduce the likelihood of developing dental caries without staining the teeth.[3]

It is vital to understand, as students of public health, the importance of oral health and its close relationship to the rest of the body and the overall health of an individual. Physiological mechanisms to ward off diseases and conditions throughout the rest of the body are similar to those involved in fighting oral diseases. For example, acute inflammation and chronic immunological intervention by the body to fight *H. pylori* infection in the gastrointestinal tract is similar to the inflammation and immunological response observed in periodontal disease. The etiology that applies to oral cancer is also similar to other cancers that occur throughout the body.

Because it is considered a "neglected epidemic," preventive measures for oral disease such as lowering sucrose intake, reducing acidic beverage consumption, and routinely brushing and flossing teeth to maintain good oral hygiene must adequately be promoted with as much attention as with other diseases that manifest in other parts of the body. It is important to understand these diseases as multifactorial in which there is no single cause for the specific condition. Predisposing, precipitating, and perpetuating factors also must be observed to understand the genetic and environmental **cofactors** that lead to an oral condition. Understanding the biological basis of these oral conditions is integral in helping people understand key preventive measures to keep the oral cavity free from diseases and to encompass the notion of "well-being" in an individual.

PUBLIC HEALTH OVERVIEW/CONCLUSION

This chapter has focused entirely on oral health and its significant contribution to the systemic health of an individual. The concept of the oral craniofacial complex must not be interpreted as a separate entity, but more as a part of the body that must be maintained and taken care of adequately to improve the quality of life of an individual and to lessen the risk of developing potentially fatal conditions. Oral health has a major impact on the number of school/workdays missed as well as disturbing the mental well-being of an individual as a result of physiological complications. Oral diseases are also closely associated with other diseases in the body. For example, research has shown periodontal disease to be linked with other health problems including: cardiovascular disease, neurological conditions, diabetes, low birth weight in babies, and more.[10] Routine preventive measures performed on the oral cavity will

CASE STUDIES

CASE STUDY #1

Data are from *The Washington Post*, Wednesday, February 28, 2007:
"Twelve-year-old Deamonte Driver died of a toothache Sunday.
A routine, $80 tooth extraction might have saved him.
If his mother had been insured.
If his family had not lost its Medicaid.
If Medicaid dentists weren't so hard to find.
If his mother hadn't been focused on getting a dentist for his brother, who had six rotted teeth."[11]

Clinical Perspective

Deamonte's death has received a great deal of media attention, and not just because it is shocking to hear that an otherwise healthy child died as a result of a toothache. From a purely clinical perspective, Deamonte's death could have easily been prevented had his abscessed tooth been treated in a timely manner. Unfortunately, by the time the severity of his condition was recognized and he was finally admitted to the hospital where he could receive adequate medical attention, the bacterial infection was too far advanced for doctors to be able to save his life.

Deamonte's tooth decay may also be linked to the poor diet he and his brother received either at the household or at school. Six rotted teeth in his brother and an untimely death of Deamonte clearly indicate the availability of foods with high sugar and acid content these children were accustomed to ingesting. Poor oral hygiene also may have increased bacterial concentrations in his mouth that spread to other parts of his body. Protective factors such as saliva to remineralize his teeth were inadequate, as the constant build-up of *S. mutans* that increased lactic acid production in his mouth, demineralizing his teeth at a faster pace than they could remineralize, and led to an oral infection and an unfortunate death due to his tooth abscess.

Public Health Perspective

From a public health perspective, a combination of several factors prevented Deamonte from receiving timely dental care:

- Deamonte's mother did not get adequate health insurance through her job.
- It was difficult for the family to find a dentist to treat them—less than 1/6 of Maryland dentists accept Medicaid because of low reimbursement rates.[11]
- Their family Medicaid coverage had lapsed because they had missed some paperwork during a stay in a homeless shelter.
- Deamonte's mother did not have access to information about preventive dental care and did not understand the threat to her son's health. Deamonte did not complain about his teeth and was admitted to the hospital because of a headache. Furthermore, she was faced with the difficulty of trying to get dental care for Deamonte's younger brother, who had six abscessed teeth himself and complained about them frequently.

CASE STUDY #2

Latisha G. is an 18-year-old girl with rampant dental caries, including especially aggressive forms of both "smooth-surface" caries and "root" caries. This young patient resides with her grandmother who raised her. She graduated from high school and hopes to be a beautician. Her overall health is good but her dental health has recently been deteriorating rapidly.

At first glance, a physician might describe her as a "WDWNF" (a well-developed, well-nourished female). Closer introspection into her history and her oral health reveals that she is very inadequately nourished. In addition, her continuous snacking, frequent consumption of sucrose-laden, carbonic acid-containing beverages, her limited dental awareness, her poor oral hygiene, and her lack of professional dental hygiene treatment have put her at high risk for poor oral health.

Latisha has been to a dentist who accepts Medicaid but the extent of her dental caries requires aggressive and extensive treatment. She has multiple dental and periodontal lesions and the decay has advanced sufficiently to involve her pulp tissue. She is in constant pain. The optimal treatment of her condition requires several endodontic procedures (root canal treatments) followed by fabrication of post-cores and crown placement. Medicaid will not cover this type of service and—even if it did—her eligibility ends this year due to her age. The treatment plan she may have to settle for is an urgent referral to her family physician (for a blood sugar and lipid panel, and nutrition counseling) coupled with an expedient dental solution: pretreatment with an antibiotic regimen, extractions of all posterior (back) teeth, and a fitting for dentures or partial dentures. She says that her dreams of becoming a beautician are fading because of how she feels about her teeth and what others think of her because of her oral health.

Clinical Perspective

Similar to the case of Deamonte and his untimely death due to dental abscess, Latisha was negligent in practicing proper oral hygiene, leading to the accumulation of plaque that significantly resulted in the loss of tooth structure that serves as a protective barrier to her teeth. Improper eating habits also contributed to the build-up of S. mutans in plaque that eventually was able to adhere and colonize on the surface of Latisha's teeth. Routine brushing and flossing are very important in maintaining a proper level of microorganisms present in the oral flora. Plaque is constantly building in the mouth and can remain invisible without the suspicion of having elevated amounts of bacteria in the oral cavity.

Emotional and mental well-being is also critical to discuss with Latisha's treatments because of her desire to become a beautician. In fact, oral diseases can affect the emotional well-being of many individuals who suffer from a certain oral condition, as pain and agony in the oral cavity can serve as a stressor that may complicate the way an individual may think or act. Encompassing the notion of well-being should not only involve physiological aspects, but should also include the mental health of an individual and their overall mental capabilities.

The clinical issues and treatment options for Latisha are determined by her ability to pay; the optimal treatment for her condition seems beyond her financial means. The choice to have her teeth extracted and getting dentures is more financially viable for her but a less attractive alternative, especially for a young adult.

Public Health Perspective

From a public health standpoint, people who find themselves in Latisha's situation do not seem to have many options. In this specific case, Latisha seems to have received little or no preventive care or education about oral health. Understanding the different risk factors that increased her likelihood of developing rampant dental caries could have helped Latisha in preventing this condition from occurring.

An individual who looks and feels healthy may necessarily not be free of disease, as evidenced in Latisha's care. She does not seem well informed about her own propensity to engage in behaviors that are negatively affecting her oral health, not only in terms of her teeth but also in terms of her future aspirations and her self-esteem.

not only reduce the likelihood of developing oral diseases, but would also contribute in a reduction of conditions that manifest in other parts of the body.

Different aspects must be observed to understand the importance of receiving health care involving the oral cavity. First, proper health insurance is necessary in providing a better scope of access to care, including receiving more services and having an adequate amount of resources available for the beneficiaries' needs. Much of this dilemma deals with political aspects involving the amount of services available either through the private or government sector, the latter being of great importance in terms of providing dental coverage to low-income families through Medicaid who would otherwise not be able to afford coverage in the private market.

Issues must also be addressed and improved to allow low-income individuals, especially children, to gain adequate dental coverage to prevent diseases such as dental caries, the single most chronic disease of childhood. According to the Health Resources and Services Administration of the U.S. Department of Health and Human Services, about one quarter of all children in the United States receive health coverage through **Medicaid**, a state-run health program designed for low-income families.[12] The same children receiving coverage through Medicaid have three times the amount of unmet needs for dental care compared to children in higher income families.[13] Factors that have impeded dental care coverage among the poor include: a decline in dentists participating in state Medicaid programs, Medicaid coverage and reimbursement rates are inadequate compared to private dental insurance as a result of state budget limitations, and there is a substantial decline in the number of dentists for the general population, especially in urban and rural areas.[12] Public health programs must work closely with Medicaid to increase dental coverage and to broaden the scope of services provided by each state.

Two major government-produced documents have provided blueprints for improving oral health in the United States. They are known as Healthy People 2010 and the Surgeon General's Report on Oral Health in America (2000).[1,14] Healthy People 2010 identifies seventeen objectives (with specific quantitative targets) to help achieve their stated goal of preventing and controlling oral and craniofacial diseases, conditions, and injuries as well as improving access to related services. Some of these objectives include:

The Surgeon General's Report on Oral Health in America (2000) recommends the development of a National Oral Health Plan with the following principal objectives:

- Change perceptions regarding oral health and disease so that oral health becomes an accepted component of general health.
- Accelerate the building of the science and evidence base and apply science effectively to improve oral health.
- Build an effective health infrastructure that meets the oral health needs of all Americans and integrates oral health effectively into overall health.
- Remove known barriers between people and oral health services.
- Use public-private partnerships to improve the oral health of those who still suffer disproportionately from oral diseases.[1]

While the Healthy People 2010 document delineates more specific and quantifiable objectives than the Surgeon General's Report and focuses more on the oral health of children and underserved groups, both represent attempts at major comprehensive public health initiatives. It remains to be seen how quickly the objectives identified in these reports can be achieved.

Throughout the history of oral health, great accomplishments have been made to reduce oral diseases among the general population. For example, the fluoridation of drinking water remarkably decreased the incidence of tooth decays. According to the most recent statement issued by Surgeon General Richard Carmona in 2004 on community water fluoridation, a $1 investment in fluoridation saves roughly $38 in costs of treatment.[15] Still, much more can be done to further decrease oral health issues, especially among low-income individuals. Education on the prevention of oral diseases in schools and community centers would serve as a great asset in combating these diseases or preventing them from occurring. Raising awareness on oral health issues will only help the fight and not hurt it. Take the initiative, go out, and make a difference by intervening in the field of oral public health!

Healthy People 2010

Indicator:

Focus Area: Oral Health

Goal: Prevent and control oral and craniofacial diseases, conditions, and injuries, and improve access to related services.

Objectives:

21-1. Reduce the proportion of children and adolescents who have dental caries in their primary or permanent teeth.

21-2. Reduce the proportion of children, adolescents, and adults with untreated dental decay.

21-5. Reduce periodontal disease.

21-7. Increase the proportion of adults who, in the past 12 months, report having had an examination to detect oral and pharyngeal cancers.

21-8. Increase the proportion of children who have received dental sealants on their molar teeth.

21-9. Increase the proportion of the U.S. population served by community water systems with optimally fluoridated water.

21-10. Increase the proportion of children and adults who use the oral health-care system each year.

21-12. Increase the proportion of low-income children and adolescents who received any preventive dental service during the past year.

21-13. Increase the proportion of school-based health centers with an oral health component.

21-17. Increase the number of Tribal, State (including the District of Columbia), and local health agencies that serve jurisdictions of 250,000 or more persons that have in place an effective public dental health program directed by a dental professional with a public health training.[14]

KEY TERMS

Biology/Clinical Terms

Dental Caries: Destruction of the tooth by a formation of plaque in the oral cavity.

Dental Plaque: Oral flora that adheres to the surface of teeth and initiates the breakdown of the tooth enamel.

Fluoroapatite: Structural element of teeth composed of mineralized calcium, phosphate, and fluoride ions, causing tooth surface to become harder and less prone to decay.

Gingivitis: The first stage of gum disease characterized by inflammation and infection of the oral soft tissue (gums).

Hydroxyapatite: Structural element of teeth composed mainly of mineralized calcium and phosphate ions.

Periodontitis: A more severe form of gum disease characterized by the breakdown of alveolar bone and connective tissue surrounding and supporting the teeth.

Streptococcus mutans: Highly cariogenic microorganism involved in the breakdown of teeth, causing dental caries.

Public Health Terms

Cofactors: Factors that influence the effect of other conditions.

Medicaid: A state-run health insurance program intended for low-income individuals.

Oral Health: Freedom from diseases and disorders that affect the craniofacial complex.

Protective Factors: Certain conditions that increase the health and well-being of an individual and decrease the likelihood of developing a disease or condition.

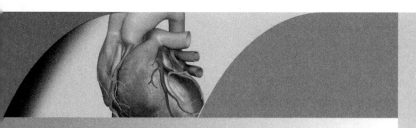

Questions for Further Research, Study, Reflection, and Discussion

For the Individual Student

In order to answer these questions, it may be necessary to research the primary literature.

- What are the causes of dental caries? What are the causes of periodontal disease? What behaviors put people at risk for these diseases?
- Why does fluoridating public water supplies improve oral health? What is considered the optimal amount of fluoride in water? What is the result if there is too much fluoride in drinking water?

For Small Group Discussion

- Why has oral health historically been considered separate from overall health? What are the implications of this distinction? Has it impacted the development of the field or access to oral health care?
- The oral health benefits of community water fluoridation have been well documented for more than 60 years. Yet, there is still some opposition to this practice because it can be viewed as government sponsored, forced medication. From a public health perspective, what are the best ways to overcome such opposition?
- Consider the first case study mentioned above (concerning the untimely death of Deamonte Driver). What steps could have been taken to prevent this boy's death? What interventions would you recommend to prevent similar deaths from occurring in the future?
- Consider the second case study mentioned above (Latisha G.). How does oral health, or lack of it, contribute to psychological and mental health or an overall sense of well-being?

For Entire Class Discussion

- Consider the oral health objectives outlined by Healthy People 2010 and the recommendations in The Surgeon General's Report on Oral Health in America listed above. Are these objectives and recommendations desirable? Practical? Realistic? If so, what would be the best way to implement them and what would be the major obstacles to their implementation? Which demand should be implemented most urgently? Why have they not yet been implemented?

EXERCISES/ACTIVITIES

Promotion: How to Brush Your Teeth

- The use of education to teach individuals proper oral hygiene has tremendously helped in the decline of dental caries, especially among children who are most susceptible to tooth decay. Obtain permission to attend a preschool class and come up with a presentation demonstrating correct brushing techniques. Get acquainted with the proper techniques of brushing teeth by researching correct methods from a reliable source. Include statistics, toothbrushes, and model teeth to help illustrate the process of tooth brushing.

Exposing Plaque: Using an Egg to Demonstrate Plaque Growth

- Constantly forming in your teeth, plaque plays a major role in tooth decay by adhering to the surface of teeth to initiate the dissolution of tooth substance. Try this activity at home to expose stains on an egg similar to plaque formation in your teeth. You will need the following items:

  - One hard-boiled egg
  - Carbonated soda with high sugar content
  - Toothbrush
  - Toothpaste containing fluoride

Directions: Submerge the hard-boiled egg into a cup of carbonated soda (keep it submerged for one day). Next, take the stained egg out and observe the stain formed on its surface, similar to plaque formation in teeth. Brush the stain off with a toothbrush and toothpaste and observe the fluoridated toothpaste's effects in removing stains. Write a 250-word response on its effects, and discuss the importance of flossing and mouthwash

rinsing and their role in removing extra plaque that a toothbrush cannot reach.

REFERENCES

1. U.S. Department of Health and Human Services. *Oral Health in America: A Report of the Surgeon General.* Rockville, MD: U.S. Department of Health and Human Services, National Institute of Dental and Craniofacial Research, National Institutes of Health; 2000: iii, 285–286.

2. Allukian M. The neglected epidemic and the Surgeon General's Report: a call to action for better oral health (editorial). *Am J Public Health* 2000;90:843–845.

3. *Milestones in Public Health: Accomplishments in Public Health over the Last 100 Years.* New York: Pfizer Global Pharmaceuticals, Pfizer Inc. 2006: 169, 171, 176, 178–179, 181, 184–185.

4. American Dental Association. *About the ADA.* Chicago: ADA. Available at http://www.ada.org/ada/about/index.asp. Accessed April 4, 2008.

5. American Dental Association. *History of Dentistry.* Available at http://www.ada.org/public/resources/history/index.asp. Accessed April 4, 2008.

6. Allukian M. The neglected American epidemic. *The Nation's Health.* May-June 1990:2.

7. Allukian M. Oral diseases: the neglected epidemic. In: Scutchfield FD, Keck CW, eds. *Principles of Public Health Practice,* Albany, NY: Delmar Publishers Inc; 1996:261–279.

8. *The Oral Health of California's Children: A Neglected Epidemic.* San Rafael, CA: Dental Health Foundation; 1997.

9. Gotsch AR. The neglected epidemic. *The Nation's Health.* September 1999:2.

10. World Health Organization. *The World Oral Health Report 2003: Continuous improvement of oral health in the 21st century—The approach of the WHO Global Oral Health Programme.* Geneva, Switzerland: WHO. Available at http://www.who.int/oral_health/media/en/orh_report03_en.pdf. Accessed April 4, 2008.

11. Otto M. "For Want of a Dentist: Pr. George's Boy Dies After Bacteria From Tooth Spread to Brain." *Washington Post* February 28, 2007: p. B01.

12. U.S. Department of Health and Human Services, Human Resources and Services Administration. *Opportunities to Use Medicaid in Support of Access to Health Care Services.* Washington, DC: DHHS. Available at http://www.hrsa.gov/medicaidprimer/oral_part3only.htm. Accessed April 4, 2008.

13. Newachek P, Hughes DC, Hung YY, Wong S, Stoddard JJ. The unmet health needs of America's children. *Pediatrics* 2000;105:989–997.

14. Centers for Disease Control and Prevention, Health Resources and Research Administration, Indian Health Services, National Institutes of Health. Healthy People 2010. *Chapter 21: Oral Health.* Available at: http://www.healthypeople.gov/Document/HTML/Volume2/21Oral.htm. Accessed April 4, 2008.

15. Department of Human and Health Services, Centers for Disease Control and Prevention. *Surgeon General's Statement on Community Water Fluoridation, 2004.* Available at http://www.cdc.gov/fluoridation/fact_sheets/sg04.htm. Accessed April 4, 2008.

RESOURCE

Medline Plus. *Gum Disease.* Available at http://www.nlm.nih.gov/medlineplus/gumdisease.html. Accessed April 4, 2008.

CROSS REFERENCE

Inflammation

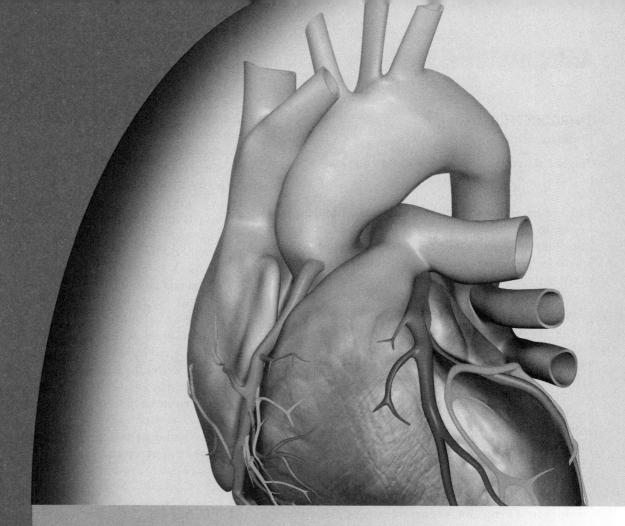

PART III

Concepts of Pathophysiology

Constance Battle

INTRODUCTION

Constance Battle

Happy is the person who is able to discern the cause of things.

—Virgil (37 BC)

Part 3 addresses some of the basic concepts of pathophysiology, the study of the biological and physical manifestations of disease that result from underlying abnormalities and physiological derangements. These five chapters describe mechanisms of self-defense and of cellular proliferation.

An area of intense research today, the inflammation response can be regarded as an immediate, transitory life-saver, or as the cause of chronic disease states such as atherosclerosis or diabetes (Chapters 16 and 17). Perhaps the inflammatory process, necessary as an evolutionary adaptation for survival, is no longer necessary and results in chronic diseases.

The immune response, the body's ability to respond in a specific manner to a specific organism and to recognize it with memory on the next encounter, albeit in a more desultory fashion, is the second line of defense. *Both* these lines of defense are necessary for *both* immediate and long-term protection against diseases.

Protecting against disease by inducing the self-defense mechanism of immunity, vaccines are extremely effective and are safe. Arguably, immunization is the major achievement of public health in the 20th century and one of the most cost-effective of all health investments.

Chapter 18 on scientific integrative medicine presents a framework, a way of thinking (like other chapters in Part I) that applies systems concepts in order to understand acute and chronic complex diseases and builds on systems biology, yet differs in several important ways.

Chapter 19 describes cancer and cancer development from the perspective of what is known about its biology. Colon cancer in Chapter 20 illustrates aspects of cancer development and its relationship to family history and to inflammation. Both Chapters 19 and 20 emphasize what scientists understand: most cancer is not born but made.[1]

Chapters 16 through 20 attempt to explore mechanisms with the aim of explaining the occurrence of disease for therapeutic as well as theoretical purposes. Thagard says our confidence that a factor really is a major cause of a disease is greatly increased if we can describe in detail the biochemical process by which the cause produces the disease and its symptoms.[2] Thus he reiterates the importance of studying biochemistry first presented by Elliot in Part 1.

Elaborating on the mechanism of disease is the final step in really understanding disease causation. Over the past centuries the multistep process of *disease understanding* has required as many as several hundred years or as few as three to five. The evolution of our understanding of human diseases is an important foundation throughout this book.

REFERENCES

1. Davis D. Off tangent in the war on cancer. *The Washington Post* 2007; November 4: pp. B1, B4.
2. Thagard P. *How Scientists Explain Disease*. Princeton: Princeton University Press; 1999: 132.

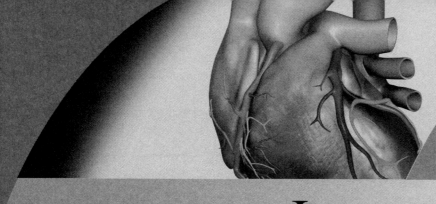

CHAPTER 16

Immunizations and Immunity

Carol A. Smith

An estimated 2.1 million people around the world died in 2002 of diseases preventable by widely used vaccines.[1] With an investment of 3 billion USD a year, every child in the developing world could receive complete immunization coverage.[2]

LEARNING OBJECTIVES

By the end of this chapter, the student will be able to:

- Differentiate the two systems of immunity.
- Identify elements of the innate immune system.
- Compare and contrast humoral and cell-mediated immunity.
- Explain B cell immunity as it relates to first antigenic exposure and subsequent exposure.
- Differentiate active and passive immunity giving examples of each.
- Explain how a vaccine works to achieve resistance to an infectious organism.
- List five types of vaccines giving examples of each.
- Define the term toxoid.
- List the currently recommended childhood and adult immunizations in the United States.
- Define the term herd immunity and explain how it provides protection for the nonimmunized person.

HISTORY

Immunization is believed by many to be one of the most successful applications of immunologic principles. **Immunization**, or **vaccination**, is a procedure in which an infectious disease is prevented by prior exposure to a microorganism adminis-

tered in a form that will not cause illness. The first widespread use of vaccination occurred during the late 18th century against smallpox, an infectious disease that was widespread in Europe. In 1796, Edward Jenner, an English physician, observed that individuals who had been infected by cowpox appeared to be resistant to smallpox, a similar disease in humans. Jenner injected fluid from a pustule of a young dairymaid infected with cowpox into the eight-year-old son of his gardener. Six weeks later, he injected the young boy with fluid from a smallpox pustule. As Jenner anticipated, the boy did not develop smallpox. Jenner repeated his experiment with others during the following years and published his findings. Unknown to Jenner, he had discovered a fundamental principle of immunization. By using a relatively harmless foreign agent, he had invoked an immune response that protected someone from an infectious disease.

Although immunization against smallpox spread rapidly, vaccination against other agents did not occur until the latter part of the 19th century when Louis Pasteur accidentally discovered a means for protecting against cholera. Pasteur had grown the organism that caused fowl cholera in culture. After returning from a summer vacation, he injected some chickens with an old culture of the organism and to his surprise, the chickens became ill with cholera but recovered. To save resources, he injected these recovered chickens with a fresh culture of the organism. The chickens that had been previously exposed to the organism did not develop cholera; however, chickens that had not previously been exposed did develop the disease. Pasteur hypothesized that the aging of the bacterial culture had altered the virulence of the organism, rendering it incapable of causing disease. In recognition of Jenner's earlier work, he named the aged culture a **vaccine**, which was derived from the Latin word *vaccinus* meaning "pertaining to cows." Pasteur subsequently experimented with other infectious organisms and developed more vaccines including one for rabies. Although Jenner and Pasteur showed that immunization was effective in preventing disease, they did not understand how this was done. It was not until elucidation of the mechanisms of immunity in the 20th century that the how became known.

BASIC SCIENCE FACTS/KEY CONCEPTS REVIEW

Mechanisms of Immunity

The human body has a variety of mechanisms that provide protection against infectious agents. This is accomplished by complex processes that require detection of changes in an individual's cells or the presence of infectious organisms. There are two systems of **immunity** that work together to provide protection:

- innate immune system
- adaptive immune system

The innate system that is present from birth provides the first line of defense against infectious agents. The response of the innate system is nonspecific in that it does not differentiate between different challenges. It reacts in the same manner no matter the organism. A wide range of anatomical and physiological barriers create an environment inhospitable to invading organisms (Table 16-1). The physiological processes of inflammation and phagocytosis facilitate movement of cells to infected sites where engulfment and clearance of microorganisms can occur (Figure 16-1).

When the innate immune response is insufficient to protect the individual from the invading organisms, the second form of immunity—**adaptive immunity**—is stimulated to respond to the challenge. Adaptive immunity, also known as *acquired* or *specific immunity*, involves the activation of immune cells and development of substances that will aid in the elimination of the organisms and facilitate the development

---

TABLE 16-1 Host Defenses of the Immune System

Innate Immunity

Anatomical barriers
   Skin and mucosal membranes: provide mechanical barriers preventing entry of organisms

Physiological barriers
   Acid environment of stomach: kills ingested organisms
   Chemical mediators: lysozymes and other enzymes in secretions destroy organisms

Phagocytic cells
   Neutrophils and macrophages with the aid of complement engulf and destroy ingested organisms

Inflammatory processes
   Produce antibacterial activity and stimulate phagocytosis

Natural killer cells
   Possess cytotoxic activity against tumor cells and some virus-infected cells

Adaptive Immunity

Humoral
   B lymphocytes: production of antibodies and memory cells

Cell-mediated
   T lymphocytes: cell-to-cell contacts, secretion of soluble products and memory cells

---

FIGURE 16-1 Phagocytosis.

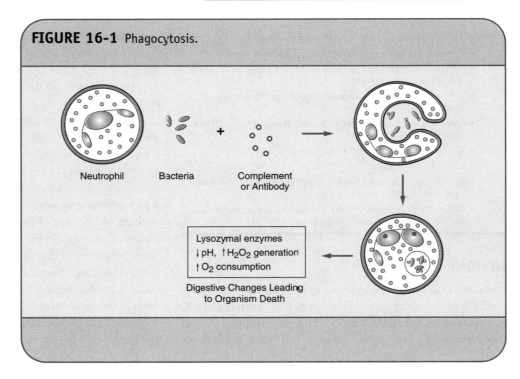

Neutrophil   Bacteria   Complement or Antibody

Lysozymal enzymes
↓pH, ↑H_2O_2 generation
↑O_2 consumption

Digestive Changes Leading to Organism Death

of immunological memory. It is this immunological memory that is crucial to the success of a vaccine.

Unlike **innate immunity**, adaptive immunity demonstrates specificity for the foreign agent. Microorganisms possess surface molecules capable of stimulating an immune response. These molecules are known as **antigens**. Interactions between antigens and the cells of the adaptive system help clear the organism from the body.

Two Types of Immunity: Humoral and Cell Mediated

There are two major types of adaptive responses: humoral and cell-mediated (cellular) immunity. Each type involves different cells and molecules that help rid the body of extracellular and intracellular organisms. Although humoral and cell-mediated immunity are often discussed as separate entities, there is a great deal of cooperation between the two. The major cells involved in the adaptive response are T and B lymphocytes. **Cell-mediated immunity** primarily involves T lymphocytes (T cells), which are derived from the bone marrow but undergo differentiation in the thymus. T lymphocytes develop into cells with specific functions (Figure 16-2). T lymphocytes are important in eliminating intracellular organisms such as viruses and certain types of bacteria. T cells also play an important role in presenting protein antigens to B cells in a form that the B cell can recognize. Activation of T cells leads to secretion of

substances known as *cytokines*, soluble proteins that mediate the functions of the cells that secrete them and of other cells. Some cytokines play amplification roles while others are involved in regulation and communication of cells within the immune system.

Humoral immunity is a function of B lymphocytes (B cells) and is the primary defense against extracellular organisms. When B cells encounter an organism, they recognize parts of the antigens on the surface called antigenic determinants or **epitopes**. These are smaller portions of the antigen that the cells recognize as foreign. Binding of the antigen to the B lymphocyte triggers the cell to transform into an antibody-producing cell known as a *plasma cell*. Plasma cells manufacture antibodies that are specific for the antigen that induced their production. **Antibodies**, which are proteins of the immunoglobulin class, are secreted by the plasma cell into plasma and function to help eliminate the foreign organisms. The five classes of antibodies produced by plasma cells are: IgM, IgG, IgA, IgD, and IgE. Each plays a role in supporting the immune system's functions, but their chief functions are to:

- neutralize bacterial toxins
- neutralize viruses
- attach to bacteria promoting phagocytosis
- activate components involved in the inflammatory response

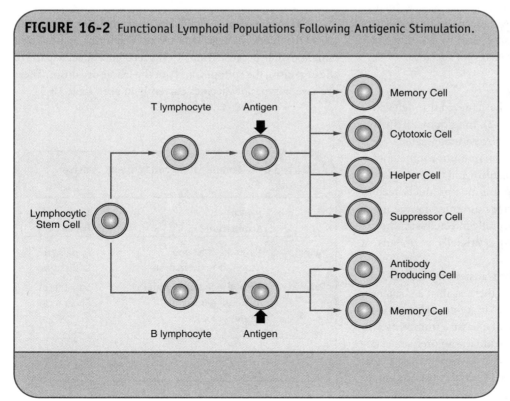

FIGURE 16-2 Functional Lymphoid Populations Following Antigenic Stimulation.

T lymphocyte   Antigen
Memory Cell
Cytotoxic Cell
Helper Cell
Suppressor Cell
Lymphocytic Stem Cell
Antibody Producing Cell
Memory Cell
B lymphocyte   Antigen

Antibodies at Work

When the body encounters a particular antigen for the first time, a primary immune response is initiated (Figure 16-3). The adaptive immune system becomes activated and antibody production occurs. A few days to a week after exposure to the antigen, IgM antibody that is specific for the antigen that stimulated its formation begins to appear in the blood. A short time later, IgG specific for the antigen appears. The antibody titer then rises in the blood, reflecting the antibody production. Levels will plateau and eventually decline over time as the antibody is used up in helping to clear the invading organisms. Any excess antibody will be broken down into simpler molecules (catabolized). If the immune system

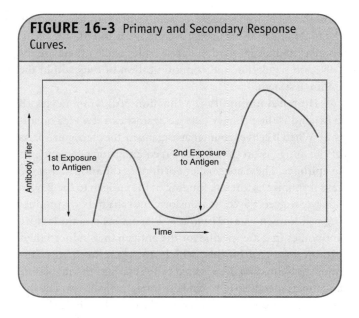

FIGURE 16-3 Primary and Secondary Response Curves.

encounters the same organism again in the future, memory cells that were formed during the first encounter will "remember" the organism and the response of the immune system will be much quicker than during the first encounter (Figure 16-3). Antibodies will be made much faster and in greater amounts so they will be readily available to assist in clearing the organism quickly. Should an individual be exposed to the antigen a third time, the antibody response will be further amplified because of previously having seen the antigen. These memory responses as well as the specificity of the antibodies produced are crucial to the effectiveness of vaccines.

Active and Passive Immunity

Immunity to microorganisms can be achieved through active or passive immunization (Table 16-2). In both cases, the immunity can be acquired or attained by natural means.

Active immunity occurs when an immunocompetent individual is exposed to a foreign organism and the person's immune cells respond by producing immune products such as antibodies and memory cells. Active immunity may be naturally developed if the person is naturally infected with the organism. It also may be acquired artificially by means of vaccination.

Passive immunity involves the transfer of preformed antibodies to an individual to protect them against a challenge. The transfer of maternal antibodies to a fetus in utero is an example of natural passive immunity. Passive immunity also can be achieved by injecting an individual with preformed antibodies to an organism. This is used primarily when someone who was not previously immunized becomes exposed to an

organism for which an immunoglobulin product is available. An example of this is the use of hepatitis B immunoglobin for someone who may have been exposed to the disease.

Development of active immunity to an organism generally provides long-term protection against future exposure to the organism. Because the individual's immune system is activated, memory cells are formed. Re-exposure to the organism will result in a rapid response of the immune system to clear the organism before illness can develop. Passive immunity provides short-term protection. Memory cells are not formed and when the antibodies have been consumed or catabolized, there will be no remaining protection against future exposure.

Vaccines

Vaccines attempt to stimulate the immune system by mimicking a natural infection. The success of a vaccine depends on two key elements: immunological memory and specificity. These elements allow the immune system to mount a much stronger response on a second encounter with the organism.

The aim in vaccine development is to alter the organism in such a way that it does not cause disease but maintains its immunogenicity. The goal is to stimulate memory T and B cells in an individual to:

- induce specific immunity
- eliminate organisms that enter the host
- neutralize bacterial toxins

A vaccine contains a killed or weakened form or derivative of the infectious organism. Use of such forms of the organism is possible because B and T cells recognize specific parts of the organism, the epitopes, and not the whole organism. There are several types of vaccines currently in use (Table 16-3).

TABLE 16-2 Comparison of Active and Passive Immunity

	Type of Acquisition	Length of Protection
Active	Natural—infection	Long term
	Acquired—vaccination	Long term
Passive	Natural—transfer in utero	Short term
	Acquired—injection of immunoglobulin	Short term

TABLE 16-3 Types of Vaccines

Vaccine Type	Examples of Vaccines
Live, attenuated vaccine	Measles, mumps, rubella, polio (Sabin) vaccine, varicella
Inactivated (killed) vaccine	Cholera, rabies, influenza, hepatitis A, polio (Salk) vaccine
Toxoid vaccine	Tetanus, diphtheria
Subunit vaccine	Hepatitis B, pertussis, pneumococcus (*Streptococcus pneumoniae*)
Conjugate vaccine	*Haemophilus influenzae* type B, pneumococcus (*Streptococcus pneumoniae*)

Live, attenuated vaccines contain a weakened form of the microorganism. This weakening process, known as **attenuation**, occurs in the laboratory by growing the organism under abnormal culture conditions. The resultant vaccine retains similar characteristics to the original organism but lacks its pathogenicity. Because a live attenuated vaccine contains an altered organism similar to the causative organism, it is the closest thing to an actual infection and tends to produce strong cellular and humoral responses resulting in long-term protection after just a few doses. Two disadvantages to using attenuated vaccines are the remote chance that the organism could mutate back to a virulent form and the need for refrigeration of the vaccine.

Inactivated or killed vaccines are created by treating the microorganism with chemicals or heat. These types of vaccines are usually more stable and safer than live vaccines but tend to stimulate a weaker response. They do not require refrigeration and can often be shipped in freeze-dried form, which is an advantage in developing countries.

Some bacteria produce toxins that cause illness in an individual. These toxins can be made harmless by treating them with **toxoid** vaccines, created by treating bacterial toxins with formaldehyde. This treatment renders the toxin harmless but maintains its immunogenicity. Thus, the resultant toxoid can stimulate a strong antibody response that will help eliminate the harmful toxin.

Subunit vaccines are composed of selected epitopes from the organism rather than the entire antigen. This contributes to the specificity of the immune response that is mounted by T cells and antibodies. Because the vaccine is composed of only certain parts of the antigens, the chances of adverse reactions to the vaccine are lessened. The difficulty in creating subunit vaccines is identifying the epitopes from the organism that will best stimulate an immune response. Subunit vaccines and toxoids often contain **adjuvants**. Vaccine adjuvants, usually aluminum salts, increase the length of stay of the antigen in the body so that the immune system has more time to respond to the antigen.

Conjugate vaccines attempt to strengthen the immunogenicity of some organisms with polysaccharide capsules. Polysaccharide antigens associated with these organisms may be difficult for the immature immune system of infants and younger children to recognize. Conjugate vaccines couple these antigens to a protein carrier. The antigen-protein complex becomes more readily recognizable by the immune system so that a strong response is made.

Mechanisms of protection stimulated by vaccines can be affected by many factors including nutritional status, underlying diseases, and age. Immunization never confers absolute protection, so there will always be individuals who will not respond (poor responders). The size of the poor responder group will vary with the individual vaccine and the number of booster shots given.

Future Vaccines

Several other types of vaccines are in experimental stages. DNA vaccines use the organism's own genetic material. When an organism's genes are introduced into the host, the DNA becomes incorporated in the host's cells where it can instruct the cells to make antigens that are secreted and displayed on the cells. The displayed antigens can then stimulate the host's immune system. Somewhat similar to DNA vaccines are recombinant vector vaccines. These experimental vaccines use an attenuated virus or bacterium to introduce the microbe's DNA into the host's cells. These newer techniques are being tested for diverse diseases such as influenza, malaria, rabies, and measles.

One of the biggest hurdles faced by vaccine researchers is the ever changing nature of many microorganisms. The organism responsible for human immunodeficiency virus (HIV) infection is a classic example of this problem. HIV often mutates, creating new forms of the virus and making it much more difficult to develop a single vaccine that is effective against all forms of the virus. Development of an effective malarial vaccine also has suffered from the fact that the malarial parasite is genetically complex and presents thousands of antigens. Determining which of these many antigens would be most effective in stimulating an immune response complicates the development of a vaccine. Despite these problems,

CASE STUDY
Scenario

Maria Gonzalez, a native of Washington, D.C., is a 21-year-old pre-med student at George Washington University. She has decided to take a year off before her senior year at college to travel to South Africa and work as a relief worker in the war-torn country of Darfur, to gain insight to the effects of war on the health and well-being of villagers. During her year-long visit, she will be assisting local clinicians in providing health services, including assisting in the immunization clinics provided in local villages, performing basic health assessments, and assisting the local hospitals run by visiting physicians treating those injured in the war. In addition, she will teach hygiene and first aid classes to local schoolchildren in the villages.

In planning for her trip, Maria scheduled a check-up with her primary care physician to discuss possible health risks and preventive strategies necessary when traveling to foreign countries. During her visit, Maria's physician reviewed her immunization records, which had been accurately maintained since she was born. At the end of the visit, her physician informed her that because of the proposed overseas travel and healthcare work, she should receive vaccinations for hepatitis A and hepatitis B prior to her travel date. Her physician also recommended that as a precaution while she was abroad, Maria should wear bug spray and refrain from drinking untreated water and eating uncooked vegetables.

According to her immunization records, Maria has never received these vaccinations herself, but she recalled that her newborn niece, Lucy, age 2 months old, was given hepatitis B vaccinations as part of her routine childhood vaccination program at her local health center. She also knew that her three-year-old nephew, Luis, received both the hepatitis A and B series as part of his routine childhood immunization.

Maria asked her physician why hepatitis A and B vaccinations are recommended for overseas travel and why it is standard protocol for healthcare workers to be vaccinated against these viruses. She also wondered why both her niece and nephew have received these immunizations as part of their childhood immunization program. She is interested in learning who and why others receive these immunizations.

Defining the Issues

Maria is a healthy young women and therefore receiving immunizations does not place her at risk as it might for an immunocompromised patient. As a healthy person, she must still take precautions for international travel.

Many diseases that have been eradicated from the developed world still plague other parts of the globe, so travelers that may be exposed to diseases uncommon in the United States should pay particularly close attention to recommended international immunization guidelines. Maria was wise to consult a primary physician to inquire about what shots she may need. She should also check other sources such as the U.S. Department of State's Web page to discover for herself which shots she should receive (http://travel.state.gov/travel/tips/tips_1232.html; accessed April 7, 2008).

Immunization guidelines are dynamic, changing in accordance with the latest scientific knowledge as well as shifting patterns of disease. The most common types of changes are relatively minor and involve administering the same vaccines but at different intervals or ages. Very rarely, an immunization prescribed during earlier periods may be phased out entirely, as was the case with smallpox. Also, new immunizations may be introduced. Changing guidelines can make it difficult for physicians and their patients to stay educated about which immunizations they should receive. Maria was confused because her niece and nephew both received hepatitis vaccines as a part of their regular schedule of immunizations, yet she had not.

Patient's Understanding

As a pre-medical student, Maria most likely understands why she may need certain vaccinations but not others. She also knows her own clinical history and is aware of which vaccinations she has received, which helps the physician confidently prescribe needed immunizations without unnecessarily administering redundant treatments.

CLINICAL PERSPECTIVE FOR THE INDIVIDUAL PATIENT

Immunizations are arguably the single most cost-effective intervention available. The cost of immunizing a patient against a disease is negligible compared to the potential cost of treatment, medicine, and hospitalization as well the personal and emotional cost should they become infected. In the case of Maria, by counseling her to get immunized for hepatitis A and B, the physician could be saving her from an even larger health burden down the road. Because the disease protection conferred by some types of vaccines may weaken after several years, physicians also should make sure that their patients are aware of the importance of keeping their immunizations up to date. Although the vaccines for hepatitis A and B will provide protection for over 20 years, if Maria were to travel abroad 30 years down the line, she would need to be vaccinated again. Physicians should help their patients stay current by encouraging them to take the initiative to research immunization guidelines and schedules.

many researchers believe it is only a matter of time before these challenges are conquered.

PUBLIC HEALTH PERSEPCTIVE FOR THE HEALTH OF THE GENERAL POPULATION AND OF HIGH RISK GROUPS

Immunization of Selected Groups

Immunization has proven to be a cost-effective means of preventing infectious diseases. Successful immunization programs have been responsible for the eradication of smallpox worldwide. The last reported case of a naturally acquired smallpox infection occurred in 1977. The success of this program led the World Health Organization (WHO) to call for a cessation of vaccination for smallpox in 1979 in all countries. Immunization programs against polio also have been successful. Although childhood vaccination for polio is currently recommended, many believe that polio will be eradicated in the near future.

Immunizations play a central role in the U.S. Department of Health and Human Service's Healthy People 2010 framework.[3] In the project, immunization has been designated one of the ten leading health indicators, which is reflected by the fact that out of the 467 specific objectives included, 23 of them concern improving and expanding immunization coverage. All 23 objectives are listed at the end of this chapter.

Exhibit 16-1

Vaccine-Preventable Diseases

The number of reported cases of vaccine-preventable diseases has generally decreased over the past several decades. In 2004, there were no reported cases of diphtheria, rubella, or polio in the entire U.S. population and no cases of tetanus among children under five years of age.

From 2003 to 2004, the number of reported cases of *H. influenzae* and hepatitis B decreased among children under five years of age. Rates of hepatitis B infection have steadily declined with the implementation of a national strategy to eliminate the disease. This strategy includes routine screening of pregnant women for the hepatitis B virus and routine vaccination of infants and children. It is important to note that because most hepatitis B infections among infants and young children are asymptomatic, the reported number of cases likely underestimates the **incidence** in these age groups.

While the number of reported cases of several vaccine-preventable diseases decreased from 2003 to 2004, the number of reported cases of measles, mumps, hepatitis A, and pertussis increased over the same period. In 2004, the incidence of reported pertussis among the entire U.S. population increased for the third year in a row, and the number of cases was the highest reported since 1959. Of cases for which age was reported, 10 percent occurred among children under six months of age who were too young to have received the full schedule of acellular pertussis vaccine. The highest reported rate of the disease (136.5 per 100,000) occurred among this age group. With regard to hepatitis A, although the number of cases among children under five years increased from 2003 to 2004, the overall incidence of the disease has dropped dramatically since routine vaccination for children living in high-risk areas was recommended starting in 1996.

Source: Health Resources and Services Administration. Child Health USA 2006. Available at http://www.mchb.hrsa.gov/chusa_06/. Accessed April 7, 2008.

Childhood immunization programs have played an important role in reducing infection and deaths among children. In the United States, childhood immunizations are recommended starting at birth. The Centers for Disease Control and Prevention (CDC) publishes recommended immunization schedules on their Web site. These schedules are approved yearly by the CDC, the American Academy of Pediatrics, and the American Academy of Family Physicians. Figure 16-4 shows the schedule for children from birth to six years of age. Similar charts exist for other age groupings, and charts are available in Spanish.

Vaccination too early following birth may be ineffective for some vaccines due to protective effects of passively transferred maternal antibodies. Efficacy depends on the vaccine and whether booster doses are administered. Most of these vaccines require multiple doses over a period of time. The heightened immune response that occurs with each exposure to the vaccine contributes to the development of effective immunity.

Recommendations for adult immunizations are dependent on the risk group. Recommendations for older adults, those with underlying medical conditions, and those whose immune systems may be compromised include yearly influenza vaccine and immunization with pneumococcal vaccine.

Other vaccines may be recommended for travelers and those exposed to certain microorganisms through their work environment. The threat of bioterrorism has concerned many in recent years. Governmental and military agencies have ongoing research and development programs for vaccines against biological threats. Anthrax and smallpox vaccines are currently licensed but only recommended for select groups such as military personnel, individuals working in research labs with these

FIGURE 16-4 Recommended Immunization Schedule for Persons Aged 0 to 6 Years.

Recommended Immunization Schedule for Persons Aged 0–6 Years – United States · 2007

Vaccine ▼ Age ►	Birth	1 month	2 months	4 months	6 months	12 months	15 months	18 months	19–23 months	2–3 years	4–6 years
Hepatitis B[1]	HepB	HepB				HepB				HepB Series	
Rotavirus[2]			Rota	Rota	Rota						
Diphtheria, Tetanus, Pertussis[2]			DTaP	DTaP	DTaP		DTaP				DTaP
Haemophilus?influenzae type b[4]			Hib	Hib	Hib[4]	Hib		Hib			
Pneumococcal[5]			PCV	PCV	PCV	PCV				PCV PPV	
Inactivated Poliovirus			IPV	IPV		IPV					IPV
Influenza[6]						Influenza (Yearly)					
Measles, Mumps, Rubella[7]						MMR					MMR
Varicella[8]						Varicella					Varicella
Hepatitis A[9]						HepA (2 doses)				HepA Series	
Meningococcal[10]										MPSV4	

- Range of recommended ages
- Catch-up immunization
- Certain high-risk groups

Source: Department of Health and Human Services. Centers for Disease Control and Prevention National Immunization Program. Available at: http://www.cdc.gov/nip/recs/child-schedule.htm. Accessed April 8, 2008.

agents, and first-responders. The vaccines are not available to the general public.

Vaccination is not always effective. A small group of individuals will respond poorly or not at all. Generally, these poor responders are not of concern when looking at the effectiveness of an immunization program. If most of the individuals who have been exposed to an infectious organism through vaccination have responded adequately, the chances of a poor responder encountering an infected person is small. Herd (community) immunity is the term often used to describe the immunity to an infectious organism developed by the large group of vaccinated individuals; the goal of **herd immunity** is to stop the transmission of the infectious disease. Impediments to the achievement of herd immunity include concerns regarding adverse side effects and costs, especially costs of newer vaccines.

Barriers to Achieving Widespread Coverage

In the Developed World

Expanding immunization coverage faces distinct barriers in the developed and developing world. In developed nations, immunizations are widely available but access issues still occur among marginalized populations. Education materials may not exist for non-English speaking populations, and immigrants are especially vulnerable to a lack of access to primary care. In general, new parents are very cautious about a newborn's health, so vaccine coverage for infants is not a large problem. However, as children age, they are less likely to come in for follow-up boosters and other immunizations.

Parents' fears and misunderstandings about immunizations also may prevent them from having their children vaccinated. Many people believe that a "bad batch" of a vaccine can actually cause the disease it is designed to prevent. Although certain vaccines are made from attenuated viruses that can mutate into a virulent form, none of the immunizations prescribed in the United States carries this risk. Patients may underestimate their risk for contracting a disease, which can prevent them from seeking immunizations.

In Developing Countries

Although many developing countries have achieved impressive child immunization rates, some other countries fail to meet their vaccination goals. Although providing vaccine coverage costs relatively little, logistical issues can present a significant hurdle. Several types of vaccines must be refrigerated at all times, a feat that is difficult to accomplish in areas without electricity. In countries with large rural populations, poor infrastructure and a lack of roads pose problems to developing consistent supply chains. Many developing countries also suffer from a huge shortage of health care workers, which serves as a bottleneck to expanding vaccine coverage.

KEY TERMS

Biology Terms

Adaptive Immunity: An immune response developed following exposure to a foreign agent that results in antigen recognition by T and B lymphocytes with subsequent development of specificity and memory.

Active Immunity: Adaptive immunity developed after exposure to an infection with a microorganism or following vaccination.

Adjuvant: A substance that enhances an immune response by prolonging exposure to the antigen within the body.

Antibody: A protein made in response to exposure to a foreign antigen that can bind to the antigen to facilitate elimination of the antigen.

Antigen: A foreign agent that can stimulate an immune response and bind to antibodies and T cells.

Attenuation: A process in which a pathogen is altered so it is less virulent.

Cell-Mediated Immunity: Immunity mediated by antigen-specific T lymphocytes and other cells that are involved in protecting against challenges such as intracellular organisms, viruses, and tumor cells.

Epitope: A small portion of an antigen that can stimulate an immune response and serve as a binding site for antibody.

Humoral Immunity: Immunity that involves antibody-mediated responses.

Immunity: A state of protection from disease created by innate and specific mechanisms.

Immunization: Protection of individuals against disease by vaccination.

Innate Immunity: Nonspecific mechanisms involved in the early response to pathogens that lacks specificity and involves anatomical, physiological, phagocytic, and inflammatory mechanisms.

Passive Immunity: Immunity acquired by natural or acquired transfer of preformed antibodies.

Toxoid: An altered toxin capable of inducing production of antibodies.

Vaccination: Injection of a vaccine in order to establish resistance to an infectious disease.

Vaccine: A preparation of antigenic material designed to induce an immune response and immunological memory when injected.

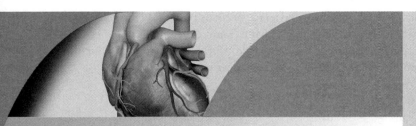

Questions for Further Research, Study, Reflection, and Discussion

For the Individual Student

In order to answer these questions, it may be necessary to research the primary literature.

- Why must individuals be inoculated against influenza every year?
- How would you develop an immune globulin for passive protection of someone exposed to rabies?
- What are the impediments to creating a vaccine for the common cold?
- How are the Sabin and Salk polio vaccines different? Why does the U.S. recommended immunization schedule no longer include the Sabin vaccine?

For Small Group Discussion

- Develop a time line showing the changes in the U.S. immunization schedule over the last 30 years.

- How does the U.S. immunization schedule differ from the schedules of other developed nations?

For Entire Class Discussion

- Despite evidence that immunizations are a cost-effective means of preventing specific infectious diseases, many people do not receive the recommended immunizations. Discuss possible reasons for the resistance to vaccination. Suggest means of overcoming these obstacles and to increase the percentage of the immunized population.

EXERCISES/ACTIVITIES

- A previously undeveloped island in the South Pacific has been designated for development as a resort destination. Two tribes of people inhabit this island but have never intermingled. The people of both tribes have rarely, if ever, encountered anyone from outside their island home. Develop an immunization program that will protect the inhabitants against any diseases to which they may be exposed.
- Community influence campaign: Select a focused population and develop a community campaign plan, including handouts and flyers, to promote community-based influenza clinics. How will you determine the success of the immunization process?

Public Health Terms

Herd Immunity: Ability of a group to resist specific pathogens either through widespread natural exposure or through vaccination.

Incidence: Number of specified new events during a specified period on a specified population.

ACKNOWLEDGMENTS

Special acknowledgment to Richard Billingsley and Daniel Webb for contributing to the Case Study and Chapter Questions.

REFERENCES

1. World Health Organization. Immunization Against Diseases of Public Health Importance. Geneva, Switzerland: WHO; March 2005. Available at http://www.who.int/mediacentre/factsheets/fs288/en/index.html. Accessed April 7, 2008.

2. United Nations Children's Fund (UNICEF). Immunize Every Child: GAVI Strategy for Immunization Services. New York: UNICEF; February 2000. Available at http://www.unicef.org/immunization/files/immunize_every_child.pdf. Accessed April 7, 2008.

3. Office of Disease Prevention and Health Promotion, U.S. Department of Health and Human Services. Washington, DC: DHHS. Healthy People 2010. Available at http://www.healthypeople.gov/. Accessed April 7, 2008.

Healthy People 2010

Indicator: Immunization

Focus Area: Immunization and Infectious Diseases

Goal: Prevent disease, disability, and death from infectious diseases, including vaccine-preventable diseases.

Objectives:

14-1. Reduce or eliminate indigenous cases of vaccine-preventable diseases.

14-2. Reduce chronic hepatitis B virus infections in infants and young children (perinatal infections).

14-3. Reduce hepatitis B.

14-4. Reduce bacterial meningitis in young children.

14-5. Reduce invasive pneumococcal infections.

14-6. Reduce hepatitis A.

14-7. Reduce meningococcal disease.

14-8. Reduce Lyme disease.

14-15. Increase the proportion of international travelers who receive recommended preventive services when traveling in areas of risk for select infectious diseases: hepatitis A, malaria, and typhoid.

14-22. Achieve and maintain effective vaccination coverage levels for universally recommended vaccines among young children.

14-23. Maintain vaccination coverage levels for children in licensed day care facilities and children in kindergarten through the first grade.

14-24. Increase the proportion of young children and adolescents who receive all vaccines that have been recommended for universal administration for at least 5 years.

14-25. Increase the proportion of providers who have measured the vaccination coverage levels among children in their practice population within the past 2 years.

14-26. Increase the proportion of children who participate in fully operational population-based immunization registries.

14-27. Increase routine vaccination coverage levels for adolescents.

14-28. Increase hepatitis B vaccine coverage among high-risk groups.

14-29. Increase the proportion of adults who are vaccinated annually against influenza and ever vaccinated against pneumococcal disease.

14-30. Reduce vaccine-associated adverse events.

14-31. Increase the number of persons under active surveillance for vaccine safety via large linked databases.

RESOURCES

Centers for Disease Control and Prevention National Immunization Program. Available at http://www.cdc.gov/vaccines/. Accessed April 7, 2008.

National Institute of Allergy and Infectious Diseases. Understanding Vaccines. What They Are. How They Work. Available at http://www.niaid.nih.gov/publications/vaccine/pdf/undvacc.pdf. Understanding the Immune System. How It Works. Available at http://www.niaid.nih.gov/publications/immune/the_immune_system.pdf. Accessed April 7, 2008.

World Health Organization. Immunizations, Vaccines and Biologicals. Geneva: WHO. Available at http://www.who.int/immunization. Accessed April 7, 2008.

Centers for Disease Control. 2007 Child & Adolescent Immunizing Schedules. Available at http://www.cdc.gov/vaccines/recs/schedules/child-schedule.htm#printable. Accessed April 7, 2008.

CROSS REFERENCES

Infectious Disease Chapters

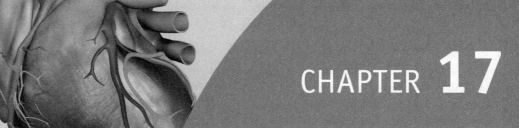

CHAPTER 17

Inflammation: Understanding Its Role in Acute and Chronic Disease

Patricia S. Latham

Inflammation destabilizes cholesterol deposits in the coronary arteries, leading to heart attacks and potentially even strokes. It chews up nerve cells in the brain of Alzheimer's victims. It may even foster the proliferation of abnormal cells and facilitate their transformation into cancer. In other words, chronic inflammation may be the engine that drives many of the most feared illnesses of middle and old age.[1]

LEARNING OBJECTIVES

By the end of this chapter, the student will be able to:

- Describe the basic sequence of events that occur in the vessels and tissues as a nonspecific response in acute inflammation.
  - Describe the five classic clinical signs.
  - Describe the changes that occur within the vessels and surrounding tissues.
- Name the two key phagocytic cells responsible for antimicrobial activity in the acute inflammatory cell.
  - Describe the mechanism, major chemical mediators, and temporal sequence of events that bring each of the two cell types to the site of bacterial invasion or injury.
  - Define an opsonin and name three that are important in the antimicrobial function of these cells.
  - Describe the mechanism of anaerobic antimicrobial function in these cells.
  - Describe the mechanism of aerobic antimicrobial function in these cells.
  - Name the phagocytic cell that predominates in tissues during the first 24 to 48 hours of the acute inflammatory response.
- Define **granulation tissue** and name three key cells involved in its composition and their function in wound healing.
- Name the major chemical mediators involved in wound healing; which ones are most important to angiogenesis and to scar formation?

- Describe the similarities and differences between wound healing by first intention and second intention.
- Describe what tissue capabilities are necessary for injured tissue to heal completely with return to a normal appearance and function after injury, and what factors ensure formation of scar.
- Describe two cell types that are most important in mediating chronic inflammation in tissues and their function.
- Define a granuloma and discuss how it is formed and the etiologies most commonly associated with its occurrence in chronic inflammation.

HISTORY

Inflammation has been recognized as an integral component of the body's response to injury from the time of the Egyptian Pharaohs. Figures carved in early temples showed men reflecting physical signs of injury including pain, swelling, and redness. These signs were later documented by Celsus of Rome as the four cardinal signs of inflammation—calor, rubor, dolor, and tumor—with functio laesa added as a later manifestation. In the absence of a true understanding of the physiological mechanism, the signs were at first considered the works of the Gods, but it is now clear that inflammation is an integral part of a person's **innate immunity**, defined as a mechanism of nonspecific first response to any of a number of pathogens, toxins, pollutants, and inhalants.

It is now apparent that chronic inflammation exists to some extent in almost all chronic illnesses in the body. The role of inflammation continues to expand as research reveals more details of its pathogenesis. In addition to chronic diseases in which inflammation has an obvious role, such as osteoarthritis, rheumatoid arthritis, or chronic hepatitis, increasing evidence suggests that inflammation also has a potentially significant role in atherosclerosis and cardiovascular disease, Alzheimer dementia, and even in the natural process of aging. Inflammation is also a common component of many injuries that result from a multitude of diverse environmental hazards important to the field of public health. For example, trauma or infection can cause direct injuries to skin and tissue that are associated with an acute inflammatory response, and alcohol, pollutants and many other toxins cause a more chronic injury to cells and tissues that are associated with progressive loss of organ function and accumulation of scar tissue.

An understanding of the role of acute and chronic inflammation in disease informs health policy in the regulations that are established to control exposure to many environmental hazards. An understanding of pathogenesis in inflammation also informs the treatments that are in everyday use for relief of the cardinal signs and symptoms of inflammation that we all experience. These treatments include antihistamines, aspirin, nonsteroidal anti-inflammatory agents, and steroids.

BASIC SCIENCE FACTS/KEY CONCEPTS REVIEW

Inflammation can be defined as the body's local vascular and cellular response to injury caused by factors that invade and injure the body from the outside (*exogenous factors*) or factors within the body that result in cellular or tissue injury (*endogenous factors*). Examples of exogenous factors are foreign bodies or bacteria. Examples of endogenous factors are those released from cells that are stressed or that have died, perhaps due to ischemia or even a complete loss of blood supply (infarction), or damage to cells and tissues that can occur as a result of traumatic injury such as kidney or gallstones or by activation of complement due to the formation of immune complexes.

Inflammation is part of an innate immune response that requires no previous exposure to the insult. It is designed to be a rapid first response that can neutralize or destroy injurious agents, create a barrier to limit injury and prevent its spread to normal tissue, and that can set in place the required cells and elements that can remove the debris and heal the wound. Most commonly, the reaction is the result of exogenous factors such as bacteria that threaten the integrity and survival of the host. However, endogenous factors also can stimulate an acute inflammatory response, such as injury caused by antigen-antibody complexes that activate the complement cascade and damage cells, or the trauma to tissue that a gallstone or kidney stone might cause, or necrosis of cells due to loss of blood and oxygen supply (*infarction*).

Acute Inflammation

Acute inflammation is short term and can be measured in hours or days. It is usually abrupt in onset, with five prominent clinical signs and symptoms: 1) warmth and 2) redness in the area of injury due to an increase of blood flow (hyperemia) and dilation of arterioles and capillaries; 3) pain, often described as throbbing, due to the pulse of blood flow; 4) localized swelling that results from fluids that weep out of vessels made more permeable by effects of the injury; and, 5) a loss of function in the site of injury if the pain and swelling are severe enough to limit motion.

Vascular Response

The clinical signs of acute inflammation are due to an initial **vascular response** localized to the area of injury. The increased blood flow and dilatation of vessels is caused by relaxation of vascular smooth muscle, particularly in pre-capillary arterioles. The increased permeability of vessels is caused by contraction of endothelial cells that line vessels, particularly in post-capillary venules, resulting in intercellular gaps. At first, only water and electrolytes can pass through the endothelial gaps, but as the gaps widen, larger proteins such as immunoglobulins and fibrinogen follow to result in an accumulation of extravascular, protein-rich fluid referred to as an *inflammatory exudate*.

The stimuli for this vascular response can be immediate (within minutes) in response to direct injury or IgE-mediated effects on tissue mast cells, causing the cells to release preformed histamine from intracellular granules. Histamine is the predominant stimulus to vascular smooth muscle relaxation and increased permeability in the first 30 minutes after direct injury, but other mediators of the vascular response will come from plasma and be synthesized by other cells in the area of the injury in the following hours and days. In addition to the vascular response, these mediators orchestrate other clinical features of the acute inflammatory response. These factors and the major cell types that produce them are summarized in Table 17-1.

Cellular Response: Neutrophils, Monocytes, and Macrophages

The second phase of the acute inflammatory response is marked by the accumulation of a **cellular exudate** of neutrophils in the early phase of acute inflammation within the area of injury. Neutrophils are the first line of defense against foreign invaders such as bacteria. These cells are always at the ready as they are the predominant cell type in normal circulation. Neutrophils are uniquely adapted to the task, because they contain a cytoskeleton and actin-myosin filament network that allows the cells to move in an ameboid fashion out of blood vessels and through tissue to the site of injury. The cells also are capable of engulfing particulate matter, such as bacteria, to prevent the

TABLE 17-1 Major Mediators of Acute Inflammation

Major cell-derived mediators include histamine that is preformed in mast cells and platelets and released immediately. Other major cell-derived mediators must be synthesized largely by macrophages, but also in neutrophils and endothelial cells during acute inflammation.

Major plasma-derived mediators include bradykinin, complement factors, and products of the coagulation cascade and fibrinolytic system.

Major Mediators of Vascular Effects
- Histamine: immediate release of preformed mediator
- Prostaglandin
- Nitric oxide
- Platelet-activating factor
- Cytokines, predominately interleukin-1 and tumor necrosis factor
- Bradykinin: activation of kinin metabolism in plasma
- Complement 3a and 5a: activation of complement cascade in plasma

Major Mediators of Chemotaxis
- Leukotriene B4
- Complement 5a
- Chemokines, such as interleukin-8
- Bacterial components

Fever
- Prostaglandin
- Interleukin-1

Pain
- Prostaglandin
- Bradykinin

---

organisms from causing further harm, a process called **phagocytosis**. The particulate matter is engulfed within a vacuole that isolates it from the cytoplasm of the cell. Lysosomes containing lysozyme and granules containing proteases can then be mobilized from within the cell to fuse with the membrane of the vacuole containing the bacterium or other matter, forming a phagolysosome. The enzymes and proteases can break down many proteinaceous materials and they are capable of destroying most bacteria. This entire process can be made even more efficient if the matter to be engulfed is associated with ligands that can bind to receptors on the surface of the neutrophils, such as mannose receptors that can bind to terminal mannose

residues found in some microbial walls, scavenger receptors that can bind oxidized and degraded, low-density lipoprotein and some microbial glycolipids, receptors to the Fc fragment of immunoglobulin, and receptors to C3b that are generated by activation of the complement cascade. When these factors coat particulate matter to enhance phagocytosis, they are referred to as **opsonins**.

The entire process of phagocytosis and antimicrobial activity is illustrated in Figure 17-1. The initial binding of matter, phagocytosis, formation of the phagolysosome, and killing of bacteria by action of lysosomal and protease enzymes can be accomplished in an anaerobic environment without oxygen. Thus, the neutrophils can perform these functions even in settings where tissue damage has compromised oxygen supply. However, the microbicidal activity of neutrophils is much greater when oxygen is present, because the cell can then use oxidative metabolic pathways to generate oxygen and hydroxyl free radicals. Myeloperoxidase enzyme in the cell can be used to generate hypochlorite free radicals. These free radicals are much more potent than those antimicrobials available in the absence of oxygen.

Although the normal life of neutrophils is three to five days and less in tissue, the body can rapidly replace these cells from the bone marrow. Neutrophils commonly arrive in an area of injury within hours of the acute event and will become maximal within 24 to 48 hours in tissue and then disappear if the inciting agent is not sustained. The benefit of neutrophils in the area of injury is great, especially if the injury is due to a pathogen such as bacteria, but the secondary damage to tissue also can be significant. As the enzymes are released within cells, there is some leakage out of the cell that increases as the cells reach the end of their lifespan in tissue. The leakage of these enzymes can result in damage and necrosis within the surrounding tissue. This injury must be healed and repaired during the healing phase of the acute inflammatory response.

In addition to neutrophils, monocytes in circulation and macrophages in tissue can be stimulated to have ameboid motion and to be phagocytic. Monocytes and macrophages have the same receptors for Toll-ligands and opsonins that are expressed on neutrophils. Toll-like receptors are receptors present on the plasma membrane of neutrophils and macrophages, which allow them to recognize and bind common antigens, such as endotoxin lipopolysaccharide (LPS) in the walls of Gram-negative bacteria. Binding of ligands to Toll-like receptors activates the leukocytes to increase phagocytic activity and to stimulate the synthesis and release of proinflammatory cytokines. Macrophages are much longer lived than neutrophils (they may live one or more months in tissue) and can synthesize many cytokines that are essential in regulating the inflammatory

FIGURE 17-1 Antimicrobial Activity in Phagocytic Cells.

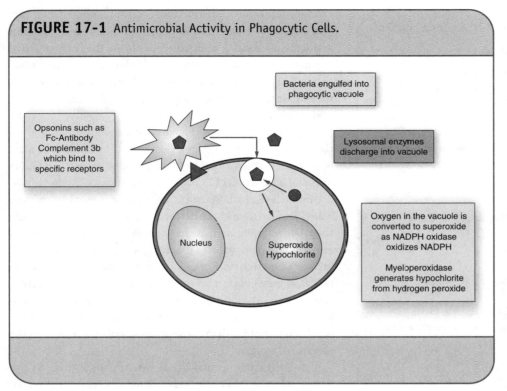

Bacteria engulfed into phagocytic vacuole

Opsonins such as Fc-Antibody Complement 3b which bind to specific receptors

Lysosomal enzymes discharge into vacuole

Nucleus

Superoxide Hypochlorite

Oxygen in the vacuole is converted to superoxide as NADPH oxidase oxidizes NADPH

Myeloperoxidase generates hypochlorite from hydrogen peroxide

and β-integrins on leukocytes, which allows the circulating leukocytes to bind and anchor the neutrophils against the inner wall of the post-capillary venule. Once fixed in that position, the neutrophil can be exposed to other mediators called **chemoattractants** that are synthesized by cells in the area of injury and released from the cells to diffuse into the surrounding tissue. Chemoattractants pass through the gaps in the endothelial cells to bind to the surface of the neutrophils and monocytes as well as stimulate contraction of their cytoskeleton, causing the cell to move in an ameboid-like fashion in the direction of maximal chemoattractant binding. In this way, the neutrophils will be drawn to move out of the post-capillary venules through the gaps

response and in orchestrating the phases of healing and repair that follow. The antimicrobial metabolism includes the production of oxygen and other free radicals. Although myeloperoxidase is a less important factor in generating free radicals than it is in neutrophils, macrophages have the ability to up-regulate production of nitric oxide synthetase, which can be used to generate nitric oxide, a potent free radical derived from arginine metabolism. Macrophages also have a critical role in processing foreign material for "presentation" to lymphocytes in generating the immune response. Monocytes in the circulation differentiate into macrophages in the tissue and contribute to the second wave of cells at sites of injury in acute inflammation.

Neutrophils and monocytes migrate out of the circulating blood into the injured tissue through a series of steps referred to as margination, adherence, and emigration, illustrated in Figure 17-2. The early mediators cause circulating neutrophils, monocytes that will become macrophages in tissue, and endothelial cells to synthesize selectins, such as endothelial (E-) and leukocyte (L-) selectins, and to express them on their cell surfaces. Expression of selectins causes the neutrophils and monocytes to become sticky, so they roll along the surface of the endothelial cells instead of gliding past in the stream of blood. The more prolonged contact stimulates the synthesis and expression of integrins, such as intercellular- and vascular-adhesion molecules (ICAM and VCAM) on endothelial cells

between endothelial cells and through the tissues along a positive concentration gradient of chemoattractant that is maximal at the specific site of injury. Major chemoattractants include the C5a component generated by activation of the complement cascade, leukotriene B4 generated by arachidonic acid metabolism through the action of lipoxygenase, and chemokines such as interleukin-8.

Accumulation of protein-rich fluid exudate is one of the most recognizable clinical features of acute inflammation in patients and is referred to as a *suppurative exudate* or *pus*. Pus is a well-recognized hallmark of infection, consisting of a dense exudate of neutrophils and necrotic tissue. Other exudates in acute inflammation may contain lesser numbers of neutrophils and they are named by their major component as serous (rich in edema fluid alone), fibrinous (rich in fibrin) or hemorrhagic (rich in blood), and so forth.

Manifestations and Complications of Acute Inflammation

In many cases of acute inflammation, the inciting agent is short-lived and the body is able to heal itself with no additional intervention. When the swelling and pain create too much discomfort, medications can be used to counteract the effect of inflammatory mediators. For example, antihistamines or nonsteroidal inflammatory drugs (NSAIDs) can be used to block

FIGURE 17-2 Emigration of Neutrophils from Vessels in Acute Inflammation. (A) Schematic drawing of steps (B) Photomicrograph of Neutrophils Emigrating from a venule (at arrowhead) during an acute inflammatory response in tissue.

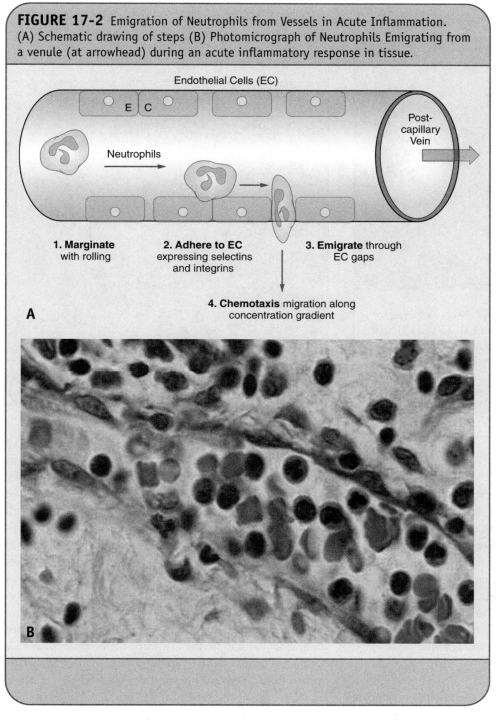

ticularly noteworthy: an abscess and an ulcer.

An **abscess** is a compartmentalized collection of suppurative exudate and tissue necrosis that is enclosed by tissue such as skin or by a body cavity (Figure 17-3). Abscesses are often difficult to heal because the inner core is dead tissue that has no vascular supply. The danger of an abscess is the risk of ongoing tissue injury and seeding of bacteria from the abscess into the bloodstream where it can cause widespread infection (*sepsis*). Abscesses must often be lanced or unroofed to release bacteria and give the tissue a chance to heal.

An **ulcer** is a localized site of inflammation and necrosis at the surface of skin or the inner surface of an organ such as the stomach (Figure 17-4). In the case of an ulcer, there has been sufficient damage to tissue to cause a gap or hole to appear at the surface of the tissue. Suppurative exudate fills the gap. In the case of the ulcer, it is possible to remove bacteria or other injurious agents from the tissue, although infectious agents that are not removed can go on to penetrate deeper into tissue and cause systemic infection. In other settings, such as an ulcer in the stomach, there is an increased risk for tissue necrosis that extends deep into the wall of the stomach, possibly causing erosion of a major artery with resultant hemorrhage, or perforation

the effects of histamine and prostaglandin, respectively, on the vascular response. The greater danger of acute inflammation lies in the risk that infection or injury will result in so much tissue damage that function is lost or that associated infection can extend beyond the localized area of injury to the rest of the body. Two distinctive manifestations of acute inflammation are par-

of the ulcer through the organ's wall tissue that can result in the escape of gastric acid into the body of the pancreas, liver, or peritoneal space.

When mediators of acute inflammation enter the circulation, more generalized systemic signs of inflammation can appear, including leukocytosis and fever. Leukocytosis applies

FIGURE 17-3 Pulmonary Abscess.

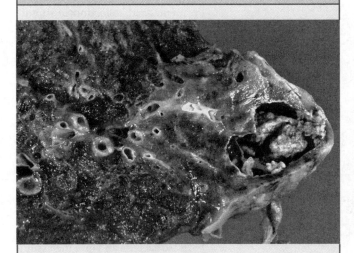

A Cut section of lung in which an abscess cavity can be seen. The abscess is also cut in half to show that it is filled with a suppurative or purulent exudate

Source: From the University of Alabama at Birmingham Department of Pathology Library © (http://peir.net)

FIGURE 17-4 Gastric Ulcer.
Notice the hemorrhagic gastric ulcer in the fundus of the stomach creates a deep hole in the mucosal surface of the stomach lining.

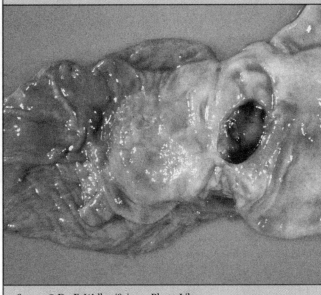

Source: © Dr. E. Walker/Science Photo Library.

to an increase of circulating leukocytes, usually neutrophils (granulocytosis), often occurring within hours of a stimulus, mobilized from bone marrow and other reservoirs. In proportion to demand, the marrow can also generate new cells (granulopoiesis) to meet the need when marrow is stimulated by cytokines such as colony stimulating factor (CSF), produced especially in this setting by macrophages. Fever results from stimulation of the hypothalamic thermoregulatory center by cytokines released from activated macrophages and other cells, especially interleukin-1 (IL-1) and prostaglandin (PG).

Healing and Repair

Healing and repair are necessary for the resolution of acute inflammation. The body will try to restore integrity as quickly as possible. If there is a wound in the skin, for example, the body will try to close and fill the wound as quickly as possible to prevent loss of blood and body fluids as well as the entry of infectious agents. At first, fibrin-rich exudate and blood from a local hemorrhage will form a gel-like clot that will fill the gaps in the tissue. As the clot dries, a scab will form to protect

the underlying tissue. The gel-like clot forms a scaffold, a temporary architecture to which macrophages and regenerating connective tissue cells can attach. As edema fluid is reabsorbed into lymphatics, the phagocytic macrophages work to engulf and dissolve dead cells and cell debris in the phagolysosomes. Macrophages are also one of the most important cell types to synthesize and release the many cytokines involved in cell regeneration and the proliferation of endothelial cells to form new vessels and fibroblasts that form new connective tissue. Fibroblasts synthesize collagen that will give the tissue at least temporary support during healing and, if necessary, will form the scar required to fill the gap when the original tissue cells cannot regenerate. Wounds typically heal from the edges where normal tissue is present toward their center. The sequence of events in healing and repair can be considered in three overlapping phases: 1) influx of macrophages and clearance of debris; 2) influx and regeneration of endothelial cells and new vessel formation (angiogenesis); 3) proliferation of fibroblasts and myofibroblasts that produce a progressive accumulation of collagen, as required by the extent of the wound. The loose matrix of regenerating connective tissue cells has a characteristic appearance in microscopic tissue sections that is referred to as *granulation tissue*. When granulation tissue is present, the wound is said to be *organizing* or *organized*.

The process of healing from a single insult in time usually proceeds along a characteristic time table in which gel-like clot and neutrophils predominate at 24 to 48 hours, to be replaced by macrophages that predominate from two to five days. During this two- to five-day time interval, tissue necrosis is often maximal and connective tissue regeneration has just begun, so the tissue is least strong at this time and most in danger of tearing open (*dehiscence*). Sutures are often used to bring the edges of a wound together to give it strength during this vulnerable interval. Thereafter, there is an increasing influx of endothelial cells that form new vessels and fibroblasts that produce collagen, giving the tissue ever greater strength and integrity as the days and weeks progress. The collagen and fibroblasts are at first randomly positioned in the wound, but gradually align themselves along lines of stress to provide the strength in function that is required. As the wound heals, the myofibroblasts contract to pull the edges of the wound together in order to minimize the impact of lost tissue on the function and strength of the organ. The myofibroblasts and fibroblasts produce collagen that can replace lost tissue and form a scar. Collagen and the scar hold tissue together against forces that might pull it apart. The cytokine mediators that orchestrate these events are produced largely by macrophages, as well as other cell types, summarized in Table 17-2.

Wounds on the skin are often described as healing by *first* or *second intention*. These terms refer to the extent of healing and repair required to close the wound. A wound that can heal by first intention is one in which the edges of the wound can be brought together, usually by stitches. The amount of tissue regeneration required to restore continuity of such a wound is relatively little. Sutures support the wound when it has the least integrity in the early days of healing, but need to be removed sometime before dense collagen traps the sutures in the tissue (usually at 10 days or so). Wounds of the skin that heal by second intention are those that are so large that the edges cannot be approximated, so scar formation is the inevitable result. These wounds may require skin grafts to provide closure to the exposed wound and to minimize the appearance of scar.

Complete healing without loss of function or scar after tissue injury and acute inflammation requires that the architecture of the tissue remain intact, so that cells that are able to regenerate can orient themselves in a way that allows them to function appropriately. Superficial injuries to the skin can heal without a scar, because epidermal cells can rapidly regenerate from the basal layer to replace the cells that were lost. Superficial injuries to intestinal mucosa can also heal rapidly because these cells have a normal turnover on a near-weekly basis. On the other hand, a myocardial infarct will heal with a scar, because myocytes cannot regenerate to replace the cells lost by necrosis.

Healing will be delayed or absent if there are host factors that prevent the regeneration or function of native and new connective tissue cells. If the area of injury is too large and/or the stimulus for inflammation cannot be removed, then healing will not be effective. If the blood supply is inadequate, as in the case of diabetes or after ionizing radiation, healing may be slow or incomplete. Systemic factors also can impair wound healing; for example, malnutrition may result in inadequate protein for synthesis of needed tissue components; suppression of the immune response can blunt the production of cytokines needed to mediate healing and repair; and vitamin C deficiency can prevent adequate collagen synthesis.

Chronic Inflammation

Chronic inflammation occurs most commonly when the inciting stimuli for inflammation cannot be removed from the body. Because many chronic inflammatory stimuli are chronic infections, tissue irritants, or altered proteins, the immune response becomes activated and contributes to the inflammation.

TABLE 17-2 Major Mediators of Chronic Inflammation and Wound Healing

Major mediators are synthesized by macrophages as well as fibroblasts and other cells that may be present in new connective tissue. Plasma-derived mediators continue to be important in chronic inflammation, but are not as prominent as in acute inflammatory reactions. Lymphocytes have a role in cytokine production by their production of interferon-gamma (IFN-γ) that can activate macrophages and by their role in adaptive immunity as it comes into play in chronic inflammatory processes.

Major Mediators of Angiogenesis

- Vascular Endothelial Growth Factor (VEGF)
- Fibroblast Growth Factor (FGF)

Major Mediators of Fibroblast Proliferation and Collagen Production

- Fibroblast Growth Factor (FGF)
- Transforming Growth Factor-Beta (TGF-β)
- Platelet-Derived Growth Factor (PDGF)

Lymphocytes and macrophages predominate in the inflammatory infiltrate. In chronic inflammation, there is a shift in macrophage chemoattractant production that favors the migration of lymphocytes, rather than neutrophils, to the area of injury. The stimulus for inflammation and the body's response to it is more subdued in chronic inflammation than in the acute inflammatory response. The more dramatic tissue effects associated with neutrophils are not part of most chronic inflammatory responses. However, the ongoing tissue injury does incite efforts to heal that are seen as a progressive increase in the accumulation of collagen and scar formation in the tissue.

Chronic inflammation is associated with most of the major chronic organ system diseases. The progressive loss of functional tissue and the increase of scar tissue in the organ impact on the function of the organ and ultimately results in its failure. For example, infection by the hepatitis C virus leads to chronic inflammation in the liver in most persons who are infected. In these persons, infection with the hepatitis C virus is associated with an ineffective immune response and failure to eliminate the virus from the body. The resulting ongoing hepatocellular injury is referred to as *chronic hepatitis*. The danger to these patients is as much due to the gradual accumulation of scar tissue as it is to the functional loss of hepatocytes. Eventually, the scar tissue is sufficient to result in cirrhosis with a loss of liver architecture. The scar tissue distorts and impedes blood flow through the liver, resulting in a marked increase in pressure within the portal venous circulation, referred to as *portal hypertension*. Cirrhosis caused by hepatitis C is now the most common reason for liver transplantation in the United States. In addition, the constant stimulus to regenerate liver cells caused by ongoing injury promotes the development of hepatocellular carcinoma; hepatitis C is recognized worldwide as one of the leading causes of hepatocellular carcinoma. A few other examples of major diseases associated with chronic inflammation, progressive tissue damage, loss of function, and variable scar include: atherosclerosis, chronic bronchitis, rheumatoid arthritis and other collagen vascular diseases, and inflammatory bowel disease.

The most common microscopic appearance of chronic inflammation in tissue such as that seen in chronic hepatitis is evidence of tissue injury and scar associated with an infiltrate of lymphocytes, lesser numbers of macrophages, and occasional antibody-producing plasma cells. However, certain etiologies of chronic inflammation can be associated with a distinctive inflammatory infiltrate that contains increased numbers of macrophages in a characteristic cluster referred to as a **granuloma**. A classic granuloma is approximately 1 to 2 mm in size and consists of a nodule-like aggregate of macrophages surrounded by an outer rim of lymphocytes (Figure 17-5). When activated and stimulated by lymphocyte cytokines, macrophages in granulomas become *epithelioid* in their microscopic appearance, that is, they take on some features reminiscent of epithelial cells. Their nuclei develop a characteristic elongation and pallor and there is an increase in cytoplasm. It is thought that granulomas form when macrophages are unable to kill certain organisms or degrade certain proteins that are resistant to their antimicrobial defenses and digestive enzymes. Macrophages are then recruited to form aggregates and some may fuse together to form multinucleated *giant cells* (also called *Langhans giant cells*). In the United States, *Mycobacterium tuberculosis* and sarcoidosis are two major causes of chronic inflammation associated with granulomas, although fungal infections, parasitic infections, and some inorganic substances also can be associated with the finding. In the case of *Mycobacterium tuberculosis*, the granulomas often show a characteristic central necrosis, called *caseous necrosis*, which is rarely seen in other etiologies of granulomas. There is no progressive disease in most cases, unless there is overwhelming infection or the body is unable to mount an effective immune response. As in other causes of chronic granulomatous disease, however, the potential exists for the chronic infection to be associated with chronic inflammation that can go on to damage tissue and result in accumulation of scar. In the case of tuberculosis, it is important to remember that latent *Mycobacteria* can remain in quiescent granulomas and become reactivated in conditions of immunosuppression, a

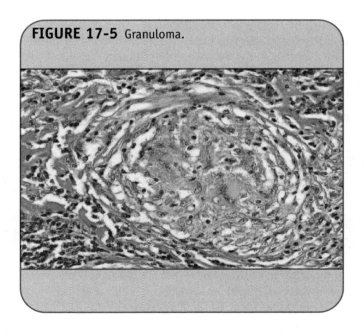

FIGURE 17-5 Granuloma.

CASE STUDY
Scenario

A 55-year-old man is seen in clinic with complaints of moderate pain and swelling in his right calf for two days. He says that it is now painful to walk. He does not remember any injury to the leg, but his work as a research associate requires him to stand for hours each day as he does his experiments in the laboratory. He does have varicose veins in his legs, and he states that he did have a similar episode of calf pain one year ago, which was treated with rest and elevation of his leg, elastic stockings, gentle, non-weight bearing exercises, and a nonsteroidal anti-inflammatory drug (NSAID). His only other medical problems are obesity of 30 years and hypercholesterolemia for which he takes a statin medication.

> Physical exam: Weight 250 lbs, Height 5'8"
> Body Mass Index (BMI): 38
> BP 150/85, pulse 72 per minute
> Respirations 14 per minute
> Temperature 99.8°F
> Cardiopulmonary exam: Normal breath sounds on auscultation and normal cardiac exam.

> Extremities:
> - The skin over the right calf is intact, but it is erythematous (red). The calf is tender to touch and to dorsiflexion of the foot. The skin feels tense on palpation (pressure) and there is swelling in the right calf, which measures 2-cm more in circumference than the left calf. There are no palpable nodules or cords in the calf.

Defining the Issues
- What is the pathogenesis of the inflammatory process that is causing painful swelling in the leg of this patient?
- What is phlebitis?
- What are the potential complications of phlebitis?
- What are some risk factors for the development of phlebitis and for the formation of blood clots or venous thrombi?

Patient's Understanding

During the time of his previous episode, the patient was told that pain and swelling in his leg can be caused by *phlebitis*. Furthermore, he was told that phlebitis can be associated with the formation of blood clots that can travel to his lungs with serious consequences. He was told to call the doctor if he experienced similar signs in the future. The patient understands that phlebitis is a type of inflammation that requires treatment, but he does not know exactly what it is or how it might be a cause of blood clots.

CLINICAL PERSPECTIVE FOR THE INDIVIDUAL PATIENT

This case highlights the common inflammatory condition of phlebitis and the risks that it poses for complications of thrombosis and embolization. The case underscores the often overlooked contribution that occupational and environmental factors can have in causing inflammatory conditions. In other settings, the contribution of these factors may have even greater impact. For example, phlebitis and thrombosis can occur as a complication of intravenous lines and therapy in the hospital setting or intravenous drug abuse on the street. A tendency to form clots and deep vein thrombosis (DVT) can occur as a complication of prolonged sitting or standing with limited movement, such as that occurring during postoperative recovery or prolonged bed rest in hospitals or during long airline flights in confined seating in the course of everyday life.

Level of Intervention Now

The patient's symptoms suggest that he has a phlebitis of superficial veins (superficial phlebitis, but the previous episode increases the risk for formation of venous clots (thrombi) in larger and deeper veins (DVT). Current treatment of phlebitis in this patient should be directed at reducing inflammation in order to decrease any further injury to the veins of the legs, to ease the pain and swelling, and to increase mobility. Specific interventions might include resting the leg and raising and straightening the knee and lower leg to increase venous drainage out of the lower extremity and back to the heart. Elastic stockings can help to support tissue tone and lessen edema accumulation. If heart failure or other conditions are believed to be contributory to the edema, diuretics to induce fluid loss may be added. A nonsteroidal anti-inflammatory medication can be given to lessen the accumulation of additional edema and to ease the pain associated with inflammation. Additional studies of the leg, such as Doppler ultrasonography, should be done to determine if thrombus is present in the deep leg veins (DVT), because blood clots can break free and lodge in distant capillaries (embolize) particularly in the lung. Anticoagulants may have been added to this patient's regimen, because he has a prior history of phlebitis, but certainly would be added if the patient has multiple risk factors for thrombosis or clot is identified. It also will be important to monitor for fever and other signs of increasing evidence for infection, since infection can also occur as another potential complication of phlebitis.

Potential Level Earlier

Interventions at the time of the first episode of phlebitis would be the same as those described for the current episode. In the previous instance, clots were not identified and anticoagulants were not used, but it is likely that the patient was advised to lose weight and to continue the use of elastic stockings. Supportive shoes can help to soften the trauma to the legs, as will the use of rubber mats in areas where prolonged standing might be necessary. Frequent movement and periodic breaks to relieve positional stress also can help to diminish the chance of injury. It would be important to identify health problems such as heart failure that might predispose to the formation of edema, or hypercoagulable states such as that induced by smoking or cancer (or use of oral contraceptives in women) that might predispose to clot formation in blood.

common concern in the setting of cancer chemotherapy or HIV infection.

In summary, the inflammatory response can be a double-edged sword in the body's effort to protect itself from injury and infectious threat. In acute inflammation, the rapid and nonspecific response is critical to contain the damage, neutralize or kill invading organisms, and repair tissue damage. In chronic inflammation on the other hand, prolonged activation of the inflammatory response and the formation of scar can cause permanent damage to tissues and loss of function, forming the basis for much of the pathology that is seen in many chronic active disease processes in the body.

PUBLIC HEALTH PERSPECTIVE FOR THE HEALTH OF THE GENERAL POPULATION AND OF HIGH RISK GROUPS

Inflammation and the Shifting Burden of Disease

As discussed in this chapter, the inflammatory response is a critical component of the immune reaction to injury and infection. Before the advent of modern medicine, infectious disease accounted for the majority of **disability adjusted life years** (DALYs), and in that era, the body depended on rapid inflammatory responses to survive. As medical knowledge progressed and general living conditions improved, however, the most burdensome infectious diseases became either treatable or preventable, and as a result, people began to live for a longer and

longer time. Lengthening life spans led to increases in the rates of chronic diseases, which eventually began to account for a much larger share of the total disease burden than infectious disease. Because chronic disease is now the major source of DALYs, improving public health will depend on scientists' ability to understand the risk factors, disease mechanisms, and health consequences of chronic conditions.

Although it plays an important role in battling infections and injury, inflammation is an example of an evolutionary adaptive response that has become maladaptive in today's environment. Despite its beneficial role battling infectious disease, researchers have recently discovered that chronic inflammation, even at low levels, is quite injurious and contributes to many chronic conditions including heart attack, stroke, Alzheimer disease, and cancer, all of which are some of the largest killers affecting the middle-aged and elderly populations. Unlocking the process by which inflammation affects those diseases will be necessary not only for improving patient outcomes, but also for safeguarding the public's health.

KEY TERMS

Abscess: A localized pocket of suppurative exudate and liquifactive necrosis that is entirely within, and surrounded by, tissue of an organ or body cavity.

Cellular Exudate: An accumulation of protein-rich fluid in an extravascular space or tissue; also referred to as *inflammatory edema*. When the exudate includes an influx of leukocytes, neutrophils, or other leukocytes, it is referred to as a *cellular exudate*.

Chemotaxis and **Chemoattractants:** In the inflammatory response, chemotaxis describes the ameboid movement of cells, particularly neutrophils, monocytes, and macrophages, out of vessels and toward a site of injury in response to a chemoattractant signal. Chemoattractant factors include some bacterial products and products released from necrotic cells, fibrinopeptides, [C5a derived from activation of the complement cascade], and factors produced by stimulated macrophages and other cells, including leukotriene B4 and the chemokine interleukin-8 (IL-8).

Disability Adjusted Life Year (DALY): A method of measuring disease burden based on a quantification of years of potential life lost through death and years of life expected to be lived with disability.

Granulation Tissue: The histological appearance of tissue during the early healing phase of acute inflammation when there is an influx of macrophages and a proliferation of connective tissue cells and matrix disproportionate to the predominance of fibrosis and scar, which are seen in the later stages of healing. The new connective tissue is loosely woven and includes many macrophages, proliferating endothelial cells, and new blood vessels (angiogenesis), and an increasing number of myofibroblasts producing fine collagen strands.

Granuloma: An aggregate of macrophages surrounded by a rim of lymphocytes. Although granulomas can be formed as a nonspecific response to indigestible matter (i.e., suture material), it is necessary to consider infectious and immune-mediated causes. Immune-stimulated macrophages take on a distinctive appearance referred to as *epithelioid* and may form giant cells with multiple nuclei ringing the periphery of the enlarged macrophage (*Langhans giant cell*). Tuberculosis is the most likely etiology of the granulomas if caseous necrosis is seen within the granulomas.

Inflammation: A vascular and cellular host response that marshals leukocytes and essential proteins into tissues affected by infection or injury in order to kill or neutralize organisms, contain damage, and set in place those factors that can result in healing and repair.

Innate Immunity: Host defenses that are in place or immediately available to respond to infection or injury and that do not require prior immune sensitization, including physical barriers such as mucosa or skin; leukocytes such as neutrophils and monocytes in circulation or macrophages in tissue; natural killer (NK) cells, eosinophils; and many proteins and cytokines such as complement, tumor necrosis factor (TNF), interleukin-1 (IL-1), and many others.

Opsonin: A protein that coats particulate matter in a way that enhances uptake in phagocytic leukocytes through binding of that protein to specific receptors, such as the C3b receptor in the case of complement factor C3b or the Fc receptor in the case of an antibody.

Phagocytosis and Phagosomal Antimicrobial Activity: The process by which neutrophils and macrophages engulf particulate matter (i.e., microbes) into a vacuole formed by an in-folding of the plasma membrane within the cytoplasm. The vacuole is called a *phagosome* when cytoplasmic granules containing acid hydrolase enzymes and lysozymes discharge into the vacuole for the purpose of killing the organism and digesting the protein. A potent mechanism of antimicrobial activity also occurs in the phagolysosome in the presence of oxygen.

Ulcer: An ulcer is an area of suppurative exudate and liquifactive necrosis in a tissue or organ that extends into the body of the organ or tissue, but that remains open at an outer or inner surface of that organ or tissue.

Vascular Response: In acute inflammation, the vascular response refers to the increase of blood flow and permeability that can occur within minutes in an area of injury or infection.

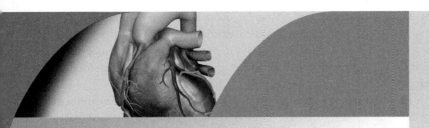

Questions for Further Research, Study, Reflection, and Discussion

For the Individual Student

In order to answer these questions, it may be necessary to research the primary literature.

- Protection of the body from pathogens is the most obvious role for acute inflammation and innate immunity. However, oxidant stress in cells is another important stimulus for the acute inflammatory response. What is oxidant stress and how does it stimulate inflammation?

- In considering what factors are necessary for complete healing after acute inflammation, what sequence of cellular changes would you expect to find in the tissue of the heart after complete ischemic necrosis (a myocardial infarct due to a coronary artery occlusion)? What would you expect to be the final appearance of the tissue after the inflammatory sequence is complete?

- Chronic inflammation is associated with concurrent acute inflammation and tissue destruction with efforts of the tissue to heal and to repair the ongoing damage. What complications in organs can result from chronic inflammation? Provide a few examples.

For Small Group Discussion

- The redness, swelling, and pain that occurred in the calf of this patient are signs and symptoms of phlebitis, an inflammation of veins. Consider how inflammation might occur in this setting. Can you think of other conditions that might cause phlebitis?

- What is(are) the most likely cause(s) of the swelling in the calf?

- Formation of thrombus in the veins of the leg is a very common complication of phlebitis. What factors in acute inflammation of veins predispose to the formation of thrombi?

- Can you think of a life-threatening complication of phlebitis that might occur in this patient?

- In addition to possible toxicity of an infusate, what concern(s) would you have if you saw the signs of phlebitis at the site of an intravenous line or catheter?

- This patient had an earlier episode of phlebitis that was treated with rest and elevation of his leg, elastic stockings, gentle, non-weight bearing exercises, and an NSAID. What favorable effects were intended by each component of therapy?

For Entire Class Discussion

- Given what you now know about inflammation and its role in chronic diseases, what would be an appropriate public health response? What are some common behaviors that could be targeted with a national education program that could help people dampen their inflammatory response?

EXERCISE/ACTIVITY

Small groups of five students each should select an acute or chronic inflammatory disease and explore at least one anti-inflammatory medication that has been used in treatment of that disease. Each group should create a five to ten slide PowerPoint presentation that reports on the following features of the disease and the anti-inflammatory treatment that they have chosen:

- What are the major clinical problems associated with the disease?

- What is the leading theory to explain the acute or chronic inflammation that occurs in the disease (in general terms, without the need for very specific details)?

- How common is the disease, and what is the impact of the problem on the health system?

- What is one medication that has been used to subdue or eliminate inflammation in the disease, and what is the target for its action and the presumed benefit?

Examples of chronic inflammatory diseases include: chronic bronchitis or pneumonitis, chronic viral hepatitis, chronic inflammatory bowel disease (Crohn disease and ulcerative colitis), rheumatoid arthritis, gout, tendonitis, sarcoidosis, among others.

REFERENCE

1. Gorman C, Park A. "The Fires Within." *TIME Magazine* 2004;163:39–46.

RESOURCES

Kumar V, Fausto N, Abbas A, eds. *Robbins and Cotran Pathologic Basis of Disease*, 7th ed. Philadelphia: Elsevier Saunders; 2005.

Rubin R, Strayer DS. *Rubin's Pathology: Clinicopathologic Foundations of Medicine*, 5th ed. Philadelphia: Lippincott Williams & Wilkins; 2008.

Barrington R, Zhang M, Fischer M, Carroll MC. The role of complement in inflammation and adaptive immunity. *Immunol Rev* 2001;180:5–15.

Botting RM, Botting JH. Pathogenesis and mechanisms of inflammation and pain: an overview. *Clin Drug Invest* 2000;19(Suppl 2):1–7.

Broughton G, Janis JE, Attinger CE. The basic science of wound healing. *Plast Reconstr Surg* 2006;117(Suppl 7):12S–34S.

Charo IF, Ransohoff RM. The many roles of chemokines and chemokine receptors in inflammation. *N Engl J Med* 2006;354:610–621.

Co DO, Hogan LH, Kim S, Sandor M. Mycobacterial granulomas: keys to a long-lasting host-pathogen relationship. *Clin Immunol* 2004;113:130–136.

Dandona P, Aljada A, Chaudhuri A, Mohanty P, Garg R. Metabolic syndrome: a comprehensive perspective based on interactions between obesity, diabetes, and inflammation. *Circulation* 2005;111:1448–1454.

Hansson GK. Inflammation, atherosclerosis, and coronary artery disease. *N Engl J Med* 2005;352:1685–1695.

Medzhitov R, Janeway C Jr. Innate immunity. *N Engl J Med* 2000;343:338–344.

Muller WA. Leukocyte-endothelial cell interactions in the inflammatory response. *Lab Invest* 2002;82:521–533.

Schottenfeld D, Beebe-Dimmer J. Chronic inflammation: a common and important factor in the pathogenesis of neoplasia. *CA Cancer J Clin* 2006;56:69–83.

Segal AW. How neutrophils kill microbes. *Annu Rev Immunol* 2005;23:197–223.

Tracey KJ. The inflammatory reflex. *Nature* 2002;420:853–859.

CROSS REFERENCES

Alzheimer Disease
Atherosclerosis
Diabetes
Infectious Disease Chapters
Oral Health and Disease

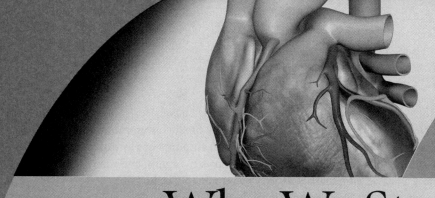

CHAPTER 18

Why We Stay Well: Stress, Allostasis, and Scientific Integrative Medicine

David S. Goldstein

> Inside every person is an inner world, full of comings and goings and the beautiful paradox of seeming constancy despite continuous change.
>
> D.S.G.

LEARNING OBJECTIVES

By the end of this chapter, the student will be able to:

- Describe the profound shift from our understanding of unifactorial disease to multifactorial disorders over the past century.
- Discuss the concept of allostasis and its significance.
- Describe how the brain coordinates steady states in order to maintain apparent constancy despite the continual changes to which humans are subjected.
- Define scientific integrative medicine and distinguish it from systems biology.

HISTORY

The past century has seen a profound shift in diseases of humankind. Acute, unifactorial diseases, such as from infection by a single bacterial strain, are being replaced increasingly by multifactorial disorders that arise from complex interactions among genes, environment, concurrent morbidities and treatments, and time. This complexity applies in acute critical illness as well as in chronic degenerative diseases, involving dysfunction of multiple body systems in somewhat overlapping syndromes, although those syndromes are usually diagnosed and treated based on the most prominent symptoms or signs within a single system. Researchers must acquire and apply fundamentally new concepts to take into account this develop-

ment, by appreciating the multidisciplinary, integrative, and even "mind–body" aspects of acute and chronic disorders.

According to the concept of **allostasis**, there is no single, ideal set of steady-state conditions in life. Allostasis reflects active, adaptive processes that maintain apparent steady states, via multiple, interacting effectors regulated by homeostatic comparators called **homeostats**. **Stress** can be defined as a condition or state in which a sensed discrepancy between afferent information and a setpoint for response lead to activation of effectors, reducing the discrepancy. **Allostatic load** refers to the consequences of sustained or repeated activation of mediators of allostasis. From the analogy of a home temperature control system, the temperature can be maintained at any of a variety of levels (*allostatic states*) by multiple means (*effectors*), regulated by a comparator thermostat (*homeostat*). Allostatic load and risks of system breakdown increase when, for example, the front door is left open in the winter. Applying these notions can aid in understanding how stress might exert adverse health consequences via allostatic load. This presentation describes models of homeostatic systems that incorporate **negative feedback** regulation, multiple effectors, effector sharing, environmental influences, intrinsic obsolescence, and destabilizing positive feedback loops. These models can be used to predict effects of environmental and genetic alterations on allostatic load and therefore on the development of multisystem disorders and failures.

The Seed and The Soil

The great French physiologist, Claude Bernard, introduced the idea of the "inner world" of the body, when he theorized that body systems function as they do to maintain a constant internal environment, what he termed the *milieu intérieur*. Near the end of his life, in about 1876, he postulated that the body maintains the constant internal environment by myriad, continual, compensatory reactions, which would tend to restore a state of equilibrium in response to any outside changes, enabling independence from the external environment. *Bernard's Lectures on the Phenomena of Life Common to Animals and Vegetables* (Vol. 1, translated by Hoff HE, Guillemin R, Guillemin L. Springfield, IL: Charles C Thomas Publisher; 1974) contains famous passages in the history of physiology: "The constancy of the internal environment is the condition for free and independent life" (p. 84), and: "All the vital mechanisms, however varied they might be, always have one purpose, that of maintaining the integrity of the conditions of life within the internal environment" (p. 89). This view might seem straightforward or even simpleminded today, but it was revolutionary in the history of medical ideas.

Bernard's views sometimes conflicted with those of his contemporary, Louis Pasteur, the father of microbiology and the germ theory of disease. According to Pasteur's followers, diseases would result mainly from external threats to the well-being of the organism, such as exposure to germs; the body's responses would be relatively unimportant. According to Bernard's followers, diseases would result from inappropriate or inadequate responses of the body; the actual threats would be relatively unimportant. To paraphrase the great physician, William Osler, the debate was over whether disease is caused by the "seed" or caused by the "soil."

During the era of ascendance of the germ theory of disease, at the end of the 1800s, the importance of the equilibrium of the organism receded. Today, however, with increasing recognition that diseases often stem from deleterious interactions between heredity and environment, or from genetic flaws outright, Bernard seems vindicated. Pasteur on his deathbed is said to have conceded, "Bernard was right. The microbe is nothing: the soil is everything."

BASIC SCIENCE FACTS/KEY CONCEPTS REVIEW

Inside every person is an inner world, full of comings and goings and the beautiful paradox of seeming constancy despite continuous change. We are born, we develop and mature, we reproduce, we live out our lives, we get old, we get sick, and we die. Yet for most of our existence, we believe in our essential sameness day to day.

For most of the amazing longevity that characterizes us humans, we rarely notice the internal workings that constitute the political affairs of the inner world. Cells of the body "turn over"—we literally replace ourselves over time—yet things inside seem to stay in a steady state so well, for so long. Body temperature, blood levels of key fuels, concentrations of red blood cells in the bloodstream, amounts of electrolytes, the rate of the heartbeat, blood flows to organs, and many more variables normally vary by remarkably little.

These steady states do not happen by chance. In higher organisms, they depend on complex coordination by the brain. This chapter introduces a way of thinking about how the brain regulates the inner world, to maintain apparent constancy despite continual changes.

In a single word, the brain does so via *systems*. Just as the brain receives information from sense organs and determines our interactions with the outside world, the brain also receives information from internal sensors and acts on that information to regulate the inner world. For most of our lives, we can cling to our belief in sameness only because the brain tracks many monitored variables, by way of internal sensory information, and acts on this information to maintain levels of monitored variables at controlled, steady values by modulating numerous effectors that work simultaneously, in parallel.

Scientific Integrative Medicine

Scientific integrative medicine is not a treatment method or discipline but a way of thinking that applies systems concepts to understand acute and chronic complex disorders.

Scientific integrative medicine builds on systems biology but is also distinct in several ways: 1) Scientific integrative medicine recognizes that in higher organisms, including us humans, the brain dominates regulation of the "inner world" of the body. The brain regulates the many internal monitored variables of the body in parallel, which is analogous to a computer's multitasking. 2) The brain has plasticity, enabling modifications in algorithms for cellular, tissue, organ, and systemic processes. According to the concept of allostasis, set points and other elements of these algorithms vary, depending on recollections, sensations, and anticipations by the brain. 3) Scientific integrative medicine is medical, its overall mission to understand and rationally treat disorders and diseases. Clinicians rarely cure; rather, they manage, in particular by exploiting negative feedback loops and attempting to forestall or counter positive feedback loops. 4) The medications and treatments clinicians prescribe interact with their patients' internal systems. Multiple, simultaneous degenerations, combined with multiple effects of multiple drugs and remedies, and myriad interactions between the degenerations and the treatments, constitute the bulk of modern medical practice. The scientific integrative medicine approach provides a framework for understanding highly complex and dynamic challenges to our integrity as organisms.

Characteristics of Homeostatic Systems

Negative Feedback Regulation

Levels of multiple monitored variables are kept stable by negative feedback loops. By analogy to a home heating system, a decrease in outside temperature would lead to a decrease in inside temperature, except for the thermostat directing the furnace to turn on (Figures 18-1 and 18-2). A (−) sign indicates a negative relationship.

If a homeostatic loop has an odd number of minus (−) signs, then during exposure to a continuous perturbing influence, the monitored variable will attain a stable level. Physiological homeostatic systems entail negative feedback regulation of monitored variables, such as core temperature, blood pressure, serum osmolality, and metabolic rate. Conceptually,

each system depends on a comparator—a homeostat—to compare afferent information about the monitored variables with set points or other criteria for responding.

Disruption of a negative feedback loop, whether by preventing afferent information from reaching the brain, inability to process the information and regulate effector functions correctly, or dysfunction or loss of effectors, leads to fluctuations in the level of the monitored variable. A clinical example of this phenomenon is labile blood pressure as a late sequela of neck irradiation due to interference with the carotid sinus baroreflex.

Multiple Effectors

The key monitored variables of the body are regulated by multiple effectors (Figure 18-3). This extends the range of control, allows some regulation of the monitored variable if a

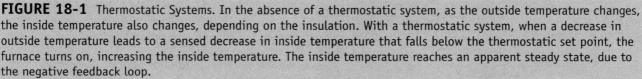

FIGURE 18-1 Thermostatic Systems. In the absence of a thermostatic system, as the outside temperature changes, the inside temperature also changes, depending on the insulation. With a thermostatic system, when a decrease in outside temperature leads to a sensed decrease in inside temperature that falls below the thermostatic set point, the furnace turns on, increasing the inside temperature. The inside temperature reaches an apparent steady state, due to the negative feedback loop.

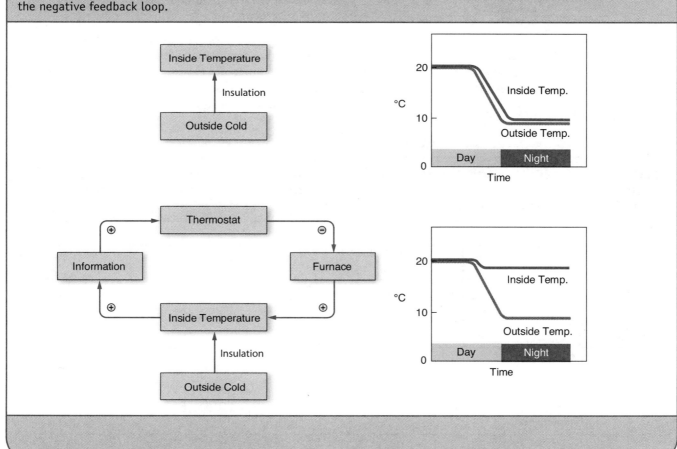

FIGURE 18-2 A Physiological Homeostatic System. As the level of the monitored variable changes, afferent information is compared with a set point or other algorithm for responding, and the sensed discrepancy leads to altered activities of effectors. Note the odd number of minus (−) signs, indicating a negative feedback loop. In response to a continuous perturbation, the level of the monitored variable reaches an apparent steady state.

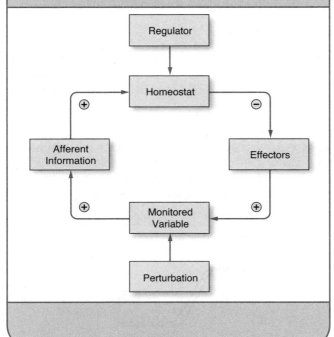

particular effector fails (via compensatory activation), improves cost efficiency, and enables elaboration of specific effector patterns. For instance, the sympathetic noradrenergic system (SNS), adrenomedullary hormonal system (AHS), and hypothalamic-pituitary-thyroid axis (THY) are effectors for regulation of core temperature. Hypophysectomy, thyroidectomy, and hypothyroidism are all associated with compensatory activation of the SNS. Because of compensatory activation, exposure of a thyroidectomized individual to cold results in exaggerated SNS activation.

Effector Sharing

An air conditioner not only cools the air but also dries it, and a dehumidifier not only dries the air but also warms it. An air conditioner and a dehumidifier therefore can function as shared effectors for both temperature and humidity control. Analogously, different physiological homeostats can share effectors (Figure 18-4). Effector sharing can explain hyperglycemia in gastrointestinal hemorrhage and, as illustrated in the figure, hyponatremia in congestive heart failure.

Homeostatic Definitions of Stress, Allostasis, and Allostatic Load

In physiological homeostatic loops regulated by negative feedback, *stress* is a condition in which there is an error signal, reflecting the difference between afferent information about actual conditions as sensed and the set point for responding, determined by a regulator (Figure 18-5).

FIGURE 18-3 Compensatory Activation. One advantage of multiple effectors is compensatory activation of alternative effectors if one effector fails, enabling control of the monitored variable. For instance, thyroidectomy augments sympathetic nervous system (SNS) responses to cold exposure.

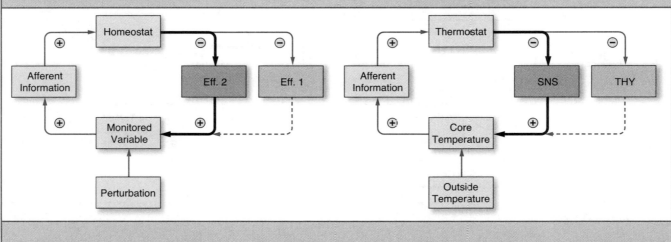

FIGURE 18-4 Effector Sharing. Sharing of an effector by multiple homeostats can explain unpredicted consequences and syndromic features of disease processes. For instance, in heart failure, decreased aortic filling increases levels of vasopressin (AVP), which, as the antidiuretic hormone, promotes retention of free water, explaining hyponatremia attending heart failure.

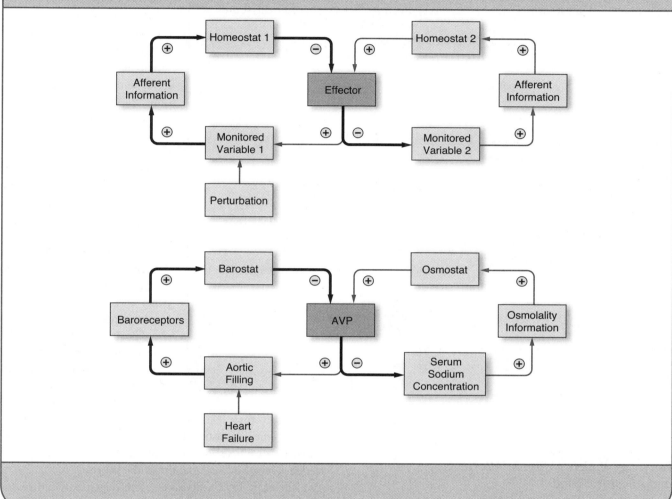

Although levels of monitored variables in a system regulated by negative feedback attain apparent steady-states, the actual level of the monitored variable can be adjusted by changing the set point or other instructions for responding. Allostasis refers to this "other sameness." This flexibility comes at the cost of wear and tear: allostatic load (Figure 18-5). For instance, one can set the thermostat at a high temperature in the winter. Maintaining the high temperature at an apparent steady state accelerates wear and tear on the furnace. Moreover, as wear and tear progress, furnace efficiency declines, requiring it to be on more of the time to maintain the temperature, in turn accelerating the wear and tear on the furnace. In other words, allostatic load can lead eventually to a positive feedback loop, with rapid failure of the system.

Computer Models of Stress, Allostatic Load, and Acute and Chronic Diseases

Computerized kinetic models to illustrate the above concepts and produce quantitative predictions can be generated using Stella II (isee Systems, Inc., Lebanon, NH), an icon-based model-building and simulation tool. Briefly, Stella models consist of "stocks," represented by a rectangle, "flows" among them, represented by conduit pipes with transparent arrowheads in

FIGURE 18-5 Homeostatic Definitions of Stress and Allostatic Load. In stress, the organism senses a discrepancy between afferent information about a monitored variable and a set point and other instructions for responding, altering activities of effectors to decrease the discrepancy. Allostatic load reflects wear and tear, which, if sustained and substantial enough, decreases effector efficiency, further activating the effector and accelerating wear and tear. Allostatic load therefore can eventuate in a destabilizing and pathological positive feedback loop.

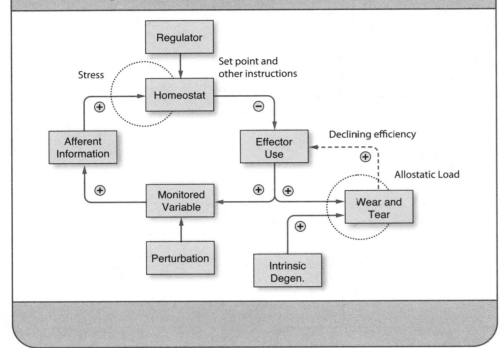

Computer Models of Stress, Allostasis, and Allostatic Load

Computer models can generate predictions about effects of stress and allostatic load on levels of physiological monitored variables (Figure 18-6). By taking into account relatively straightforward principles such as negative feedback regulation, multiple effectors, effector sharing, and homeostat resetting, one can model complex, multisystem disorders.

In the depicted model (in this case of internal temperature), in response to a continuous perturbation, the error signal drives the effector (in this case the furnace), and actions of the effector alter the level of monitored variable in a direction opposite to the perturbation. The model therefore predicts a change in the level of the monitored variable in the direction of the perturbation, with a new apparent steady state attained that depends on the instructions to the effector and the efficiency of the effector. In the home heating model, stress is identical to the error signal driving the furnace. It can be shown

the direction of positive flow, and valve-like flow regulators determining the flow rate (Figure 18-6).

that if the error signal alone drives the furnace, the final inside temperature will be lower than the thermostatic setting, with the difference depending on the outside temperature. Addition of the integrated error signal as a second determinant of furnace heating rate results in the inside temperature reaching the same stable level, regardless of the outside temperature.

In the computer model, allostasis reflects the regulator changing the set point or other components of algorithms for responding. For the same continuous perturbation, the amount of change in effector activation then depends on the change in the error signal, and the change in the error signal in turn depends on the change in the allostatic setting.

Allostatic load in the model reflects long-term effects of allostasis. The amount of wear and tear on the furnace would depend on intrinsic obsolescence and usage history. The usage history depends on the error signal over time. If allostatic load were large enough to decrease the furnace's efficiency, this would set the stage for a positive feedback loop and rapid failure of the system.

Allostatic load links stress with degenerative diseases (Figure 18-7). Activation of effectors to counter threats to **homeostasis** produces wear and tear on the organs determining the level of the monitored variable and on the effectors themselves. Wear and tear, combined with planned obsolescence, decreases effector efficiency. The same perturbation then results in greater wear and tear and further decreases effector efficiency. Eventually, even with the effectors activated continuously, the monitored variable drifts from the allostatic setting. Finally, when the effectors fail, the organism can no longer mount a stress response at all.

PUBLIC HEALTH PERSPECTIVE FOR THE HEALTH OF THE GENERAL POPULATION AND OF HIGH RISK GROUPS

Consider diseases of senescence. Aging-related increases in susceptibilities to cardiovascular, neurological, oncological, and

FIGURE 18-6 Computer Model of a Thermostatic System and Loci of Stress (the Error Signal) and Allostatic Load.

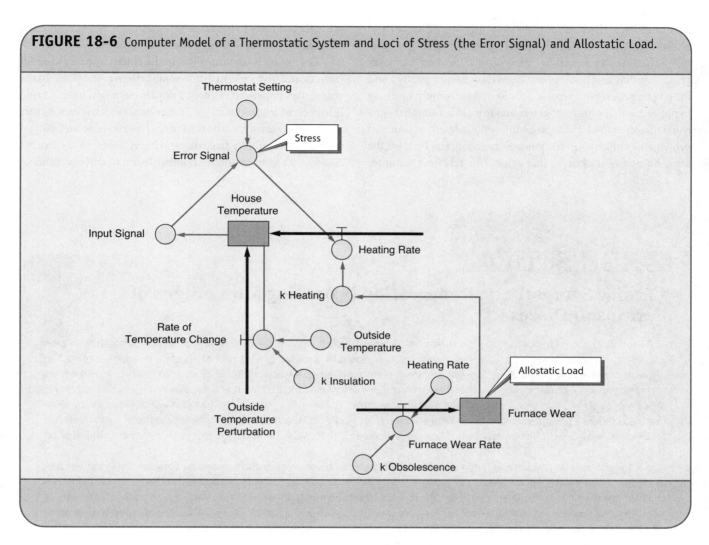

FIGURE 18-7 Model-predicted Affects of Stress and Aging on Allostatic Load on an Individual's Wellness. According to the model, chronic stress can lead to sufficient allostatic load to eventuate in symptomatic disease as an individual ages.

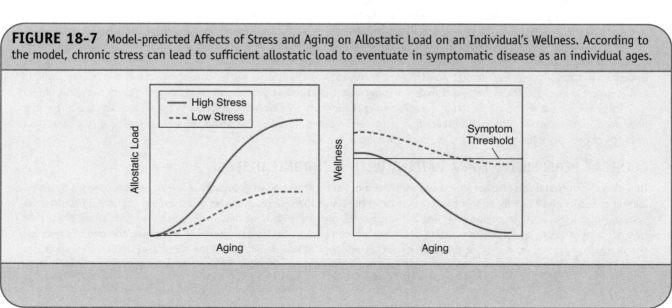

immunological diseases have always limited our lifespan and always will. One may search for rare genetic mutations causing premature degeneration. Alternatively, however, one may recognize that our bodies have been designed to protect and propagate genes, not to live indefinitely. Accordingly, one may hypothesize that groups of genes bias toward accelerated neuronal loss in the elderly because they enhance protection and propagation of genes in the younger reproducers. Perhaps the same homeostatic systems that organisms rely on to counter acute threats early in life cause senescence by the accumulation of toxic by-products of the actions of those systems.

For instance, parkinsonism in the elderly appears to result from cumulative injury to dopamine cells over the years. In the young, this enhanced release of dopamine might enable rapid initiation of locomotion or of other behaviors relevant to survival. Analogously, cardiovascular hypertrophy, and consequently susceptibility to stroke and heart failure in the elderly, could result from prolonged bombardment of adrenoceptors or

CASE STUDY
Cardiac Sympathetic Denervation Preceding Motor Signs of Parkinson Disease

In Parkinson disease (PD), by the time the movement disorder develops, most of the nigrostriatal dopamine terminals have been lost. Identification of biomarkers of PD should improve early diagnosis and spur development of effective treatments. Consistent with early involvement of peripheral autonomic or lower brainstem centers, several studies of *de novo* PD have reported evidence of cardiac noradrenergic denervation or of decreased baroreflex-cardiovagal function. Whether these abnormalities can actually precede symptomatic PD has been unknown. The following describes the case of a patient who had cardiac noradrenergic denervation, detected by 6-[^{18}F]fluorodopamine positron emission tomography (PET), and decreased baroreflex-cardiovagal gain, detected by abnormal beat-to-beat blood pressure and heart rate responses to the Valsalva maneuver, four years before the clinical onset of PD.

A 56-year-old man was referred for possible pheochromocytoma, based on episodic hypertensive episodes and symptoms suggesting excessive catecholamine effects. In July 2001, 6-[^{18}F]fluorodopamine PET scanning and plasma levels of metanephrines excluded pheochromocytoma. Over several months in 2005, the patient noted progressive slowing of movement and inability to relax the arms, small handwriting, decreased facial expression, and decreased voice volume. Neurological consultation noted stooped posture and axial instability, cogwheel rigidity in all four extremities, paucity of spontaneous movements, masked face with infrequent blinking, and monotone voice, but with normal speed of gait and no resting tremor. The patient was diagnosed with mild PD. 6-[^{18}F]fluorodopamine PET revealed severely decreased 6-[^{18}F]fluorodopamine-derived radioactivity throughout the left ventricular myocardium. In retrospect, the scan from 2001 showed the same severely decreased radioactivity.

In this patient, clinical laboratory findings indicated cardiac sympathetic denervation four years before the clinical onset of PD. Considering that in PD loss of cardiac noradrenergic innervation progresses slowly over years, and that the patient already had evidence for markedly decreased cardiac noradrenergic innervation at the time of initial evaluation, loss of cardiac sympathetic nerves probably preceded the movement disorder by many more than the four years between initial testing and the onset of PD.

This case teaches that a clinical laboratory biomarker can identify a pathogenetic process in the presymptomatic phase of a neurodegenerative disease. One might expect that treatment initiated in this phase would be more effective, at less cost, than after the patient develops symptoms and much of the damage has already been done.

CLINICAL PERSPECTIVE FOR A PATIENT WITH A CHRONIC DISEASE

In patients with chronic diseases of almost any sort, the inner world breaks down eventually; a key way this happens is by development of positive feedback loops. Heart failure stimulates the **sympathetic nervous system** and the renin-angiotensin-aldosterone system, which increases fluid retention, growth of heart muscle, and the work of the heart, worsening the heart failure. Chest pain from coronary ischemia evokes **distress**, stimulating the adrenomedullary hormonal system and increasing the rate of consumption of oxygen by the heart, worsening the ischemia. Orthostatic hypotension from failure of the sympathetic nervous system causes lightheadedness, a fall, fracture of a hip, and prolonged bed rest in traction, worsening the orthostatic hypotension when the patient tries to get up. A footballer practicing in full uniform in the heat releases **adrenaline**, which constricts skin blood vessels and augments heat production in the body, producing heat exhaustion, which releases more adrenaline, bringing on heat shock and death. Loss of **dopamine** terminals in the nigrostriatal system in the brain increases pathway traffic to the remaining terminals, accelerating dopamine turnover and thereby production of toxic by-products of dopamine metabolism, increasing the rate of loss of dopamine terminals, eventually manifesting clinically as **Parkinson disease.**

The timing and rapidity of system failure from positive feedback loops depend on dynamic interactions between usage experience of the system and built-in manufacturing and design characteristics. Analogously, in the body, the occurrence, timing, and rapidity of progression of degenerative diseases would depend on interactions between environmental exposures and genetic predispositions. The kinetic model of allostasis and allostatic load provides a nice framework for linking stress, distress, allostatic load, and degenerative diseases.

continuous "rev-ing" of vesicular engines, enhancing adaptive **fight-or-flight** responses in the young at the cost of chronic changes in cardiovascular architecture.

This genetic-evolutionary perspective also leads to therapeutic hypotheses. If chronic production and metabolic breakdown of dopamine led to toxic injury to the cells, then long-term decrease in that breakdown in individuals with a genetically determined high rate could prolong the average useful life of human nervous systems. Analogously, disconnecting genetically determined hyperreactivity of catecholamine systems from chronic cardiovascular hypertrophy could prolong the average useful life of human circulatory systems.

CONCLUSION

As noted earlier, scientific integrative medicine focuses on prevention and treatment in the presymptomatic phase of organ dysfunction. The goal is to prevent positive feedback loops that would cause premature system failure. In general, it is in the pediatric age group that genetic or biochemical testing would have the greatest chance of success in revealing the existence of diseases before symptoms occur. If a patient had a mutation, a typo in the genetic encyclopedia, then correcting that typo with some form of gene therapy might make sense, as in gene therapy for adenine deaminase deficiency. If a patient had absent activity of an important enzyme, replacing that enzyme could work, as in enzyme replacement therapy for Gaucher disease. In a disease such as Menkes disease, prenatal or early neonatal biochemical diagnosis offers the only hope of survival, by initiation of treatment with copper. After the neonatal period, the baby is doomed, with or without the treatment.

For adult medicine, the future of clinical science is neither in molecular genetics nor in integrative pathophysiology but in building bridges between the two. Common, but complex, modern-day diseases will be found to be mainly disorders of regulation, only indirectly related to genetic changes. Most of the genetic contribution to disease in adults will be found

to result not from direct genetic orders but from subtle genetic advice, which has afforded a survival advantage in evolution.

To the end, there is hope. In the presymptomatic, stable phase, there is hope of prevention. In the presymptomatic, unstable phase, there is hope of curative treatment. In the symptomatic, unstable phase, there is hope of alleviating symptoms. Even in the terminal phase, there is hope of allaying anxiety and distress, reducing pain, and offering commiseration.

A person's genes link that person not only with his or her family, and not only with the family of man, but with all things that have ever lived. This surely is a basis for the fascination of genetics. As amazing as is the detail of the genetic instructions revealed by the Human Genome Project, we must now turn to the uses to which those instructions are put by living things to maintain organismic integrity so well for so long. Genes are life's blueprint; ongoing information processing and compensatory adjustments enable life to go on. Scientific integrative medicine focuses on how that processing and those adjustments go awry and on means to predict and prevent premature system failures. Future development of scientific integrative medicine will require redirection of molecular genetics, molecular biology, and integrative physiology to focus on the real first causes of many modern diseases of adults: the loss of "wellness," where both health and disease depend on genetic algorithms determining the development and adaptive regulation of homeostatic systems.

Conducting integrative medical research—especially in patients—is difficult. Studying one drug or one gene is always easier, cheaper, and more conclusive than studying more than one simultaneously. Studying the effects of a single gene knockout for an endogenous substance is always easier, cheaper, and more conclusive than studying the homeostatic systems that use that substance. Nevertheless, studying multiple homeostatic systems that operate in parallel and interact, according to influences of multiple genes, life experiences, drug treatments, and time, offers unique opportunities for early detection of presymptomatic system failure and optimal timing of interventions for prevention, cure, or effective treatment of chronic diseases of adults. Because of the availability of genomic information and computer software for database mining and kinetic modeling, the time seems ripe for development of scientific integrative medicine in research, teaching, and practice.

ACKNOWLEDGMENTS

Reprinted with permission of the Johns Hopkins University Press. From Goldstein, David S., M.D., Ph.D., *Adrenaline and the Inner World: An Introduction to Scientific Integrative Medicine.* pp. 271–291. © 2006 The Johns Hopkins University Press.

Special acknowledgement to Daniel Adam Lyons for contributing Questions and Exercises/Activities.

KEY TERMS

Biology Terms

Adrenaline (Epinephrine): The main hormone released from the adrenal medulla.

Allostasis: A concept according to which organisms maintain stability through change. By analogy, one can keep home temperatures at different but constant levels by changing the thermostat setting.

Allostatic Load: A concept according to which prolonged activation of effectors involved in allostasis contributes to wear and tear. This idea provides a basis for studying the long-term health consequences of stress.

Distress: A form of stress that is consciously experienced in which the individual senses an inability to cope, attempts to avoid or escape the situation, elicits instinctively communicated signs, and has activation of the adrenal gland.

Dopamine: One of the body's three catecholamines. Dopamine is converted to norepinephrine and norepinephrine to adrenaline.

Fight-or-Flight: A phrase coined by Walter Cannon that refers to the adrenaline-mediated response the body produces when confronted with an external stress that threatens homeostasis. Although Cannon believed the "fight" and "flight" responses to be physiologically identical, further research has proven there are significant differences between them.

Homeostat: A physiological comparator, analogous to a thermostat, that senses discrepancy between a setting and information about a monitored variable, the discrepancy leading to changes in activities of effectors that tend to reduce the discrepancy.

Homeostasis: State of equilibrium of the internal environment of the body that is maintained by dynamic processes of feedback and regulation. Homeostasis is a dynamic equilibrium.

Negative Feedback: A way in which homeostatic systems keep levels of monitored variables stable. If the sensed level is too high, the system directs changes in effectors that bring the level down; if the sensed level is too low, the system directs changes bringing the level up.

Parkinson Disease: A progressive nervous system disease that produces slow movements, a form of limb rigidity called "cogwheel rigidity," and a "pill-roll" tremor that is present when the patient is at rest and decreases with intentional movement. Other features of Parkinson disease include a masklike facial expression, stooped posture, difficulty initiating or stopping movements, small handwriting, and improvement of the movement disorder by treatment with levodopa.

Stress: A condition in which the organism senses a challenge to physical or mental stability that leads to altered activities of body systems to meet that challenge.

Sympathetic Nervous System: One of the main components of the autonomic nervous system, responsible for many "automatic" functions such as constriction of blood vessels when a person stands up.

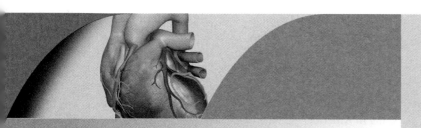

Questions for Further Research, Study, Reflection, and Discussion

For the Individual Student

In order to answer these questions, it may be necessary to research the primary literature.

- Within the text, there are several examples of ways in which positive feedback loops might be able to rapidly increase the severity of a medical situation. For example, the adrenaline produced by an overheated football player can lead to heat shock and possibly death. What other examples, outside of the text, can you find that may illustrate positive feedback loops and the rapid effects they bring about?

- The concept of allostatic load can link stress with degenerative diseases. Find and explain examples outside of this text that may correlate chronic stress levels with disease.

For Small Group Discussion

- Cardiovascular hypertrophy could result from prolonged bombardment of adrenoceptors, enhancing adaptive fight-or-flight responses in the young at the cost of chronic changes in cardiovascular architecture. What therapeutic hypotheses are available to curtail this damage and prolong the average life of human circulatory systems?

- How could the identification of biomarkers of Parkinson disease improve early diagnosis and spur development of effective treatments?

- In the case study, what early symptoms and warning signs preceded the eventual diagnosis of mild Parkinson disease?

- What does the case study teach about clinical laboratory biomarkers?

- How would treatment in the presymptomatic stages of the patient's disease progression be beneficial to both patient and caregiver?

- What role, if any, could scientific integrative medicine play in the case study?

For Entire Class Discussion

- In what ways do you believe scientific integrative medicine will impact the traditional practice of medicine in the United States, if at all?

- How will the availability of genomic information from the Human Genome Project, as well as emerging computer software for kinetic modeling, impact the advancement of scientific integrative medicine?

EXERCISES/ACTIVITIES

1. Within your group, create an argument either for or against increasing the prevalence of scientific integrative medicine into the medical school curriculum and in the clinical setting. Depending on your group's viewpoint, present to the class how scientific integrative medicine could revolutionize the way that doctor's practice medicine or, conversely, how its benefits are still speculative.

2. After reading about the effects of positive feedback loops and how they can hasten the degeneration of an individual's health, imagine that you are a doctor in a hospital and have just diagnosed a patient with type 2 diabetes. The patient adamantly refuses any type of future treatment. Describe the possible feedback loops that could arise from the diabetes if the patient does not accept treatment.

ACKNOWLEDGMENTS

Special acknowledgement to Daniel Adam Lyons for contributing Questions and Exercises/Activities.

RESOURCES

Goldstein DS. *Adrenaline and the Inner World: An Introduction to Scientific Integrative Medicine.* Baltimore: The Johns Hopkins University Press; 2006.

Goldstein DS. *Stress, Catecholamines, and Cardiovascular Disease.* New York: Oxford University Press; 1995.

Goldstein DS. *The Autonomic Nervous System in Health and Disease.* New York: Marcel Dekker, Inc.; 2001.

High Performance Systems, Inc. *An Introduction to Systems Thinking.* Hanover, NH; 1993.

CROSS REFERENCES

Aging in America
Chapters on Chronic Diseases

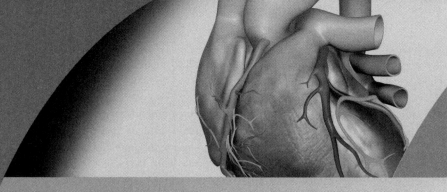

CHAPTER 19

Cancer Prevention from a Biologist's Perspective

Jackie A. Lavigne
Stephen D. Hursting

In 2007, it is estimated that there will be close to 560,000 cases of cancer diagnosed in the U.S. Cancer is therefore poised, for the first time, to overtake heart disease as the number one cause of death in America.

American Cancer Society[1]

LEARNING OBJECTIVES

By the end of this chapter, the student will be able to:

- Describe cancer and cancer development from the perspective of what is known about the biology of cancer.
- Illustrate and explain the multistage **carcinogenesis** model of cancer.
- Describe some of the targets of cancer prevention with respect to this model.
- Explain how diet and obesity are emerging as major public health challenges due to the associated increased risk of numerous chronic diseases, including cancer, in overweight and obese individuals.
- Illustrate how emerging technologies are being used in laboratory animals to provide insight into places along the carcinogenesis pathway that may serve as potential targets for preventing cancer in at-risk individuals.

HISTORY

Cancer prevention research historically has been focused on reducing the incidence or mortality from cancer. More recently, however, as we learn more about the cancer process, it has become clear that prevention can also occur via the delay of cancer development. As presented below, cancer development, or *carcinogenesis*, is a multistage process, and thus, delaying or

blocking one or more steps in this process could contribute to cancer prevention. As cancer generally takes years to develop, opportunities for cancer prevention exist as early as in utero and usually continue throughout the life course. Recently, a newly emerging public health challenge, overweight and obesity in both children and adults, is stimulating new research into the area of cancer prevention as it has become evident that overweight and obese individuals are at an increased risk of developing tumors in multiple organ systems.

BASIC SCIENCE FACTS/KEY CONCEPTS REVIEW

What Is Cancer?

Cancer is currently poised to overtake heart disease as the number one cause of death in America. It is estimated that there will be close to 560,000 new cases diagnosed in 2007.[1] The good news is that, overall, cancer deaths have been declining for the past several years in the United States, perhaps in part due to the application of tools developed from recent advances in our knowledge about cancer. However, despite this good news, as the U.S. population ages, cancer diagnoses will likely continue to rise, and this complex disease will continue to challenge our research establishment and tax the resources of our healthcare system.

Webster's dictionary defines cancer as: "a **malignant** tumor of potentially unlimited growth that expands locally by invasion and systemically by metastasis."[2] In this view, cancer is defined by its ability to grow indefinitely and propagate itself in other areas of the body by sending out malignant cells from the original mass using the body's vascular system. These aspects of cancer are certainly critical to its description but only broadly define a highly complex process.

Others have come to view cancer as more of an evolutionary problem.[3] In this scenario, cancer begins with a heterogeneous population of mutant clones. These clones are cells that have acquired some mutation(s) in their DNA, and they are able to divide and pass on their mutation(s) to their progeny, which is similar to evolution at the organismal level where mutations already existing in the egg or sperm of any individual can be passed on to his or her progeny. Again, similar to evolution at the organismal level, inheritance of variant mutant genes can influence survival and reproduction rates of the mutant clones' cellular "offspring." Importantly, this passing on of mutant genes occurs in the context of limited resources in the body; thus, mutations continue to occur that will give the growing mass of cells an advantage over other cells in gathering these resources and in continuing to grow. The end result is that tumor evolution is working against us in our efforts to treat cancer as the mass of cells constantly evolves and is never really a fixed target.

In addition to what is described above, cancer biologists also generally take into account the known molecular details of the cancer cell when defining cancer so that the targets for treating and/or preventing cancer become evident. Many have chosen to depict cancer via a structural framework that describes cancer as developing in a stepwise manner over time and that incorporates specific changes required by the growing mass to continue growing. This cancer growth continuum divides the cancer into three stages, referred to as **initiation, promotion** and **progression,** and has come to be known as multistage carcinogenesis (Figure 19-1).[4–6] Though the multistage carcinogenesis framework itself continues to evolve and is open to differential interpretation, it is very useful for describing general concepts of carcinogenesis and targets for cancer prevention.

Ultimately, regardless of how cancer is defined, the end result is that tumors are heterogeneous masses of cells, and each tumor can have unique profiles of mutations. Tumors can arise from both inherited and spontaneous mutations, and the latter can result from **endogenous** and/or **exogenous** exposures to chemicals (natural and industrial), infectious agents, and radiation among other things. With this and the above descriptions of cancer in mind, we asked: what are the targets along the multistage carcinogenesis pathway for cancer prevention and what is the role of diet, and especially calorie intake, in carcinogenesis? However, before delving into these questions, we begin with a brief review of the multistage carcinogenesis framework.

Multistage Carcinogenesis: Overview

The model for multistage carcinogenesis has undergone much revision over the last four decades as scientists have learned and incorporated information about the genetic basis for cancer, but, as presented in Figure 19-1, the multi-step nature of the process is still the basis for our understanding of how cells go from normal to **neoplastic.** Tumor initiation begins after a cell has divided and incorporated DNA damage resulting from spontaneous or carcinogen-induced genetic or **epigenetic** alterations.[7,8] As mentioned earlier, mutations also may be inherited from a germ cell; thus, a cell may already be "initiated" and at increased risk for becoming a tumor cell from birth.

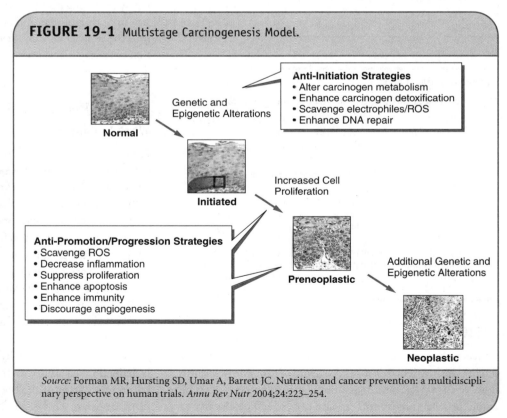

FIGURE 19-1 Multistage Carcinogenesis Model.

Normal

Genetic and Epigenetic Alterations

Anti-Initiation Strategies
• Alter carcinogen metabolism
• Enhance carcinogen detoxification
• Scavenge electrophiles/ROS
• Enhance DNA repair

Initiated

Increased Cell Proliferation

Anti-Promotion/Progression Strategies
• Scavenge ROS
• Decrease inflammation
• Suppress proliferation
• Enhance apoptosis
• Enhance immunity
• Discourage angiogenesis

Preneoplastic

Additional Genetic and Epigenetic Alterations

Neoplastic

Source: Forman MR, Hursting SD, Umar A, Barrett JC. Nutrition and cancer prevention: a multidisciplinary perspective on human trials. *Annu Rev Nutr* 2004;24:223–254.

The incorporated DNA damage then must have an impact on what is occurring at the RNA and/or protein level of the cell, either by changing the expression of genes or the actions or quantities of their resulting proteins. These changes must then modify cellular behavior such that the cell has a growth advantage relative to normal cells. The subsequent tumor promotion stage is characterized by clonal expansion of the initiated cell caused by hyperproliferation, altered programmed cell death (**apoptosis**), tissue remodeling, and/or increased inflammation.[9,10] Finally, during the tumor progression stage, preneoplastic cells develop into neoplastic, invasive tumors through further expansion associated with the accumulation of additional alterations in the genome caused by progressive genomic instability.[11] Within this framework, intervention to prevent cancer can occur at multiple places and can occur via a variety of mechanisms. Several of these are discussed below.

Multistage Carcinogenesis and Targets for Prevention

Two Strategies

We present the two major approaches for cancer prevention in the context of the multi-stage carcinogenesis pathway: anti-initiation and anti-promotion/progression strategies.[4,7] Much has been learned about various events and processes that can contribute to initiation, promotion, and progression of cancer, and these inform us about potential places where prevention interventions may have an impact. As cancer is a very complex disease, the discussion below aims to cover several potential prevention strategies but is not meant to be completely comprehensive.

Anti-Initiation

Anti-initiation strategies include the following: alteration of **carcinogen** metabolism and detoxification; scavenging of **electrophiles** and **free radicals** such as some of the reactive oxygen species; and enhancement of DNA repair.[7] These processes are all linked, but they can be treated somewhat separately given the different genes/proteins involved. With regards to carcinogens and their metabolism and detoxification, we are all exposed to carcinogens (cancer-causing agents) primarily from our diet and environment. Carcinogens entering our bodies from our diet and/or environment, or sometimes produced within our bodies through the course of normal metabolism, are typically further metabolized by what are referred to as phase I and phase II enzymes in order to enhance excretion.[12] The aim of phase I metabolism is to oxidize the carcinogen, which often results in the activation of that compound to a very reactive state. This reactive molecule often has the capability of damaging cellular molecules such as DNA, RNA, or proteins. DNA damage in the form of **adducts** can cause mutations that potentially contribute to carcinogenesis. On the other hand, the role of phase II metabolism is to conjugate and excrete the activated compound. Conjugation is simply the process of attaching the activated compound to another molecule in order to give rise to a larger, deactivated (in most cases) molecule that can then easily be excreted via one of the excretion systems (e.g., urine, feces, etc.). Phase I metabolism is primarily accomplished by the cytochrome P450 enzyme system, and phase II metabolism is primarily accomplished by a smaller number of phase II enzymes, including glutathione-S-transferases, sulfotransferases, UDP-glucuronosyltransferases, methylases, N-acetyl-transferases, and quinone reductase.

Logically then, two prevention strategies that target this process are: 1) reducing the activation of dangerous carcinogens by decreasing transcription, translation or activity of phase I enzymes; and 2) increasing the deactivation of dangerous carcinogens by increasing the transcription, translation, or activity of phase II enzymes. Both are achieved by sulforaphane, a compound found in broccoli, radishes, and other cruciferous vegetables.[13] Among other things, this compound can inhibit some phase I enzyme **isozymes** and increase the phase II enzymes glutathione-S-transferase and quinone reductase. These activities are then thought to contribute to the cancer preventive properties ascribed to eating cruciferous vegetables.

The removal of DNA-reactive electrophiles or free radicals is another anti-initiation strategy. These molecules are highly reactive due to either an electron deficiency (electrophiles) or an unpaired electron (free radicals) and can come from exogenous exposures or be produced endogenously from normal processes such as phase I metabolism (see above) and respiration. Respiration produces several reactive oxygen species (ROS) that are either electrophiles or free radicals. These two types of highly reactive molecules can damage macromolecules like DNA, and ROS can induce cell signaling pathways, modulate gene expression, and/or suppress immune competence.[7] Our bodies have enzymes responsible for reacting with, or "scavenging," and therefore decreasing both electrophiles and free radicals, and increasing the levels of these enzymes is another prevention strategy. Examples of the enzymes include the phase II enzymes mentioned above and superoxide dismutase, catalase, and glutathione peroxidase.[14] Alternatively, nonenzymatic antioxidants available from many dietary sources, especially fruits and vegetables, also potentially contribute to cancer prevention by scavenging and reducing the number of reactive species.

Though molecules activated by the cytochrome P450 system, reactive electrophiles, and other reactive species have the ability to damage DNA, the body has evolved systems to repair the damage to DNA, because faithful maintenance of genomic stability and integrity is important to keeping a cell alive, performing its necessary functions, and avoiding diseases such as cancer. Some examples of endogenous and exogenous factors that induce DNA damage are mentioned above, but they also include ultraviolet light, ionizing radiation, cigarette smoke, and many dietary factors. There are three major types of DNA repair pathways and each has a specific role in repairing the various types of DNA damage that our cells encounter.[15] These include: the homologous recombinational and non-homologous end joining repair pathway; the nucleotide excision repair pathway; and the mismatch repair pathway. These pathways and the types of DNA repair for which they are responsible will not be presented in depth here, but one important point bears mentioning. Each pathway is made up of multiple enzymes and, once again, a potential means of preventing cancer is maintaining, or possibly increasing, the levels of these enzymes.

Anti-Promotion/Anti-Progression

In addition to the anti-initiation strategies presented thus far, several anti-promotion/anti-progression strategies bear mentioning. They include, among others, scavenging electrophiles and ROS, decreasing inflammation, suppressing proliferation, enhancing apoptosis, and decreasing **angiogenesis** (or the process of creating new blood vessels).[4,7] The first in the list, the scavenging of electrophiles and ROS, was described earlier and is mentioned again here as these highly reactive molecules can contribute to heritable DNA damage along the entire multistage carcinogenesis pathway, and ultimately be involved in the genomic instability that characterizes neoplastic cells. ROS also can serve as cell signaling molecules that can influence pathways regulating cell proliferation and survival.[16] Next in the list is decreasing inflammation. Inflammation has been described by many as a double-edged sword; it is required by our bodies to kill invading **pathogens** and remove damaged cells and tissue, but it also can cause tissue damage and scarring and contribute to cancer.[17,18] Chronic inflammation, which itself results in the generation of a variety of free radicals, is thought to result in a cycle of cell death and replacement by proliferation of remaining cells. The evidence that inflammation contributes to cancer comes from a host of diseases in which an inflammatory condition of a particular organ has been associated with increased risk of developing cancer in that organ. For example, individuals with ulcerative colitis, pancreatitis, and gastritis are at increased risk for colorectal, pancreatic, and stomach cancer,

respectively. Chronic skin irritation also has long been known to increase the risk of developing skin cancer. There are many mediators of inflammation in our bodies, and one well-studied example is arachidonic acid and its metabolic products prostaglandins.[19] Prostaglandins are generated from arachidonic acid by two enzymes known as cyclooxygenase-1 and -2. These enzymes have become the targets of many cancer prevention studies, as they can be inhibited by nonsteroidal anti-inflammatory drugs, like aspirin, which have been shown to decrease colorectal cancer risk in individuals at increased risk for this type of cancer. Though the role of inflammation in cancer has been most closely studied in colon cancer, it is thought that decreasing inflammation or certain mediators of the inflammatory process could potentially decrease the risk of many other types of cancer.

Cells in our bodies that are not terminally differentiated have the ability to divide, and this ability can be exploited to contribute to promotion and progression of cancer cells. Though cell division is an important component of carcinogenesis, normal cell division is critical at the cellular, tissue, and organismal levels and can be contributed to by many sources, including hormones and growth factors. Hormones are responsible for such processes as reproduction, growth and development, energy production and utilization, and maintenance of our internal environment. Growth factors, such as insulin-like growth factor-1 (IGF-1), contribute to normal growth and development and processes such as apoptosis.[20] However, steroid hormones like estrogen and growth factors like IGF-I can act alone or in concert to lead to cell proliferation with the potential for subsequent increased cell survival and cancer development. Therefore, minimizing the generation of or decreasing existing levels of these compounds also could contribute to cancer prevention. In addition, there has been much focus on developing drugs that prevent the interaction of hormones and/or growth factors with the cellular receptors through which many of their biological activities occur. One example is the development of tamoxifen, which has been shown to inhibit the binding of estrogen to its receptor in breast tissue and reduce the risk of breast cancer.[21]

Cell division of course can be stopped if a cell senesces or dies, but the complex processes by which cells stop dividing or die via necrosis or apoptosis[22] will not be discussed here. Additionally, a developing tumor requires a large supply of oxygen and nutrients to grow and therefore exploits the normal process by which new blood vessels form (angiogenesis) to develop its own blood supply.[23] Again, this process will not be addressed here. The reader is encouraged to learn about these important processes from the extensive literature that is available for each topic.

Diet and Obesity as Emerging Issues for Cancer Prevention

The contribution of diet to carcinogenesis has long been of interest to scientists involved in cancer prevention research. A variety of dietary compounds are known carcinogens and are thus targets for minimizing exposure or impact, if possible, to prevent cancer. On the other hand, other dietary compounds have been shown to possibly decrease the risk of cancer (sulforaphane, described above) and have therefore been the targets of intense research to understand how they can best be used to prevent cancer. Studies in animals also have long shown that the simple consumption of excess calories through the diet, leading to overweight and obesity, increases the risk of cancer, and, conversely, limiting calorie intake decreases the risk of cancer compared to overweight controls that consume calories freely [ad libitum (AL)].[24] Animal models have proved useful in the analysis of associ-

ations between energy intake and carcinogenesis, and the early studies of this relationship have been followed up in many animal models of cancer, both induced and naturally occurring, and at many different tissue sites. The findings from these studies consistently demonstrate that animals who receive fewer calories (20%–40% fewer) as compared to AL controls have a dramatically decreased risk of cancer (Tables 19-1 and 19-2).[24–26] Importantly, the groups for which calories are reduced continue to grow and thrive because they are provided with a diet that affords complete nutrition and does not allow the animals to become malnourished. Understanding the relationship between reduced calorie intake and cancer prevention therefore may provide insights into how to prevent cancer at a variety of tumor sites, regardless of the root cause.

Recently, the study of excess caloric intake by humans has become a major focus of public health interest. The prevalence of obesity has risen steadily for the past several decades in the United States, and, currently, almost two thirds of American adults are considered overweight (defined as having a **body mass**

TABLE 19-1 The Effect of Dietary Restriction on the Incidence of Spontaneous Tumors in Mice

Tumor Type	Animal Model	% DR	Relative Tumor Incidence[a]	Reference
Mammary	dba mice	33	44.0	[3]
	Wistar rats	20	5.0	[103]
	H:NMRI mice	20	2.3	[104]
	C3H mice	33	44.0	[5]
	Swiss mice	20	7.0	[103]
	Swiss mice	25	4.0	[105]
Lung adenoma	ABC mice	33	2.0	[3]
	Swiss mice	33	6.0	[4]
	Swiss mice	25	3.5	[105]
	Strain A mice	20	1.6	[106]
Leukemia	AKR mice	25	6.5	[6]
Dermis	Wistar rats	20	6.0	[103]
Pituitary	Wistar rats	20	1.7	[103]
	SD rats	30	5.0	[107]
	Swiss mice	20	7.0	[103]
	H:NMRI mice	20	4.1	[104]
Pancreas	SD rats	30	4.0	[107]
Testes	F344 rats	40	1.7	[108]

[a]Ratio of tumor incidence in *ad libitum* animals/diet restricted animals.

Source: Reprinted from Mutation Research, 443 (1–2): Hursting SD, Kari FW, The anti-carcinogenic effects of dietary restriction: mechanisms and future directions, 235–249. Jul 15 1999, with permission from Elsevier.

TABLE 19-2 The Effect of Dietary Restrictions on the Incidence of Experimentally Induced Tumors in Mice, Rats, and Hamsters.

Tumor Type/Induction	Animal Model	Route of Exposure	% DR	Relative Tumor Incidence[a]	Reference
Chemically induced					
Skin	ABC mice	BP skin paint	33	2.3	[3]
	C57 BL mice	BP injection	20	1.5	[3]
	DBA/2 mice	BP skin paint	40	3.0	[4]
	C57BL mice	BP skin paint	40	1.7	[4]
Intestinal	SD rats	MAM injection	25	4.5	[10]
Mammary	SD rats	DMBA injection	50	4.8	[109]
	F344 rats	DMBA injection	16	10.4	[8]
Liver	Swiss mice	DEN injection	30	> 100.0	[9]
Cheek pouch	Hamster	DMBA injection	25	3.9	[7]
Physically induced					
Skin	C57 mice	UV light	30	12.4	[110]
Mammary	SD rats	X-ray	66	3.3	[111]
Leukemia	SD rats	g-radiation	50	17.0	[112]

[a] Ratio of tumor incidence in *ad libitum* animals/diet-restricted animals.

Source: Reprinted from Mutation Research, 443(1–2): Hursting SD, Kari FW, The anti-carcinogenic effects of dietary restriction: mechanism and future directions, 235–249, Jul 15 1999, with permission from Elsevier.

index [**BMI**= weight in kg/height in m^2] $\geq 25 \text{ kg/m}^2$) and approximately half of the **overweight** individuals (~30% of all Americans) are classified as **obese** (defined as having a BMI $\geq 30 \text{ kg/m}^2$) according to definitions put forth by the U.S. Department of Agriculture.[27] Obesity has been steadily on the rise in the United States since the late 1980s, and it is commonly believed that it has now reached epidemic proportions. Particularly alarming are the increasing rates of obesity among children and adolescents, portending further increases in the rates of adult obesity and obesity-related illnesses. The underlying cause of the obesity epidemic is thought to be a combination of excess caloric intake and insufficient physical activity.[28]

In 2003, Calle et al.[29] published data from a large prospective cohort study of men and women that provided strong evidence for a connection between obesity and increased mortality from most forms of cancer. This study illustrated that, as compared to normal weight controls, as BMI increased, so did cancer risk. Considering the wide spectrum of cancers associated with overweight and/or obesity in this study—by far the largest prospective cohort study to date of the association between weight and cancer—these findings suggest that a broadreaching biological mechanism underlies the relationship between excess calorie intake and carcinogenesis, and certainly support the findings in the large number of animal studies done to date.

Studying the Role of Diet and Obesity in Cancer Development

Despite the interesting findings described above and the reproducibility and breadth of the beneficial anti-cancer and other anti-aging effects of limiting energy intake, the underlying biological mechanisms of the energy balance–cancer relationship are not well understood. Some attempts have been made to describe what is known about how the cancer processes can be inhibited at multiple points by energy restriction,[30] but further research is urgently needed to fill in the gaps in our understanding and facilitate the development of new cancer prevention strategies. The recent availability of several new technologies holds the promise of providing new insights into the calorie intake–cancer relationship. These technologies include new animal models of cancer and genetic and protein array technologies that provide information on thousands of targets that are being affected by calorie intake at a single time, targets that may be exploitable for cancer prevention in overweight and obese individuals.

CASE STUDY

Targets for Prevention Emerging from Animal Studies in Diet and Obesity

Two groups of female laboratory mice are put on specific diets. One group is allowed to eat freely (*ad libitum* [AL]), and the other is allowed only 70% of what the AL animals eat on average (30% calorie restricted [CR]). After four weeks of these dietary interventions, the two groups are seen to be different with respect to overall weight. After eight weeks of the interventions, the animals are sacrificed and their livers harvested. Gene expression studies are done on the livers of the animals using RNA **microarrays** that assess the expression of 12,000 genes, and many genes are found to have changed in the CR group relative to the AL group (Table 19-3).

TABLE 19-3 Hepatic Gene Expression Changes in 30% Calorie Restricted Versus Ad Libitum-Fed Mice

Biological Process	Genes Upregulated	Genes Downregulated
Xenobiotic Metabolism	Gst alpha; Gst tau	CYP450s
Other Metabolism	Cytosolic acyl-CoA thioesterase	Fatty acid elongation enzyme
ROS Detoxification	Metallothionein 1 and Metallothionein 2	
Estrogen Metabolism	Sulfotransferase	Hydroxysteroid dehydrogenase 17 beta 2
Insulin-Like Growth Factor-1 (IGF-1) Pathway	IGF Binding Protein 1	IGF-1
Receptor Tyrosine Kinases		Epidermal Growth Factor Receptor; Leukemia Inhibitory Factor Receptor

Source: Data are from Lavigne et al., unpublished.

SCIENTIFIC PERSPECTIVE AND ISSUES

Though CR has been shown in many models of cancer to reduce tumor number and/or size and to delay cancer development, the case study was done without a cancer endpoint. However, because cancer takes some time to develop as described earlier in the multistage carcinogenesis model, changes that reduce the risk of cancer should likely be occurring before there are any signs of cancer. Given the cancer prevention

Exhibit 19-1

Key Unanswered Questions

A. Does reversal of obesity through diet, exercise, or pharmacologic regimens decrease cancer risk or impact existing cancers?

B. Are there important differences between anti-obesity regimens (caloric restriction, exercise, drugs) in terms of anti-cancer effects, or is weight reduction/maintenance the key irrespective of the means?

C. Which, if any, of the hormonal changes (such as IGF-1, insulin, leptin, sex steroids) or biosystem changes (such as weight, adiposity, insulin resistance, inflammation, alterations in energy metabolism) accompanying energy imbalance are causally linked to carcinogenesis?

D. Can specific inhibitors of the IGF/insulin/Akt signaling pathway (such as rapamycin and its newer derivatives), of the leptin/JAK/STAT signaling pathway (such as STAT3 inhibitors), or of the inflammatory cascade disrupt the link between obesity and cancer in the absence of weight loss, which for many individuals is very difficult?

E. What is the impact of different energy balance states and their associated effects on physiology (i.e., lean vs. obese; insulin resistant vs. insulin sensitive; high vs. low postmenopausal estrogen levels) on the response to cancer prevention or cancer therapy regimens?

strategies described in this chapter, the gene expression changes seen are in line with what one might expect if cancer risk were to be decreased. They include changes in transcripts encoding phase I and II enzymes that metabolize **xenobiotics** and estrogen and changes in transcription of other metabolic enzymes, genes involved in growth factor signaling, and genes that play a role in ROS generation (Table 19-3).

To date, no microarray studies of CR or exercise in the context of cancer have been reported. Weindruch, Prolla, and colleagues as well as Spindler, Dhahbi, and coworkers were among the first to use microarray technology to investigate the anti-aging effects of CR in mice.[31–34] A recent review by Han and Hickey of the nearly 25 reports of microarray analyses in various organisms that included some aspect of CR in their work suggests that no specific genes were altered in common across all the studies, possibly due to differences in microarray platform, species/strain, and tissue differences, etc.[35] However, consistent with the arguments put forth in this review, several functional categories of genes universally emerge as responsive to the negative energy balance associated with CR, particularly energy metabolism (including components of the IGF and insulin signaling pathways), stress responses (such as heat shock and oxidative), and inflammation pathways.

Although the *associations* between overweight/obesity and several cancers are becoming well defined, the *causal relationships* between energy balance, hormones, and other biological mediators and cancer risk are still not well established and are therefore an area of continuing active research. As discussed above and illustrated in Figure 19-1, the components of several interacting pathways associated with carcinogenesis are likely altered by perturbations in energy balance, such as physical activity and CR. One approach to deciphering the complex network of mediators underlying the energy balance and cancer link is to incorporate genomic (such as the array studies described above), proteomic, and metabolomic analyses into studies of some of the key unanswered questions in this area of research (Exhibit 19-1). Progress in understanding the relationship between diet and cancer will certainly require a mul-

tidisciplinary approach, and these and other key questions will only be answered through well-designed studies in both animals and humans that incorporate molecular, genetic, and metabolic/nutritional tools and expertise.

PUBLIC HEALTH PERSPECTIVE

As the prevalence of obesity and overweight continues to rise worldwide, the search for strategies to prevent the associated diseases and healthcare costs will become ever more urgent. Finding the mechanistic targets that link calorie intake and diseases such as cancer is therefore an important strategy for avoiding the disastrous public health impact that will occur as the number of overweight and obese individuals continues to rise. This fact has been recognized by the United State's largest research establishment, the **National Institutes of Health (NIH)**. In 2003, NIH director Elias Zerhouni, who was also aware that obesity impacts numerous human diseases, established the NIH Obesity Research Task Force part of an overall effort to accelerate progress in obesity research across the NIH's many institutes. The task force was charged with the development of a Strategic Plan for NIH Obesity Research, the result of which was published in 2004 (available at http://obesityresearch.nih.gov/About/strategic-plan.htm. Accessed April 10, 2008). The document lays out a dynamic plan for guiding coordinated research on obesity and various diseases across the NIH.

We already know several mechanisms by which interventions, including obesity prevention, may contribute to cancer prevention. They can: a) reduce the mutation and/or proliferation rate of cells; b) reduce the ability of tumor cells to multiply and gather limited resources from the host; and/or c) result in increased death of tumor cells. However, truly achieving cancer prevention in human populations will require a transdisciplinary approach combining findings from animal, molecular and cellular, clinical/epidemiological, and behavioral studies to identify the best possible ways to prevent or delay cancer onset in humans and ensure that they are effectively translated into strategies for human health promotion.

KEY TERMS

Biology/Science Terms

Adduct: A new chemical species AB, each molecular entity of which is formed by direct combination of two separate molecular entities A and B in such a way that there is change in connectivity, but no loss, of atoms within the moieties A and B.

Angiogenesis: Blood vessel formation. Tumor angiogenesis is the growth of blood vessels from surrounding tissue to a solid tumor. This is caused by the release of chemicals by the tumor.

Apoptosis: Programmed cell death ("cell suicide"); a form of cell death in which a controlled sequence of events (or program) leads to the elimination of cells without releasing harmful substances into the surrounding area.

Carcinogen: Material that causes cancer in humans, or, because it causes cancer in animals, is considered capable of causing cancer in humans.

Carcinogenesis: The generation of cancer from normal cells; correctly, the formation of a carcinoma, but often used synonymously with transformation or tumorigenesis.

Electrophile: An atom, molecule, or ion able to accept an electron pair.

Endogenous: Developing or originating within the organisms or arising from causes within the organism.

Epigenetic: Refers to the state of the DNA with respect to heritable changes in function without a change in the nucleotide sequence. Epigenetic changes can be caused by modification of the DNA, such as by methylation.

Exogenous: Produced outside of, originating from, or due to external causes.

Free Radical: A highly chemically reactive atom, molecule, or molecular fragment with a free or unpaired electron. Free radicals are produced in many different ways such as normal metabolic processes and UV radiation from the sun. Free radicals have been implicated in aging, cancer, cardiovascular disease, and other kinds of damage to the body.

Initiation: Preneoplastic change in the genetic material of a cell.

Isozyme: Multiple forms of an enzyme that catalyze the same reaction but whose synthesis is controlled by more than one gene.

Malignant: Refers to cells or tumors growing in an uncontrolled fashion. Such growths may spread to and disrupt nearby normal tissue, or reach distant sites via the bloodstream.

Microarray: A technology using a high-density array of nucleic acids, protein, or tissue for examining complex biological interactions simultaneously, which are identified by specific location on a slide array.

Neoplastic: Characterized by the presence of new and uncontrolled cellular growth.

Pathogen: An organism that causes disease in another organism.

Progression: The process by which a growing mass of initiated cells undergoes qualitative changes, potentially including a transition from benign to malignant behavior. The process is characterized by the accumulation of new genetic changes in and continued expansion of the tumor.

Promotion: The process by which an initiated cell develops into an overt neoplasm; characterized by proliferation under permissive host conditions.

Xenobiotic: Chemical substances that are foreign to the biological system. They include naturally occurring compounds, drugs, environmental agents, carcinogens, insecticides, etc.

Public Health Terms

Body Mass Index (BMI): Weight in kilograms divided by height in meters squared (kg/m^2).

National Institutes of Health (NIH): Federal agency responsible for overseeing government-sponsored biomedical research. It is divided into 27 institutes and research centers (NIH Web site available at http://www.nih.gov. Accessed April 10, 2008).

Obese: Having a BMI $\geq$ 30 kg/m^2.

Overweight: Having a BMI $\geq$ 25 kg/m^2.

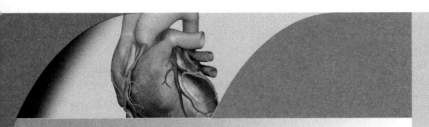

Questions for Further Research, Study, Reflection, and Discussion

For the Individual Student

In order to answer these questions, it may be necessary to research the primary literature.

- What role will the genes listed in Table 19-3 have in cancer prevention by calorie restriction? Do you see any as potential targets for drug development for future studies in humans?

- What cancers are linked to both obesity and hormone exposure? How would you treat a patient who was both obese and at risk for a steroidal hormone-associated cancer due to a strong family history? What aspect of their profile, family history or obesity, do you think would have the strongest impact on their cancer risk and why?

- Exercise is another way to decrease the risk of obesity. What is the animal evidence that exercise interventions reduce the risk of cancer? Is it as strong as the evidence that CR reduces cancer risk?

For Small Group Discussion

- Do you think that the impact of CR seen on liver gene expression would be the same in other tissues such as breast and colon? Why or why not?

- What are some of the aspects of the animal diet that must be considered when designing such a study? How would these translate to a human intervention if a similar study were designed for an adult population (if a sample of tissue could be obtained for gene expression analysis in humans)? Would this study be much more complicated to do in humans (even if you could easily obtain a sample of liver tissue)?

- The study described above was done in animals that had just reached reproductive age. If CR has

an impact on cancer risk, at what age(s) do you think that starting CR no longer has any effect? Do you think that calorie restricting a mother will have an impact on her unborn offspring's cancer risk?

For Entire Class Discussion

- Discuss key unanswered questions A and B listed above. What are your hypothesized answers? Can you design a human study that would address questions A and B? What markers would you measure?

- If you were responsible for trying to impact obesity in the United States, how would you begin to address the problem? What would be your first target group and why? How do you think this target group could best be reached?

- Individuals who might try to get the public to eat less battle a heavily funded food industry that benefits financially if the U.S. population eats more. What regulations do you think would be fair to put in place to try to limit the food industry's power to convince us all to eat, eat, eat?

EXERCISE/ACTIVITY

Energy balance, the interplay of total calories in and total calories out, has been associated with increased cancer risk. One way to impact the expanding waistlines of U.S. citizens is to encourage more exercise, thereby increasing the "calories out" part of the equation. This exercise is designed to make you think about ways to make this happen:

- Sketch out some typical road map patterns of three types of neighborhoods: urban, suburban (cul de sac type), and rural. Include things like stores, restaurants, and schools on your maps. Think about what features of these different neighborhood layouts might encourage or discourage walking or other types of exercise. Given that most of the U.S. population now lives in suburban-type neighborhoods, how would you design your ideal neighborhood if you wanted to encourage participation in exercise by the neighborhood residents? What would be the most important aspects of your neighborhood in this respect; i.e., if you had limited funds to spend, what would be your top priorities?

Healthy People 2010

Focus Area: Cancer

Goal: Reduce the number of new cancer cases as well as the illness, disability, and death caused by cancer.

Objectives:

3-1. Reduce the overall cancer death rate.

3-15. Increase the proportion of cancer survivors who are living 5 years or longer after diagnosis.

REFERENCES

1. American Cancer Society. *Cancer Facts and Figures, 2007.* Atlanta: ACS. Available at http://cancer.org/downloads/STT/CAFF2007PWSecured.pdf. Accessed April 10, 2008.

2. *Merriam-Webster's Collegiate Dictionary,* 10th ed. Springfield, MA: Merriam-Webster, Inc.; 1999.

3. Merlo LM, Pepper JW, Reid BJ, Maley CC. Cancer as an evolutionary and ecological process. *Nat Rev Cancer* 2006;6:924–935.

4. Forman MR, Hursting SD, Umar A, Barrett JC. Nutrition and cancer prevention: a multidisciplinary perspective on human trials. *Annu Rev Nutr* 2004;24:223–254.

5. Foulds L. Some general principles of neoplastic development. *Acta Unio Int Contra Cancrum* 1964;20:663–666.

6. Slaga TJ, Fischer SM, Weeks CE, Klein-Szanto AJ. Multistage chemical carcinogenesis in mouse skin. *Curr Probl Dermatol* 1980;10:193–218.

7. Hursting SD, Slaga TJ, Fischer SM, DiGiovanni J, Phang JM. Mechanism-based cancer prevention approaches: targets, examples, and the use of transgenic mice. *J Natl Cancer Inst* 1999;91:215–225.

8. Weir HK, Thun MJ, Hankey BF, et al. Annual report to the nation on the status of cancer, 1975–2000, featuring the uses of surveillance data for cancer prevention and control. *J Natl Cancer Inst* 2003;95:1276–1299.

9. Slaga TJ. Can tumour promotion be effectively inhibited? *IARC Sci Publ* 1984(56):497–506.

10. Slaga TJ. Multistage skin carcinogenesis: a useful model for the study of the chemoprevention of cancer. *Acta Pharmacol Toxicol (Copenh)* 1984;55(Suppl 2):107–124.

11. Pitot HC. Progression: the terminal stage in carcinogenesis. *Jpn J Cancer Res* 1989;80:599–607.

12. Sheweita SA, Tilmisany AK. Cancer and phase II drug-metabolizing enzymes. *Curr Drug Metab* 2003;4:45–58.

13. Keck AS, Finley JW. Cruciferous vegetables: cancer protective mechanisms of glucosinolate hydrolysis products and selenium. *Integr Cancer Ther* 2004;3:5–12.

14. Valko M, Rhodes CJ, Moncol J, Izakovic M, Mazur M. Free radicals, metals and antioxidants in oxidative stress-induced cancer. *Chem Biol Interact* 2006;160:1–40.

15. Thoms KM, Kuschal C, Emmert S. Lessons learned from DNA repair defective syndromes. *Exp Dermatol* 2007;16:532–544.

16. Trush MA, Kensler TW. An overview of the relationship between oxidative stress and chemical carcinogenesis. *Free Radic Biol Med* 1991;10:201–209.

17. Goodman JE, Hofseth LJ, Hussain SP, Harris CC. Nitric oxide and p53 in cancer-prone chronic inflammation and oxyradical overload disease. *Environ Mol Mutagen* 2004;44:3–9.

18. Hussain SP, Hofseth LJ, Harris CC. Radical causes of cancer. *Nat Rev Cancer* 2003;3:276–285.

19. Khanapure SP, Garvey DS, Janero DR, Letts LG. Eicosanoids in inflammation: biosynthesis, pharmacology, and therapeutic frontiers. *Curr Top Med Chem* 2007;7:311–340.

20. Yu H, Rohan T. Role of the insulin-like growth factor family in cancer development and progression. *J Natl Cancer Inst* 2000;92:1472–1489.

21. Dunn BK, Ford LG. Hormonal interventions to prevent hormonal cancers: breast and prostate cancers. *Eur J Cancer Prev* 2007;16:232–242.

22. Thompson HJ, Strange R, Schedin PJ. Apoptosis in the genesis and prevention of cancer. *Cancer Epidemiol Biomarkers Prev* 1992;1:597–602.

23. Noonan DM, Benelli R, Albini A. Angiogenesis and cancer prevention: a vision. *Recent Results Cancer Res* 2007;174:219–224.

24. Hursting SD, Lavigne JA, Berrigan D, Perkins SN, Barrett JC. Calorie restriction, aging, and cancer prevention: mechanisms of action and applicability to humans. *Annu Rev Med* 2003;54:131–152.

25. Hursting SD, Kari FW. The anti-carcinogenic effects of dietary restriction: mechanisms and future directions. *Mutat Res* 1999;443:235–249.

26. Zhu Z, Haegele AD, Thompson HJ. Effect of caloric restriction on premalignant and malignant stages of mammary carcinogenesis. *Carcinogenesis* 1997;18:1007–1012.

27. U.S. Department of Agriculture ARS, Dietary Guidelines Advisory Committee. *Report of the Dietary Guidelines Advisory Committee on the Dietary Guidelines for Americans, 2000, to the Secretary of Health and Human Services and the Secretary of Agriculture.* Beltsville, MD: USDA; 2000.

28. Hill JO, Wyatt HR, Reed GW, Peters JC. Obesity and the environment: where do we go from here? *Science* 2003;299:853–855.

29. Calle EE, Rodriguez C, Walker-Thurmond K, Thun MJ. Overweight, obesity, and mortality from cancer in a prospectively studied cohort of U.S. adults. *N Engl J Med* 2003;348:1625–1638.

30. Vainio H, Kaaks R, Bianchini F. Weight control and physical activity in cancer prevention: international evaluation of the evidence. *Eur J Cancer Prev* 2002;11(Suppl 2):S94–S100.

31. Cao SX, Dhahbi JM, Mote PL, Spindler SR. Genomic profiling of short- and long-term caloric restriction effects in the liver of aging mice. *Proc Natl Acad Sci U S A* 2001;98:10630–10635.

32. Lee CK, Klopp RG, Weindruch R, Prolla TA. Gene expression profile of aging and its retardation by caloric restriction. *Science* 1999;285:1390–1393.

33. Lee CK, Weindruch R, Prolla TA. Gene-expression profile of the aging brain in mice. *Nat Genet* 2000;25:294–297.

34. Weindruch R, Kayo T, Lee CK, Prolla TA. Microarray profiling of gene expression in aging and its alteration by caloric restriction in mice. *J Nutr* 2001;131:918S–923S.

35. Han ES, Hickey M. Microarray evaluation of dietary restriction. *J Nutr* 2005;135:1343–1346.

CROSS REFERENCES

Colon Cancer

Exercise

Genetics

Inflammation

The Nutrition Transition

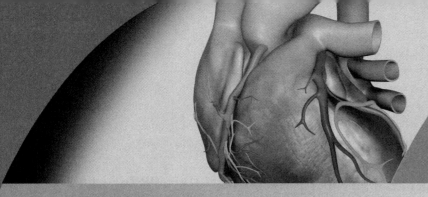

CHAPTER 20

Colon Cancer: A Common, and Yet Preventable, Cancer

James F. Cawley

Research indicates that a glass of alcohol a day increases your risk of colon cancer by 10%.[1]

LEARNING OBJECTIVES

By the end of this chapter, the student will be able to:

- Describe the known factors that increase the risk of colon cancer.
- Name the hereditary syndromes and inflammatory colonic diseases that confer a high risk of colon cancer.
- List the major signs and symptoms of colon cancer.
- Identify the clinical stages of colon cancer.
- Discuss the approaches to screening for colon cancer.
- Indicate strategies of prevention for colon cancer.

HISTORY

Colon cancer is a neoplasm that starts in the large intestine (colon) or the rectum (end of the colon). This category of cancer is typically referred to as *colorectal cancer*. Other types of cancer affecting the colon such as lymphoma, carcinoid tumors, melanoma, and sarcomas are rare. In this chapter, use of the term *colon cancer* refers to colon carcinoma (**adenocarcinoma**) and not these rare types of colon cancer. Colorectal cancer is one of the leading causes of cancer-related deaths in the United States. In many cases, early diagnosis can lead to a complete cure.

BASIC SCIENCE FACTS/KEY CONCEPTS REVIEW

What Causes Colon Cancer?

There is no single cause for colon cancer. Nearly all colon cancers begin as benign polyps, which slowly develop into cancer. Certain genetic syndromes also increase the risk of developing colon cancer.

Most colorectal cancers arise from an adenomatous polyp. A **polyp** is defined as a tissue protuberance from the colon mucosa. Several genes are associated with an increased risk of colorectal cancer. As many as 25% of patients with colorectal cancer have a family history of the disease, which suggests the involvement of a genetic factor.[2]

Such inherited colon cancers can be divided into two main types: the well-studied but rare familial adenomatous polyposis (FAP) syndrome, which accounts for approximately 1 percent of cases of colon cancer annually, and the increasingly well-characterized, more common hereditary non-polyposis colorectal cancer (HNPCC), which accounts for 5 percent to 10 percent of cases.[3]

Hereditary Non-Polyposis Colorectal Cancer

HNPCC, sometimes called **Lynch syndrome**, accounts for approximately 5 percent to 10 percent of all colorectal cancer cases. The risk of colorectal cancer in families with HNPCC is 70 percent to 90 percent, which is several times the risk in the general population. In HNPCC, the average age for a person to be diagnosed with colorectal cancer is 45. Women with HNPCC also have an increased risk of uterine (50 percent) and ovarian (10 percent) cancers. In addition, people with HNPCC are also at increased risk for cancers of the stomach, small intestine, and kidney. There may also be some increased risk of breast cancer.

Several genes have been identified that are linked to HNPCC. Mutations in the *MLH1, MSH2,* and *MSH6* genes are the most frequent cause of HNPCC. The HNPCC genes are part of a group of genes called *mismatch repair genes.* They make proteins that repair DNA mistakes that occur as cells divide. If one of these genes has a mutation, the mistakes cannot be repaired, which leads to damaged DNA and an increased risk of cancer.

Because colorectal cancer is one of the most treatable forms of cancer if identified early, people diagnosed with HNPCC, or those considered at increased risk based on their family history, often benefit from increased screening. Individuals who are found to be at increased risk can benefit from screening with annual **colonoscopy** examinations.

Women at risk for HNPCC may benefit from additional screening for uterine and ovarian cancers with pelvic examinations, ultrasound, endometrial **biopsy**, and a CA-125 blood test. However, the exact effectiveness of these screening methods is unknown.

To prevent colorectal cancer, a prophylactic **colectomy** (surgical removal of the colon) is often recommended and can significantly decrease the risk of colorectal cancer in patients who are at high risk.[4]

Familial Adenomatous Polyposis

FAP accounts for about 1 percent of colorectal cancer cases. People with FAP typically develop hundreds to thousands of colon polyps (small growths). The polyps are initially benign (noncancerous), but there is nearly a 100 percent chance that the polyps will develop into cancer if left untreated. In FAP, colorectal cancer usually occurs by age 40. Most people with FAP develop polyps while they are in their 20s or 30s, although polyps can be found as early as the teenage years. Individuals with FAP are also at risk for other types of cancer including stomach, small bowel, pancreas, thyroid, and hepatoblastoma (liver cancer seen mainly in early childhood). Although FAP is inherited in an autosomal dominant pattern, approximately 30 percent of people with FAP have no family history of the condition.

> **The Science: Key Points**
> - There is evidence that there is activation of certain tumor-promoting genes or oncogenes (*K-ras, c-myc*) and an inactivation of tumor-suppressor genes (*MCC, DCC, p53*).
> - Colon cancers arise from commonly-occurring polyps of the inner lining of the colon (mucosa).
> - In FAP, polyps will always develop into cancer if left untreated.

> - While most cases occur sporadically, there is a strong genetic basis to this disease.

PUBLIC HEALTH PERSPECTIVE FOR THE HEALTH OF THE GENERAL POPULATION AND OF HIGH RISK GROUPS

Colorectal cancer is the second most common cancer among both men and women in the United States and the third most common cause of cancer death among men and women in the United States.[4] In 2007, approximately 153,760 adults (79,130 men and 74,630 women) in the United States will be diagnosed with colorectal cancer. These numbers include 112,340 new cases of colon cancer and 41,420 new cases of rectal cancer. An estimated 52,180 deaths (26,000 men and 26,180 women) will occur. Colon cancer is rare in Africa and Asia, primarily because of environmental differences. A diet high in meat and animal fat and low in fiber are believed to be important etiological factors.[7] There are, however, studies that show that the risk does not drop when one adopts a high-fiber diet, so the cause of the link is not yet clear.[8]

In the United States, the lifetime risk of colon cancer is 1 in 17, but this statistic is higher in those with one affected first-degree relative. The risk of colorectal cancer is increased in those with:

- Colorectal polyps
- A family history of colon cancer
- Ulcerative colitis
- Crohn's disease
- History of breast cancer

Generally, colorectal cancer is uncommon in persons under the age of 60 years. People free of a family history of colon cancer may however, still be at risk of the disease. In fact, about 80 percent of new colon cancer cases are diagnosed in people who would not be identified as "high risk." Studies of colon cancer cases found that lifestyle factors can put a person at higher risk. These factors include: a diet high in fat and red meat but low in fruits and vegetables, high caloric intake, low levels of physical activity, and obesity. In addition, smoking and excessive alcohol intake may play a role in colon cancer development. Despite avoiding all of these factors, some people will still develop colon cancer. With screening and early detection, these patients can be effectively treated in a majority of the cases.

Screening

Mortality from colon cancer has dropped in the last 15 years, likely due to increased awareness and screening by colonoscopy.

CASE STUDIES
Scenario

Case 1

Beth M.'s father died of colon cancer, as did her grandmother. Now, two of her brothers, both in their 40s, have been diagnosed with colon cancer. Beth, age 37, feels that a curse is hanging over her family and is worried about her future and that of her children.

Case 2

Paul C. was 35 when his doctor told him the grim news: He had advanced colon cancer. As far as he knew, Paul had no family history of the disease. But after checking, Paul learned that several aunts and uncles had died of colon cancer at an early age.

Further research revealed that some members of both Beth and Paul's families carried an altered gene, passed from parent to child, which predisposes them to a form of inherited colon cancer (HNPCC). Sometimes difficult to diagnose, HNPCC is believed to account for one in six of all colon cancer cases.

Cancers arise from a multistep process that involves the interplay of multiple changes, or *mutations*, in several different genes, in combination with environmental factors such as diet or lifestyle. In the most common, noninherited forms of cancer, the genetic changes are acquired after birth. But individuals who have a hereditary risk for cancer are born with one altered gene; in other words, they are born one step into the cancer process. In hereditary nonpolyposis colorectal cancer, for instance, children who inherit an altered gene from either parent face a 70 percent to 80 percent chance of developing this disease, usually at an early age. Women also face a markedly increased risk of uterine and ovarian cancer.

The earliest beneficiaries will be those families facing a very high risk of colon cancer. First, for those who choose to take it, a simple blood test in these cancer-prone families can determine who does or does not carry the altered genes. The consequences could be enormous, for as many as 1 in 200, or 1 million Americans, may carry one or the other of these altered genes.

Defining the Issues and Patients' Understanding

Individuals found to carry an altered gene would likely be counseled to adopt a high-fiber, low-fat diet in the hope of preventing cancer. They would also be advised to start yearly examinations of the colon at about age 30. Such exams should help physicians to detect any benign polyps, which are wart-like growths on the colon, early in the disease process, and then remove them before they turn malignant. For those individuals who turn out not to carry the altered genes, the diagnostic test may be a huge relief, removing the fear they have lived under and sparing them the need for frequent colonoscopies.

Despite the life-saving potential of such diagnostic tests, numerous issues need to be resolved before they are introduced into general medical practice. Genetic testing is not as simple as drawing blood and telling someone the results. For one thing, the best way to test large numbers of individuals is by no means clear. In deciding whether or not to be tested, individuals need information not only about the disorder and its risk but also about the test and its limitations. Equally important, genetic testing must be accompanied by counseling to help people cope with information about their future risk, whatever the outcome of the test. Those who test positive and who are trying to decide what course to pursue will need to know how effective various strategies (such as frequent colonoscopy and polyp removal) actually are at preventing colon cancer.

Definitive answers are still lacking for these questions. Broader, societal issues arise as well, such as how to protect the confidentiality of genetic information and ensure that it is not used to discriminate against individuals in employment or insurance.

Even before these colon cancer susceptibility genes were discovered, the Human Genome Project had begun planning pilot studies to address these and other questions about testing for cancer risk. Careful attention to these social and ethical issues now will help prepare the public and the medical profession for the choices that lie ahead.[5]

CLINICAL PERSPECTIVE FOR THE HEALTHCARE PROVIDER

Signs and Symptoms

Many people with colon cancer experience no symptoms in the early stages of the disease. When symptoms appear, they tend to vary, depending on the cancer's size and location in the large intestine.

Signs and symptoms of colon cancer may include:

- A change in bowel habits, including diarrhea or constipation or a change in the consistency of stool for more than a couple of weeks
- Rectal bleeding or blood in stool (**melena**)
- Persistent abdominal discomfort, such as cramps, gas, or pain
- Abdominal pain with a bowel movement
- A feeling that your bowel doesn't empty completely
- Weakness or fatigue
- Unexplained weight loss

Blood in your stool (**melena**) may be a sign of cancer, but it can also indicate other conditions. Bright red blood you notice on bathroom tissue more commonly comes from hemorrhoids or minor tears (fissures) in your anus, for example. In addition, certain foods, such as beets or red licorice, can turn your stools red. Iron supplements and some anti-diarrheal medications may make stools black. Still, it's best to have any sign of blood or change in your stools checked promptly by your doctor because it can be a sign of something more serious.

Clinical Staging

Like many cancers, there is a staging classification of colorectal cancers. Colon cancer staging is an estimate of the amount of penetration and spread of the cancer. Staging is performed for diagnostic and research purposes, and to determine the best method of treatment. The systems for staging colorectal cancers largely depend on the extent of local invasion, the degree of lymph node involvement and whether there is distant metastasis.

Definitive staging only can be done after surgery has been performed and pathology reports reviewed. An exception to this principle would be after a colonoscopic polypectomy of a malignant pedunculated polyp with minimal invasion. Preoperative staging of rectal cancers may be done with endoscopic ultrasound. Adjuncts to staging of metastasis include abdominal ultrasound, CT, positron emission tomography (PET) scanning, and other imaging studies.

Dukes' staging classification, first proposed by Cuthbert E. Dukes in 1932, identifies the stages as (Figure 20-1)[5]:

A: Tumor confined to the intestinal wall
B: Tumor invading through the intestinal wall
C: With lymph node(s) involvement
D: With distant metastasis

Treatment

Surgery

Surgery is the most common treatment for colon cancer. If the cancer is limited to a polyp, the patient can undergo a polypectomy (removal of the polyp) or a local excision, where a small amount of surrounding tissue is removed also. If the tumor invades the bowel wall or surrounding tissues, the patient will require a partial resection (removal of the cancer and a portion of the bowel) and removal of local lymph nodes to determine if the cancer has spread into them. After the tumor is removed, the two ends of the remaining colon are reconnected, allowing normal bowel function. In some situations, it may not be possible to reconnect the colon, and a **colostomy** is needed.

Chemotherapy

Despite the fact that a majority of patients have the entire tumor removed by surgery, as many as 50 percent to 60 percent will develop a recurrence. Chemotherapy is given to reduce this chance of recurrence. There is some controversy over whether or not patients with stage II disease should receive chemotherapy. Studies have not consistently shown a benefit in treating these patients. Generally, patients with stage II disease who present with a bowel perforation or obstruction, or who have poorly differentiated tumors (determined by a pathologist looking at the tumor under a microscope), are considered at higher risk for recurrence and are treated with six months of fluorouracil (5-FU) and leucovorin (LV; both chemotherapy agents). Other patients with stage II disease are followed closely but generally receive no chemotherapy. Patients who present with stage III colon cancer are typically treated

FIGURE 20-1 Stages of Colon Cancer.

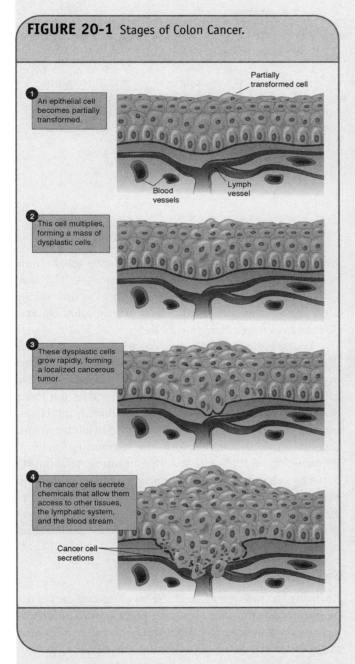

① An epithelial cell becomes partially transformed.

Partially transformed cell

Blood vessels

Lymph vessel

② This cell multiplies, forming a mass of dysplastic cells.

③ These dysplastic cells grow rapidly, forming a localized cancerous tumor.

④ The cancer cells secrete chemicals that allow them access to other tissues, the lymphatic system, and the blood stream.

Cancer cell secretions

with a regimen of 5-FU and LV for six months, resulting in improved survival rates when compared with surgery alone.

Forty to fifty percent of patients have metastatic disease (cancer that has spread to other organs) at the time of diagnosis, or have a recurrence of the disease after therapy. Unfortunately, the prognosis for these patients is poor. The standard therapy for patients with advanced disease is a combination of fluorouracil, leucovorin, and irinotecan (CPT-11 or Camptosar) or oxaliplatin (Eloxitin). Regimens adding either irinotecan or oxaliplatin to fluorouracil and leucovorin were found to be more effective than using the fluorouracil and leucovorin alone. With this therapy, an average of 39 percent of patients have a response, but the average survival is still only 20 months.

Bevacizumab (Avastin) is a new type of treatment called anti-angiogenic therapy. Tumors need nutrients to survive and are able to get these nutrients by growing new blood vessels. This medication works by attacking the new blood vessels the tumor has formed, in other words, by cutting off its food source. Bevacizumab is used in combination with chemotherapy.

Cetuximab is a new type of monoclonal antibody that targets cancer cells specifically, sparing the normal cells and therefore causing fewer side effects. The drug causes the patient's immune system to recognize the cancer cells as foreign and attack them. Cetuximab is given either alone or in conjunction with chemotherapy agents. Capecitabine, an oral form of 5-FU, is being used also in the treatment of colon cancers when the patient cannot tolerate or has progressed on the above therapies.

Patients and their physicians must weigh the benefits of therapy versus the side effects of the treatment. Patients who are younger and/or in better physical shape are more likely to tolerate therapy, but elderly patients should not be excluded from chemotherapy based on age alone.

Radiotherapy

Colon cancer is not typically treated with radiation therapy. If the cancer has invaded another organ or attached itself to the abdominal wall, radiation therapy may be a treatment option. One reason for the limited role of radiation is that it is a local treatment typically aimed at a "target." Once the colon cancer has been surgically resected, the targeted high-risk area for disease recurrence is not very easy to define. Furthermore, if the cancer has spread to other organs, chemotherapy (rather than radiation therapy) is able to reach all the distant areas of tumor cells.

Follow-Up Testing

Once a patient has completed chemotherapy, they must be followed closely for recurrence. Guidelines for follow-up surveillance written by the National Comprehensive Cancer Network are: physical exam (including digital rectal exam) every three months for two years, and then every six months for three years; carcinoembryonic antigen (CEA) level (if elevated preoperatively) checked every three months for two years, then every six months for three years; and colonoscopy in one year with a repeat in one year if abnormal, or every two to three years if no polyps are found. There is not enough evidence to support or refute the use of chest x-ray or computed tomography scan for surveillance at this time, so this varies from physician to physician and is more likely to be used in higher risk cases.

Clinical trials have played and continue to play an important role in the treatment of colon cancer. In the past 20 years, considerable improvements have been made in colon cancer therapy, with overall survival rates increasing from 45 percent to 75 percent. The treatments we have today were refined through the research and analysis of clinical trials, and many new avenues continue to be explored. Talk with your physician about current clinical trials for colon cancer in your area or visit our clinical trials matching service.

Colon cancer almost always can be caught in its earliest and most curable stages by colonoscopy. Men and women age 50 and older should have a colonoscopy. Colonoscopy is usually painless and most patients are asleep for the entire procedure.

Underuse of Screening

As many as 60 percent of deaths from colorectal cancer could be prevented if everyone age 50 and older were screened regularly. Colorectal cancer screening remains underused, despite the availability of effective screening tests. Screening for colorectal cancer lags far behind screening for breast and cervical cancers. Findings from the National Health Interview Survey (NHIS), which is administered by CDC, indicate that in 2000, only 42.5 percent of U.S. adults aged 50 or older had undergone a sigmoidoscopy or colonoscopy within the previous 10 years or had used a fecal occult blood test (FOBT) home test kit within the preceding year. Screening for colorectal cancer was particularly low among those respondents who lacked health insurance, those with no usual source of health care, and those who reported no doctor's visits within the preceding year.

Prevention Levels

Primary Prevention

Dietary and lifestyle modifications are important. Evidence suggests that low-fat and high-fiber diets may reduce the risk of colon cancer. It has been observed that persons taking certain drugs also have lower rates of colon cancer.[9] Chemoprophylaxis, also known as, chemoprevention, refers to the administration of medications which inhibit the enzyme cyclooxygenase-2 (COX-2). These drugs have been approved for reducing polyps in FAP and are currently being tested for the prevention of HNPCC-related colon cancers. The U.S. Preventive Services Task Force recommends against taking other anti-inflammatory medicines to prevent colon cancer if one has an average risk of the disease.

Taking more than 300 mg a day of aspirin and similar drugs may cause dangerous gastrointestinal bleeding and heart problems. Although low-dose aspirin may help reduce the risk of other conditions, such as heart disease, it does not lower the rate of colon cancer.[10] Calcium may indirectly inhibit colorectal cancer by binding bile acids into insoluble soaps, thereby blocking contact with the luminal epithelium. Epidemiological studies have shown an inverse relationship between calcium intake and cancer risk. A randomized, placebo-controlled trial tested the effect of calcium supplementation (3 g of calcium carbonate daily, which is equivalent to 1,200 mg of elemental calcium) showed a modest effect on the risk of recurrent adenoma.[11]

Secondary Prevention

Reducing the number of deaths from colorectal cancer depends on detecting and removing precancerous colorectal polyps as well as detecting and treating the cancer in its early stages. Colorectal cancer can be prevented by removing precancerous polyps or abnormal growths, which can be present in the colon for years before invasive cancer develops. When colorectal cancer is found early and treated, the five-year relative survival rate is 90 percent. Because screening rates are low, less than 40 percent of colorectal cancers are found early. One U.S. clinical trial reported a 33 percent reduction in colorectal cancer deaths and a 20 percent reduction in colorectal cancer incidence among people offered an annual FOBT.

KEY TERMS

Clinical Terms

Adenocarcinoma: A type of cancer that arises from glandular tissue.

Biopsy: Surgical removal of a small amount of tissue for examination under a microscope.

Colectomy: Surgical removal of the colon; performed in patients with high risk forms of the disease.

Colostomy: An opening in the abdominal wall to allow passage of stool.

Colonoscopy: Visual examination of the inner surface of the colon using a flexible lighted scope passed into the body while under sedation.

Chemoprophylaxis: Prevention of disease by use of chemicals or drugs.

Lynch Syndrome: Hereditary form of colon cancer characterized by multiple polyps that accounts for 5 percent to 10 percent of all cases.

Melena: Blood in the stool.

Polyp: A tissue protuberance from the colon mucosa.

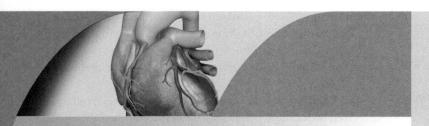

Questions for Further Research, Study, Reflection, and Discussion

For the Individual Student

In order to answer these questions, it may be necessary to research the primary literature.

- Should all persons over the age of 50 take aspirin or nonsteroidal anti-inflammatory drugs (NSAIDs) to prevent the occurrence of colon cancer?
- Describe how diet and lifestyle may influence the risk of developing colon cancer.
- Discuss the advantages and disadvantages of the screening modalities for colon cancer. Identify the current recommendations (guidelines) for screening for colon cancer?

For Small Group Discussion

- Ask the group if they are aware of their parents or older relatives having been screened for colon cancer.
- If a person has a first-degree relative who had colon cancer, how often should he or she be screened for this disease beginning at what age?
- Discuss some of the reasons that explain why it is so difficult to identify a dietary origin (cause) for a disease like colon cancer.

- Because the prevalence of colon cancer is common, and many public health students choose this career path due to personal experience, ask for volunteers in the class who have had family members with the disease to describe their feelings.

For Entire Class Discussion

- Ask class members how many have a friend or relative who has had colon cancer. Ask how many of them are survivors and, if they know, at what stage was the disease identified. Did their friend or relative undergo surgery for the disease?
- Ask students in the class what they would view as the characteristics of an ideal screening test for colon cancer.

EXERCISE/ACTIVITY

The Giant Walk-Through Colon

An exhibition featuring a giant 100-foot long replica of a human colon has been travelling throughout the United States and Canada for the past year. The exhibition was prepared by the Cancer Research and Prevention Foundation to promote screening for a cancer that is 90 percent curable when detected early. Learn about the travelling colon exhibition and determine where it is currently being held. If possible, visit the exhibition and take a walk through the colon. What is your impression? Do you think this exhibition will have an impact in encouraging persons to schedule a colonoscopy when they understand better how a polyp develops and can be easily removed? Research information about whether documentation exists about the impact of such an educational experience.

Healthy People 2010

Focus Area: Cancer

Goal: Reduce the number of new cancer cases as well as the illness, disability, and death caused by cancer.

Objective:

3-5. Reduce the colorectal cancer death rate.

3-12. Increase the proportion of adults who receive a colorectal cancer screening examination.

REFERENCES

1. Burke CA. Colorectal cancer. In: Lang RA, Hensrud DD, eds. *Clinical Preventive Medicine*, 2nd ed. Chicago: AMA Press; 2004.

2. Abeloff M, Armitage J, Niederhuber J, Kastan M, McKenna G, eds. *Clinical Oncology*, Philadelphia: Elsevier; 2004.

3. American Cancer Society. *Cancer Facts and Figures 2006*. Atlanta, GA: American Cancer Society; 2006.

4. National Institutes of Health, National Center for Human Genome Research. The Human Genome Project: From Maps to Medicine. Bethesda: U.S. Department of Health and Human Services; 1995. Genetic Discoveries Offer Hope for Prevention. Available at http://www.accessexcellence.org/RC/AB/BA/Case_Hereditary_Colon.html. Accessed April 14, 2008.

5. Dukes CE. The classification of cancer of the rectum. *J Pathol Bacteriol* 1932;35:323–332.

6. Chao A, Thun MJ, Connell CJ, McCullough ML, Jacobs EJ, Flanders WD, Rodriguez C, Sinha R, Calle EE. Meat consumption and risk of colorectal cancer. *JAMA* 2005;293:172–182.

7. Park Y, Hunter DJ, Spiegelman D, Bergkvist L, Berrino F, et al. Dietary fiber intake and risk of colorectal cancer: a pooled analysis of prospective cohort studies. *JAMA* 2005;294:2849–2857.

8. Baron JA, Cole BF, Sandler RS, et al. A randomized trial of aspirin to prevent colorectal adenomas. *N Engl J Med* 2003;348:891–899.

9. U.S. Preventive Services Task Force. Routine aspirin or nonsteroidal anti-inflammatory drugs for the primary prevention of colorectal cancer: U.S. Preventive Services Task Force Recommendation Statement. *Ann Intern Med* 2007;146:361–364.

10. Flossmann E, Rothwell PM. Effect of aspirin on long-term risk of colorectal cancer: consistent evidence from randomized and observational studies. *Lancet* 2007;369:1603–1613.

11. Ferrari P, Jenab M, Norat T, et al. Lifetime and baseline alcohol intake and risk of colon and rectal cancers in the European Prospective Investigation into Cancer and Nutrition (EPIC). *Int J Cancer* 2007;121:2065–2072.

CROSS REFERENCES

Cancer Prevention from a Biologist's Perspective

Genetics

The Nutrition Transition

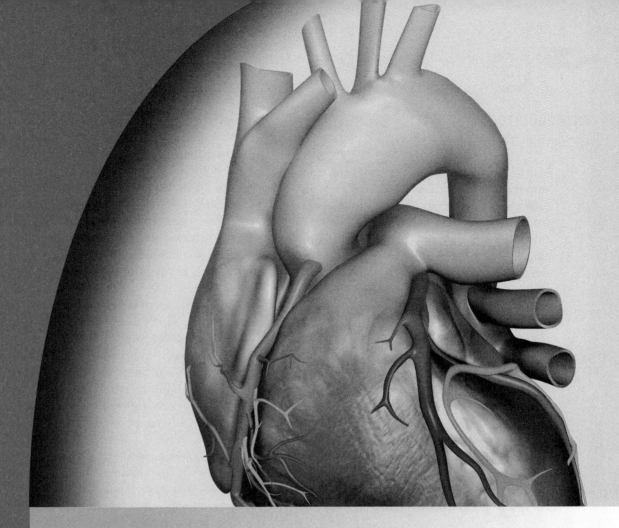

PART **IV**

The Public Health Burden of Infectious Disease

Constance Battle

INTRODUCTION

Constance Battle

"For so it had come about, as indeed I and many men might have foreseen had not terror and disaster blinded our minds. These germs of disease have taken toll of humanity since the beginning of things—taken toll of our prehuman ancestors since life began here. But by virtue of this natural selection of our kind we have developed resisting power; to no germs do we succumb without a struggle, and to many—those that cause putrefaction in dead matter, for instance—our living frames are altogether immune. But there are no bacteria in Mars, and directly these invaders arrived, directly they drank and fed, our microscopic allies began to work their overthrow. Already when I watched them they were irrevocably doomed, dying and rotting even as they went to and fro. It was inevitable. By the toll of a billion deaths man has bought his birthright of the earth, and it is his against all comers; it would still be his were the Martians ten times as mighty as they are. For neither do men live nor die in vain."

Herman George Wells (1866–1946)
The War of the Worlds[1]

In 1898, H.G. Wells' science fiction novel creatively described a time when humans believed they had an invincible immune system. Apparently they did, but 21 days after Martians landed on Horsell Common near London, all of the invaders were found dead, having succumbed abruptly to terrestrial pathogenic bacteria to which they had no immunity. In 2007, just over 100 years later, another space story ironically was reported in the *Proceedings of the National Academy of Sciences*. Researchers documented gene expression changes that occurred in bacterial cells (and any microbial pathogens) during space flight, thus demonstrating that a microgravity growth condition provides an environmental signal that can induce molecular changes in bacterial cells.[2] As a result of these changes, a microbe becomes more virulent, causing it to increase the risk of infectious disease during a long-term mission in crew members who may already demonstrate immune dysfunction. Such new information has tremendous significance for the risk of infectious diseases during a long-duration space mission and more generalizably might provide insight into how pathogens cause infection on earth.

Of several hundred possibilities, these chapters on infectious disease have been selected to illustrate the past, the present, and the future of public health. The criteria I used for selection were: global importance; the oldest infectious diseases in history, which continue to present extraordinary challenges to control; diseases that can infect the students reading this textbook; the alarming rise of microbial resistance globally; *the* epidemic disease of the twentieth century; and two frightening categories of disease that have not yet been fully recognized or understood. These last categories may or may not be inevitable at this point, but we understand enough to appreciate that avian flu or various bioterrorism agent diseases could be devastating to national and global health.

To conclude this introduction to the chapter on infectious diseases, it is educational to explore ways of looking at the meaning of the term *epidemic*.[3] It is particularly revealing to review the exposition of the evolution of the term over 2,500 years by Martin and Martin-Granel.[4] Limiting the view of epidemic to its relationship to infectious diseases, these authors describe four stages throughout history.[4] To Hippocrates, epidemic meant a collection of symptoms occurring at a given place over a given period. During the Middle Ages, waves of plagues enabled physicians to identify epidemics of the same well-characterized disease. Pasteur and Koch recognized epidemics caused by the same microbe. Finally, it has been recognized that most epidemics were due to the clonal expansion of an epidemic strain as defined with molecular markers. This semantic evolution provides us a brief look at the history of infectious disease.

REFERENCES

1. Wells HG. *The War of the Worlds*. New York: Barnes & Noble Books; 1898:195.

2. Wilson JW, Ott CM, Höner zu Bentrup, et al. Space flight alters bacterial gene expression and virulence and reveals a role for global regulator Hfq. *Proc Natl Acad Sci U S A* 2007;104:16299–16304.

3. Gladwell M. "The Tipping Point. Why Is the City Suddenly So Much Safer—Could It Be That Crime Really Is an Epidemic? *The New Yorker*, June 3, 1996. Available at: http://www.gladwell.com/1996/1996_06_03_a_tipping.htm. Accessed April 14, 2008.

4. Martin PMV, Martin-Granel E. 2,500-year evolution of the term epidemic. *Emerging Infectious Diseases* [serial on the Internet]. 2006 Jun. Available at: http://www.cdc.gov/ncidod/EID/vol12no06/05-1263.htm. Accessed April 14, 2008.

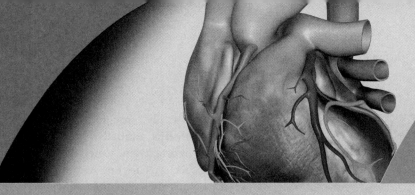

CHAPTER 21

Soil-Transmitted Helminths: Worms Are the Most Common Pathogens of Mankind

Ami Shah Brown, Sophia Raff, & Peter Hotez

In 1947, a paper titled *This Wormy World* showed that intestinal helminths, or worms, were one of the most prevalent infections in humans.[1] Today, over one billion people, or almost one-third of the world's poorest people living on less than U.S. $2 per day, harbor parasitic worms in their intestines.[2]

LEARNING OBJECTIVES

By the end of this chapter, the student will be able to:

- Provide historical context for soil-transmitted helminths and other neglected tropical diseases.
- Describe the life cycles of roundworm, whipworm, and hookworm in human hosts and the clinical manifestations of infection.
- List the major epidemiological features of soil-transmitted helminth infection, especially with relation to age, geographical region, socioeconomic status, re-infection rates, and polyparasitism.
- Discuss the long-term health impacts of chronic helminth infection, including childhood nutritional deficiencies, anemia, delays in cognitive development, poor pregnancy outcomes, and decreased worker productivity.
- Discuss major global approaches to the control of helminth infections.

HISTORY

Intestinal worms are a major public health problem in the developing world. At least one billion people worldwide harbor at least one, two, or all three major types of these parasites. The intestinal worm infections occur predominantly in impoverished areas of sub-Saharan Africa, Southeast Asia, India, and parts of Central and South America and the Caribbean.[3] Helminth species thrive in tropical areas where warm, moist soil provides an ideal environment for the maintenance of helminth eggs and **larvae**.[4] Helminth eggs are passed from a human host through feces, and underdeveloped environments with poor sanitation promote continuous transmission of the worm infections. Intestinal worm infections are primarily caused by three different types of these soil-transmitted helminths (Table 21-1):

- The human roundworm, *Ascaris lumbricoides*,
- The human whipworm, *Trichuris trichiura*, and
- The human hookworms, *Necator americanus* and *Ancylostoma duodenale*.

As opposed to newly emerging infectious diseases such as HIV/AIDS and severe acute respiratory syndrome (SARS), soil-transmitted helminth infections are ancient parasitic diseases that have existed for centuries. Ancient Greek and Roman medical writings include descriptions of roundworm infections.[5] Roundworms are the largest of the soil-transmitted helminths, and can grow up to 45 cm in a human host's intestine.[6] Their large size may explain why roundworms were one of the first helminth infections to be discovered and described in ancient medical writings.

Through the beginning of the 20th century, hookworm infection was actually a public health problem in the southern United States, especially in coastal areas along the Atlantic seaboard and the Gulf of Mexico. In 1905, Southern medical doctors reported that over 40 percent of residents in some areas were infected with hookworm.[7] The warm, tropical-

TABLE 21-1 Most Prevalent Soil-Transmitted Helminth Infections Worldwide: Ascariasis, Trichuriasis, and Hookworm Infection

Infection	(Most Prevalent) Species	Common Name	Worldwide Prevalence[1]
Ascariasis	*Ascaris lumbricoides*	Roundworm	1.2 billion
Trichuriasis	*Trichuris trichiura*	Whipworm	795 million
Human hookworm infection	*Necator americanus* and *Ancylostoma duodenale*	Hookworm	740 million

Source: Prevalence data are from Hotez PJ, Bundy DA, Beegle K, et al. Helminth infections: soil-transmitted helminth infections and schistosomiasis. In: Jamison DT, Breman JG, Measham AR, et al., eds. *Disease Control Priorities in Developing Countries*, 2nd ed. New York: Oxford University Press; 2006:467–482.

like environment in the American South allowed hookworm larvae to thrive in the soil. Moreover, hookworm eggs are passed through feces, and poor sanitation in Southern states permitted continuous transmission. The anemia, stunted growth, and developmental delays caused by hookworm took a devastating toll on those infected. One economic analysis indicates that children growing up in the American South lost up to 43 percent of their future wage-earning capacity because of hookworm.[8] In 1910, the Rockefeller Foundation undertook a campaign to eradicate hookworm from the South.[8] The foundation started a free treatment program, and distributed deworming pills throughout the Southern states. The antihelminthic medication, however, only provided temporary relief from current infection and could not prevent future re-infection with hookworm. Therefore, the Rockefeller Foundation also instituted health education programs to improve personal hygiene and sanitation facilities.[8] Ultimately, improvements in the economy and poverty reduction, together with urbanization, led to the elimination of hookworm as well as other tropical diseases such as malaria, pellagra, and typhoid fever from the United States by the 1970s.[7]

Despite their prevalence in developing countries, their centuries-long existence, and their presence in American public health history, many public health professionals are unaware of the global health impact of soil-transmitted helminths. Instead, most of the recent global health efforts to curb infectious diseases in developing countries have centered on the "Big Three" diseases: HIV/AIDS, tuberculosis, and malaria. The "Big Three" are important causes of infectious disease mortality: the diseases contributed to 2.8 million, 1.6 million, and 1.3 million deaths in 2004, respectively.[9] By comparison, the World Health Organization reported only 12,000 deaths worldwide due to soil-transmitted helminths in 2004.[9] Although some estimates show that helminth infections may

actually cause up to 135,000 deaths annually,[10] the low mortality due to helminth infections are one reason they are often overlooked by policy makers and public health professionals.[4]

Despite their low mortality rates, soil-transmitted helminths cause severe morbidity in infected persons. Long-term health impacts of chronic helminth infection include compromised nutritional status, poor iron absorption, anemia, stunted physical growth, impaired cognitive development, and decreased worked productivity. Historically, quantifying the effects of disease morbidity has been difficult and unrefined. Over the past fifteen years, researchers have developed a measurement known as the **disability-adjusted life year (DALY)**, which is the number of healthy life years lost to disability or premature death. The DALY measurement allows systematic quantification of the morbidity and the mortality caused by a disease. Researchers calculate DALY measurements by estimating the number of healthy, productive years of life lost due to morbidity or premature mortality from a disease.[11] The morbidity estimates for DALY calculations are derived by applying disability "weights" to different conditions and multiplying that weight by the number of years that an infected person is affected by that condition.[12]

Due to the severe disability caused by soil-transmitting helminths, the DALY is a more robust measure for quantifying their burden of disease as compared to mortality estimates. Soil-transmitted helminths cause an estimated 39.0 million DALYs annually, and as shown in Table 21-2, the morbidity due to these diseases rivals other major infectious diseases including tuberculosis and malaria.[13]

Along with soil-transmitted helminths, there are other lesser-known infectious diseases that primarily affect people in the developing world and cause significant morbidity. For example, lymphatic filariasis ("elephantiasis") is parasitic disease caused by thread-like worms that invade a human host's lymphatic system. The infection leads to blockage within the lymphatic system that causes severe and disfiguring swelling of limbs, genitals, and/or breasts.[14] Schistosomiasis is a waterborne parasitic infection caused by fluke worms (schistosomes) that can penetrate the skin. Chronic schistosomiasis infection can damage the lungs, bladder, and intestines. The morbidity caused by lymphatic filariasis and schistosomiasis leads to 5.8 million and 4.5 million DALYs, respectively, per year.[15]

TABLE 21-2 Disability-Adjusted Life Years (DALYS) Estimates for Infectious Diseases Worldwide

Disease	DALY Estimate (Annually)
HIV/AIDS	84.5 million
Diarrheal diseases	62 million
Malaria	46.5 million
Soil-transmitted helminths	
Total	39.0 million
Hookworm infection	22.1 million
Ascariasis	10.5 million
Trichuriasus	6.4 million
Tuberculosis	34.7 million

Source: Modified from Table 2, World Health Organization. *Prevention and Control of Schistosomiasis and Soil-Transmitted Helminths.* (2002). WHO Technical Report Series 912. Geneva, Switzerland, with data from HIV/AIDS, diarrheal diseases, malaria, and tuberculosis estimates from World Health Organization (2004). The World Health Report 2004, Annex Table 3: Burden of disease in DALYs by cause, sex, and mortality stratum in WHO regions, estimates for 2002. Available at http://www. who.int/whr/2004/annex/topic/en/annex_3_en.pdf. Accessed April 14, 2008. Also, Chan MS. Global Burden of Intestinal Nematodes—Fifty Years On. *Parasitology Today* 1997;13:438–443.

Historically, public health researchers have examined soil-transmitted helminths and other lesser-known infectious diseases as individual components. Recognition of the similar characteristics of these diseases led to the creation of a unifying term: the neglected tropical diseases (NTDs).[15] Despite their different causes and pathologies, NTDs such as soil-transmitted helminth infections, lymphatic filariasis, and schistosomiasis share many similar epidemiological characteristics. First, NTDs are chronic and disabling ancient conditions that have infected humans for centuries. NTDs are poverty-promoting diseases that occur primarily in underdeveloped, tropical areas of the world.[15] As demonstrated in the DALY estimations above, most of the NTDs are diseases of severe morbidity but not significant mortality.[15] Finally, in some areas of the world people suffer from multiple NTDs concurrently.[15] Other diseases that fall into the category of NTDs include trachoma, leprosy, Buruli ulcer, African trypanosomiasis, leishmaniasis, and onchocerciasis. Based on DALY estimates, the major NTDs result in a global disease burden equivalent to malaria and almost as great as HIV/AIDS.[13]

A barrier to the control and elimination of soil-transmitted helminths and other NTDs is access to essential medicines to combat these diseases.[13] In the case of soil-transmitted helminths, the major approach to control is through **mass drug administration** of so-called **anthelminthic drugs**. It is common to refer to mass treatments of soil-transmitted helminth infections as *deworming*. Deworming of children has a number of proven health benefits including improvements in catch-up growth and physical fitness as well as improved cognition and educational performance. In 2001, the 54th World Health Assembly adopted a resolution that recommends as a goal to deworm at least 75 percent and up to 100 percent of all at-risk school-aged children.[16] Deworming is carried out by administering on an annual basis a single dose of either albendazole or mebendazole (although in areas of intense parasite transmission sometimes two or three doses annually are required). In some areas, drug administration is conducted together with improvements in sanitation. However, in the absence of an overall improvement in economic development, environmental control measures that include sanitation have been surprisingly ineffective or prohibitively expensive.[17] Therefore, frequent and periodic deworming of children is currently the major public health intervention practiced worldwide.

Today, in many countries, the antihelminthic drugs are administered in schools and by teachers because of the cost-effectiveness of this approach, and because in many African countries deworming is linked to school-feeding programs.[18] In addition to cost-effectiveness, the advantage of having schoolteachers administer the medicines is that this school-based deworming does not rely on bringing in trained microscopists to conduct fecal examinations, which is very expensive. The disadvantage of school-based deworming is that some children in any given endemic area do not have worms and therefore they do not require treatments. Also, in some developing countries children do not attend school and it is difficult to reach these individuals. Accordingly, some national health ministries prefer to administer the antihelminthics during child health days with mobile teams of individuals trained in deworming. Many preschool-age children, that is, children between the ages of 1 and 5, are also being dewormed through child health day programs.

Since 2001, antihelminthic drugs have been administered to millions of school-aged children and many preschool children. However, even these stepped-up measures fall short in meeting the ambitious targets set forth by the World Health Assembly. Some estimates indicate that as few as 10 percent of eligible populations have so far received treatments. One approach to improve access to medicines is to link school-based deworming with other public health control measures, such as the distribution of vitamin A, antimalaria bednets, or childhood vaccinations. In 2005, it was proposed that deworming of soil-transmitted helminth infections could be linked to mass drug administration for other NTDs.[15]

But who will pay for the NTD drugs? Almost everyone suffering from NTDs lives on less than U.S. $2 per day, and therefore have no funds to pay for drugs. In 1988, Merck and Co., a major U.S. pharmaceutical company, announced a large-scale donation initiative with a drug they produce called ivermectin.[19]

Though originally created as a veterinary deworming treatment, ivermectin was shown to treat onchocerciasis ("river blindness"), a neglected tropical disease that can lead to partial or complete loss of vision. Merck pledged to donate the drug for free for as long as necessary to treat the disease.[19] Pfizer also created an azithromycin drug donation program for treatment of blinding trachoma, and GlaxoSmithKline created a donation program for albendazole, which treats soil-transmitted helminth infection, and, in combination with ivermectin, can also treat lymphatic filariasis.

Within the last two years the most common NTDs—the three soil-transmitted helminth infections, schistosomiasis, elephantiasis, trachoma and river blindness—have started to be simultaneously tackled by mass drug administration. In many low-income countries in sub-Saharan Africa, Asia, and the tropical regions of the Americas, the soil-transmitted helminth infections occur in the same geographic location with other important NTDs including elephantiasis, river blindness, schistosomiasis, and trachoma. Many people living in rural poverty in the developing world may have several of these NTDs at the same time. Accordingly, it has been proposed that mass drug administration of albendazole or mebendazole can include a package of additional NTD drugs including praziquantel (for schistosomiasis), ivermectin or diethylcarbamazine (for river blindness and elephantiasis), and azithromycin (for trachoma).[15] This integrated control approach is now being advocated by WHO and other international organizations as a means to maximize efficiency and minimize costs.[17] Because many of the drugs are being donated some estimates indicate that administration of the so-called "rapid impact" drug package can be delivered for around U.S. $0.50 per person.[13,17] This means that a group of diseases causing disease burden almost as great as HIV/AIDS could be controlled or eliminated for under U.S. $1 per person. Beginning in 2006, a Global Network for NTDs[20] (available at http://www.sabin.org/gnntdc; accessed April 14, 2008) was established to help coordinate the major public and private partnerships currently involved in mass drug administration and to provide advocacy and resource mobilization to support the scale-up of the rapid impact package for 56 countries at risk for multiple NTDs.[17] As a result, integrated control of the NTDs (including the soil-transmitted helminth infections) has now begun in several African countries.

Another new and innovative approach to control soil-transmitted helminth infections is through the development of preventative vaccines. In areas of intense transmission, children can become re-infected with hookworm within just a few months after treatment. It would be ideal if a vaccine could be given after deworming to prevent posttreatment reinfection. Through the support of the Bill and Melinda Gates Foundation, the Human Hookworm Vaccine Initiative[21] (available at http://www.sabin.org/hhvi; accessed April 14, 2008) was established in 2000. The Human Hookworm Vaccine Initiative (HHVI) is a non-profit product development partnership that is developing a recombinant protein vaccine for human hookworm infection. Its goal is to develop a safe, efficacious, and low-cost vaccine in order to reduce the burden of disease caused by human hookworm infection. Because hookworm occurs exclusively among people who live on less than $2 per day, there is no commercial market for a hookworm vaccine. To be cost-effective, the hookworm vaccine that HHVI is developing must be manufactured and distributed for less than $1 a dose. Through support by the Gates Foundation, and a network of carefully selected partnering organizations, HHVI has utilized a unique approach to manufacture and deliver this vaccine product to the countries and areas where it is needed most.

Organizations such as the Global Network for Neglected Tropical Disease Control and the HHVI have created new opportunities for the control and elimination of helminth infections. The landscape of infectious diseases is changing, and increased recognition of NTDs as a major global health problem is leading to increasing funding for control programs, research, and development. At an international conference on NTDs at the George Washington University in October 2006, Dr. Tony Fauci, Director of the National Institute of Allergy and Infectious Diseases, affirmed that the global public health community must now look beyond the "Big Three" to the new "Gang of Four": HIV/AIDS, malaria, tuberculosis, and NTDs.

BASIC SCIENCE FACTS/KEY CONCEPTS REVIEW

Ascariasis, trichuriasis, and hookworm infection are of great public health importance due to their worldwide prevalence and their effects on human development.[3] Table 21-1 shows the parasite, common name, and prevalence of each infection.

A. lumbricoides, T. trichiura, N. americanus, and *A. duodenale* are the most prevalent soil-transmitted helminths worldwide, but there are additional soil-transmitted helminths that will not be discussed in detail in this chapter. Other soil-transmitted helminth infections include *Strongyloides stercoralis,* which causes threadworm infections, and *Enterobius vernicularis,* which causes pinworm infections.[4] Roundworms, whipworms, and hookworms are categorized as "soil-transmitted" helminths because soil is their primary reservoir and their vehicle for infecting humans. Humans can ingest *A. lumbricoides* or *T. trichiura* eggs through accidentally ingesting contaminated soil. *N. americanus* and *A. duodenale* larvae infect humans through penetrating the skin. Other helminth species have other routes of infection. For example, schistosomiasis is a water-borne parasitic disease in which cercariae penetrate the skin of humans when they have contact with infected water, such as when bathing or washing clothes.

Life Cycle

Ascaris, trichuris, and hookworm eggs are passed out of infected humans through feces. In areas with poor sanitation, feces are deposited onto the ground and the eggs are able to thrive in warm soil.[4] Eggs are the infective stage of *A. lumbricoides* and *T. trichiura*; humans become infected with ascariasis or trichuriasis by ingesting these eggs. Hookworm eggs, however, must first develop into larvae in the soil, and the larvae infect humans by penetrating their skin. Therefore, the larva is the infective stage of hookworm disease (Figure 21-1).

Once in the human host, *A. lumbricoides* eggs migrate to the small intestine where they develop into larvae. *A. lumbri-coides* larvae undergo a complex travel pattern through organs of the human host before fully developing into an adult worm.[22] From the small intestine, *A. lumbricoides* larvae enter the bloodstream by piercing the wall of the small intestine. The larvae travel through blood vessels to the liver. In the liver, the larvae continue to develop and then re-enter the bloodstream to travel to the human host's heart and then to the lung capillaries. Once in the lungs, the larvae enter the bronchi, the trachea, and the epiglottis, where they are swallowed and are reintroduced to the small intestine. During this second visit to the small intestine, the larvae develop into adult helminths within six weeks.[22] *A. lumbricoides* worms can grow up to 45

FIGURE 21-1 *Ascaris lumbricoides.*

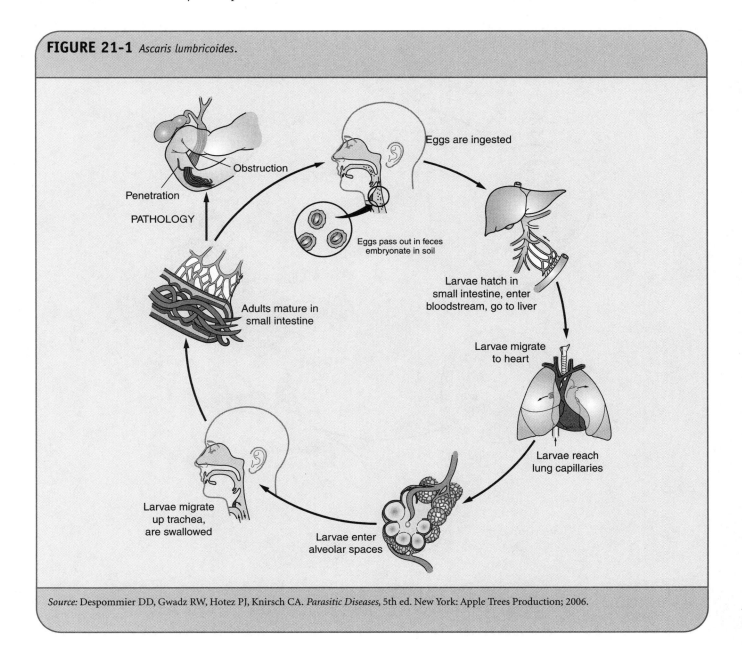

Source: Despommier DD, Gwadz RW, Hotez PJ, Knirsch CA. *Parasitic Diseases*, 5th ed. New York: Apple Trees Production; 2006.

cm, and are the largest of the soil-transmitted helminths.[22] Adult worms undergo sexual reproduction in the small intestine and their eggs are passed out of humans through feces.

After being ingested, *T. trichiura* also travel to the small intestine. From there, *T. trichiura* undergoes a simpler life cycle than *A. lumbricoides*. In the small intestine, the eggs develop to larvae that then migrate to the large intestine. There the *T.*

trichiura larvae develop to mature adult worms, which can measure up to 50 mm in length.[22] The adult worms mate in the large intestine, and eggs are passed out of the human through feces (Figure 21-2).

Hookworm eggs develop to larvae in the soil, and then attach to blades of grass, where they can easily penetrate human skin, sometimes through a hair follicle.[22] Once in the

FIGURE 21-2 *Trichuris trichiura.*

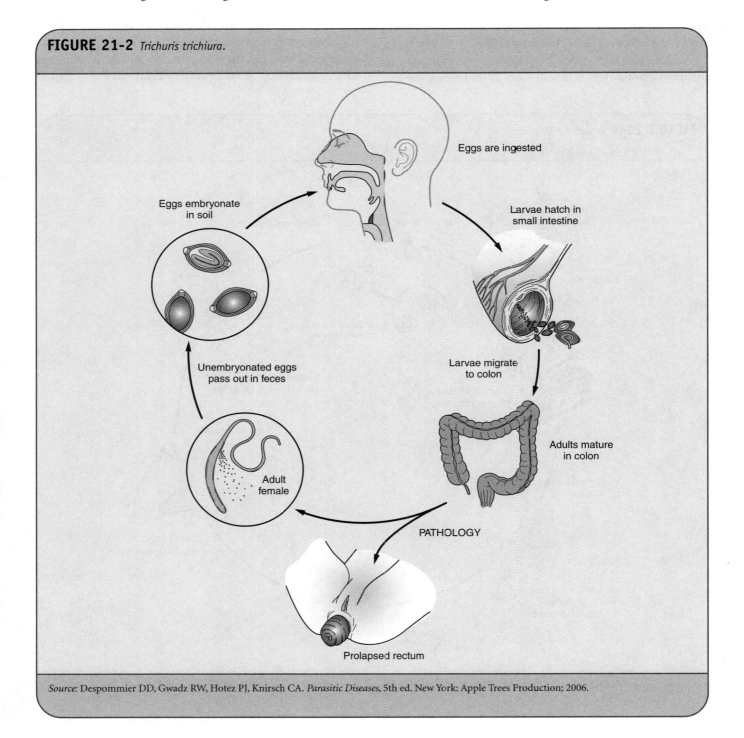

Source: Despommier DD, Gwadz RW, Hotez PJ, Knirsch CA. *Parasitic Diseases,* 5th ed. New York: Apple Trees Production; 2006.

human host, hookworm larvae move through the bloodstream to the heart, where they travel into the lungs and then into the trachea. They are then swallowed and taken to the small intestine, where they mature to adults, mate, and produce eggs which are carried out of the host through feces.[22]

Both species of hookworm—*A. duodenale* and *N. americanus*—follow a similar life cycle, but there are some distinctions. While *N. americanus* worms grow up to between 7 and 11 mm in length, *A. duodenale* worms grow slightly larger to between 8 and 13 mm.[23] Also, *A. duodenale* worms produce more eggs than *N. americanus*: adult *A. duodenale*

worms can produce about 28,000 eggs per day, while *N. americanus* adults only produce around 10,000 eggs per day.[22] Another important variation between the two hookworm species is their geographic location. Kucik, Martin, and Sorter refer to *A. duodenale* as "Old World" hookworm because it is primarily found focally in parts of Africa, India, and Asia. *N. americanus* is often considered "New World" hookworm because it is primarily found in the Americas, although it is also the major hookworm found in sub-Saharan Africa and Southeast Asia.[24] *N. americanus* is the most common hookworm worldwide (Figures 21-3 and 21-4).

FIGURE 21-3 *Necator americanus.*

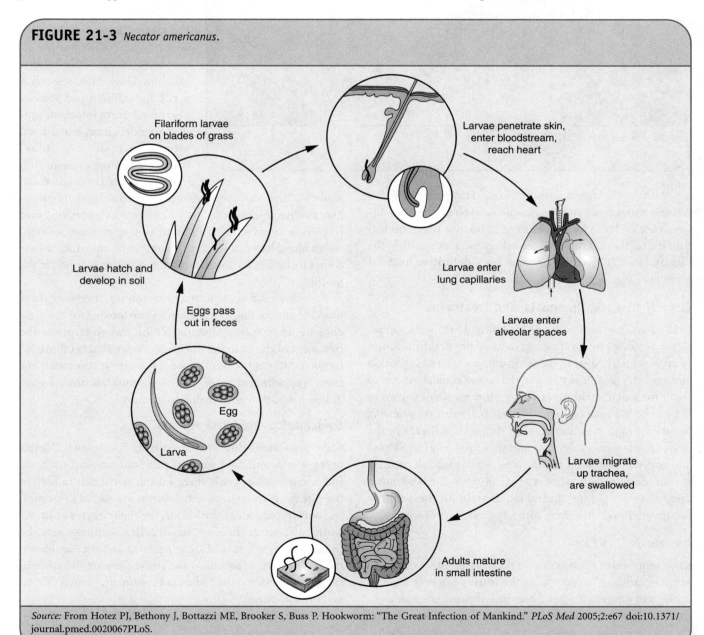

Source: From Hotez PJ, Bethony J, Bottazzi ME, Brooker S, Buss P. Hookworm: "The Great Infection of Mankind." *PLoS Med* 2005;2:e67 doi:10.1371/journal.pmed.0020067PLoS.

FIGURE 21-4 Adult Hookworm.

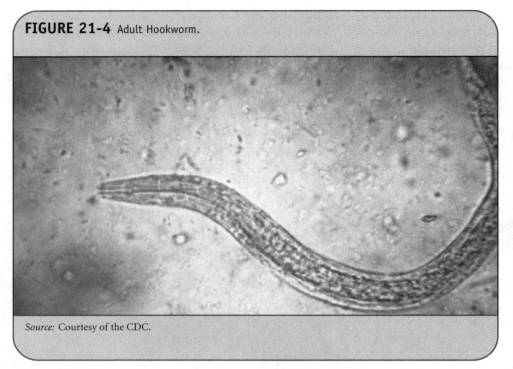

Source: Courtesy of the CDC.

Although *Ascaris lumbricoides, Trichuris trichiura, Necator americanus*, and *Ancylostoma duodenale* undergo different life cycles in human hosts, a distinctive common feature is that they all undergo sexual reproduction within the human hosts. Therefore, humans are a **definitive host** for these parasites.

Clinical Disease, Diagnosis, and Treatment

In children, infection with soil-transmitted helminths can result in physical growth stunting, reduced physical fitness, and neuropsychiatric disturbances including impaired cognition and memory loss. It is possible that these clinical outcomes result from malnutrition caused by the presence of worms in the intestine. In the case of ascariasis, malnutrition probably occurs through malabsorption of nutrients, whereas in the case of hookworm, malnutrition results primarily from blood loss caused by the blood-feeding behavior of the adult parasite.

In addition, each major type of soil-transmitted helminth causes its own unique clinical manifestations; these mostly occur with heavy infections with large numbers of worms.

Ascariasis

Large numbers of adult worms in the small intestine can cause acute intestinal obstruction, or the worms can migrate into the liver or pancreas to cause hepatitis or pancreatitis, respectively. Also, as the larvae migrate in the lungs before reaching the intestine they can cause wheezing that resembles asthma.

Trichuriasis

The adult worms cause inflammation in the large intestine (also known as the colon) to produce colitis. Very heavy infections in young children result in bloody diarrhea, a condition known as the *Trichuris* dysentery syndrome, as well as a prolapse of the rectum.

Hookworm

Hookworm disease results when large numbers of hookworms simultaneously produce significant blood loss.[25] Because blood is rich in both iron and protein, heavy hookworm infections produce **iron deficiency anemia** and protein malnutrition. Hookworm is a leading cause of iron deficiency anemia in children and women of reproductive age. These two populations are particularly vulnerable because they often have low underlying iron reserves to begin with. In addition, during pregnancy, hookworm blood loss can result in a number of unfortunate outcomes including low birth weight and severe anemia for the mother.

All three soil-transmitted helminth infections are diagnosed by conducting a fecal examination looking for the presence of worm eggs. Albendazole or mebendazole is the treatment of choice for all three soil-transmitted helminth infections. Although a single dose is used most commonly for mass drug administration, sometimes multiple doses are required in order to achieve full deworming.

Epidemiology and Risk Factors

Soil-transmitted helminth infections are diseases of the developing world, and the people of sub-Saharan Africa, China, India, and Southeast Asia share a disproportionate burden of the disease. Although these helminths are found in tropical and sub-tropical areas worldwide, the highest rates of hookworm infection are in sub-Saharan Africa, Southeast Asia, the Indian subcontinent, and Latin America and the Caribbean; the highest rates of ascariasis and trichuriasis are in East Asia, sub-Saharan Africa, the Indian subcontinent, Latin America, and the Caribbean.[26]

Poverty is perhaps the greatest risk factor for infection with a soil-transmitted helminth. Worldwide, infection is primarily limited to individuals who live on under $2 per day.[4,17] This phenomenon is primarily explained by environmental conditions in the developing world. Globally, the "poorest of the poor" live in areas with inadequate sanitation, scarce water supply, and insufficient health systems.[26] Combined with a tropical climate, these factors contribute to ongoing transmission in many developing countries.

Age is another important risk factor for soil-transmitted helminth infections, with school-aged children being at greatest risk. In endemic areas, prevalence of infection sharply increases from birth and peaks between the ages of five and ten. After this initial peak, prevalence of infection in an endemic community will remain high in all age groups if no efforts are made to reduce transmission, such as through mass drug administrations. In terms of intensity of infection (roughly defined as the number of worms per person), school-aged children tend to have the highest intensities of infection in a population until the adolescent years. This age disparity is important because intensity of infection is directly related to morbidity; therefore, children experience anemia, malnutrition, and other health effects of infection during a crucial period of cognitive and physical development. Intensity of infection will slowly decrease throughout the adolescent years and then will sharply decrease during adulthood.[3] The gradual decrease of individual worm burden throughout adulthood indicates that humans may develop protective immune mechanisms after continuous exposure to intestinal helminths.[27,28] This age distribution is also likely influenced by behavioral factors. Children tend to place dirty fingers in their mouths and run around barefoot, which are both routes of worm exposure.[28]

A related epidemiological aspect of helminth infections is that a minority of the people infected harbor the majority of infection. This phenomenon is sometimes referred to as the 80/20 rule: 20 percent of the infected population harbor 80 percent of the helminths.[3] The reason behind this aggregation of parasites within hosts is not well understood. Possible explanations include exposure factors, increased susceptibility to infections in certain persons, and immunological differences within a population.[3]

Infection with soil-transmitted helminths can be treated using albendazole or mebendazole. Mass drug administration with these drugs is typically conducted on an annual basis. However, in areas of high transmission, such treatment is simply a short-term solution. Studies of **reinfection rates** in endemic regions have shown that individuals can become reinfected months or even weeks after treatment. This cycle of reinfection occurs because individuals are constantly exposed to the parasites. Helminth reinfection has special implications

for school-aged children, who typically harbor the highest infection intensities in a community. Research suggests that in very high transmission areas children may need to receive albendazole or mebendazole every four to six months to keep their worm burdens down or effectively reduce the prevalence of infection.[29]

Another important characteristic of the epidemiology of helminth infections is that individuals are often infected with two or more helminth infections concurrently. A survey of over 1,500 schoolchildren on Pemba Island, Tanzania, found that over 90 percent were infected with more than one helminth infection, and 58% were infected with A. lumbricoides, T. trichiura, and hookworm concurrently.[30] Polyparasitism in endemic regions is linked to individual predisposition to helminth infections and environmental influences.[31] Also, emerging evidence on polyparasitism indicates that the multiple concurrent parasitic infections may have a synergistic effect. A study conducted in Americaninhas, a rural village in Minas Gerais, Brazil, found that 50.3 percent of the population harbored two concurrent helminth infections, and 23.0 percent of individuals were infected with three helminths.[32] Furthermore, researchers found that the intensity of hookworm infection correlated with increasing co-infections from other parasites, suggesting that hookworm infection may promote immunological pathways for increased susceptibility to other helminth infections.[32]

Long-Term Health Impacts

Parasitic infections exert a strong influence on the host's nutritional status. Children with heavy helminth infections have decreased appetite as compared with children with light helminth infections or uninfected children, even if food is readily available.[28] Studies of children with roundworm infection have shown that children's' appetites increase after their helminth load is reduced following antihelminthic treatment.[27] Also, adult worms reside in humans' small and large intestines and these infections negatively impact the body's ability to absorb some nutrients.[27] For example, ascariasis has been linked to poor vitamin A, iodine, and protein absorption.[27]

A significant nutritional deficiency caused by helminth infections is intestinal blood loss, which is associated with decreased iron stores. Anemia develops because blood loss leads to a decrease in circulating red blood cells in the infected individual. Among the soil-transmitted helminths, hookworms are the major cause of intestinal blood loss. This blood loss occurs when adult hookworms suck blood from their host in the small intestine.[23] In addition, Trichuris adult worms cause bleeding in the large bowel, and bleeding in the rectum for children who develop Trichuris dysentery syndrome.[33] Physically,

iron deficiency and anemia are two separate conditions; however, the majority of people with anemia in the developing world also suffer from iron deficiency.[34] Therefore, the term iron deficiency anemia is often used to describe the intersection of these two conditions.[34]

Impaired physical growth is another health impact of soil-transmitted helminth infections, and this is likely mediated by nutritional deficiencies. Physical growth deficits have been seen in infected individuals through a variety of anthropometric methods, including weight-for-age, height-for-age, tricep skinfold, and middle arm circumference measurements.[35] It is difficult, however, to definitively link the helminth infections as the direct cause of physical growth impairment because infected individuals live in impoverished environments where a host of other influences also affect physical growth.[35] Despite the lack of direct causal evidence, researchers have documented that treating children with antihelminthic drugs leads to improvements in their physical development, especially with weight gain. In an intervention trial among Kenyan schoolchildren, researchers found that children who received albendazole treatments showed improvements in several anthropometric measurements as compared to children who did not receive the treatment.[36] A study in Guatemala showed that deworming medication reduced the intensity of ascariasis and trichuriasis in infected children and led to significant improvements in weight gain six months after treatment.[37]

Helminth infections are also linked to poor cognitive development among children. Delays in cognitive development correlate with intensity of infection; high intensities of helminth infection are associated with poorer cognitive development in children as compared to uninfected children or children with light burdens of infection.[38] Early randomized experimental studies provided the initial evidence for the link between helminth burden and cognitive deficits, which were typically measured by performance on standardized tests. A study in the early 1900s in the United States found that children who received treatment for hookworm infection showed larger improvements in arithmetic and handwriting skills as compared to children who did not receive treatment.[38,39] More recently, a double-blind placebo study of 159 school children in Jamaica in 1992 found that children with moderate to severe whipworm infection who received antihelminthic treatment showed significant improvements on some tests of cognitive function as compared to children who received a placebo.[40] The improvements were primarily evident on tests that assessed the child's attention or memory.[40]

Ethical considerations in designing health studies have progressed to the current belief that if researchers provide deworming pills for a study, they must provide them to all infected subjects. Therefore, more recent studies on the association between helminth infection and cognitive functioning have a cross-sectional design, or a quasi-experimental design, in which cognitive performance is measured before and after mass drug administrations. In a 1999 study, Sakti and colleagues measured the association between helminth infection and cognitive function among 432 schoolchildren in Indonesia. The researchers found that hookworm infection was associated with lower scores on tests of working memory.[41] A cross-sectional study of over 300 children in the Philippines in 2005 demonstrated that moderate or high roundworm infection was associated with poor performance on memory tests and all intensities of infection with whipworms were associated with lower scores on tests of verbal fluency.[42] As compared to earlier experimental studies, the design of cross-sectional analyses does not allow strong evidence to support a causal relationship between helminth burden and cognitive functioning. However, when consideration is given to the earlier experimental studies and later cross-sectional analyses, the combined evidence points to a strong association between high burdens of helminth infection and impaired cognitive development in children.

Several biological mechanisms are hypothesized to cause this delayed cognitive functioning in infected children. Nutritional deficiencies, including low iron stores, lead to low energy levels in children, and therefore children have less energy to pay attention in school.[38] Children may experience discomfort as a result of worm migration in their bodies, such as the ground itch that often occurs when hookworm larva penetrate the skin or when A. lumbricoides worms migrate through the lungs.[38] This acute physical discomfort can also distract a child from being fully alert and ready to learn. Also, chronic helminth infection leads to continuous stress by the host immune system, which can contribute to slower reaction times in children.[38]

The highest prevalence and intensities of hookworm, whipworm, and roundworm infections are in children; therefore, studies on nutritional deficiencies, physical growth, and cognitive development have focused on this age group. New attention is being given to how these ill health effects manifest from childhood to adulthood. For example, studies of adult workers with chronic iron deficiency anemia have shown that they have less energy for work and produce less work output as compared to their healthier counterparts.[43] Moreover, cognitive deficits and poor performance in school are associated with decreased financial earning later in adulthood.[43] The long term effects of helminth infections show that these are not just conditions of poverty—soil-transmitted helminth infections are also poverty-promoting diseases.[13]

CASE STUDY
Scenario

Eduardo is an eight-year-old boy who lives in a rural town in the northeast corner of the state of Minas Gerais, Brazil, called Americaninhas. He is very thin and is underdeveloped compared to other children his age. He used to attend school periodically, but now he is needed by his family to work in the fields. Sometimes at night, Eduardo has trouble falling asleep because he has a mild stomachache. Eduardo does not like to wake up early in the morning to accompany his older brothers to the field because he always feels tired. While there, he is not quite as productive as his brothers as he always works a bit slower than everyone else. His parents notice that Eduardo sometimes scratches his skin, including his feet.

Defining the Issues

The major clinical symptoms of hookworm infection may include dermatitis when filarial hookworm larvae penetrate the skin in a condition called "ground itch." Larvae passing through the lungs after entering the circulation may cause pulmonary symptoms such as cough, wheezing, and pulmonary infiltrates. Some individuals infected with hookworm also may experience gastrointestinal discomfort as a result of the adult hookworms residing in the intestine.

The long-term health effects of chronic hookworm infection common to rural areas in developing country settings are of major concern. Blood loss caused by adult worms living in the intestine can result in the development of anemia and protein deficiency. In areas where children like Eduardo are continually exposed to hookworm larvae (and to other helminth infections), the loss of iron and protein can stunt growth and cognitive development. As a result, children infected with hookworm are often thin, anemic, and lethargic.

Patient's Understanding

While Eduardo has the signs and symptoms associated with chronic hookworm infection, he may not even know he is infected because the symptoms are often mild and nondescript. He just knows that he feels tired, sluggish, and may have some gastrointestinal discomfort at times. Eduardo's hookworm infection status is determined by examining a stool sample. When there are hookworm eggs present in the stool, he is definitely diagnosed with hookworm infection.

CLINICAL PERSPECTIVE
Current Interventions

The standard treatment for hookworm infection includes a class of drugs called benzimidazoles. Albendazole, a synthetic nitroimidazole, has broad spectrum antinematodal activity. A single dose of albendazole is often effective treatment for most forms of intestinal helminthiasis, though multiple doses may be needed to treat heavy infections. However, in areas such as Americaninhas where the prevalence of hookworm infection is very high, several doses must be given in order to effectively treat individuals with heavy hookworm infections. Mebendazole is another similar drug used to treat hookworm that must be given for three days. In addition, iron supplementation is also required for individuals such as Eduardo who may have iron-deficiency anemia.

Prevention Initiatives

The transmission of hookworm infection is aided by poor sanitary practices in which infected persons defecate in areas where others may walk without shoes. Like for many other infectious diseases, the primary prevention measure includes improved sanitation initiatives. In addition, educational interventions targeted towards individuals in hookworm-endemic areas should focus on prevention of transmission through improved sanitation practices.

PUBLIC HEALTH PERSPECTIVE FOR THE HEALTH OF THE GENERAL POPULATION AND OF HIGH RISK GROUPS

Many school-aged children worldwide experience similar symptoms as Eduardo. In tropical regions of the developing world, poverty is the greatest risk factor for hookworm and other helminth infections. Economic development, combined with improved sanitation, greater access to medical care, and health education programs, would greatly impact public health outcomes in Eduardo's village. Even if Eduardo and other children are treated for helminth infections with albendazole or mebendezole, they are likely to be reinfected due to continuous transmission in the area. From a public health perspective, a vaccine against hookworm infection, such as the one being developed by the Human Hookworm Vaccine Initiative, could provide protection from infection and reinfection. From an epidemiological standpoint, it is important to consider that Eduardo and his peers are likely afflicted by several helminth infections, and they may also have other neglected tropical diseases, such as schistosomiasis. Public health interventions should aim to address all of these multiple concurrent infections.

The public health impacts of helminth infections should be considered over the entire course of Eduardo's life. Helminth infections are associated with poorer cognitive development among children, and this is likely due to the nutritional deficiencies caused by helminth infections. As a result, Eduardo and other children in the developing world will experience greater difficulties in learning and school performance. When he grows older, Eduardo may find that he cannot perform job functions as quickly or efficiently as others who were not continuously exposed to hookworm in childhood.

KEY TERMS
Biology Terms

Anthelminthic Drugs: Medicine used to treat intestinal helminth infections. Albendazole or mebendazole are currently the standard anthelminthic treatments. Although anthelminthic drugs are used to treat current infection, they do not prevent future reinfection.

Definitive Host: Location where parasites undergo sexual reproduction.

Iron Deficiency Anemia: The intersection of two health conditions: iron deficiency, caused by inadequate iron absorption and/or iron loss, and anemia, which is caused by insufficient circulating red blood cells. Many individuals in the developing world infected with helminth infections suffer from both iron deficiency and anemia.

Larva: Immature stage of helminth prior to developing to adult worm.

Public Health Terms

Disability-Adjusted Life Year (DALY): An estimate of the number of healthy, productive years of life lost due to morbidity or premature mortality from a disease. The estimates are derived by applying disability "weights" to different conditions and multiplying that weight by the number of years that an infected person is affected by that condition.

Mass Drug Administration (MDA): Treating an entire community for a condition, as opposed to only treating infected individuals.

Reinfection Rate: Number of times an individual is infected with a disease over a particular time period. In areas endemic with helminth infections, unless interventions, such as regular mass drug administrations, improved sanitation infrastructure, and health education, reinfection rates are implemented.

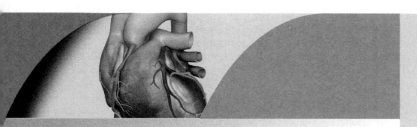

Questions for Further Research, Study, Reflection, and Discussion

For the Individual Student

In order to answer these questions, it may be necessary to research the primary literature.

- Review the life cycles of *A. lumbricoides*, *T. trichiura*, and hookworm. What are some similarities and differences in their life cycles?
- Why do you think having multiple helminth infections (*polyparasitism*) may have different health effects in humans than only having one helminth infection?
- What are some issues that may arise with drug distribution programs such as semi-annual distribution of albendazole or mebendazole?

For Small Group Discussion

- Imagine that your group is responsible for delivering a vaccine to a small village in a rural location. What are some challenges that your team may face?
- Although soil-transmitted helminths are one of the most prevalent diseases on Earth, they are not well known by the lay public. What factors do you think contribute to their neglected status?
- What are some differences in quantifying the burden of a disease using mortality estimates versus morbidity estimates, such as the disability-adjusted life year (DALY) estimate? Discuss which diseases one type of estimate may be more useful for than the other.

For Entire Class Discussion

- In what ways are helminth infections and poverty interrelated?
- Albendazole and mebendazole are drugs that are currently effective in treating soil-transmitted helminths. The Human Hookworm Vaccine Initiative is developing a vaccine against hookworm infection. If we have these drug treatments, then why is the development of a hookworm necessary? What are some advantages and disadvantages of drug treatments versus vaccines?
- Philanthropic organizations such as the Bill and Melinda Gates Foundation have revolutionized neglected tropical disease (NTD) research and control programs by providing large-scale financial support for such initiatives. What other types of organizations also need to be involved in order to promote long-term, sustainable solutions in NTD-afflicted areas? Consider a broad range of institutions, including national and local governments, international organizations, private industry, and academic institutions.

EXERCISES/ACTIVITIES

- Break into small working groups. Conduct a literature search for academic publications on other neglected tropical diseases such as lymphatic filariasis, schistosomiasis, onchocerciasis, and trachoma. Which features of these diseases are similar to soil-transmitted helminths? How are these diseases different?
- Visit the Web site of The Global Network for Neglected Tropical Disease Control (GNNTDC; http://www.gnntdc.org), a partnership of neglected tropical disease control programs and initiatives. Research the different partner organizations to learn about each organization's work in the fight against NTDs. How do you think initiatives like GNNTDC will aid in reducing the prevalence and burden of NTDs worldwide?

REFERENCES

1. Norman NR. This wormy world. *J Parasitol* 1947;33:1–18.

2. Montressor A, Crompton DWT, Gyorkos TW, Savioli L. Helminth control in school-age children: a guide for managers of control programmes. Geneva: World Health Organization Press; 2002.

3. Hotez PJ, Bundy DA, Beegle K, et al. Helminth infections: soil-transmitted helminth infections and schistosomiasis. In: Jamison DT, Breman JG, Measham AR, et al., eds. *Disease Control Priorities in Developing Countries*, 2nd ed. New York: Oxford University Press; 2006:467–482.

4. Bethony J, Brooker S, Albonico M, Geiger SM, Loukas A, Diemert D, Hotez PJ. Soil-transmitted helminth infections: ascariasis, trichuriasis, and hookworm. *Lancet* 2006;3671:1521–1532.

5. Cox FEG. History of human parasitology. *Clin Microbiol Rev* 2002;15:595–612.

6. World Health Organization. *Prevention and Control of Parasitic Diseases: Report of a WHO Expert Committee.* WHO Technical Report Series 749. Geneva: WHO; 1987.

7. Marin MG, Humphreys ME. Social consequences of disease in the American South, 1900–World War II. *South Med J* 2006;99:862–864.

8. Bleakley H. Disease and development: evidence from hookworm eradication in the American South. *Quart J Economics* 2007;122:73–117.

9. World Health Organization. The World Health Report 2004, Annex Table 21-2: Deaths by cause, sex, and morality stratums in WHO regions, estimates for 2002. (2004). Available at http://www.who.int/whr/2004/annex/topic/en/annex_2_en.pdf. Accessed April 15, 2008.

10. World Health Organization. *Prevention and Control of Schistosomiasis and Soil-Transmitted Helminths.* WHO Technical Report Series 912. Geneva: WHO; 2002.

11. Murray CJ, Lopez AD. Global mortality, disability, and the contribution of risk factors: Global Burden of Disease Study. *Lancet* 1997;349:1436–1442.

12. Chan MS. Global burden of intestinal nematodes—fifty years on. *Parasitol Today* 1997;13:438–443.

13. Hotez PJ, Molyneux DH, Fenwick A, Ottesen E, Sachs SE, Sachs J. Incorporating a rapid-impact package for neglected tropical diseases with programs for HIV/AIDS, tuberculosis, and malaria. *PLoS Med* 2006;3:e102 doi:10.1371/journal.pmed.0030102.

14. World Health Organization (2007). Lymphatic filariasis: Fact Sheet. Available at http://www.who.int/mediacentre/factsheets/fs102/en/. Accessed April 15, 2008.

15. Molyneux DM, Hotez PJ, Fenwick A. "Rapid-impact interventions": how a policy of integrated control for Africa's neglected tropical diseases could benefit the poor. *PLoS Med* 2005;2:e336 doi:10.1371/journal.pmed.0020336.

16. World Health Organization. 54th World Health Assembly Resolution (2002). Available at http://www.who.int/wormcontrol/documents/wha/en/. Accessed April 15, 2008.

17. Hotez PJ, Molyneux DH, Fenwick A, Kumaresan J, Sachs SE, Sachs JD, Savioli L. Control of neglected tropical diseases. *N Engl J Med* 2007;357:1018–1027.

18. World Bank. *School Deworming at a Glance.* Washington, DC: World Bank Publications; 2003.

19. Hotez P, Ottesen E, Fenwick A, Molyneux D. The neglected tropical diseases: the ancient afflictions of stigma and poverty and the prospects for their control and elimination. *Adv Exp Med Biol* 2006;532:23–33.

20. The Global Network for Neglected Tropical Diseases. (2006). Available at http://www.sabin.org/gnntdc. Accessed May 5, 2008.

21. The Human Hookworm Vaccine Initiative. (2007). Available at http://www.sabin.org/hhvi. Accessed May 5, 2008.

22. Despommier DD, Gwadz RW, Hotez PJ, Knirsch CA. *Parasitic Diseases*, 5th ed. New York: Apple Trees Production; 2006.

23. Crompton DW. The public health importance of hookworm disease. *Parasitology* 2000;121:S39–S50.

24. Kucik CJ, Martin GL, Sortor BV. Common intestinal parasites. *Am Fam Physician* 2004;69:1161–1168.

25. Hotez PJ, Brooker S, Bethony JM, Bottazzi ME, Loukas A, Xiao S. Hookworm infection. *N Engl J Med* 2004;351:799–807.

26. de Silva NR, Brooker S, Hotez PJ, Montresor A, Engels D, Savioli L. Soil-transmitted helminths: updating the global picture. *Trends Parasitol* 2003;19:547–51.

27. O'Lorcain P, Holland CV. The public health importance of *Ascaris lumbricoides*. *Parasitology* 2002;121:S51–S71.

28. Bundy DA, Del Rosso JA. Making nutritional improvements at a low cost through parasite control: Guidelines for designing and implementing mass treatment interventions. *The World Bank, Human Resources Development and Operations Policy #7*, 1993.

29. Albonico M, Smith PG, Ercole E, Hall A, Chwaya HM, Alawi KS. Rate of reinfection with intestinal nematodes after treatment of children with mebendazole or albendazole in a highly endemic area. *Transact Royal Soc Trop Med Hygiene* 1995;89:538–541

30. Booth M, Bundy DA, Albonico M, Chwaya HM, Alawi KS, Savioli L. Associations among multiple geohelminth species infections in schoolchildren from Pemba Island. *Parasitology* 1998;116(Pt 1):85–93.

31. Booth M, Bundy DA. Estimating the number of multiple-species geohelminth infections in human communities. *Parasitology* 1995;111(Pt 5):645–653.

32. Fleming FM, Brooker S, Geiger SM, Caldas IR, Correa-Oliveira R, Hotez PJ, Bethony JM. Synergistic associations between hookworm and other helminth species in a rural community in Brazil. *Trends Parasitol* 2003;19:547–551.

33. Stephenson LS, Holland CV, Cooper ES. The public health significance of *Trichuris trichiura*. *Parasitology* 2000;121:S73–S95.

34. World Health Organization. Iron deficiency anemia: assessment, prevention and control. Geneva: WHO; 2001. Available at http://www.who.int/nutrition/publications/en/ida_assessment_prevention_control.pdf. Accessed April 15, 2008.

35. De Silva NR. Impact of mass chemotherapy on the morbidity due to soil-transmitted nematodes. *Acta Tropica* 2003;86:197–214.

36. Adams EJ, Stephenson LS, Latham MC, Kinoti SN. Physical activity and growth of Kenyan school children with hookworm, *Trichuris trichiura* and *Ascaris lumbricoides* infections are improved after treatment with albendazole. *J Nutr* 1994;124:1199–1206.

37. Watkins WE, Pollitt E. Effect of removing *Ascaris* on the growth of Guatemalan schoolchildren. *Pediatrics* 1996;97:871–876.

38. Watkins WE, Pollitt E. "Stupidity or worms": do intestinal worms impair mental performance? *Psychol Bull* 1997;121:171–191.

39. Strong EK. Effects of Hookworm Disease on the Mental and Physical Development of Children. New York: Rockefeller Foundation's International Health Commission; 1916.

40. Nokes C, Grantham-McGregor SM, Sawyer AW, Cooper ES, Robinson BA, Bundy DA. Moderate to heavy infections of *Trichuris trichiura* affect cognitive function in Jamaican school children. *Parasitology* 1992;104:539–547.

41. Sakti H, Nokes C, Hertanto WS, Hendratno S, Hall A, Bundy DA, Satoto. Evidence for an association between hookworm infection and cognitive function in Indonesian school children. *Trop Med Int Health* 1999;4:322–334.

42. Ezeamama AE, Friedman JF, Acosta LP, et al. Helminth infection and cognitive impairment among Filipino children. *Am J Trop Med Hygiene* 2005;72:540–548.

43. Guyatt H. Do intestinal nematodes affect productivity in adulthood? *Parasitol Today* 2000;16:153–158.

CROSS REFERENCES

Nutrition Transition

The Public Health Triad

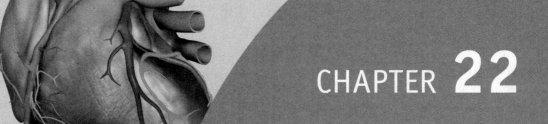

Malaria:
The Challenge of Scaling-Up
Multiple Effective Tools

Lawrence Barat

The World Health Organization (WHO) estimates that 250 million to 550 million cases of malaria occur each year, resulting in more than one million deaths. More than 90 percent of deaths are in children less than five years of age in Sub-Saharan Africa. In other words, about 2,700 African children die every day from malaria, or about two each minute. The devastation caused by malaria continues to occur despite the availability of a number of effective tools for control.[1]

LEARNING OBJECTIVES

By the end of this chapter, the student will be able to:

- Outline the lifecycle of malaria and its effect on clinical disease.
- Describe the global burden of malaria and factors that affect those who bear that burden.
- Detail the range of available effective malaria control measures.
- Discuss some of the challenges that impede the scaling up of effective malaria control interventions and propose some possible solutions to these problems.

HISTORY

Malaria is considered one of the oldest human diseases. Descriptions are found in Egyptian hieroglyphics and other ancient texts written thousands of years ago. Despite this, the causative agents of malaria, parasites of the genus **Plasmodium**, were not discovered until the late 19th century by researchers in India.

As recently as the middle of the 20th century, malaria transmission was common in Italy and southern Europe, the Caucases, and the Southeast United States. Effective control efforts during the middle of the 20th century interrupted malaria transmission in all of Europe, the Soviet Union, and the United States. The break-up of the Soviet Union, though, saw a re-introduction of malaria into the Caucases and the Korean Peninsula, where it persists today.

BASIC SCIENCE FACTS/KEY CONCEPTS REVIEW

Malaria is caused by infection with a single-celled, nucleated protozoan of the genus *Plasmodium*. There are four species of *Plasmodium* that cause disease in humans: *P. vivax, P. falciparum, P. ovale, and P. malariae. P. vivax* and *P. falciparum* are far more prevalent, accounting for almost 90 percent of all cases worldwide. Almost all severe disease and death from malaria is the result of *P. falciparum* infection.

Like most parasites infecting humans, malaria goes through both asexual and sexual reproduction during its lifecycle. Different from almost all other such parasites, asexual reproduction occurs in the human and sexual reproduction in the gut of **Anopheles** spp. mosquito, meaning that mosquitoes are the final host for malaria and humans are intermediate hosts.

Only mosquitoes from the genus *Anopheles* can transmit human malaria and only female mosquitoes bite. Different *Plasmodium* species infect other animals, particularly birds. In fact, penguins in zoos must be kept on malaria treatment to prevent them from being infected with a type of bird malaria that is fatal to them. Female anophelines take "blood meals" to get heme, an iron-containing compound found in hemoglobin. Heme is required for the mosquito eggs to complete maturation but the blood meal does not provide the mosquito with nourishment. When an infected female *Anopheles* mosquito takes a blood meal, parasite sporozoites in the mosquito's mouthparts are released into the bloodstream and travel immediately to the host's liver (Figure 22-1). These sporozoites infect hepatocytes (liver cells), mature, multiply, and are released back into the bloodstream. This "extra-**erythrocytic cycle**" takes from 9 to up to 30 days, depending on the species of infecting parasite. Once released from the hepatocytes, the parasites then infect red blood cells and go through a second round of asexual reproduction (that is, the erythrocytic cycle). These parasites mature, multiply, and ultimately rupture the red blood cells. The released parasites go on to infect other red blood cells, repeating the cycle.

For reasons that are unclear, a small percentage of parasites that infect red blood cells will not go through the asexual cycle, but rather differentiate in female or male gametocytes. When another *Anopheles* spp. mosquito bites that person, the mosquito must take up both male and female gametocytes for the lifecycle to be completed. These gametocytes will mature into gametes and then fuse to form a zygote in the wall of the mosquito's gut. The zygote differentiates and produces multiple sporozoites, which then travel to the mosquito's mouthparts. When the mosquito takes its next blood meal, these sporo-

zoites will be passed into the bloodstream of the next host, thereby completing the lifecycle.

In *P. vivax* and *P. ovale* infections, there is a variation in the **exo-erythrocytic cycle**. With these two species, a small percentage of parasites that infect hepatocytes do not mature and multiply, but instead become dormant. These so-called hypnozoites reactivate weeks to months later, completing their lifecycle and causing a second parasitemia. This is known as a **relapse**. Relapses have symptoms identical to those of the initial parasitemia and can be treated in the same way as the initial infection.

PUBLIC HEALTH PERSPECTIVE FOR THE HEALTH OF THE GENERAL POPULATION AND OF HIGH RISK GROUPS

Malaria is transmitted in more than 100 countries, mostly in tropical and subtropical regions (Figure 22-2). Sub-Saharan Africa bears more than 80 percent of the global burden. Other heavily affected areas include South and Southeast Asia, many Indian and Pacific Islands, Central and South America, particularly the Amazon basin and Guyana Shield (Guyana,

FIGURE 22-1 Life Cycle of *Anopheles* Mosquito.

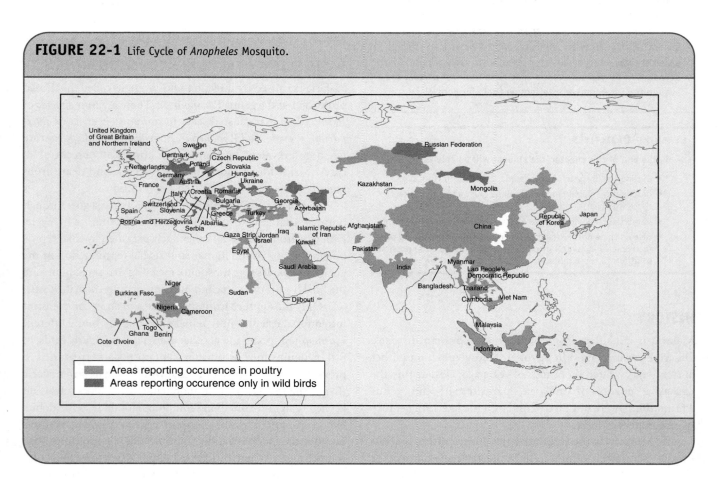

CASE STUDY

ATTACKING THE MOST VULNERABLE

Scenario

Malaria transmission has been interrupted in almost all of North America, Europe, and East Asia. A typical person with malaria in the United States, therefore, would be an immigrant from a country with malaria transmission or his or her children who return to their home country to visit family. Even such cases are rare.

The most typical person affected with malaria is a child in Sub-Saharan Africa during their second year of life. Such a child can have up to eight or more episodes of malaria during that year. Malaria will manifest with fever, irritability, decreased appetite, and sometimes diarrhea. Anemia is also common, although malaria is usually one of several causal factors.

Left untreated, the illness can progress. The child may develop coma, seizures, severe anemia, and/or respiratory distress. In rare cases, the child's kidneys or liver may fail.

If a full-course of correct treatment is provided before severe disease develops, the sick child should recover fully and be cured. Treatment is possible for those with severe disease, but up to 40 percent will die nonetheless.

Defining the Issues

For a person with malaria, the keys to survival are rapid detection and treatment. A delay of even a few hours can mean the difference between life and death.

Rapid detection requires that mothers quickly identify when their child has fever and immediately seek care from a trained medical professional. That professional must assess the child to rule out other causes of illness, look for signs and symptoms of severe disease, and do the appropriate diagnostic testing to confirm malaria infection.

Once malaria has been diagnosed, the clinician must prescribe the correct treatment at an appropriate dose, based on the child's age or weight. The prescribed medicines must be in stock at the pharmacy and dispensed correctly. The mother must then administer the correct dose at appropriate times for the prescribed duration of treatment. If the child is severely ill, he or she must be properly referred for inpatient treatment.

The steps just outlined for successful diagnosis and treatment would appear to be easy to carry out. When the infected person is a young African child, though, many challenges arise. Weak health systems, an uneducated population, cultural beliefs and norms, and the financial and opportunity costs of care and treatment pose significant barriers to the rapid diagnosis and treatment of children with malaria in Sub-Saharan Africa.

Patient's Understanding

An African child, or more specifically her/his mother, seeking treatment for malaria faces numerous choices and challenges. The symptoms of malaria, particularly in a young child, are identical to those of influenza, diarrheal disease, and any number of other infectious diseases. The mother, therefore, may decide to wait a day or two to see if the child improves before seeking care for her sick child, hoping to avoid the financial and opportunity costs involved in obtaining healthcare services.

In cases where the child develops severe disease, particularly when it manifests with coma or recurrent seizures, local cultural beliefs may lead the mother to believe the child is the victim of possession or a curse. Rather than seek medical care, this child would be brought to the local religious leader or shaman.

Once the mother has determined that the child needs treatment, many factors will affect her decisions about where such treatment should be sought. Public health facilities may be several hours away on-foot and take the mother away from her work in the fields and her other children. There frequently are fees for both the examination and laboratory tests, and treatment that can be beyond the mother's ability to pay.

The mother may first try administering leftover drugs from a previous illness. Alternatively, the mother's cultural upbringing may lead her to first use a traditional healer or traditional remedies. Only if the child fails to improve will the mother look for care outside the home.

She may then decide to purchase medicine from a nearby informal (that is, unlicensed) drug seller or shop. Although these drug sellers are often more easily accessible and less expensive, they usually lack even basic medical training and can sell medicines that are of poor quality or completely counterfeit.

For those mothers who decide to invest the time and money to bring their child to a health facility, the nearest health facility is unlikely to have a laboratory. Their child will be diagnosed and treated based solely on the clinical grounds, leading many children to be misdiagnosed. Poorly trained clinicians also may miss signs and symptoms of **severe malaria** and send the mother home with oral medication when hospital care is warranted.

Even for those mothers whose child is correctly diagnosed with malaria, they will often be handed a prescription and told to go buy the medicines in a private pharmacy, because the clinic pharmacy has run out. No doubt, this must leave many mothers to wonder why they spend the time and money to seek care at a facility, when they could have gone directly to a drug seller in the first place.

Until recently, if a mother was lucky enough to bring her child to a health facility where drugs were in stock, the treatment that was likely to be dispensed was chloroquine, despite extensive evidence of high levels of treatment failures to this drug. Fortunately, this and other ineffective drugs are rapidly being phased out and replaced with more effective treatments.

CLINICAL PERSPECTIVE FOR THE INDIVIDUAL PATIENT

As stated in the case study, the symptoms of **uncomplicated malaria** are indistinguishable from a number of common infectious and even some noninfectious causes of febrile illness. High fever with body ache, headache, and sometimes diarrhea are typical symptoms of malaria. Classical cyclical fever develops late in the course of illness and rarely occurs with falciparum malaria. The nonspecific nature of these symptoms poses a significant challenge for clinicians who often confuse other causes of febrile illness with malaria.

A careful examination of the lifecycle provides us with an understanding of the timing and array of symptoms typically seen with malaria. For example, the symptoms of malaria generally begin from 9 to 30 days after the infective mosquito bite, which correlates with the period during which the parasite is maturing and reproducing in the liver. The release of parasites into the bloodstream causes the first symptoms of malaria.

Malaria can only be definitively diagnosed by laboratory testing. The "gold standard" remains the examination under a microscope a drop of giemsa-stained, capillary blood, obtained from a finger prick (Figure 22-3). In the last decade, a series of rapid diagnostic tests (RDTs) that use antibodies to specific parasite proteins have been developed and are increasingly being used to diagnose malaria in locations where malaria microscopy is not available.

Persons infected with falciparum malaria, particularly those who are non-immune, risk developing severe malaria, which can manifest in a number of ways, including:

- Cerebral malaria, which can manifest as coma or recurrent seizures
- Severe anemia
- Acute respiratory distress syndrome (ARDS)
- Kidney or liver failure
- Systemic acidosis and other metabolic disorders

Cerebral malaria and severe anemia are the most common manifestations of severe malaria. Uncomplicated malaria often progresses to severe disease when care and treatment are delayed. Mortality from severe malaria can exceed 40 percent in many settings where malaria is endemic.

The clinical manifestations of malaria vary significantly depending on the intensity of transmission. In areas outside of Sub-Saharan Africa, malaria is a disease of all ages.

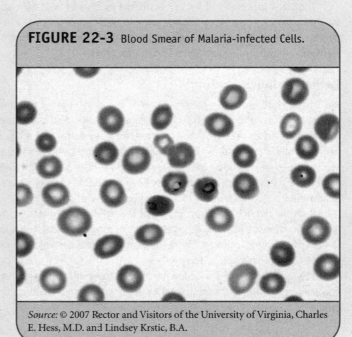

FIGURE 22-3 Blood Smear of Malaria-infected Cells.

Source: © 2007 Rector and Visitors of the University of Virginia, Charles E. Hess, M.D. and Lindsey Krstic, B.A.

Anyone infected with malaria in these areas is at risk of developing severe disease and possibly dying from malaria, particularly if treatment is delayed or inadequate. In Sub-Saharan Africa, malaria manifests quite differently. Almost all the severe disease and death from malaria occur in children less than five years of age. Adults and older children in this region are protected from severe disease and death by acquired immunity.

Unlike many childhood diseases, like measles and varicella (chicken pox), people can be infected repeatedly with malaria. In areas of intense transmission, particularly tropical Africa, children receive up to one infective bite per night and will develop as many as eight episodes of symptomatic malaria in a year. If a child is infected repeatedly, as occurs in most parts of Sub-Saharan Africa, they slowly develop a partial immunity to malaria during the first two to five years of life. If they survive to their fifth birthday, the immunity they have developed protects them from developing severe disease or dying from malaria. Older children and adults can still develop fever, body aches, headache, and diarrhea, but their illness will not progress further.

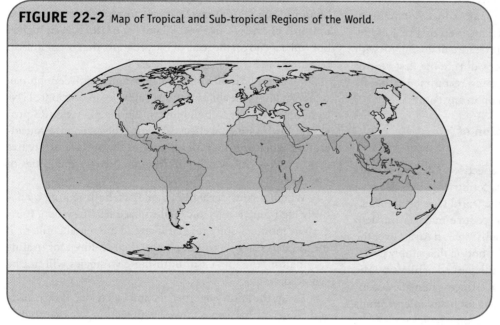

FIGURE 22-2 Map of Tropical and Sub-tropical Regions of the World.

from getting infected. Prevention can take the form of preventing human-mosquito contact or providing preventive treatment. Each of these strategies has its costs, benefits, and challenges for full implementation.

Fortunately, effective treatments for malaria are available. In most countries today, **Artemisinin-based combination therapies** (ACTs) are the gold standard for treatment of uncomplicated malaria. These ACTs rapidly clear infection even when the parasite is resistant to other drugs, such as chloroquine. These drug combinations also are thought to slow the development of drug resistance.

Suriname, and French Guiana). Malaria results in more than one million deaths each year, of which about 90 percent are among children less than five years in Sub-Saharan Africa. Most of the remaining 10 percent are occur in South Asia.

Malaria is also a leading cause of school and work absenteeism. Recent research also shows that malaria can impede a child's ability to learn. Household expenditures on malaria treatment and prevention can consume upwards of 30 percent of disposable income of the poorest of the poor. Therefore, malaria's impact is not just on public health but also on the capacity of countries to develop out of poverty.

Existing Anti-Malarial Tools and Public Health Interventions

The approach to controlling malaria focuses on two strategies, treating people infected with malaria and preventing people

For the treatment of severe malaria, intravenous or intramuscular treatment is recommended either with quinine, which has been used to treat malaria for more than a century, or injectable **artemisinins**. Drug treatment must be accompanied by supportive care including hydration, blood transfusion (if severely anemic), monitoring of glucose, and electrolytes.

Two primary tools prevent mosquitoes from biting: **insecticide-treated bed nets** (ITNs) and **indoor residual spraying** (IRS). Developed and extensively tested during the 1990s, ITNs have been proven to reduce child mortality by an average of 20 percent. IRS has been used very successfully to reduce and in some cases eliminate malaria burden, particularly outside of Africa and in the subtropical zones of southern Africa and the Horn of Africa. Its effectiveness on a large scale in tropical Africa has been variable.

The final category of intervention is preventive treatment. **Intermittent preventive treatment** of pregnant women (IPTp) has been in use in some parts of Africa for more than a decade. Sulfadoxine-pyrimethamine (SP), a single dose treatment for malaria, is given to pregnant women at antenatal clinic visits after quickening (the moment during a pregnancy when the mother first feels the baby move). Unlike most other malaria control interventions (IPTp) primary effect is not on the person being treated (the pregnant women) but rather on her developing fetus. Malaria is a leading cause of low birth weight in Sub-Saharan Africa; low birth weight is a leading risk factor for infant mortality. IPTp has been shown to reduce the frequency of low birth weight, thereby lowering infant mortality.

Recent studies have demonstrated that intermittent preventive treatment of infants (IPTi) can reduce both clinical episodes and anemia in children during their first year of life. This strategy involves giving a single treatment dose of SP with scheduled childhood immunizations during the first year of life. This strategy is currently awaiting recommendation by WHO and has not yet been scaled up in any country.

Barriers to Widespread Adoption of Existing Treatments

Despite the existence of multiple effective tools for preventing and treating malaria, numerous countries in Sub-Saharan Africa and other poor regions of the world have been unsuccessful in utilizing these tools to reduce malaria burden. Experiences in malaria control in Sub-Saharan Africa over the last decade should serve to dispel the notion that simply developing effective control tools is sufficient to achieve public health impact. This explains why investments in malaria control have now shifted to taking existing tools and interventions to scale, rather than focusing on developing better tools.

As an example, many challenges exist in getting ACTs to those who most need it. Being made from a plant extract, supplies of ACTs have been limited by the available amount of harvestable Artemesia. Developing high-quality products is also challenging when dealing with a plant extract. Even when ACTs are available, their price is 10- to 20-fold higher than previously used first-line treatments such as chloroquine, placing a major burden on already overstretched government and household budgets. Beyond the drug itself, weak public health infrastructures in most malaria-affected countries limit the ability of governments to deliver ACTs to rural areas, where people are a greatest risk of malaria.

Access to health services is limited by distance, staff shortages, the cost of services, and opportunity costs of time lost from work. Because laboratories capable of carrying out definitive diagnosis for malaria are scarce, most people are treated for malaria based solely on clinical grounds, which tend to be highly nonspecific (that is, most people treated for malaria don't have malaria). Those laboratories that are functioning frequently lack quality equipment, sufficient supplies, and quality control procedures to ensure the accuracy of their test results. In addition, as stated earlier, most people seek treatment for malaria in the private sector, buying drugs of uncertain quality from untrained or poorly trained personnel in largely unregulated markets.

Barriers to the use of both ITNs and IRS are often related to the cost and logistics and infrastructure requirements. ITNs can cost from about U.S. $4.00 for a single sized, net bundled with an insecticide treatment kit to more than $7.00 for a long-lasting insecticide treated net (LLIN), where the insecticide is bound to the netting material extending its effectiveness to upwards of three to five years. The cost of IRS is even higher, but will depend on the scale of the program, the cost of human resources, and what insecticide is used.

Weak public health infrastructure and insufficient human resources limits the ability of most countries to distribute ITNs to remote areas or to build and sustain large-scale IRS programs. Environmental effects also must be taken into consideration whenever insecticides are used, but are of greater concern with IRS, which requires much larger quantities of insecticides.

Whether considering IPTp or IPTi, both require a relatively high functioning and well-utilized health system. If expectant mothers don't regularly attend antenatal clinic or if the mothers of newborns don't take their children for routine vaccination, the impact of both these strategies will not be achieved.

Lastly, the knowledge, beliefs, and behaviors of caretakers and clinicians have an enormous impact on whether and to what extent any of the above interventions will be adopted and how effective they will be. For example, if a mother stops treatment because the child has improved, the infection may not be completely cleared and symptoms may recur. Even if an ITN is properly hung in a sleeping space or the house may be properly sprayed with insecticide, the benefits will be lost if children sleep outdoors. If a clinician doesn't trust the results coming from the laboratory, he may decide to treat a child for malaria even if the test is negative. Clinicians may also be skeptical of newer treatments, choosing instead to prescribe older, less effective medicines.

KEY TERMS

Biology Terms

Anopheles: The genus of mosquito that is capable of transmitting malaria to humans.

Erythrocytic Cycle: The part of the parasite lifecycle in humans that occurs in blood cells.

Exo-Erythrocytic Cycle: The part of the parasite lifecycle in humans that occurs in the liver, prior to release of parasites into the bloodstream.

Plasmodium: The genus of single-celled parasites that cause malaria. Four species—*Plasmodium falciparum, P. vivax, P.ovale,* and *P. malariae*—are the causative agents in human malaria.

Relapse: A second parasitemia caused when dormant parasite cells, call hypnozoites, residing in the host's liver, reactivate weeks to months later and cause a second infection of the blood cells. Relapses only occur with *P. vivax* and *P. ovale.*

Public Health Terms

Artemisinins: A class of antimalarial drugs developed originally in China, which is derived from the sweet wormwood plant (*Artemisia annua*).

Artemisinin-Based Combination Therapy (ACT): Treatment for malaria that combines an artemisinin-based compound with a drug or drugs from a different class. WHO now recommends this drug combination as the first-line treatment for malaria in most regions.

Indoor Residual Spraying (IRS): The spraying of insecticide on the interior walls of a house, which leaves a residue on the walls that remains for three to six months depending on the housing construction and the type of insecticide used.

Insecticide-Treated Bed Net (ITN): A mosquito net that has been treated with insecticide. Bed nets can be treated by dipping in an insecticide mixture (traditional ITN) or the insecticide can be bound to the fabric, allowing it to remain on the netting for periods of three to five years (long-lasting insecticide-treated net or LLIN).

Intermittent Preventive Treatment (IPTi/p): Administration of treatment doses of an antimalarial drug or drug combination to persons who do not have the symptoms of malaria in order to prevent the onset of clinical malaria. The "i/p" designation denotes IPT given to infants or pregnant women.

Severe Malaria: Symptomatic malaria infection which is complicated by coma or recurrent seizures (that is, cerebral malaria), severe anemia, respiratory distress, kidney or liver failure, systemic acidosis, or other associated life-threatening conditions.

Uncomplicated Malaria: Symptomatic infection with the malaria parasite manifesting as fever, body aches, headache, diarrhea, and possibly other symptoms not associated with severe illness.

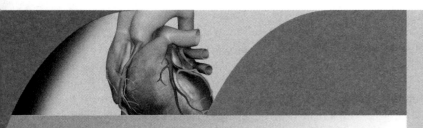

Questions for Further Research, Study, Reflection, and Discussion

For the Individual Student

In order to answer these questions, it may be necessary to research the primary literature.

- What are the four species of *Plasmodium* that cause disease in humans? List some of the features that distinguish each species from the others.
- What are the available effective tools for malaria control? How effective are they for controlling malaria? What are the advantages and disadvantages of each tool? Are there settings or clinical situations where one tool is more or less appropriate?
- What groups are currently researching a malaria vaccine? What progress are they making? What barriers are there to vaccine development?

For Small Group Discussion

- For any of the malaria control tools described in this chapter, what strategies have been used to scale-up these interventions? How do these strategies differ? Which is best for rapid scale-up? Which is better for long-term sustainability? Do you think any one strategy is superior to the others?
- What types of information would be useful when deciding which tool or tools to use for controlling malaria in a given country?
- Current global malaria control goals focus on reducing malaria-associated mortality by 50 percent by the year 2010. Would your malaria control strategy, and particularly the choice of tools, differ if your goal was to reduce morbidity rather than mortality? If yes, how would it differ?

For Entire Class Discussion

- Consider some recent public health emergencies or mass casualty event and how much attention it received in the media. Given its scale in comparison to the toll of malaria, why do you think malaria does not receive more public attention?
- What are some of the trade-offs that you can envision when deciding among the range of available and effective malaria control tools?

EXERCISE/ACTIVITY

Have the class divide in four to six groups. Each group should be assigned a malaria-affected country with different characteristics (for example, one post-conflict country, one poor country with a stable government, one middle income country, one country in a sub-tropical area, etc.) and imagine that they are the staff of the national malaria control program for that country. A benefactor has approached the NMCP staff. She is donating U.S. $20 million dollars to that country for malaria control. Assume the following costs:

Confirmatory laboratory test for malaria	$0.60
ACT treatment provided at a public health facility	$2.00
Traditional ITN with delivery costs	$5.00
LLIN with delivery costs	$7.00
IRS application to one house	$6.00
Single dose of IPTp administered at antenatal clinic	$0.20
Media campaign to promote use of treatment and prevention tools	$0.40

Based on the published effectiveness of each of these tools and their cost, how would you allocate this money to achieve the greatest impact? What factors did you take into account in deciding how to allocate these resources?

REFERENCE

1.   World Health Organization. *Fact Sheet on Malaria.* May 2007. Available at http://www.who.int/mediacentre/factsheets/fs094/en/index.html. Accessed April 16, 2008.

CROSS REFERENCES

Disease Versus Disease
The Public Health Triad

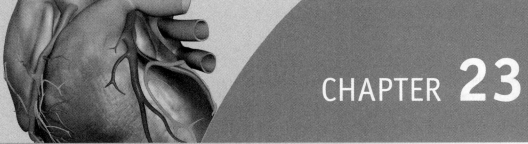

CHAPTER 23

Tuberculosis: The Deadly Comeback of an Old Infectious Disease

Yanis Ben Amor

Tuberculosis (TB), one of the world's oldest infectious diseases, has plagued humans since the fourth millennium BC. TB still claims 5,000 lives *every day*, which is more than severe acute respiratory syndrome (SARS; 774 deaths), Marburg (150 deaths), and avian flu (76 deaths) combined throughout history. However, during the last 40 years, advances in treatment and control have stopped the disease from posing a significant public health threat in wealthy nations. Consequently, tuberculosis rarely makes the headlines.[1-4]

LEARNING OBJECTIVES

By the end of this chapter, the student will be able to:

- Describe the difference between latent tuberculosis infection and active tuberculosis disease.
- Describe the transmission of TB and the natural history of infection.
- Describe the symptoms of tuberculosis and the diagnosis of the disease.
- Describe the TB treatment and the drug resistance problem.
- Define key terms necessary to discuss tuberculosis and public health.

HISTORY

Tuberculosis (TB) originally spread from animals to humans, probably from cows, about 80,000 or 100,000 years ago when people first settled down in communities to tend their cattle. More recently, TB afflicted the Ancient Egyptian civilization: characteristic scars of tuberculosis have been found in the bones of ancient Egyptian mummies. In 460 BC, the Greek physician Hippocrates described tuberculosis as "an almost always fatal disease of the lungs." The Greeks called the disease *phthisis*, which may be derived from the Greek word for wasting or decay.

Introduction of the sanatorium cure provided the first public health step against TB (the disease was then referred to as *consumption*). In the United States, the sanatorium movement was started by Dr. Edward Trudeau, who had become dangerously ill with TB. He helped found the National Association for the Study and Prevention of Tuberculosis, now the American Lung Association, still the most important voluntary organization dealing with TB. We know today that sanatoriums had no effect in curing TB. Sanatoriums did not affect the death rate: whether TB patients were treated in a sanatorium or not treated at all, half of them died. But sanatoriums did accomplish one critical thing: they removed people with active, infectious tuberculosis from their communities, effectively isolating them and preventing new infections.

In the early 1880s, the German microbiologist Robert Koch developed a technique—still used to this day—to visualize the TB agent under a microscope, and destroyed the myth that tuberculosis was a hereditary disease (it was noticed that TB would usually strike whole families and therefore was assumed that the disease was hereditary rather than transmissible).

The first vaccine against tuberculosis, the **Bacille de Calmette et Guérin (BCG)**, was developed in France in the 1920s and proved to be successful in preventing TB first in cattle, and then in humans. It has since been administered to over three billion people. Even though it was shown to be protective in severe forms of TB in children, the protective effect against pulmonary TB in adults is questioned and the vaccine is not used in the United States.

Finally, the disease became curable in the 1940s when the first antibiotic, streptomycin, was discovered by Selman Waksman. Several other antibiotics followed and, in the 1960s, after the discovery of rifampicin, the most potent antibiotic, tuberculosis was deemed under control.

BASIC SCIENCE FACTS/KEY CONCEPTS REVIEW

TB, a disease forgotten by many, re-emerged in the mid-1980s as a major global public health problem. Its resurgence resulted initially from the global health community's assumption that effective therapy alone would control the disease, and more recently from the impact of the global HIV epidemic. With the return of TB, we face the paradox of a well-defined disease, caused by a well-defined agent (*Mycobacterium tuberculosis*), which is treatable with effective and affordable drugs according to internationally recommended guidelines, but yet causes increasing human suffering and death. Indeed, the World Health Organization (WHO) has determined that one new person becomes infected with the tubercle bacilli every second, resulting in eight million new cases of TB disease and over two million deaths annually. It is estimated that one third of the world's population (or two billion people) is infected with *M. tuberculosis*, but most of these latently infected persons show no symptoms of disease.

Tuberculosis Disease and Tuberculosis Infection

Tuberculosis exists under two manifestations: tuberculosis infection (also referred to as **latent tuberculosis infection**), which is the state of people infected with *M. tuberculosis* (two billion people worldwide) but who are not sick, do not present symptoms, and are not contagious; and tuberculosis disease (also referred to as **active tuberculosis**), which characterizes patients who are sick (eight to nine million new cases worldwide), frequently symptomatic, and, very often, contagious. TB is mostly a lung disease, but the bacteria can infect other organs as well. TB disease is therefore divided in two categories: **pulmonary TB**, which represents 85 percent of all TB cases and **extrapulmonary TB** (EPTB). Examples of EPTB sites are the skin (lupus), the cervical lymph nodes (scrofula), the spine (Pott disease), or the brain (meningeal TB), which occurs most frequently in children. Only pulmonary TB is contagious.

Not everyone exposed to a significant source of infection develops tuberculosis disease. Most people whose immune systems are not depressed are able to contain the infection at the initial site (the lungs). Only 5 percent will develop TB disease within the first two years of infection, whereas 95 percent be-

come latently infected, meaning the bacteria are not actively multiplying and therefore not causing lung and other organ damage. However, throughout an infected patient's lifetime, there is an additional 5 percent risk of reactivation, when the patient goes from TB infection to TB disease. That rate of reactivation increases dramatically in HIV-positive patients, reaching 10 percent to 15 percent a year. This explains why the recent HIV pandemic has reinstated tuberculosis as a major public health threat when worldwide, before the 1980s, the TB rates had been steadily decreasing.

Transmission of Tuberculosis

TB is an airborne disease. Transmission can occur every time a patient with pulmonary TB speaks, sings, coughs, sneezes, or spits. Microscopic droplets filled with TB bacteria are then vaporized in the air, and people in close vicinity breathing the contaminated air can become infected. It is estimated that each person with active TB who is not put on appropriate TB treatment will infect an average of ten to fifteen people annually.

Natural History

Every time a person coughs, a spray of moisture erupts from the nose or mouth. If the person has active TB, that spray may include millions of droplets loaded with TB bacteria as their nuclei. Even though the moisture in the droplets dries up quickly, the nuclei can hang in the air for hours. These lethal nuclei can then infect anyone who breathes them in. It is still not clear how many mycobacteria are needed to start a human tuberculosis infection: while it has been shown that a single droplet nucleus can indeed start an infection, an infection is far more likely to occur after lengthy exposure, such as when sharing a confined space with a contagious patient for more than six to eight hours. Genetic differences between human beings also may play a role in determining who will become infected after exposure to TB bacteria as does the virulence of a particular strain of TB.

If infection does occur, macrophages are attracted to the area to try to contain the invading mycobacteria by phagocytosis. TB bacteria are encircled and enclosed in a vesicle inside the phagocytes. Unfortunately, *M. tuberculosis* has developed ways to evade the toxic environment inside the macrophage vesicle and is not always killed inside the macrophage, as demonstrated by people with latent TB infection who develop active tuberculosis when they grow older or when their immune system is weakened. If TB bacteria are not killed at the initial site of infection, they break out of the vesicles into the macrophages and begin multiplying inside them, before bursting out through the walls of the phagocytes. Successive waves of macrophages rush in to continue the phagocytosis process, but suffer the same fate. The multiplying mycobacteria stick together in a growing cluster where macrophages can no longer penetrate. After several cycles, a microscopic, tumor-like nodule is created—the tubercle—which gives its name to the disease. Occasionally, mycobacteria migrate out of the tubercle through the bloodstream and the lymph that drain the lungs, therefore spreading the infection. However, after about three or four weeks, the body's immune system usually manages to successfully contain the TB bacteria. Although the mycobacteria are not killed, they are walled off into lumps of scar tissue, the tubercle. The majority of the mycobacteria remain latent and in most people, the infection stays latent, confined within the tubercle, for the rest of their lives. A chest x-ray of these people may show very small areas of scar tissue in their lungs. In about one out of ten cases, the initial infection is never completely controlled by the body's defenses. In about half of those 10 percent, the infection progresses immediately or within the first two years to active, often infectious tuberculosis. In the other half, it does so after a delay of up to several decades, as described earlier.

Tuberculosis Symptoms

One major issue that is faced every day worldwide by thousands of healthcare workers attempting to diagnose TB accurately is that tuberculosis does not present specific symptoms. The most common symptom of pulmonary tuberculosis is a persistent cough for two to three weeks or more. Any patient with otherwise unexplained persistent cough is usually evaluated for TB by sputum smear diagnosis. However, although most patients with pulmonary TB have a cough, the symptom is not specific to the disease. It can occur in a wide range of respiratory conditions, including acute respiratory tract infection, asthma, and chronic obstructive pulmonary disease. Other nonspecific symptoms suggesting TB are chest pain, difficulty breathing, weight loss, anorexia, fever, night sweats, and fatigue.

Tuberculosis Diagnosis by Sputum Smear

Sputum examination by microscopy, the technique developed by Robert Koch, is the cheapest diagnostic method for detection of pulmonary tuberculosis. Microscopy detects the most infectious TB cases. For diagnosis, each TB suspect provides three sputum samples over the course of two days as follows:

- Sample #1: on the spot, under supervision of a nurse or diagnostician
- Sample #2: collected by the patient the next morning, at home, before the second visit to the clinic
- Sample #3: Under supervision of a nurse or diagnostician during the second visit

Unfortunately, several outcomes are possible, which complicates the diagnostic algorithm:

- If two or more samples are positive after microscopy examination, the patient is confirmed with pulmonary TB and immediately put on **directly observed therapy (DOTS)** and supervision. The patient is then classified **smear positive**.
- If only one sample is positive:
  ○ Diagnosis needs to be repeated with three more sputum samples.
  ○ If those samples still don't add up to two positive samples (between the two runs), the patient is then referred for chest x-ray examination and HIV screening. If TB is diagnosed, the patient is still classified smear positive.
- If all three samples are negative:
  ○ The patient is placed on broad spectrum antibiotics (amoxicillin) for seven days.
  ○ If symptoms persist, the patient is referred for chest x-ray examination and HIV screening. If TB is diagnosed on x-ray, the patient is classified as **smear negative**.

The chest x-ray examination specifically seeks the tubercles caused by the mycobacteria during the initial infection. The physician therefore looks for white shadows and spots in an otherwise dark lung field. Unfortunately, other respiratory infections or conditions present with the same white shadows on x-rays. A chest x-ray is therefore NOT a specific diagnostic tool for TB. As a result, treatment should never be started based on a positive chest x-ray alone.

Tuberculosis Diagnosis by Alternate Tools

Alternatives to microscopy for TB diagnosis exist: culture of sputum on solid media, the gold standard for TB detection, has high sensitivity and specificity and allows **drug susceptibility testing**, a particularly important advantage in light of the rapid spread of **multidrug-resistant TB (MDR-TB)** and **extensively drug-resistant TB (XDR-TB)**. Cultures, however, can take up to two months before a proper diagnosis can be provided to the patient. Although *M. tuberculosis* can be detected in less than four weeks in a positive culture, an incubation of six to eight weeks is often required before a culture can be classified as negative.

To address that issue, culture systems based on liquid media have been developed. Such diagnostic tools have a shorter median time to culture positivity (around 13 days), but the median time to susceptibility tests results is still relatively long (around 22 days).

Tuberculosis Treatment

Despite the recent threats of MDR-TB and XDR-TB, tuberculosis is still mostly a curable disease. The last TB antibiotic, however, was discovered in the 1960s so the worldwide rise in rates of resistance to TB drugs is a serious concern.

Control of TB rests on interruption of its transmission through the rapid identification and cure of infectious cases. The internationally recommended strategy for delivering the basics of TB cure is known as **DOTS** (originally derived from directly observed therapy, short course). **DOTS** is not simply a clinical approach to patients where drug intake is monitored daily by a nurse or a trained healthcare worker to ensure patient compliance. Rather, it is a management strategy for public health systems that includes political commitment, maintenance of adequate drug supply and sound recording and reporting systems.

Patients undergoing TB therapy are classified into two categories.

1. New cases (those who have never been treated before) are placed on a Category I regimen. It consists of a six-month therapy combining two months of four antibiotics (isoniazid, rifampicin, ethambutol, and pyrazinamide), also known as **first-line drugs**, in an intensive phase, followed by four months of two antibiotics (isoniazid and rifampicin) in a continuation phase.
2. Patients who have failed or interrupted a Category I regimen before completion or who have relapsed after being deemed cured are treated with a Category II regimen. Category II is an eight-month therapy which adds an injectable antibiotic (streptomycin) to the regimen of four standard TB drugs for the first two months. The third month's regimen combines only the four standard drugs whereas during the last five

months, the patient receives a combination of isoniazid, rifampicin, and ethambutol only.

Drug Resistance

Drug resistance is a man-made problem: when the first antibiotics for tuberculosis were used, they were often used in monotherapy rather than in combination, creating a selective pressure on the populations of mycobacteria in patients who gradually became resistant. Even if the proper combination of drugs was prescribed by the physician, often the patient would pick and choose which antibiotics to ingest based on whether they had side effects or not. There is no TB antibiotic on the market today for which at least one resistant TB strain has not been described. Even though there has been a recent interest in developing new drugs for TB, it is estimated that the earliest a new drug could be put on the market is 2012 to 2014.

The two most potent drugs currently available to treat tuberculosis are isoniazid and rifampicin. A multidrug-resistant TB strain (MDR-TB) is defined as resistant to at least both of those two antibiotics.

MDR-TB is still technically curable, but it requires the use of **second-line drugs**, which are more expensive to use, take longer to cure the patient (up to two years), and have more serious side effects.

Recently, extensively drug-resistant strains were described as TB strains that satisfy the condition for MDR-TB, and also include resistance to a fluoroquinolone (one class of second-line drugs) and at least one of the second-line injectable drugs (such as capreomycin or amikacin). XDR-TB strains are virtually untreatable.

CASE STUDY

The factual details set forth in this case study were obtained solely from newspaper articles that were published in The New York Times, The Washington Post, *and* The International Herald Tribune *from May 31, 2007, to June 15, 2007. The analysis is solely that of the author.*

Scenario

Andrew S. is a 31-year-old lawyer who has recently traveled extensively all over the world. In January 2007, Andrew suffers a fall and goes to the doctor, worried he has a bruised rib. The doctor x-rays his chest and finds an abnormality that requires further analysis. The initial tests by culture of sputum reveal that Andrew has tuberculosis, though he shows no noticeable symptoms. Sputum samples are tested further by culture to determine the drug susceptibility, but because the TB bacteria grow slowly in culture, results will only be available several weeks later. On May 11, 2007, Andrew and his fiancée are about to leave on a trip to Europe for their wedding and honeymoon. Health officials who meet with Andrew urge him not to travel, but do not specifically forbid him from doing so. Andrew doesn't think the warning is really serious, as the language used by the health officials is unclear. However, to reiterate the warning, health officials try to deliver a letter to Andrew saying in part that it is strongly recommended that he postpone his travel to see a specialist in Denver, Colorado. The letter, however, never reaches Andrew, because he has already left for his wedding. On May 12th, Andrew and his fiancée fly to Paris to begin their trip. On May 18th, Andrew is contacted by the Centers for Disease Control and Prevention (CDC) and advised not to travel home on a commercial airplane because updated test results (the culture results of his sputum samples) show that he has XDR-TB. On May 21st, however, Andrew flies to Rome where he is again warned by CDC not to fly on a commercial aircraft due to the nature of his disease. Andrew is informed that a tuberculosis clinic in Denver, the National Jewish Hospital, is awaiting him to put him on his last possible chance for treatment. Andrew and his family ask the CDC for help getting home, because to fly back on a non-commercial airline would cost him $100,000, but the CDC sends no clear information regarding options for Andrew and his family to fly back on alternative transportation, even though an air ambulance is being prepared in Atlanta for this specific purpose. On May 24th, panicked and convinced that he will die if he doesn't reach the tuberculosis clinic in Denver, Andrew flies on a commercial airline from Prague to Canada to avoid being on a no-fly list to the United States. He then drives from Canada to the United States, where he is stopped at the border in Champlain, New York. A day earlier, the CDC had alerted the Homeland Security Department that a man with a serious medical condition might try to enter the United States and the information was entered in the department's computer system. The Department instructed any border control agents who encountered the man to "**isolate**, **detain**, and contact Public Health Service." When Andrew's passport is swiped at immigration on May 24th, a computer alert warns the border inspector to stop him from entering the country. But the inspector, believing Andrew looks healthy, disregards the warning, and lets him through. On May 25th, Andrew finally checks himself into a New York hospital where he is put in isolation. On May 31st, he is flown by air ambulance to the National Jewish Hospital in Denver where doctors put him in an isolation room and he is started on oral and intravenous antibiotics. Health officials subsequently confirmed that, despite months of exposure to him, his wife and family members remained uninfected.

CLINICAL PERSPECTIVE FOR THE INDIVIDUAL PATIENT

Andrew S. has an illness that is clinically consistent with smear negative tuberculosis: his symptoms have not yet developed (persistent cough, fever, weight loss), but thanks to an unrelated accident (a fall), a doctor suspected tuberculosis while analyzing a chest x-ray that showed signs of cavities. It is not very clear how Andrew contracted the disease as TB is no longer prevalent in the United States. However, because he traveled extensively before 2007, it is very likely he was exposed to an infectious source while abroad. If Andrew had been tested by tuberculin skin test immediately upon returning to the United States, latent TB infection could have been spotted early on and Andrew's physician would have recommended that he undergo nine months of isoniazid prophylactic therapy to prevent active tuberculosis. Interestingly, in Andrew's specific case, this would have been useless, as further susceptibility testing revealed he was infected with XDR-TB, a strain that is no longer responding to isoniazid.

In Andrew's case, the diagnosis of the disease went in a way opposite to that in which it ordinarily would go. In most or all cases, TB is suspected based on symptoms, and three sputum samples are analyzed to confirm the diagnosis. If those are negative, and the symptoms do not disappear after a one-week course of broad spectrum antibiotics (to rule out other upper respiratory infections), a chest x-ray is usually necessary to rule out TB. However, when the chest x-ray shows signs of lung lesions (shadows or cavities), TB is confirmed and the patient is classified as smear negative. In the United States, this diagnosis is always confirmed by culture, which is expected to be positive even for smear-negative patients. In Andrew's case, the chest x-ray was analyzed first, the cavities were observed, and then three negative sputum smears (and subsequent positive cultures) confirmed his smear-negative classification.

This classification is relevant for two reasons: a patient who is smear negative is considered less infectious than a patient who is smear positive because there are no—or not enough—bacteria that are expelled when the patient coughs or speaks for him to be a threat to others and to infect them. This probably explains why Andrew did not infect any of his family members despite months of exposure. It could also explain why the CDC was not more firm in forbidding Andrew to travel for his wedding. However, the classification also has a downside for the healthcare professional tending to the TB patient. A patient who is smear positive at the time of diagnosis is monitored based on sputum conversion. Sputum samples are checked at the end of the second month (after the intensive phase), at the fifth month (during continuation phase) and at the end of the sixth month (end of therapy). The smear-positive patient is only considered cured if his sputum samples are negative at the end of therapy, and at least one additional time before (second or fifth month). Because a smear-negative patient is negative (by definition) at the time of diagnosis, monitoring cannot rely on sputum conversion. The healthcare practitioner therefore must monitor other indicators, such as weight (through weight gain). In the case of Andrew S., however, the disease was caught early on and there was no noticeable weight loss at the time of diagnosis. The assessment of cure would then have to be monitored by a culture of the sputum samples or bronchial secretions obtained by fiberoptic bronchoscopy at the end of therapy to verify there were no live bacteria left after the full course of treatment.

In the United States, a confirmed TB patient always has his or her sputum samples screened for drug susceptibility by culture. This allows for the screening of drug resistance and therefore the possibility to adapt the regimen of antibiotics if necessary. In most cases, thankfully, this step turns out to be unnecessary as the TB strain is drug susceptible, and the patient can therefore continue the normal drug regimen he or she was started on. Unfortunately, in Andrew's case, that extra step proved to be very useful as his TB strain was shown by culture to be extensively drug-resistant. This does not leave a lot of options for treatment. After careful analysis of the drug susceptibility profile, the experts at the TB clinic in Denver will have to select the antibiotics to which Andrew's TB strain is still susceptible and develop a tailored drug regimen. Because Andrew has XDR-TB, most or all first-line drugs can no longer be used. Most likely, the treatment will therefore take up to two years, have very serious side effects such as depression, psychosis, loss of hearing, and convulsions, to name only a few. If Andrew's TB is localized in one or few cavities in one of his two lungs, the experts can give him the option to undergo surgery. Surgery is not performed anymore in the United States if the patient has susceptible tuberculosis. However, it can be an interesting option in case of MDR-TB or XDR-TB because it removes a significant amount of bacteria. Thus, antibiotics have a higher chance of killing the remaining few bacteria that were not removed through surgery, thereby significantly decreasing the risk of relapse later in life.

Vaccinating family members of a confirmed TB case with the BCG vaccine is not a good strategy, especially if the contacts are adults. Numerous studies have shown that BCG is not effective when vaccinating adults. In the United States, it would probably only be recommended if the confirmed TB patient is a nursing mother: the baby or infant then should receive BCG vaccination, as it is effective against severe forms of TB (TB meningitis for instance) in children. In Andrew's case, it would not even be considered, as he is a smear-negative case and the risk of transmitting disease is therefore low.

PUBLIC HEALTH PERSPECTIVE FOR THE HEALTH OF THE GENERAL POPULATION AND OF HIGH RISK GROUPS

The case of Andrew S. could have become a major public health catastrophe, as all ingredients could have been combined to lead to an international outbreak of XDR-TB. The initial factor that led to the successive accumulation of misjudgments and mistakes was the smear-negative classification. This led healthcare professionals and CDC members to interact with Andrew without taking specific safety measures (wearing masks while in his presence, or requiring Andrew to wear a mask while in the presence of others). Because his sputum smear was clear of bacteria, Andrew was deemed non-infectious and therefore treated as such. This in turn led Andrew to understand (or believe) that he was not a threat to others. In reality, it is a misconception even on the part of TB experts, and studies have shown numerous times that while smear-negative cases are indeed less infectious than smear positives, they do remain infectious nonetheless. Because Andrew believed that he was not a threat to others, as he had not been a threat to his family members since his tuberculosis was diagnosed in January, he decided to carry on with his wedding projects and travel to Europe despite the warnings from the CDC.

When the final results classified Andrew as XDR-TB, his risk of infecting others was quickly reassessed. Before his drug susceptibility results were available, Andrew was a smear-negative tuberculosis patient, and his infectiousness was deemed low. After his XDR-TB status was revealed, however, the "low infectiousness" classification rapidly turned into "infectious" and, this time, the CDC sent clear restrictions to Andrew not to take a commercial airplane. In that context, it was clear to the CDC members that the closed confined environment and the re-circulating air inside the aircraft were the perfect recipe for transmission of a strain of TB that is virtually incurable.

Andrew could have followed the CDC's clear orders to remain in Europe waiting to be evacuated by a non-commercial airplane. Unfortunately, through a series of miscommunications, Andrew decided to travel back to the United States, leading to a series of potential public health concerns.

The first miscommunication has been assessed above: Andrew probably did not understand why suddenly this XDR-TB status made him more likely to be a threat to others when, for months, the CDC team members had conveyed the opposite message every time they came in contact with him. In that case, why not fly a commercial airline?

The second miscommunication seems to have been the message that reached Andrew while in Europe informing him of the specialized TB center in Denver being his "last possible chance for treatment." This most definitely led Andrew to believe that, should he follow the CDC's instructions and stay in

Europe, he would most certainly die, as only that specific center in Denver could provide him with an effective treatment (this is obviously incorrect, as there are numerous specialized centers in Europe, including in Italy where Andrew was at the time, which could have started him on an appropriate treatment based on the CDC's latest drug resistance tests). The CDC should have provided Andrew with all the contact information for that center in Italy so that he could be put in isolation and started on therapy while waiting for a means of transport to be organized to fly him back safely to the United States.

The third miscommunication between the CDC and Andrew dealt with the restriction to fly a commercial airline. Flying back to the United States on a non-commercial airline would have cost Andrew $100,000, and his family maintains that the CDC offered no help in arranging alternative transportation for Andrew to get back. The CDC should have sent clear information to Andrew while in Italy regarding the air ambulance that was being organized in Atlanta.

Andrew's misconceptions that he was not a threat to others, that only the center in Denver could provide him with an effective cure, and that the CDC was "abandoning" him in Italy led him to disregard the CDC's interdiction and to fly on a commercial airline from Prague to Canada on an eight hour flight. In most airplanes, up to half of the cabin air is re-circulated, which increases the risk of transmission of infection. Usually, the air passes through filters. In recent years, a number of airlines have installed high-efficiency particulate air (HEPA) filters that remove 99.7 percent of particles the size of most bacteria from the re-circulated air. HEPA filters reduce the risk of transmission, but they don't eliminate it. It is impossible for a passenger on a particular flight to know whether the aircraft was equipped with HEPA filters. It would therefore be sensible to test all passengers and crew members of that flight for TB infection. Following the same logic, all passengers from the flight to Europe should be found and screened as well. We know from the previous section (clinical perspective) that, in this particular case, isoniazid preventive therapy would not be effective for the passengers whose skin tests turned out to be positive. Indeed, if they were infected by Andrew during the flight, their TB strain would be XDR-TB as well, which would not respond to isoniazid treatment. Knowing their status would still prove to be useful, as they could monitor the symptoms should the TB reactivate later in life. It would also flag them as possible XDR-TB patients immediately, allowing the healthcare personnel to not only put them on effective treatment immediately (unlike Andrew) but also to isolate them if necessary to prevent further transmission.

Finally, the last misjudgment in the chain of events occurred at the point of immigration when Andrew re-entered the United States from Canada. Despite a clear warning on the Homeland Security computer system, Andrew was allowed back into the country instead of being detained and isolated. The immigration officer, basing his judgment on Andrew's healthy look, disregarded the warning. The disease control center was aware that Andrew was not symptomatic (that is, not "sick-looking") and should have specified this explicitly in their warning. On the other hand, the immigration officer should not have taken the initiative (or even have the option) to overlook the warning from Homeland Security. Andrew should have been detained and isolated (not incarcerated, despite his noncompliance with the disease control centers' restriction to travel, because he could have been a threat to fellow inmates) before being flown to Denver to initiate his therapy. Despite all the misjudgments and mistakes that could have led to an international outbreak of XDR-TB, transmission was ultimately contained successfully. However, this begs the question: for this one very high-profile case that was detected and stopped, how many are still at large, undiagnosed and untreated, and continue to unknowingly infect others and spread the virtually untreatable form of tuberculosis?

KEY TERMS
Clinical Terms

Active Tuberculosis (also, **Tuberculosis Disease**): State of people infected with *Mycobacterium tuberculosis* whose infection is not contained by the immune system and who are sick, frequently symptomatic and very often contagious.

Bacille de Calmette et Guérin (**BCG**): First vaccine developed for tuberculosis.

Extensively Drug-Resistant Tuberculosis (**XDR-TB**): Strain of TB that is at least MDR-TB, and also includes resistance to a fluoroquinolone (one class of second-line drugs) and at least one of the second-line injectable drugs (such as capreomycin or amikacin). XDR-TB strains are virtually untreatable.

Extra-Pulmonary Tuberculosis: Active tuberculosis that is localized in an organ other than the lungs.

Latent TB Infection (also, **Tuberculosis Infection**): State of people infected with *Mycobacterium tuberculosis* whose infection is contained by the immune system and who are not sick (and therefore not symptomatic) and not contagious.

Multidrug-Resistant Tuberculosis (**MDR-TB**): Strain of tuberculosis that is resistant to at least isoniazid and rifampicin, the two most potent first-line drugs. MDR-TB strains are more difficult to treat and require the use of second-line drugs.

Pulmonary TB: Active tuberculosis that is localized in the lungs.

Smear Positive: Tuberculosis patient suffering from active pulmonary disease and producing (while coughing) more than 5,000 bacteria/mL of sputum; this can be detected by microscopy. Smear-positive patients are the most infectious.

Smear Negative: Tuberculosis patient suffering from active pulmonary disease who is producing (while coughing) less than 5,000 bacteria/mL of sputum; this cannot be detected by microscopy. Complementary diagnostic tests such as chest x-ray or culture must confirm tuberculosis. Smear-negative patients are less infectious than smear-positive ones.

Public Health Terms

Detention: TB patients who fail to comply with public health orders and whose movements are being restricted to a health facility or hospital (not a prison; see **Incarceration**).

Directly Observed Therapy – Short Course (DOTS): The World Health Organization recommended strategy for delivering the basics of TB cure. DOTS combines a clinical approach (patients' drug intake is monitored daily by a nurse or a trained healthcare worker to ensure patient compliance) and a management strategy for public health systems that includes political commitment, maintenance of adequate drug supply, and sound recording and reporting systems.

Drug Susceptibility Testing (DST): Determination of the resistance profile of a specific TB strain, usually by culture on media (either solid or liquid) containing the different antibiotics and by monitoring subsequent growth. DST allows for the screening of MDR-TB and XDR-TB strains. DST can be performed for first-line or second-line drugs.

First-Line Drugs: Group of five antibiotics (rifampicin, isoniazid, ethambutol, pyrazinamide, and streptomycin) used against tuberculosis that are the most effective and potent for TB treatment.

Incarceration: TB patients who break the law (specific public health order) and are sent to prison.

Isolation: Separation of people with tuberculosis from other patients or healthy people.

Quarantine: Individuals who have been exposed to a specific disease but who are not symptomatic and sick, and who are being further assessed regarding their condition in a confined location.

Second-Line Drugs: Group of antibiotics with anti-TB activity that are less potent than the first-line drugs. Treatment with second-line drugs is usually the only option for patients with MDR-TB but treatment is expensive, very long (up to 24 months), and has many serious side effects such as depression, psychosis, loss of hearing, and convulsions. There are currently six classes of second-line drugs: aminoglycosides (amikacin, kanamycin), polypeptides (capreomycin), fluoroquinolones (ciprofloxacin), thioamides (ethionamide), cycloserine, and p-aminosalicylic acid (PAS).

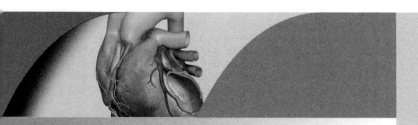

Questions for Further Research, Study, Reflection, and Discussion

For the Individual Student

In order to answer these questions, it may be necessary to research the primary literature.

- What are the two Category I TB treatment regimens (for new cases of tuberculosis) accepted by the World Health Organization, and what are the advantages and inconveniences of each?
- What vitamin deficiencies are known to be associated with TB, and how can the health practitioner use this knowledge to improve the chances of cure for his patients?
- Why is BCG vaccination not performed in the United States?
- Why is there currently no serodiagnostic test for active tuberculosis available?
- Besides Category I (new cases of TB) and Category II (retreatment), there is also a Category III, which is a regimen dedicated for children. What are the two reasons why children get a specific drug regimen?
- What first-line antibiotic should never be given to a pregnant woman and why?

For Small Group Discussion

- Isoniazid, one the first line antibiotics, kills mycobacteria that are metabolically active, which is the state of the TB bacteria in active tuberculosis. However, isoniazid preventive therapy (IPT) is recommended to treat latent TB infection (LTBI), where bacteria are dormant, and not replicating actively. Suggest reasons why IPT still works in treating LTBI.

- Drug-resistant TB strains have a phenotypic advantage over wild-type strains when growing in presence of specific antibiotics. How do drug-resistant TB strains compare to wild-type strains in the absence of antibiotics?

For Entire Class Discussion

- Multidrug-resistant tuberculosis can be caused by patients who interrupt treatment before completion. Is it ethical to refuse treating a patient who already has a history of multiple treatment interruptions, on the grounds that he/she may be generating more drug resistance?
- A secretary who works in an office with five co-workers is diagnosed with smear-positive pulmonary TB. To avoid stigmatization, the patient refuses isolation and continues to go to work, risking infecting her co-workers. She also refuses to allow her doctor to screen her colleagues for possible active TB. What should the doctor do?

EXERCISE/ACTIVITY

Class members should contact a TB clinic in their vicinity and schedule a field trip to explore TB diagnostic and treatment programs in the United States. Class members should orchestrate with the TB nurse or TB doctor a special visit (outside of regular patient visits) where each individual is a potential TB suspect, and go through all of the regular diagnostic and I.E.C (Information—Education—Communication) steps. If possible, and wherever applicable in the context of a home-based DOTS (rather than clinic-based DOTS) strategy, class members can schedule with the DOTS nurses (by small groups of 2 or 3 students) home visits to dispense the daily drug regimen (patient's consent required). Discuss with both the TB nurse and patient the challenges of the TB treatment, and the advantages/ inconveniences to the home-based DOTS versus clinic-based DOTS for either the nurse or the patient. Gather as a group and compare/discuss responses from different patients and nurses.

Healthy People 2010

Indicator: Immunization

Focus Area: Immunization and Infectious Diseases

Goal: Prevent disease, disability, and death from infectious diseases, including vaccine-preventable diseases.

Objectives:

14-11. Reduce tuberculosis.

14-12. Increase the proportion of all tuberculosis patients who complete curative therapy within 12 months.

14-13. Increase the proportion of contacts and other high-risk persons with latent tuberculosis infection who complete a course of treatment.

14-14. Reduce the average time for a laboratory to confirm and report tuberculosis cases.

14-15. Increase the proportion of international travelers who receive recommended preventive services when traveling in areas of risk for select infectious diseases: hepatitis A, malaria, and typhoid.

REFERENCES

1. World Health Organization (WHO). Avian influenza (bird flu)—Fact sheet, 2006. Geneva: WHO; 2006. Available at http://www.who.int/mediacentre/factsheets/avian_influenza/en/. Accessed April 16, 2008.

2. World Health Organization (WHO). Marburg haemorrhagic fever, 2005. Geneva: WHO; 2006. Available at http://www.who.int/mediacentre/factsheets/fs_marburg/en/index.html. Accessed April 16, 2008.

3. World Health Organization (WHO). Summary of probable SARS cases with onset of illness from 1 November 2002 to 31 July 2003. Geneva: WHO; 2006. Available at http://www.who.int/csr/sars/country/table2004_04_21/en/index.html. Accessed April 16, 2008.

4. World Health Organization (WHO). Global Tuberculosis Control—Surveillance, Planning, Financing. Geneva, WHO; 2008. Available at http://www.who.int/tb/publications/global_report/en/. Accessed April 16, 2008.

CROSS REFERENCES

Communicating Public Health Information

Immunity

Safe Medication Use

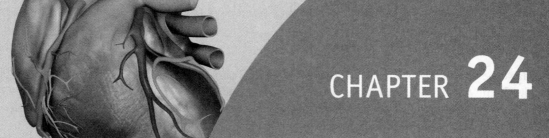

CHAPTER 24

Acquired Immune Deficiency Syndrome (AIDS): History and Time Line

Victoria A. Harden

As a global killer, AIDS now threatens to surpass the Black Death of the fourteenth century and the 1918–1920 influenza pandemic, each of which killed at least 50 million people.[1]

LEARNING OBJECTIVES

By the end of this chapter, the student will be able to:

- Explain why AIDS was first identified in male homosexual communities in the United States.
- Describe the methods used by epidemiologists to define AIDS as a new disease.
- Identify social forces that interfered with implementation of public health measures to slow or stop the transmission of AIDS.
- Discuss the public health strategies that proved most helpful in the early years of a new infectious disease outbreak and what characteristics of disease transmission help or hinder public health leaders.

INTRODUCTION

Rarely do public health practitioners face both the challenge and opportunity of addressing an infectious disease never before encountered. When **acquired immune deficiency syndrome (AIDS)** was recognized in the medical literature in 1981 as a new disease, public health workers and their colleagues who practiced medicine and conducted biomedical research were called upon to respond, simultaneously treating people who were suffering from it while attempting to define its epidemiology, etiology, and pathological physiology. The working knowledge, theories, and tools available when any new disease

strikes vary from century to century, as do the social, religious, and political contexts in which a population interprets what the disease process means in terms of class, race, gender, and other attributes. The effort against the spread of AIDS provides a case study into the historic problems medicine has faced in teasing out the causes and developing interventions in natural epidemic processes.

BASIC SCIENCE FACTS/KEY CONCEPTS REVIEW

Natural History of the Human Immunodeficiency Virus (HIV)

Before the human immunodeficiency virus (HIV) was demonstrated in 1984 as the cause of AIDS, the natural history of the disease was open to speculation and thus to all of the social and political issues that such speculation raised. Early suggestions that AIDS had its source in Africa brought strong responses from African countries, which accused Western governments of engaging in racism. Urban legends that AIDS had been created in U.S. government laboratories fanned international tensions and encouraged conspiracy theorists. In 1999, a journalist published a book alleging that AIDS had been transmitted from chimps to humans in Africa in the 1950s via trials of the polio vaccine, but subsequent scientific studies cleared the vaccines.

Scientific studies on the natural history of AIDS proceeded deliberately. In 1989, HIV-2 was linked to sooty mangabey monkeys. In 1992, some five strains of HIV were traced to west equatorial Africa as a source. By 1999, HIV-1 was traced to a few chimps, and in 2006, Beatrice Hahn at the University of

Alabama Medical School and her colleagues, testing fecal samples from wild-living chimpanzees with enhanced protein-detection techniques and HIV-1 antigen-containing strips, linked the origin of HIV-1 firmly to chimpanzees in Cameroon.[2,3]

Recognition of AIDS as a New Disease in Humans

The recognition of AIDS as a new disease in humans is much clearer in hindsight than it was as it unfolded. Knowing now that the origin of the causative virus was Sub-Saharan West Africa begs the question of why AIDS was not first identified there but instead in the gay communities of major U.S. cities. The answer undoubtedly lies in the difference between how medicine is practiced by physicians and experienced by patients in Africa and in the United States. Individuals in Africa who succumbed to AIDS in the decades before 1981 were likely poor, rural people who rarely consulted physicians who practiced Western medicine. Conversely, such physicians, seeing an African with a fever and wasting, would likely attribute the symptoms to any of a host of fevers present in tropical countries. The earliest AIDS patients in the United States, in contrast, were largely Caucasian, upper-middle class people with health insurance who regularly consulted physicians when they fell ill. Physicians who treated these individuals saw an increasing number of unusual opportunistic infections and cancers among their patients who had not experienced such problems in the past. These physicians thus recognized a disruption in the medical history of their patient populations that led them to question idiosyncratic diagnoses and wonder about the possibility of a novel disease process.

Specifically, in the late 1970s, U.S. dermatologists began seeing young men with rare cancerous lesions associated normally with elderly Mediterranean men. In early 1981, infectious disease physicians encountered patients with types of infections, especially ***Pneumocystis carinii pneumonia* (PCP)**, associated normally with patients whose immune systems had been compromised because of cancer treatments. By June 1981, several California physicians were ready to suggest that the symptoms represented a syndrome not previously seen. On June 5, Michael Gottlieb and colleagues took the lead and described the cases seen

in Los Angeles in a short paper published in the *Morbidity and Mortality Weekly Reports (MMWR)*, a weekly publication issued by the U.S. Centers for Disease Control and Prevention (CDC) in Atlanta. In July and August, two more papers linked **Kaposi's sarcoma (KS)** and/or PCP to patients in California and New York. All three of these early papers were published in the *MMWR*, indicating its centrality to monitoring disease outbreaks in the United States. More detailed studies followed in mainstream journals such as the *New England Journal of Medicine*.[4–6]

Building an Epidemiological Picture of AIDS During 1981 to 1984

Between the springs of 1981 and 1984, epidemiologists working at the local, state, and national levels made the principal contribution to understanding the new disease as they literally constructed a picture of AIDS: What did it mean to have AIDS? How was the disease transmitted? What did the epidemiological data suggest about possible etiological agents? How much morbidity and mortality did the disease exact and over what time periods? How was the disease dispersed geographically? Which populations were most at risk for contracting the syndrome? (Figure 24-1).

Just before the first *MMWR* paper was published, the CDC held conferences on sexually transmitted diseases in several U.S. cities, including San Diego, California. At the San Diego conference, James Curran and Harold Jaffe, physician-epidemiologists

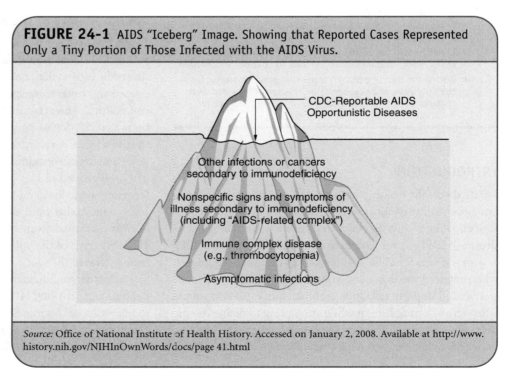

FIGURE 24-1 AIDS "Iceberg" Image. Showing that Reported Cases Represented Only a Tiny Portion of Those Infected with the AIDS Virus.

CDC-Reportable AIDS Opportunistic Diseases

Other infections or cancers secondary to immunodeficiency

Nonspecific signs and symptoms of illness secondary to immunodeficiency (including "AIDS-related complex")

Immune complex disease (e.g., thrombocytopenia)

Asymptomatic infections

Source: Office of National Institute of Health History. Accessed on January 2, 2008. Available at http://www.history.nih.gov/NIHInOwnWords/docs/page 41.html

who came to lead CDC efforts on AIDS, discussed a draft of the upcoming report on the new disease with some of their West Coast colleagues in the gay community. Initially Curran and Jaffe thought that this new outbreak might be similar to Legionnaire's disease and toxic shock syndrome, two bacterial diseases the CDC had addressed within the previous five years. They soon realized, however, that the new cases were different and would require the acquisition of much more epidemiological information before any intervention might be formulated. Shortly after the June *MMWR* publication, the CDC organized a Task Force on Kaposi's Sarcoma and Opportunistic Infections with Curran as its leader and a mandate to work for three months on the problem. A literature search by the group turned up a review article showing that pentamidine, a rare drug issued exclusively by the CDC for treatment of *Pneumocystis* pneumonia, had been requested only one time in the nine previous years for any condition not related to underlying cancer or severe **immunodepression**. This provided the Task Force with a baseline study for tracking the new disease by following new requests for the drug.

The first on-the-ground investigations of the new syndrome were done as collaborations between the CDC and state or local health agencies. The CDC places graduates from its **Epidemic Intelligence Service (EIS)** in state and local health departments. EIS officers assigned to New York City, Los Angeles, and San Francisco conducted extensive interviews with people diagnosed with the new syndrome. They followed up every case they could find of KS and PCP. From the beginning, the CDC also considered the unusual cases of KS and PCP to be a single public health problem because of the common underlying immune deficiency. Curran noted,

> "The most important thing for our case definition was that it was specific. It was not so important that it be sensitive initially. But it was important that it be specific because when you are determining whether a problem is new and looking for the etiology, you have to make sure that you do not overdiagnose it."

Over the next twelve months, epidemiologists attempted to interview every living patient with the disease across the United States. A 30-page, detailed questionnaire was developed that produced a picture of AIDS in the United States. Curran stated:

> "We could say that the average age of patients was 35, so they were not very young men. Also all of the patients were gay men, and they were living in areas of high opportunity for gay men. They were living in strong gay communities: San Francisco, New York, and Los Angeles. The other thing was

that the men were all openly gay. . . . They seemed to have large numbers of partners, and they were getting a rare condition. There were also other things associated. They all went to the same clubs. Most of them used poppers or isobutyl nitrite or amyl nitrite, and they may have been exposed to other things in their environment."

By June 1982, information about cases of AIDS outside the gay communities had been collected. A diagnosis of AIDS in newborn babies and in heterosexual patients who underwent surgery suggested a blood-borne pathogen. The next important link was the discovery of cases in hemophiliacs, which reinforced the evidence for transmission via blood, like hepatitis B. It also raised the specter of contamination of blood products, a finding that many people—including those who managed blood banks—did not want to believe. After three cases in heterosexual hemophiliacs were identified, the epidemiologists were convinced that AIDS was transmitted via blood. For hemophiliacs, the possibility of infection with hepatitis B had been tolerated because of the value of the clotting factor produced from pooling serum. With the advent of AIDS, this meant a possible death sentence for hemophiliacs and ultimately led to new rules for testing and preparing blood products.[7]

Ensuring the Safety of the Blood Supply

Blood bankers were understandably resistant to suggestions that AIDS might be transmitted via the blood supply. They had some data showing that transfusion itself could cause immune suppression. They argued that if blood products transmitted AIDS as they did hepatitis, they should have seen a much higher incidence of AIDS in hemophiliacs than had appeared by early 1983. They believed that they should have seen outbreaks of AIDS in institutions, as occurred in the hepatitis-transmitted pattern. It was known that healthcare workers were at a 15 percent to 30 percent risk of contracting hepatitis after any needlestick with a known contaminated needle. The lack of reported AIDS cases in healthcare workers thus also argued against bloodborne transmission.[8]

Blood bank administrators thus counseled restraint in response to calls from epidemiologists for new procedures in the blood products industry. They emphasized the millions of units of blood successfully transfused every year and wanted to ensure the willingness of citizens to donate blood. No technology existed in the early 1980s to screen the blood supply for AIDS, and the cost of supplying blood and blood products would increase if viruses like hepatitis had to be heat-treated or inactivated to prevent transmission to the small number of hemophiliacs as compared with the larger number of patients who received whole-blood transfusions. Without conclusive evidence that AIDS was blood borne, moreover, the U.S. Food and Drug Administration (FDA) could not act to require changes to blood banking procedure.[9,10]

The previous fall, the CDC had issued guidelines for clinical and laboratory workers to follow if they came into contact with AIDS patients or their blood. In March 1983, after a contentious conference in Atlanta at which infectious disease experts argued vehemently with blood bankers over the safety of the blood supply, the Public Health Service (PHS), parent agency of the CDC, FDA, and the U.S. National Institutes of Health (NIH), issued recommendations that high risk donors *voluntarily* defer giving blood, that autologous transfusion be encouraged, and that better methods for ensuring the safety of blood products used by hemophiliacs be developed. No penalties for noncompliance were considered at this time because no one knew what the causative agent of AIDS was and some people still argued that it was not infectious. As the evidence for a transmissible virus grew throughout 1983 and HIV was demonstrated as the cause of AIDS by mid 1984, however, the paradigm shifted. No longer were transfusion-transmitted viruses considered acceptable risks in order to reap the benefits of blood products. The enzyme-linked immunosorbant assay (ELISA) for antibodies to HIV, developed for use in laboratory research on the etiology of AIDS, was adapted in 1985 as a screening test for blood and blood products. In 1987, the FDA issued regulations requiring such screening, and in 1988 the FDA began inspecting 100 percent of FDA-regulated blood and plasma donor facilities to enforce screening regulations.[11–14]

Identification of HIV and Its Molecular Structure

With clinical evidence of drastically reduced T-cell counts in AIDS patients and epidemiological evidence for a bloodborne and sexually transmitted pathogen, virologists began searching in the fall of 1982 for a virus that attacked and destroyed **helper T-cells** in the immune system (Figure 24-2). Virological and bacteriological research at the CDC had ruled out known agents, and the only viruses known to target T cells were **retroviruses**, whose pathogenicity for humans had been demonstrated for the first time in 1980, although retroviruses pathogenic for other animals had been known for decades. The known pathogenic human retroviruses, however, caused a malignant increase in T cells rather than destroying them, so it was far from certain that a new retrovirus would cause AIDS.

Three major groups of investigators pursued retroviruses as a possible causative factor: Luc Montagnier's group at the Pasteur Institute in Paris, France; Robert Gallo's laboratory at the National Cancer Institute (NCI), Bethesda, Maryland; and Jay Levy's group at the University of California, San Francisco. In May 1983, Montagnier's group reported the isolation of a retrovirus taken from the lymph nodes of an AIDS patient. They

called it *lymphadenopathy associated virus (LAV)*. They were unable to sustain growth of the virus, however, to run further experiments. In April 1984, Gallo's group published four papers that demonstrated causation of AIDS by a retrovirus which they named *human T-cell lymphotrophic virus III (HTLV-III)*, thinking that it was in the same family of retroviruses in which they had already discovered two variants. Shortly thereafter, Jay Levy's group also identified a causative retrovirus, called *AIDS-related virus* (ARV). Subsequent genetic comparisons showed all three viruses to be the same, and in 1986, a multinational committee of scientists suggested that the virus that caused AIDS be renamed **Human Immunodeficiency Virus (HIV)**.[15–18]

As with ensuring the safety of the blood supply, the ELISA test, used by the laboratories searching for the virus to confirm the presence of antibodies to HIV in cell cultures, was adapted into a diagnostic test for AIDS in humans. The ELISA test can have false positives, however, so a second test, known as the Western blot, which assays for specific viral proteins, was used to confirm a positive ELISA test. In 1987, the FDA required that both tests be used before someone was told that he or she is infected with AIDS. Twenty-five years into the epidemic, these diagnostic tests arguably remain medicine's most useful interventions for addressing the AIDS epidemic because they provide a measurable, replicable means to identify infected individuals.

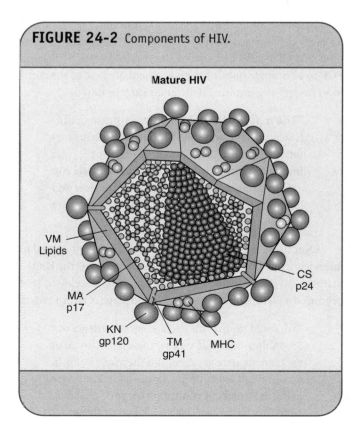

FIGURE 24-2 Components of HIV.

During the two years of intensive laboratory research when HIV was identified and characterized genetically, information also emerged about the virus that helped suggest which preventive interventions by political and public health leaders might be possible. Within just a few months after HIV was identified, molecular biologists understood that it mutated far too rapidly—up to 1,000 times as fast as influenza virus—for a traditional vaccine to be made against it. Instead of being able to vaccinate against AIDS, political and public health leaders needed to use educational methods aimed at curbing high-risk behavior to slow transmission, a much harder task.

Molecular and genetic studies also identified the key points in the virus's life cycle, which, if interrupted, would halt the spread of the virus (Figure 24-3). The first was the CD-4+ receptor on the cell wall of the host cell to which the virus attached. Second was the point at which the enzyme reverse transcriptase caused the single-strand RNA virus to make a complementary copy that transformed it into double-stranded DNA. Third, the enzyme integrase caused the viral DNA to be spliced into the genome of the host cell. Finally was the point at which the enzyme protease cut newly constructed polypeptides into viral proteins in the final assembly of new virus particles. By 1986, intellectual strategies were in place to intervene in each of these four steps, but scientists were not technologically capable of implementing most of them, and a great deal of molecular information about HIV, such as the existence of necessary co-receptors in step 1, was not yet known.[19,20]

Therapeutic Intervention Efforts

Beginning in 1984, scientists at the National Cancer Institute (NCI) utilized an anti-cancer drug screening program to identify drugs known to inhibit the enzyme reverse transcriptase. One of these that showed promise in vitro was **azidothymidine**, commonly called **AZT**. After truncated clinical trials in which AIDS patients showed a clear response to ATZ, it was approved for use by the FDA in record time and sold under the brand name Retrovir or the generic name zidovudine. Within a few more years, two additional reverse transcriptase

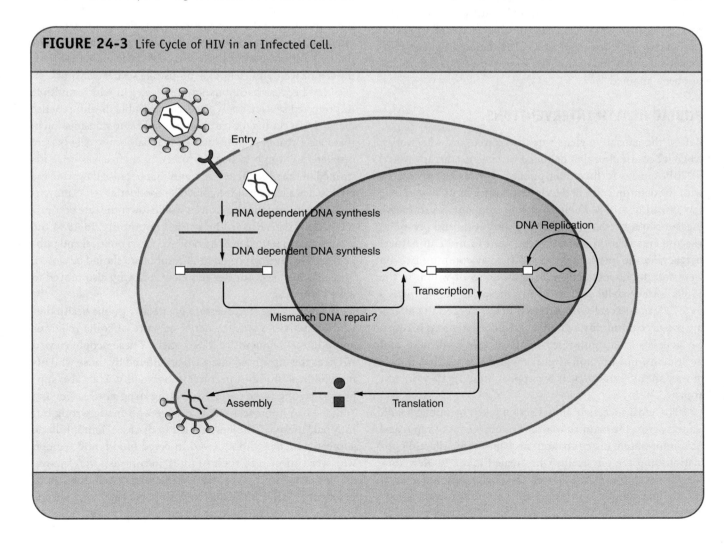

FIGURE 24-3 Life Cycle of HIV in an Infected Cell.

inhibitors, known in chemical shorthand as ddI and ddC, were approved by the FDA for treating AIDS. The reverse transcriptase inhibitors improved the condition of AIDS patients but had a number of toxic side effects and were subject to the development of resistance by HIV.

Other than these anti-retroviral drugs, treatments for AIDS focused on existing drugs for treating the opportunistic infections and cancer that people with AIDS developed. In 1995, the first of a new class of anti-retroviral drugs was introduced. Known as protease inhibitors, these drugs interfered with the final enzymatic step in the viral assembly process. For a brief period, there was optimism that the protease inhibitors would "cure" AIDS because viral loads—the number of virus particles in a quantity of blood—disappeared. It soon became apparent, however, that HIV was only suppressed and that it rapidly rebounded if the drugs were withdrawn. These drugs, too, caused unpleasant side effects. The combination of reverse transcriptase inhibitors and protease inhibitors known as **Highly Active Anti-Retroviral Therapy (HAART)** is nevertheless the most effective "cocktail" of drugs for long-term therapy against AIDS. Pharmaceutical research still works toward a rationally designed, molecularly based drug with minimal toxicity as a therapy for AIDS, but at present, that goal has not been attained.[21–25]

PUBLIC HEALTH INTERVENTIONS

Before the causative virus was discovered and afterwards, when it became clear that neither a vaccine nor therapy would likely be quickly forthcoming, public health leaders were faced with the daunting task of developing strategies to slow or stop the spread of AIDS. Their efforts to implement preventive measures not needed since the pre-antibiotic and pre-polio vaccine eras were hindered by the need to unite unnatural partners in the quest: members of the gay community, who were socially liberal, and politicians, many of whom in the 1980s were socially conservative. The social stigma carried by AIDS as a sexually transmitted disease especially affecting the gay community, required careful negotiations between gay activists intent on preserving hard-won civil rights and politicians and religious figures who believed that public money should not be spent to support lifestyles they did not approve.

The most successful initial action taken by public health leaders across the country was the establishment of rapid and clear information dissemination mechanisms for affected populations and the physicians who treated them. In New York City, for example, David Sencer, the city's Commissioner of Health, inaugurated in February 1982 monthly meetings with physicians in New York City who treated AIDS patients.

Continued for the next four years, these meetings always included an exchange of information between these two groups. Information exchange also proved important in minimizing irrational fear of infection by healthcare workers. Especially in the period of 1983 to 1987, when public fear and panic were at their most destructive, accurate communications often made the difference between keeping and losing staff at hospitals, fire houses, police departments, and other public service agencies. On the national level, Surgeon General C. Everett Koop issued an informational report on AIDS in 1986, and two years later, mailed a flier entitled, "Understanding AIDS," to every household in the United States.[26–29]

A second and more politically vexed public health policy was the decision about whether to close bathhouses in the gay communities of San Francisco, Los Angeles, and New York. These bathhouses represented for many in the gay community a civil rights triumph. After years "in the closet" for fear of losing jobs or being physically attacked, they could openly declare their gay identities and socialize in public at gay bathhouses and bars. Advocates of gay rights vehemently opposed closing the bathhouses in the years before a viral etiology for AIDS was established. Others in the gay community, bolstered by some public health leaders, believed that the epidemiological findings alone were sufficient to demonstrate sexual transmission, and that because bathhouses were locales in which multiple unprotected sex acts took place, classic public health practice dictated that closing the bathhouses would stop transmission in that locale. Another group argued that bathhouse clients were intelligent enough to begin protecting themselves once informed of the need for safe sex, and that because they were the principal population at risk for AIDS, conducting AIDS prevention education at the bathhouses would lower the rate of transmission of the virus in the entire community. In 1984 the argument was settled in San Francisco when political and public health leaders agreed that the bathhouses should be closed. The next year, Los Angeles and New York City also moved to close bathhouses.

Hovering over the question of effective public health prevention activities was the active censure of some religious and political segments of U.S. society. These people viewed AIDS as the punitive consequence suffered by those who offend biblical prohibitions on homosexuality. They also supported strong laws against injecting drug abuse, viewing addicts, like homosexuals, as people who made wrong but rational "lifestyle" choices that led to disease. Hemophiliacs, surgery patients who received infected blood, and women who were infected by their spouses, in contrast, were viewed as "innocent" victims of AIDS. This intellectual division of people with AIDS into guilty and innocent categories led advocates of conservative views to oppose any public expenditures to foster safe sex that involved condom distribution or needle exchange programs for drug addicts. Teaching personal responsibility—sexual abstinence and "just say no" to drugs—was their preferred approach to controlling AIDS. Social and religious reluctance to discuss sexuality in any public setting exacerbated the obstacles to effective public education about AIDS.

Public education programs in the United States about AIDS, therefore, were strongly split in content according to which group produced them. Those funded by the U.S. government emphasized "getting the facts" about AIDS and often used an image of the AIDS virus as the symbol for the disease. There was virtually no emphasis in government-funded educational campaigns on communicating specifically to the gay community or discussing safe sex in these posters. AIDS community action groups and other private-sector groups took the lead in producing stark, graphic messages that communicated the urgent need for condom use, clean needles, and the fact that AIDS was a killer disease. One segment of American society that proved particularly hard to reach with AIDS prevention messages was the African-American community. Traditionally, the black church had been the most effective vehicle for health messages to be communicated in the African-American community, but strong homophobic sentiments within the black church made safe gay sex extremely difficult to address. Furthermore, the African-American community had scant trust of health messages that came from the federal government. The abuses of the infamous Tuskegee syphilis study, in which African-American males in Alabama had been denied antibiotics to cure their syphilis infections, had seared into African-American consciousness a mistrust of all government health messages.[30,31]

International AIDS Issues

Public health leaders communicated with their counterparts in other countries around the world very early in the epidemic. The various professional communities, such as epidemiologists, virologists, cancer specialists, and infectious diseases, held meetings and published journals that fostered the exchange of knowledge. Because of this, and unlike the situation with respect to many diseases in past centuries, AIDS was rapidly recognized in all countries as a single disease entity that affected particular populations in different countries according to social, geographic, economic, and cultural factors that governed its spread. By 1983, for example, heterosexual transmission of AIDS was understood as the presenting pattern in Sub-Saharan Africa, Haiti, and Thailand, and that sex workers were a principal conduit for HIV. In countries where men were gone from home for long periods of time because of employment demands, AIDS transmission could be traced along the highways. Men infected while away from home brought the virus back to their wives and, via pregnancy, to their children. Social organizations in which women had virtually no power over the sexual contract put the women at exceptional risk for contracting AIDS.

Within a decade of the advent of AIDS, political leaders in every country were forced to choose a course of action on AIDS. They slowed or spurred the infection rate according to public health policies they supported. In Thailand, Australia, and Brazil, for example, the number of new HIV infections fell sharply under active educational campaigns in which clean needles were made available to drug addicts, condoms were distributed widely, and sex workers were educated about the need for safe sex and routinely examined for infection. In contrast, countries such as India and South Africa, which rejected proactive intervention methods for religious, social, or fiscal reasons, saw their AIDS infection rates climb through the 1990s. AIDS education sensitive to the cultural norms of different societies also proved critical to the course of the epidemic. In countries where individuals maintained networks of sexual partners, a message about the need to be faithful to one partner reduced risk better than messages warning against unsafe sex with strangers.

Treatment of infected people also varied widely around the globe. Wealthy countries provided the newest AIDS drugs to patients who could afford them as soon those new drugs were approved for medical use. Underdeveloped countries, however, were unable to fund the high cost of the drugs, and individuals with AIDS had no means to buy them individually. In 2000 at the International AIDS Conference in Durban, South Africa, pressure increased on drug manufacturers to supply AIDS drugs freely or at low cost to poor countries, and political pressures within those countries demanded that governments make the drugs available as widely as possible.[32]

The AIDS Doubters and AIDS Quackery

In 1987, Peter Duesberg, a distinguished molecular biologist, authority on retroviruses, and member of the U.S. National Academy of Sciences, published a paper asserting that HIV was merely a benign passenger virus and not the cause of AIDS. Duesburg's theory was refuted by leading scientists, but his arguments drew adherents from people who wished to believe that AIDS had no link to viral causation and could be cured by living a healthy lifestyle. Groups rejecting mainstream medical ideas have accompanied virtually every medical advance from smallpox vaccine to blood transfusions. Antivaccinationists in the 19th and 20th centuries opposed injecting "cow pus," as they termed smallpox vaccine, into healthy children. Other groups opposed the transfusion of blood from one person to another on religious grounds. Even anesthesia for surgery and childbirth was opposed when initially introduced on the grounds that humans were meant to suffer and that easing pain with anesthesia would disrupt God's plan.

The AIDS doubters came to play a large role in the AIDS epidemic because they captured the attention of Thabo Mbecki, who was elected president of South Africa in 1999. Faced with the largest number of people suffering from AIDS in the world and a very tight economy, in April 2000 Mbecki announced in a letter to world leaders that he did not believe HIV caused AIDS. Instead, he instructed his minister of health to develop alternative, "African" treatments for AIDS, which included nutrition and traditional medicine. In 2003, the South African government agreed to make antiretroviral drugs freely available, but the campaign has moved excruciatingly slowly.[33]

Questioning the cause of AIDS also fueled the industry of unorthodox treatments for AIDS. From the earliest days of the epidemic, desperate patients had been willing to try almost anything advertised as a cure. Early in the epidemic, promoters of questionable cancer treatments expanded their claims to encompass AIDS because of its link to Kaposi's sarcoma. As the underlying immune deficiency in AIDS became common knowledge, remedies purporting to boost the immune system flowered. Vitamins, "colostrum from cows, special lights, acupuncture, guided imagery, a bed containing low-amperage coils" were all promoted to enhance immunity. In Africa, a widespread myth that AIDS could be cured by having sex with a virgin increased the risk of rape for many young adolescents. The growth of the Internet and World Wide Web in the late 1990s and their concomitant ease of propagating messages around the world allowed the AIDS doubters to spread their message widely and open the door to multiple quack therapies and urban legends relating to AIDS. In 2007, the Snopes.com Web site, which chronicles urban legends, reported 231 such stories.[34,35]

CONCLUSIONS

The history of the AIDS epidemic permits public health workers to reflect on how their profession and others allied to it (practicing physicians, nurses, basic research scientists, etc.) responded to the introduction of a new disease in the late twentieth century. Scientific rationalism guided the intellectual understanding of AIDS, in contrast to the religious and astrological interpretations of earlier centuries, but religious beliefs and superstition played significant roles in shaping AIDS policies and informing unorthodox therapies. Quantitative, replicable research studies provided the persuasive scientific evidence that HIV was the causative agent of AIDS. In fact, the strongest evidence for HIV is that the disease simply does not exist when the virus is absent. Even so, arguments for a nonviral etiology of AIDS were strongly presented before persuasive evidence for retroviral causation was produced in 1984, and the AIDS denialists continue to reject quantitative evidence as proof. Understanding ebb and flow of such ideas, social forces, and political currents in the AIDS epidemic should help future public health leaders address the complexity of any epidemic they may be called upon to face.

SELECTED AIDS HISTORY TIME LINE

This time line was created from hundreds of possible entries with the interests of public health students as the selection criterion. Major developments in public health understanding of AIDS as a new disease are emphasized to illustrate how public health officials may be called upon to address any new infectious threat in the context of cultural and political constraints imposed by society and governments.

1930–1940	Monkey virus mutated into a form that could infect humans, somewhere in southeast Cameroon. In the 1930s, people hunting chimpanzees near the closest urban area (Kinshasha, Democratic Republic of Congo) probably first contracted the virus.
1978–1981	Gay men in the United States and Sweden—and heterosexuals in Tanzania and Haiti—began showing signs of what will later be called AIDS.
1981, June 5	The first paper in the medical literature describing *Pneumocystis carinii* pneumonia and linking it to underlying immune disorder was published.
1982, June 30	Persuasive evidence that the disease was caused by an infectious agent was presented at a meeting held at the New York Department of Health: cases had been reported in intravenous drug users, homosexuals, hemophiliacs, and Haitians.

July 27	At a meeting in Washington, D.C., attended by federal officials, university researchers, community activists, and others, the name *acquired immune deficiency syndrome* (*AIDS*), was selected for the new disease.
September	The Centers for Disease Control and Prevention (CDC) defined a case of AIDS as a disease, at least moderately predictive of a defect in cell-mediated immunity, occurring in a person with no known cause for diminished resistance to that disease.
November	The CDC issued guidelines for health workers with AIDS patients: The same precautions as taken with patients who had hepatitis B should be used.
December	The CDC reported a case of AIDS caused by blood transfusion in a previously healthy infant.
1983, January	The CDC met with blood banking organizations in Atlanta to discuss proposals to screen out individuals at high risk for AIDS from the blood donor pool. Self-identification through questionnaires or interviews was proposed.
January	The CDC reported cases of AIDS in the female sexual partners of males with AIDS.
May	Dr. Luc Montagnier and his collaborators at the Pasteur Institute reported in *Science* that they had isolated a new retrovirus, lymphadenopathy associated virus (LAV), associated with AIDS. They did not claim LAV caused AIDS.
October	Project SIDA, a multidisciplinary study based in Kinshasa, Zaire, was initiated jointly by the National Institute of Allergy and Infectious Diseases (NIAID), CDC, the Belgian Institute of Tropical Medicine, and the Zairean Ministry of Health.
1984, April	The U.S. Department of Health and Human Services held a press conference in which it was announced that Dr. Robert Gallo of the National Cancer Institute (NCI) had found the cause of AIDS, the retrovirus HTLV-III. The development of a diagnostic blood test to identify HTLV-III also was announced.
May	Four papers from Dr. Gallo's laboratory demonstrating that the HTLV-III retrovirus was the cause of AIDS were published in *Science*. These are the publications on which the link between HIV and AIDS was accepted by the scientific community.
June	Drs. Robert Gallo and Luc Montagnier held a joint press conference to announce that Gallo's HTLV-III virus and Montagnier's LAV were almost certainly identical.
September	A meeting between NCI investigators and Burroughs Wellcome pharmaceutical company was held to discuss plans to test potential drugs as retrovirus inhibitors. The outcome of this meeting was research and development of azidothymidine (AZT), the first anti-retroviral drug approved to treat AIDS.
November	After a protracted political battle, the director of San Francisco's Department of Public Health ordered the bathhouses closed.
1985, March	On March 7, the first AIDS antibody test, an ELISA-type test, was released.
April	The first International AIDS Conference was held in Atlanta, sponsored by NIH, CDC, and the U.S. Food and Drug Administration (FDA); the Alcohol, Drug Abuse, and Mental Health Administration; the Health Resources and Services Administration; and the World Health Organization (WHO). An international network of Collaborating Centres on AIDS was formed.
June	The CDC revised the case definition of AIDS to include additional specific disease conditions and to exclude people as AIDS cases if they had a negative result on testing for serum antibody to HTLV-III/LAV.
August	The U.S. military announced that it would screen all new recruits for the AIDS virus.
October	Actor Rock Hudson died, the first major public figure to die of AIDS. Public fear about AIDS increased dramatically.
November	U.S. officials advise against routine testing of workers (especially those such as food handlers, cosmetologists, manicurists, and other service personnel who have close contact with the public) for the AIDS virus, stating that there is no evidence that casual contact spreads the disease.
1986, May	The name of the AIDS virus was changed to human immunodeficiency virus (HIV) at the suggestion of a multinational committee of scientists.
October	The CDC reported that although the incidence of AIDS was rising for all racial/ethnic groups and in all geographic regions of the country, the cumulative incidence of AIDS among blacks and Hispanics was more than three times the rate for whites.

October	U.S. Surgeon General C. Everett Koop released his "Report on Acquired Immune Deficiency."
November	The first needle-exchange program was started by Jon Parker, a former addict, in New Haven, CT.
1987, February	The WHO's Global Programme on AIDS was started by Dr. Jonathan Mann.
March	The FDA approved AZT as the first antiretroviral drug to be used as a treatment for AIDS.
March	President Ronald Reagan and French Prime Minister Jacques Chirac announced a joint agreement settling the dispute arising from the discovery of the AIDS virus, the first international agreement relating to a biomedical research issue to be announced by heads of state.
April	FDA approved the first Western blot blood test (a more specific HIV diagnostic test).
August	The CDC revised its definition of AIDS to place a greater emphasis on HIV infection status.
Fall	FDA sanctioned the first human testing of a candidate vaccine against HIV.
	FDA published regulations that require screening all blood and plasma collected in the United States for HIV antibodies.
	FDA revised its strategy for the regulation of condoms by strengthening its inspection of condom manufacturers and repackers, strengthening its sampling and testing of domestic and imported condoms in commercial distribution, and providing guidance on labeling of condoms for the prevention of AIDS.
1988, January	The CDC published guidelines developed for educational efforts to combat AIDS.
June	The brochure, "Understanding AIDS," prepared by U.S. Surgeon General C. Everett Koop, was mailed to every household in the United States.
December	On December 1, WHO's Global Programme on AIDS instituted the first World AIDS Day as an annual event.
	FDA doubled blood facility inspection effort with the inspection of 100 percent of FDA-regulated blood and plasma donor facilities.
1995, December	FDA approved the first protease inhibitor, for use in combination with other nucleoside analogue medications.
1996	Data from clinical trials demonstrated that AZT used during pregnancy and at the time of delivery drastically reduces transmission of HIV from mother to child.
2000	The AIDS denialist movement received international attention and support when South African president Thabo Mbeki questioned the use and effectiveness of HIV medications as well as offered doubt that HIV causes AIDS. In response, the international scientific community issues the Durban Declaration, offering proof that HIV and AIDS are indeed connected.
2002	New recommendations for perinatal antiretroviral prophylaxis were issued.
2005	CDC published guidelines for antiretroviral postexposure prophylaxis in the United States.
2006, June 5	Twenty-five years ago, the first cases of AIDS were recognized.
September	CDC published universal screening guidelines for HIV infection in adults, adolescents, and pregnant women to make HIV status routine knowledge within the United States.

KEY TERMS

Acquired Immune Deficiency Syndrome (AIDS) (also, **HIV Disease**): Now known as a disease, it is the advanced form of HIV where the CD4+ count is below 200 mL. The body is immunocompromised and thus open to opportunistic infections such as *Pneumocystis carinii* pneumonia, tuberculosis, toxoplasmosis, wasting/extreme weight loss, diarrhea, meningitis, fungal infections, and tumors and malignancies (e.g., cervical cancer, lymphoma, Kaposi's sarcoma). (See *Human Immunodeficiency Virus.*)

Azidothymidine (AZT): First antiretroviral drug used to treat patients with AIDS.

ELISA test: Used by the laboratories searching for the virus to confirm the presence of antibodies to HIV in cell cultures.

Epidemic Intelligence Service (EIS): A division of the Centers for Disease Control and Prevention (Atlanta, Georgia) specializing in critical epidemiological training to combat the causes of major epidemics; alumni include top public health officials and medical leaders.

Highly Active Anti-Retroviral Therapy (HAART): A "cocktail" of reverse transcriptase inhibitors and protease inhibitor drugs used for long-term therapy in patients with AIDS.

Helper T Cells (also, **effector T cells**): A sub-group (lymphocytes) of white blood cells (leukocytes) that activate and direct other immune cells to establish and maximize the efficacy of the immune system.

Human Immunodeficiency Virus (HIV): A retrovirus containing reverse transcriptase (a viral enzyme) that allows the virus to convert its RNA to DNA and attack the human cell's own genetic material. Once the new cell is taken over by the virus (it's now HIV-infected), it replicates, attacking and taking over even more new cells; these HIV-infected cells kill helper T cells, which are the body's main defense against infection and illness. (See Helper T Cells, AIDS.)

Immunodepression: Prevention or suppression of the development of an immune response; may be caused by disease; chemical, biological, or physical agents; or be a natural immunological responsive.

Kaposi's Sarcoma (KS): A neoplasm (abnormal tissue that proliferates), usually malignant, of vasoformative tissue in the skin and sometimes in lymph nodes and viscera. Clinical appearance is characterized by reddish-purple to dark-blue cutaneous lesions; seen in AIDS patients and men over age 60.

***Pneumocystis carinii* pneumonia (PCP):** A type of inflammation of the lung due to bacterial or viral infection. In patients with AIDS, the damage is limited to pulmonary parenchyma; PCP is responsible for most morbidity in patients with AIDS.

Retroviruses: Any virus in the family *Retroviridae*. These viruses possess an RNA genome in an envelope and use a DNA intermediate to replicate. Reverse transcriptase enzyme causes the virus to perform reverse transcription of its genome from RNA to DNA, which is then integrated into the host's genome with an integrase enzyme. Then the virus genome replicates as part of the cell's own DNA.

Western blot: Assays for specific viral proteins, was used to confirm a positive ELISA test.

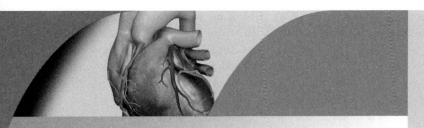

Questions for Further Research, Study, Reflection, and Discussion

In order to answer these questions, it may be necessary to research the primary literature.

1. If you were sent to deal with an outbreak of an unknown disease, what characteristics would you use to decide if it were an unusual incidence of a known disease or a wholly new disease?

2. What evidence would be necessary to convince you that a new disease was threatening the blood supply? What arguments would you present to convince political leaders that they needed to act in the face of physicians in blood banks who dismissed your concerns?

3. If the mayor of a city asked you for a recommendation about whether to close gay bathhouses to stop the AIDS epidemic, what would you advise and on what arguments would you base your recommendation?

4. You have been asked by a group of African-American ministers to organize a session for their congregations to learn about AIDS. What issues do you need to consider to make this event as successful as possible, and what items would you put on the agenda?

REFERENCES

1. Morens DM, Folkers GK, Fauci AS. The challenge of emerging and re-emerging infectious diseases. *Nature* 2004;430:242–249.

2. Hooper E, Hamilton B. *The River: A Journey to the Source of HIV and AIDS.* New York: Little Brown; 1999.

3. Keele B, Van Heuverswyn F, Li Y, Bailes E, Takehisa J, et al. Chimpanzee reservoirs of pandemic and nonpandemic HIV-1. *Science* 2006; 313:523–526.

4. Centers for Disease Control and Prevention. *Pneumocystis* Pneumonia–Los Angeles. *MMWR Morbid Mortal Wkly Rep* 1981;30: 250–252.

5. Centers for Disease Control and Prevention. Kaposi's sarcoma and *Pneumocystis* pneumonia among homosexual men–New York City and California. *MMWR Morbid Mortal Wkly Rep* 1981;30:305–308.

6. Centers for Disease Control and Prevention. Follow-up on Kaposi's sarcoma and *Pneumocystis* pneumonia. *MMWR Morbid Mortal Wkly Rep* 1981;30:409–410.

7. Harden VA, Hannaway CA. Interview with James W. Curran, 19 May 1998, Atlanta, Georgia. Retrieved 18 May 2007, from *In Their Own Words: NIH Researchers Recall the Early Years of AIDS.* Available at http://www.history.nih.gov/NIHInOwnWords/docs/curran1_01.html. Accessed April 17, 2008.

8. Harden VA, Rodrigues D. Interview with Harvey G. Klein, 29 January 1993, Bethesda, MD. Retrieved 18 May 2007, from *In Their Own Words: NIH Researchers Recall the Early Years of AIDS.* Available at http://www.history.nih.gov/NIHInOwnWords/docs/klein1_01.html. Accessed April 17, 2008.

9. Young JH. 1995 AIDS and the FDA. In: Hannaway C, Harden VA, Parascandola J, eds. *AIDS and the Public Debate: Historical and Contemporary Perspectives.* Amsterdam: IOS Press; 1995:47–66.

10. Feldman E, Bayer R, eds. *Blood Feuds: AIDS, Blood, and the Politics of Medical Disaster.* New York: Oxford University Press; 1999.

11. Centers for Disease Control and Prevention. Current trends acquired immune deficiency syndrome (AIDS): Precautions for clinical and laboratory staffs. *MMWR Morbid Mortal Wkly Rep* 1982;31:577–580

12. Centers for Disease Control and Prevention. Current trends prevention of acquired immune deficiency syndrome (AIDS): report of Inter-Agency Recommendations. *MMWR Morbid Mortal Wkly Rep* 1983; 32:101–103.

13. Centers for Disease Control and Prevention. Acquired immunodeficiency syndrome (AIDS): precautions for health-care workers and allied professionals. *MMWR Morbid Mortal Wkly Rep* 1983;32:450–451.

14. HIV AIDS Historical Time Line 1981–1990. Retrieved 18 May 2007 from U.S. Food and Drug Administration. Available at http://www.fda.gov/oashi/aids/miles81.html. Accessed April 17, 2008.

15. Gallo RC. *Virus Hunting: AIDS, Cancer, and the Human Retrovirus: A Story of Scientific Discovery.* New York, Basic Books; 1991.

16. Montagnier L. *Virus: The Co-Discoverer of HIV Tracks Its Rampage and Charts the Future.* New York: W.W. Norton; 2000.

17. Levy JA. "Animal Virology and the Discovery of the AIDS Virus," an oral history conducted in 1993 by Sally Smith Hughes in the San Francisco AIDS Oral History Series, Phase I: "The AIDS Epidemic in San Francisco: The Medical Response, 1981–1984, Volume VIII." Berkeley, CA: Regional Oral History Office, The Bancroft Library, University of California; 2001.

18. Coffin J, Haase A, Levy JA, Montagnier L, Oroszlan S, et al. Human immunodeficiency viruses. [letter] *Science* 1986;232:697.

19. Harden VA. The NIH and Biomedical Research on AIDS. In: Hannaway C, Harden VA, Parascandola J, eds. *AIDS and the Public Debate: Historical and Contemporary Perspectives.* Amsterdam: IOS Press; 1995:30–46.

20. Cohen J. *Shots in the Dark: The Wayward Search for an AIDS Vaccine.* New York: W. W. Norton; 2001.

21. Harden VA, Hannaway C. Interview with Samuel Broder, 2 February 1997, Bethesda, MD. Available at: http://www.history.nih.gov/NIHInOwnWords/docs/broder_01.html. Accessed April 17, 2008.

22. Harden VA, Hannaway C. Interview with Robert Yarchoan, 30 April 1997, Bethesda, MD. Available at: http://www.history.nih.gov/NIHInOwnWords/docs/yarchoan1_01.html. Accessed April 17, 2008.

23. Lasagna L. The history of zidovudine (AZT). *J Clin Res Pharmacoepidemiol* 1990;4:25–37.

24. Hoffmann C, Mulcahy F. ART 2006 (pp. 89–278). In: Hoffmann C, Rockstroh JK, Kamps BS, eds. *HIV Medicine, 2006.* Paris, Flying Publisher. Available at http://www.hivmedicine.com/hivmedicine 2006.pdf. Accessed April 17, 2008.

25. Hoffmann C, Rockstroh JK, Kamps BS, eds. *HIV Medicine, 2007.* Paris: Flying Publisher. Available at: http://www.hivmedicine.com/hivmedicine2006.pdf. Accessed April 17, 2008.

26. Lord K, Sencer D. New York City AIDS epidemic group oral history conducted 24–25 January 1998. New York: Commissioner's Office, Department of Health. [Manuscript given to author by Dr. David Sencer.]

27. Harden VA, Rodrigues D. Interview with David Henderson, 13 June 1996, Bethesda, MD. Available at: http://www.history.nih.gov/NIHInOwnWords/docs/henderson1_01.html. Accessed April 17, 2008.

28. Koop CE. *Koop: The Memoirs of America's Family Doctor.* New York: Harper-Zondervan; 1993.

29. Koop CE. The Early Days of AIDS as I Remember Them. In Hannaway C, Harden VA, Parascandola J, eds. *AIDS and the Public Debate: Historical and Contemporary Perspectives.* Amsterdam: IOS Press; 1995:9–18.

30. The National Library of Medicine holds an excellent collection of public education posters on AIDS collected from around the world. Search term "acquired immunodeficiency syndrome." Available at http://www.ihm.nlm.nih.gov. Accessed April 17, 2008.

31. Weatherford RJ, Weatherford CB. *Somebody's Knocking at Your Door: AIDS and the African-American Church.* Binghamton, NY: Haworth Press 1999.

32. Hunter S. *Black Death: AIDS in Africa.* New York: Palgrave McMillan; 2003.

33. Harden VA. Koch's postulates and the etiology of AIDS: an historical perspective. *Hist Phil Life Sci* 1992;14:249–269.

34. Young JH. AIDS and Deceptive Therapies. In: Harden VA, Risse GB. *AIDS and the Historian: Proceedings of a Conference at the National Institutes of Health, 20-21 March 1989.* NIH Publication No. 91-1584. Bethesda: U.S. Department of Health and Human Services, Public Health Service, National Institutes of Health; 1991:101–108.

35. Search term "Urban legends about AIDS." Available at: http://www.snopes.com/. Accessed April 17, 2008.

SUGGESTED READING

Curran JW. The CDC and the Investigation of the Epidemiology of AIDS. In: Hannaway C, Harden VA, Parascandola J, eds. *AIDS and the Public Debate: Historical and Contemporary Perspectives.* Amsterdam: IOS Press; 1995:19–29.

Engel J. *The Epidemic: A Global History of AIDS.* New York: Collins; 2006.

Grmek MD. *History of AIDS: Emergence and Origin of a Modern Pandemic.* Princeton, NJ: Princeton University Press; 1990.

Oppenheimer GM. In the Eye of the Storm: The Epidemiological Construction of AIDS. In: Fee E, Fox DM, eds.

AIDS: The Burdens of History. Berkeley: University of California Press; 1988:267–300.

Shilts R. *And the Band Played On: Politics, People, and the AIDS Epidemic*. New York: St. Martin's Press; 1987.

SELECTED TIME LINE RESOURCES

Frontline (PBS). 25 Years of AIDS. Retrieved 21 February 2007 from The Age of AIDS Web site. Available at http://www.pbs.org/wgbh/pages/frontline/aids/cron/. Accessed April 17, 2008.

New York Times. "The AIDS Epidemic." Retrieved 21 February 2007 from AIDS at 20 Web site. Available at http://www.nytimes.com/library/national/science/aids/aids-index.html.

San Francisco AIDS Foundation. Milestones in the Battle Against AIDS. Retrieved 21 February 2007 from 25 Years of an Epidemic Web site. Available at http://www.sfaf.org/custom/timeline.aspx. Accessed April 17, 2008.

CROSS REFERENCES

AIDS: An Afterward

Communicating Public Health Information

HIV Biology

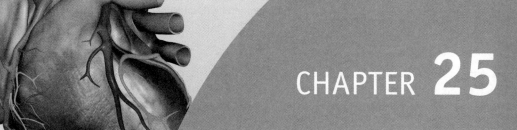

CHAPTER 25

HIV: Biology, Transmission, and Natural History in Humans

Sylvia Silver

The HIV/AIDS epidemic has taken a tremendous toll on people in the United States. From the beginning of the epidemic in 1981 through 2003, an estimated 1.3 to 1.4 million people in this country have been infected with HIV/AIDS. Of these, about one third (more than 500,000) have died.

Despite declines in new infections in the early 1990s, more people are living with HIV/AIDS than ever before. CDC estimates that about 1 million people in the United States are living with HIV or AIDS. **About one quarter of these people is unaware of their infection, which puts them and others at risk.**[1]

LEARNING OBJECTIVES

By the end of this chapter, the student will be able to:

- Explain the structure, components, and routes of transmission of HIV.
- Analyze the role of the immune system in HIV disease.
- Describe testing methods for HIV infection and status of HIV disease.
- Discuss the natural history of HIV disease.

INTRODUCTION

Humans have always shared this world with microorganisms. Bacteria, fungi, parasites, and viruses inhabited our planet long before there were humans; they developed mechanisms of adapting themselves to changing environments, and different ways of living in order to survive. These small creatures have caused an immeasurable amount of death and suffering to humans, and will continue to do so as long as we are here.

However, the microorganisms that have caused the most mortality and morbidity are but a small proportion of all living microorganisms. The smallest of these organisms are viruses, which are between 15 and 200 nanometers in diameter. To appreciate their small size, consider that there are estimated to be over 10 million virus particles in every milliliter of seawater!

When viruses were mentioned prior to the 1980s, people usually associated them with influenza, smallpox, measles, etc. However, since that time one virus—the **human immunodeficiency virus (HIV)**—claims the spotlight. During this time period and probably before this without our knowledge, HIV has killed over 25 million people worldwide. Presently, it is estimated that more than 40 million individuals are infected with the virus globally. HIV plays a prominent role in the news, sits squarely on federal, state, and local health department agendas, and factors significantly into global economic models and other relevant tools used when considering the human population. In some countries, HIV has decimated entire generations of families. Because of this, many countries will lose their economic basis, cultures will suffer, and millions of children will grow up without their parents. Although it is hard to fathom how one microorganism can be responsible for so much carnage, one has to respect its ability to make this all happen. So just what happens when HIV meets a human?

Viruses

Viruses are small, subcellular agents that may be able to survive outside of a host, but are unable to multiply or replicate outside their specific host cells; hence, they are classified as *intracellular, obligate parasites*. First, a virus must find a member of the specific species it can infect, gain entrance to that host, and then commandeer the cellular machinery of this host in order to produce new virus particles, or "reproduce." This is in essence the sole reason for its existence. Along the way, the host or parts of it may be destroyed.

Viruses are "species-specific." This means that there are viruses that can infect dogs but not cats, while others are able to infect tobacco plants but not tomato plants, etc. This occurs because there is a structure on the virus that is looking for an attachment "go-ahead" on the cell it wants to infect. This is called a *receptor*. If the virus finds its receptor, it can land, attach, and make its way inside the cell. (If the receptor is not there, the virus must do a "pass" and continue its journey. If it never finds the receptor, it will eventually cease to exist.) Viruses have a predilection for particular tissues, for example, respiratory tissue or liver tissue, and it is to these tissues that the virus will reside. Once inside its host and in residence, "all systems are set to go" for it to multiply. Sometimes (and this is what happened to the precursor of HIV), the genetic make-up of the virus is altered, and now, instead of needing monkeys to live in, it can exist and reproduce in humans (a different species).

Unlike bacteria or humans, viruses may possess either type of genetic material—deoxyribonucleic acid (DNA) or **ribonucleic acid (RNA)**—and this genetic material can be either single- or double-stranded. The genome size in viruses is rather small, ranging in size from ~2,000 to 200,000 base pairs (in contrast to over 4 million base pairs in some bacteria and over 3 billion in humans). The genome: 1) contains the genetic information that controls what the virus will have as far as proteins, nucleic acid, etc.; and 2) will control the machinery of the host cell to support viral replication. The simplest viruses are only comprised of nucleic acid and a protein coat (**capsid**). This protein coat gives a virus its structure and protects the nucleic acid from extracellular environmental insults that could destroy the virus. The protein coat also permits the attachment of the virion to the membrane of the host cell. In some cases, when viruses leave cells through **budding** from the cell, the virus picks up parts of the human cell membrane upon leaving, thereby giving it an *envelope*. Certain viruses may have spikes, composed of chemical substances, on the envelope that assist in the union between the virus and host cell.

The general steps for virus interaction with its human host are: 1) implantation of virus at the portal of entry; 2) local replication; 3) spread of the virus to target organs (disease sites); and 4) spread of the virus to sites where the virus will be shed into the environment. Specifically:

1. A virus comes in contact with a host and the first giant step is to get inside this host. This is accomplished by binding to the cell through a viral attachment protein and a specific receptor(s) on the surface of the human cell.

2. Through different mechanisms (for different viruses and which particular cell), it is able to enter the cell.

3. The genetic material of the virus then is replicated (again, different ways for different viruses) and viral proteins are produced. This step requires assistance or commandeering of host cell mechanisms.

4. The newly formed components of the virus particles are assembled into a new virion and these exit the cell. One infecting virus could actually produce more than 10,000 new virus progeny and destroy the very cell that helped it out; this is what causes destruction (symptoms) in viral diseases.

Many viruses exist within the host at levels low enough that the host is not damaged by its existence. Because the survival of the virus depends entirely on the host, most viruses tend to cause mild infections. In some instances, the virus causes death to the host in a short period of time and dies with it; examples include the Ebola virus as well as the influenza virus that caused the 1918 pandemic. However, this is not the usual mode of action for most viruses because they tend to want to stay around.

5. Once the new progeny exit or destroy the host cell, they may either enter other cells in this host and repeat the replication process, or exit this host and find their way to other susceptible hosts. This is how viruses are transmitted.

Viruses like certain specific body tissues (this is termed *tropism*) and is determined by:

- Whether the cell possesses receptors for the particular virus
- The ability of the cell to support virus replication
- Whether there are any physical barriers to the viral entrance
- Whether the cellular environment supports viral viability

For example, viruses that replicate in the respiratory tract (respiratory viruses), like influenza, are "shed" from the host through coughing or sneezing; other viruses may be shed from the intestinal tract (enteric viruses) through feces. They can enter the water supply and be transmitted by other people through ingestion. HIV is considered a bloodborne virus that replicates in human body fluid (remove the word "fluid") cells. It can survive for a period of time outside a host in body fluids, but will die if another susceptible host is not found in time.

HIV Structure and Replication

HIV is a member of the *Retroviridae* family, whose characteristics include having a single-stranded RNA as its genome and an envelope (material picked up when HIV leaves a human cell after replication). All members of the family contain three similar genes: *pol* (encodes for essential viral enzymes), *env* (encodes for a type of protein implanted in the envelope), and *gag* (encodes for proteins also found in the envelope). In addition, HIV, like all members of this family, has a particular replication cycle that is quite different from other viral families. This occurs as follows:

1. HIV has a major envelope glycoprotein, gp120, which binds to a certain type of protein (receptor), CD4, found on particular human white blood cells. This first binding then allows HIV to bind to a second receptor, which is either one of two proteins (coreceptors), CCR5 or CXCR4.

2. After binding, HIV makes its way into the cell and the viral single-stranded RNA is converted to double-stranded DNA (like human DNA), through a viral enzyme called **reverse transcriptase (RT)**.

3. The new double-stranded DNA makes its way from the cytoplasm of the cell to the nucleus, where it is inserted into the human DNA through another viral enzyme, **integrase**. At this point, the viral DNA is part of the human DNA and every time the human DNA is copied, the viral DNA is also copied.

4. When new human proteins are made from the reading and transcription of the human DNA-viral DNA, viral proteins also are being produced.

5. The new viral proteins come together to form new HIV particles.

6. These new HIV particles leave the human cell through budding from the human cell and, through maturation, become infectious.

Transmission of HIV

The goal for HIV is to find itself in close enough proximity to a human cell with the correct receptor(s) to infect. HIV is not transmitted through the air, nor can we become infected by having it contaminate a telephone, as in the case of the influenza virus. Where it is rather difficult to avoid infection from the influenza virus, which is easily transmitted through the air or by contaminated objects, HIV transmission has to occur directly through transmission of body fluids from one person to another person.

Consequently, HIV transmission is 100% preventable if proper precautions are in place as transmission demands exchange of body fluids from an infected person to an uninfected person. HIV has been found in every human body fluid; the concentration of virus depends on the length of time of infection, treatment success, etc. There are definite known routes of transmission, and, therefore, it is easy to avoid putting yourself at risk.

Sexual Transmission

HIV is in semen and vaginal or cervical fluids. In general, there is a higher concentration of HIV in semen than vaginal fluid. This changes when a women is menstruating but the degree of concentration always relies on those conditions mentioned above.

Unprotected sex, whether it occurs between two men, two women, or a man and a woman, is considered "high risk" for HIV transmission. Sexual activities that can cause trauma and therefore direct transmission of infected body fluids into the bloodstream of a recipient are the highest risk. Penile–anal intercourse is the most risky as this causes microscopic tears in the rectum. Tears in the vaginal lining also can occur in penile–vaginal intercourse but not as easily. This is not to say that an infected woman does not pose a risk to her male partner; the risk is just not considered as high. Likewise, oral sex performed on an infected partner (male or female) is risky, as HIV might enter microscopic tears in the mouth. Again, this has a lower risk but it is risky just the same. Deep kissing is theoretically possible for transmission if one partner is infected and the other has microscopic tears in their mouth; however, this activity is considered to be at very low risk.

Transmission by Blood

There are a few ways this can occur, some obvious, some not so obvious. The most apparent is through a blood transfusion with contaminated blood. Today, the risk of this happening in the United States is quite low due to probing questionnaires to blood donors and the type of testing performed on donor blood. However, in some countries around the world, having a blood transfusion might be very risky because less extensive selection criteria of donors is in place and testing is not as sophisticated. In addition, some countries can offer no guarantee of sterility of blood transfusion equipment.

Another prominent blood transmission route involves injecting chemical substances while sharing needles and other drug paraphernalia. Many drug users in the United States have become infected from this route of transmission, and unfortunately, this route of transmission continues to infect many drug users in the United States and around the world. While needle exchange programs have been shown to lower the rate of infection in this population, not all communities agree to giving drug-addicted individuals clean needles to avoid HIV transmission; rather, it is perceived as a means to supply their addiction.

Two other possibilities for infection through blood that most people do not think of as risky are body piercing/tattooing and injection of steroids. In both of these situations, individuals may share needles for piercing or someone doing the tattooing may not properly clean the needles. Improperly sterilized needles can cause transmission in these instances just as easily as in injecting drug users.

Mother-To-Child Transmission

In general, an infected woman could transmit the virus to her infant anytime during the birthing process or through breast feeding. The possibility of this occurring today in the United States and other resource-rich countries is low for a couple of reasons. Most pregnant women in these countries seek prenatal care and are tested for HIV; if found to be infected, antiretroviral therapy is given during the second and third trimesters of pregnancy, which has dramatically lowered the possibility of infection of the fetus. Also, performing a cesarean-section delivery rather than vaginal delivery lowers the percentage of risk even more. A third tactic is having the infant be fed with formula, rather than breast milk, which has been shown to transmit HIV.

Unfortunately, in resource-limited countries, where HIV infection prevalence has been shown to be as high as 40 percent in pregnant women in some countries, these options are not all available. Many countries do not have adequate counseling and testing infrastructures, adequate supplies of antiretroviral therapy, or even the possibilities for cesarean-section delivery. Also, formula is expensive and out of reach to most women in these countries. Therefore, breast feeding is the means for life for an infant in these countries but elevates the risk of infection from his or her mother with HIV.

Immunity and HIV

Immune System

Essentially, a healthy human possesses two mechanisms to resist infectious disease. *Nonspecific resistance* confers a certain ability in keeping microorganisms from gaining entry into our body or it brings about destruction of them in some way. This mechanism works against foreign invaders through the integrity of our skin, destroying them through the acidity in our tears and stomach acids, or actually washing them away with tears.

The other mechanism, the *immune system*, is more complicated and consists of several components. (A complete discussion of the HIV and the immune system is beyond the scope of this book, but an overview is necessary for understanding

HIV disease.) One component, rather nonspecific, is composed of circulating cells that are on the "lookout" for foreign invaders; these cells are capable of the recognition and destruction of foreign invaders. This broad sense of alertness to "foreignness" includes some viruses.

A more specific branch of the immune system involves the actions of principally two types of white blood cells, namely, B lymphocytes (B cells) and T lymphocytes (T cells). If we looked at these cells, they would appear identical under the microscope; however, they can be separated through chemical investigation of their surfaces and what they contain.

B cells produce particular proteins, called *antibodies,* that are produced against specific foreign substances, referred to as *antigens.* This is called our *humoral immune response* or *antibody-mediated immunity.* Antibodies surround the antigen and, either target it for destruction by other components of the immune system, or hinder it from being able to enter the cells it was going after ("neutralize it"). The production of antibodies specific to HIV starts upon the interaction of the virus with cells of our immune system.

T cells are divided on the basis of what proteins they have on their surface, and their functions. Also, after encountering a specific antigen, T cells will produce various chemical substances that can destroy the antigen or signal the production of other chemicals. This part of the immune response is called *cell-mediated immunity.* These chemical substances also are essential for other functions of the immune system, such as surveillance and looking out for foreign invaders.

Every time a B cell or T cell interacts with specific antigens, a small subset become **memory cells**, while the others go on to process information and mount a humoral or cellular response. These memory cells circulate in the body for a long time, keeping all information about specific antigens. If a memory cell again comes in contact with a previously encountered antigen, it "remembers" it and the response to that antigen this time by the immune system is placed on fast-forward. Immune system components will be quickly activated that are specific to attacking that particular antigen. This allows a rapid response in contrast to a primary "sighting" of antigen where the immune system must go though processing, etc.

One class of T cells contains the protein CD4 on their surface. This is the receptor HIV is looking for described above (*HIV Structure and Replication*). HIV infects and destroys these cells during the course of its time in a human body. Unfortunately, the CD4 cell is central to the normal functioning of the immune response; its destruction essentially causes an impaired immune response, hence the name of the virus (human immunodeficiency virus) and the name of the condition (**acquired immunodeficiency syndrome, AIDS**).

Humans are born without a "developed" immune system and our first few months of life make us dependent on what immunity is passed from our mothers through the placenta. This "maternal immunity" lasts for about three to six months before it starts deteriorating and our own immune system begins to develop. Normally, this is the status until the systems start deteriorating with "advanced age" (different in each of us). If nothing happens to harm the immune system, most of us are able to live and successfully share our environment with our microbial co-inhabitants. However, there are conditions and diseases that prematurely cause the impairment of the immune system (*immunocompromised* or *immunodeficiency*). When this occurs, some of our microbial co-inhabitants take this opportunity to invade, multiply, and cause disease (called *opportunistic organisms*), which can be fatal. This is what happens in HIV disease.

Laboratory Testing for HIV Infection

HIV testing usually determines if antibodies made specifically against HIV are present in someone's blood. However, in order for these tests to be positive, a high enough concentration of the antibodies must be present. In most people, this takes approximately three months, whereas in some it takes as long as six months before the test will show a positive result. Therefore, someone tested before there is an adequate enough concentration of antibodies present may definitely be infected, but their results will be negative.

This is why it is so important for individuals who test negative, but consider themselves to have been at-risk for HIV infection, to be retested in six months. *This means without these individuals involving themselves in any further risky behavior. If, however, they put themselves at risk between the first and second test, they must start the clock counting again for six months with no risky behavior.* Testing negative after six months from a risky behavior, without any further risky behavior in between, is a negative. If someone is found to have antibodies to HIV, they are then considered to be *seropositive* or *HIV-positive*.

The most common test used for the detection of HIV antibodies is the **ELISA** (**e**nzyme-**l**inked **i**mmuno**s**orbent **a**ssay). This test uses a sandwich-like mechanism to detect and show that antibodies to HIV are present in someone's blood. *Let's assume the person is indeed HIV-positive.* The major steps are as follows (please realize that there are numerous steps performed by a laboratory technologist in between what is described here that are part of the performance of this test; here, just the basic principle is given):

1. The test system uses a plate with many "wells" in it. In manufacturing, the wells were coated by the manufac-

turer with HIV antigens. The serum (fluid surrounding the red and white cells) of the individual being tested is placed into a well. If HIV antibodies are present in the serum of the individual being tested, they will bind to the HIV antigen. However, if this occurs, there is no way for the laboratory to detect it at this point. What we need to show is that human HIV antibodies have indeed attached to HIV antigens.

   This is how that is done (these steps were done by the manufacturer):

   - *Human HIV antibodies were injected into an animal. This animal's immune system saw these as "foreign" and its immune system made antibodies against them (hence the term "anti-HIV antibodies," which are animal antibodies made against human HIV antibodies).*
   - *In order to be able to determine that these anti-HIV antibodies find the antigen they were produced against and bind in a test system, they are tagged with a substance that can be detected by fluorescence, that can be detected under a fluorescence microscope, a radioisotope, or some other way.*

2. Anti-HIV antibodies are then added to the well. Because this person is actually infected with HIV and enough time has gone by for there to be an adequate concentration of antibodies, the anti-HIV antibodies will find its antigen and bind to it, now making a sandwich-like structure of HIV antigen, human anti-HIV, anti-HIV antibody.

   HIV antigen Antibodies to HIV Anti- HIV antibodies

3. In testing to see if the anti-HIV is present, we detect fluorescence, so the results of the test are positive. When trying to detect fluorescence, if none is found, then the results of this test would be negative.

Because the diagnosis of HIV infection is important to know so that an individual can take care not to transmit the virus and start proper management of this disease, positive results on the ELISA test must be confirmed. This is usually done by more sophisticated testing to actually show the presence of antibodies to specific proteins of the virus. If the confirmatory test comes back positive, then the individual is definitely HIV-positive. If the test comes back negative, retesting is recommended (please remember our discussion above).

The method described above is for the detection of antibodies to HIV and not the presence of the virus. To determine the actual presence of the virus and to monitor the effect of treatment, we use a test to measure the amount of HIV particles present in a sample of blood (referred to as *viral load*). These types of tests are more sophisticated, more costly, and, therefore, are usually only performed after a person has been found to be HIV-positive and has sought care of the infection. Assessing viral loads are routinely performed in management of HIV disease.

From HIV Infection to AIDS

Let's put what we have previously discussed into a sequence of events following HIV infection, and discuss what happens to the virus and the human it infects during the course of the lifetime of the person if the individual did *not* seek medical care. This is called the *natural history of HIV disease*.

Through some risky activity, a person becomes infected with the virus and is now HIV-positive. We will consider this person to be a "healthy" individual, meaning that their immune system is fully functional at the time of infection. Healthy individuals have a CD4 count of between 850 and 1,000 CD4 cells per cubic milliliter of blood. (These are just our terms for measuring the amount of these cells. Don't worry about the designation, just remember the 850 to 1,000! The numbers of circulating CD4 cells fluctuates during the course of the day, hence the range.) So, this healthy individual, who previously had no HIV particles or proteins in their body, is now exposed to a dose of virus. Let's follow the fascinating dynamics between HIV and this individual (*please remember this can be somewhat different in each individual and would be the course of events if no anti-HIV treatments are given*):

1. For a few weeks after the entrance of virus into the body the HIV viral load is high (**viremia**), but antibodies to HIV are just being produced, so their concentration is low. The individual's CD4 count is unchanged. *During this time, the individual may experience flu-like symptoms that last a short time.*

2. At several months after infection, the viral load decreases because the virus has found cells to infect, is inside them, and may not be detected. Meanwhile, antibodies to HIV are being produced so the concentration of antibodies is rising. The CD4 count may have decreased somewhat, but rebounds (but usually not to the same levels as before infection). *This is a period of no symptoms (asymptomomatic period) and may last several years. However, although there are no outward symptoms, we know that dynamics between the human and the virus are occurring:*

   a. Viral replication is occurring (it has been estimated that over a billion virus particles are produced each day!).

   b. CD4 cells are being destroyed (estimated to be over a million cells each day!) and the immune system is trying to replenish the lost cells.

   c. Eventually, the body loses the race on destruction versus replenishment and the CD4 count begins a gradual decline while the viral count climbs.

   d. With the loss of CD4 cells, the immune system becomes less able to guard the body, becomes compromised, and is unable to fight off infections. When the CD4 cell count declines to 200, the person is classified as having AIDS.

With a compromised immune system, the individual is less able to fight off infections from microorganisms, especially the opportunistic microorganisms previously mentioned. Opportunistic infections account for most of the deaths related to HIV disease. Additionally, many HIV-positive individuals may develop malignancies, again a by-product of having a compromised immune system.

Prior to the advent of antiretroviral therapy, the natural history of HIV disease from infection until death was approximately eight to ten years. Fortunately, today there are new antiretroviral drugs that can prolong the scenario described above. However, antiretroviral therapy is not a panacea, as many drugs are toxic and cause side effects. Also, these drugs must be taken under stringent requirements and because many people are unable to adhere to these requirements, they often skip doses or completely stop taking the drugs. The virus can also develop resistance to particular drugs, making choices of alternate therapies difficult. Saying all that, people infected with HIV are living longer lives than individuals infected at the beginning of the U.S. epidemic. Unfortunately, this is not true globally, as medications are only just beginning to reach some resource-poor countries or have yet to reach them.

Long Term Nonprogressors

The usual course or natural history of HIV infection in most humans is described above. However, there are some individuals who, once infected with HIV, do not progress through the steps above. These individuals are indeed infected, have measurable HIV viral loads (although low), and maintain normal CD4 counts. If their CD4 count is lowered, it is not extreme enough for them to be experiencing opportunistic infections or be classified as having AIDS. These individuals and their immune systems are being studied extensively to try to determine the mechanisms they have to control HIV so that, hopefully, the mechanisms can be adapted to therapies for others who are infected.

Treatment Issues

Because viruses use a large extent of the human cell's normal processes for its own replication, it is difficult to design drugs that will interfere specifically with just the processes of the virus and not our own. Drugs designed against HIV have been developed to interfere specifically with aspects of the entry and replication of the virus in human cells and are generally grouped by their actions. These drugs have certainly had their time in the spotlight with a great deal of hope placed on them. Unfortunately, most of these drugs have been shown to be not quite as effective as first imagined or too toxic for continued use. They also have caused problems with other human systems or the virus has managed to become resistant to them.

In addition, although many of the treatment options lower the amount of virus that can be measured, there are *reservoirs of HIV* hidden in the body that are not exposed to therapy. For this reason, HIV always rebounds and returns to high viral loads if someone discontinues therapy. Additionally, many people who have been infected for a long time and deal with many pills per day under numerous conditions (refrigeration, taking a gallon of water with each pill, taking it on an empty stomach, taking it on a full stomach, etc.) have become less compliant to adhering to the treatment regimen. This does not mean that there may be no therapeutic cure to HIV; we are just not there yet.

Much effort is under way to develop a **vaccine** that could prevent infection. Vaccines are biological substances that have similarities to a microorganism or its products. Therefore, when injected into a human body, the immune system should "recognize" it, produce some memory cells with information about the virus in them, and *be prepared* in the event the real microorganism gains entry to eradicate it.

The search for a vaccine to prevent HIV infection has been under way for quite some time, but HIV has not been an easy target. This is mainly due to the fact that the virus often *mutates*, that is, changes its antigenic fingerprint. Hence, a vaccine prepared using one HIV fingerprint will prepare the immune system against that particular HIV. However, if the HIV that someone becomes infected with has a different fingerprint, the virus is "new" and there is no immune preparation against it. Again, this is not stopping investigators from working out a solution; it will just take some more time.

KEY TERMS

Biology/Clinical Terms

Acquired Immunodeficiency Syndrome (AIDS): A condition of the immune system caused by the human immunodeficiency virus (HIV); characterized as having a CD4 cell count of less than 200 cells per cubic milliliter of blood.

Budding: Having the ability to reproduce asexually through the pinching of genetic component of a parent cell.

Capsid: A protein shell that covers the nucleic acid component of a virus.

Enzyme-Linked Immunosorbent Assay (ELISA) Test: One of the most common tests used to detect HIV antibodies in an individual's blood sample.

Human Immunodeficiency Virus (HIV): A member of the *Retrovidae* family that causes AIDS by infecting and destroying T helper cells, which are the major types of cells dedicated to maintaining the immune system. Loss of the T helper cells makes the body vulnerable to infection.

Integrase: An enzyme characteristic to retrovirals that allows viral genetic material to be integrated into the host DNA.

Intracellular: Existing within the cell.

Memory Cells: B and T cells that remember a certain antigen after an initial exposure to the antigen; if that antigen invades the body a second time, there is a faster immune response to kill it.

Retrovirus: A virus in the family of *Retroviridae* that contains RNA and replicates through a DNA intermediate.

Reverse Transcriptase: A viral enzyme converting the RNA of a virus into double-stranded DNA.

Ribonucleic Acid (RNA): A group of nucleic acids that control several forms of cellular activity.

Vaccine: A biological substance with similar characteristics to microorganisms involved in a condition that is administered to strengthen immunity to that particular condition.

Viremia: The presence of a viral load in the blood.

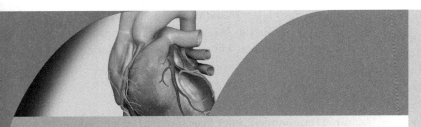

Questions for Further Research, Study, Reflection, and Discussion

For the Individual Student

- Identify prominent transmission routes in the populations that comprise the local residents of your community.
- The same number of yearly new infections with HIV has been constant throughout the years of the U.S. HIV epidemic. What do you think is the reason?
- Think back in the last six months, and determine if you have placed yourself at-risk for HIV infection.

For Small Group Discussion

- Review and discuss the HIV prevention messages you can find on television in one week.
- Visit the CDC HIV/AIDS Among Women Web site (http://www.cdc.gov/hiv/topics/women/resources/factsheets/women.htm), and discuss possible prevention messages for this population.
- Assess the effectiveness of three public HIV prevention messages you can identify seeing in the last six months.

For Entire Class Discussion

- Why do you think that there still is a U.S. HIV/AIDS epidemic?
- What is the first public health measure you would institute if you were the U.S. Global HIV Prevention czar?
- How would you ensure adequate HIV treatment to limited resource countries?

EXERCISES/ACTIVITIES

Each year, the United States spends millions of dollars researching new HIV medicines and vaccines. Identify and research which companies are currently investigating new treatments. What are the most promising areas of research and how do they differ in their basic science? Compose a presentation contrasting the various approaches, including their strengths and weaknesses.

The National Institutes of Health is one of the organizations currently researching an HIV vaccine. Their Vaccine Research Center recruits volunteers to participate in clinical trials. Research the process of becoming a volunteer in a clinical trial. What hesitations would you have about participating in the study? Many people cite fear of contracting the disease as one of their reasons for not participating. After researching the basic science, do you think that fear is well founded?

Discuss the clinical trial process with five friends, and question them on their willingness to participate. During the course of the conversation, quiz them on their knowledge of HIV, including its prevalence, paths of transmission, and risk factors. Ask them how they would rate their own risk of contracting the disease. Take notes on your conversations. Review your notes to determine which themes commonly arise. How familiar were they with the topic? How willing were they to discuss HIV? How willing were they to discuss their own lifestyle choices and risks? What was their general perception of the disease, and would they consider becoming a volunteer? After discussing the topic with friends, how would this experience inform your efforts to engage the public in a meaningful dialogue about HIV?

Healthy People 2010

Indicator: HIV

Focus Area: HIV

Goal: Prevent HIV infection and its related illness and death.

Objectives:

13-1. Reduce AIDS among adolescents and adults.

13-2. Reduce the number of new AIDS cases among adolescent and adult men who have sex with men.

13-3. Reduce the number of new AIDS cases among females and males who inject drugs.

13-4. Reduce the number of new AIDS cases among adolescent and adult men who have sex with men and inject drugs.

13-5. Reduce the number of cases of HIV infection among adolescents and adults.

13-6. Increase the proportion of sexually active persons who use condoms.

13-7. Increase the number of HIV-positive persons who know their serostatus.

13-8. Increase the proportion of substance abuse treatment facilities that offer HIV/AIDS education, counseling, and support.

13-11. Increase the proportion of adults with tuberculosis (TB) who have been tested for HIV.

13-14. Reduce deaths from HIV infection.

13-15. Extend the interval of time between an initial diagnosis of HIV infection and AIDS diagnosis in order to increase years of life of an individual infected with HIV.

13-16. Increase years of life of an HIV-infected person by extending the interval of time between an AIDS diagnosis and death.

13-17. Reduce new cases of perinatally acquired HIV infection.

REFERENCE

1. Centers for Disease Control and Prevention. HIV Prevention in the Third Decade. Atlanta GA: Centers for Disease Control and Prevention. October 2005. Available at www.cdc.gov/hiv/resources/reports. Accessed April 21, 2008.

CROSS REFERENCES

AIDS: History and Timeline

AIDS: An Afterward

Immunity

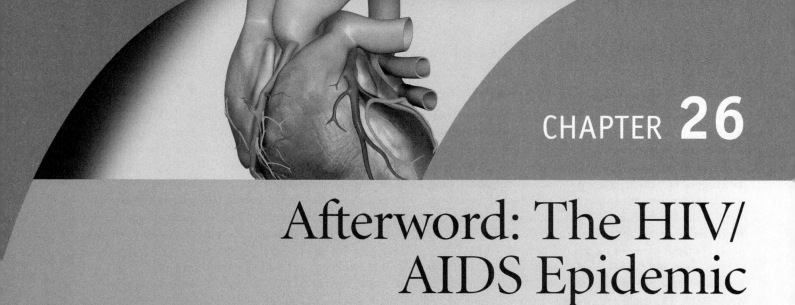

CHAPTER 26

Afterword: The HIV/AIDS Epidemic

Veronica Miller

The HIV/AIDS epidemic has been a key driver of change for public health programs and public health policy. Never before has a single disease had such an enormous impact on global public health nor illustrated the gaps so vividly. Why is this? Some of the contributors responsible for propelling the HIV/AIDS epidemic to this level of importance in global public health include the fact that we have no biological control mechanism (such as a preventive vaccine), the enormous cost (not just in terms of dollar amounts, but also in terms of expertise and required clinical and laboratory infrastructure), and the vulnerability of many of the most affected.

What are some examples of the impact of HIV/AIDS on public health programs? One example that immediately springs to mind is the effect it has had on other infectious disease programs, such as tuberculosis (TB). Although still existent, TB was very much under control in most of the world. In fact, TB surveillance and control programs, although not perfect, were considered a good example of successful public health interventions. The burgeoning HIV/AIDS epidemic has led to a complete reversal of these achievements, especially in southern Africa. This reversal is illustrated by dramatic and overwhelming rises in active TB cases and the development of multidrug resistant (as well as extremely drug resistant) strains of TB. How could this have happened? Contributing to the problem are the nature of how programs are funded and implemented, and the lack of adequate laboratory infrastructure for diagnosis and drug susceptibility testing. The "silo" approach to program funding and development makes quick adaptation, collaboration, and coordination when the setting changes—as it did when HIV arrived on the scene—very dif-

ficult. This is especially the case when one silo is old and very established, and the other silo is as new as HIV programs are in the developing world. The very obvious difference in the level of resources available to these programs adds to the tension. Although at the policy level HIV and TB programs have become more integrated (such as the WHO TB-HIV Working Group), the translation of this into on-the-ground changes will take a longer period of time.

Other examples of programs on which HIV/AIDS has had significant impact include maternal child health programs and reproductive health programs. The need for treatment of both mother and infant with antiretroviral drugs both before and after birth requires changes to program planning and infrastructure. For example, mothers need to come back with their infants for diagnostic purposes. Exposed babies will be put on prophylactic treatment for opportunistic infection, whether or not they are actually infected. The issue of breast feeding has acquired a whole new dimension if the mother is HIV infected, as HIV is frequently transmitted via breast milk. Although prevention of mother-to-child transmission of HIV by antiretroviral drugs is an intervention that has the most solid evidence base behind it, could be viewed politically as the most favorable, and is relatively straightforward to implement, the global coverage is only about 11 percent. Why is that? Could better integration of HIV programs with other existing maternal-child-health and reproductive health programs help fill this gap?

Advocacy and activism have to a large extent driven policy changes. While early on in the epidemic, activism was a United States or Western world phenomenon, groups such as the Treatment Action Campaign in South Africa have been responsible for very visible and highly effective policy changes in the areas of treatment and access to treatment in that region. Activism has been responsible for major policy changes, such as a more rapid drug approval process by the U.S. FDA and the European regulatory agency, for establishing and expanding access to treatment in many areas of the world where treatment would never have been thought possible. The international community response to the challenges of the global epidemic has been substantial, including the U.S. PEPFAR program, the Global Fund to treat AIDS, Tuberculosis, and Malaria, the Bill and Melinda Gates Foundation, and the World Bank. The challenge now is to figure out how we will control this epidemic. As has been said many times, "we cannot treat our way out of this epidemic."

Is there any chance of success? Some believe that there is none without a biological or technological intervention, whether it is a highly effective preventive vaccine or some other biological approach with similar levels of effectiveness. On the other hand, we have not really given it all-we-have-got yet. Prevention programs have been ad hoc instead of a coordinated effort, and often they have competed with each other.

What we need to implement is a complete, 100 percent public health effort that would include all the standard public health interventions but applied in a coordinated and systematic manner. These would include: routine HIV testing, acute infection case finding, partner tracing and notification, antiretroviral treatment of all infected individuals, universal implementation of prevention of mother-to-child-transmission programs, treatment of other sexually transmitted infections (which exacerbate the spread of HIV), broad availability of male circumcision services (male circumcision has been shown to decrease the risk of female-to-male transmission of HIV by about 60 percent), needle exchange programs where appropriate, condom availability, educational programs, and other efforts. This far into the epidemic, it is time to return to good public health approaches.

ACKNOWLEDGMENT

The author gratefully acknowledges stimulating discussions with Dr. Victor DeGruttola (Harvard University School of Public Health) on which some of these thoughts are based.

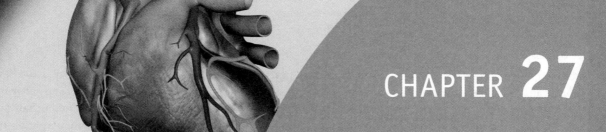

CHAPTER 27

Methicillin-Resistant *Staphylococcus aureus* (MRSA): A Deadly Superbug

Tenagne Haile-Mariam

MRSA-related deaths appear to have surpassed HIV/AIDS related deaths in the United States in 2005.[1]

LEARNING OBJECTIVES

By the end of this chapter, the student will be able to:

- Demonstrate a basic understanding of the microbiology, epidemiology, and clinical manifestations of community acquired methicillin-resistant *Staphylococcus aureus* (CA-MRSA).
- Discuss the scientific basis for some of the medical, public health, and disease control mechanisms that are being proposed to curb the spread of CA-MRSA.
- Analyze current and future scientific, public health policy, and media discourse about CA-MRSA.

OVERVIEW

***Staphylococcus aureus* (*S. aureus*)** is a commonly occurring bacterium. In fact, at any one time up to 50 percent of persons are asymptomatic carriers of *S. aureus* bacteria.[2] Although normally harmless, *S. aureus* can cause serious infection. In any given person, clinical disease due to *S. aureus* results from the complex interaction of bacterial virulence and host susceptibility factors. However, due to its widespread prevalence, *S. aureus* is a common cause of infectious disease in persons of all ages.

When penicillin was first discovered, it could be used to treat most *S. aureus* infections, but penicillin-resistant strains were quickly identified.[3] These resistant strains soon became so widespread that penicillin sensitive strains became vanishingly rare.[4] More potent antibiotics were introduced and

again, resistant bacteria emerged and flourished. For several decades, *S. aureus* species remained largely sensitive to a group of antibiotics that are referred to as the "anti-staphylococcal penicillins." *S. aureus* species that are resistant to these anti-staphylococcal penicillins are generally referred to as **methicillin-resistant *S. aureus* (MRSA)**. MRSA was rarely encountered in the general population and MRSA infections were largely restricted to hospitalized patients. MRSA infections that develop in persons who are chronically ill or have been hospitalized are classified as hospital-acquired (HA-MRSA), and those that arise in persons who are generally healthy are classified as community-acquired (CA-MRSA).

We are experiencing a global and unprecedented rise in the incidence of CA-MRSA.[5] CA-MRSA infections appear to be more aggressive and to be associated with higher degrees of host morbidity and mortality than HA-MRSA and previously encountered methicillin-sensitive *S. aureus* strains.[6]

Although it is difficult for us to imagine, there was an era before the discovery of modern antibiotics. A future when currently available antibiotics will be useless against our most common infectious diseases is just as unimaginable. Yet the medical community and the public media are reporting a growing incidence of infectious organisms that are resistant to most (and in some cases, all) known antibiotics. Infectious disease experts are warning us that such reports herald a potential return to the pre-antibiotic "dark ages" of medicine.

In this chapter, we will look at the emergence of community acquired methicillin-resistant *Staphylococcus aureus* (CA-MRSA), which has been described with terms ranging from a "growing menace" to a "public health threat."[3,7] Containment and treatment of CA-MRSA are challenging to medical practitioners and public health officials. In addition, the emergence of a "superbug" in previously healthy persons has generated concern and even fear in the general population. It is our shared responsibility to understand its causes and search for ways to halt its progression.

BASIC SCIENCE FACTS/KEY CONCEPTS REVIEW

S. aureus Microbiology and Virulence Factors

S. aureus is a Gram-positive organism that has a characteristic "grape-like" appearance on microscopic evaluation (Figure 27-1). Like other Gram-positive organisms, *S. aureus* has a thick cell wall that envelops the bacterial cell membrane (Figure 27-2). At any one time, a good proportion of the general population (up to 50 percent in some estimates) can be asymptomatically colonized with *S. aureus*. On the other hand, *S. aureus* is a common cause of a variety of diseases ranging from superficial skin infections to fulminant systemic illnesses that can lead to a rapid death.

There are several characteristics of *S. aureus* that can mediate the shift of *S. aureus* from a harmless colonizer to an agent of disease and death (Figure 27-3). These include bacterial surface proteins that can facilitate binding to host tissues and also blunt the host's immune response to the infection. *S. aureus* species may elaborate a variety of enzymes that are di-

FIGURE 27-1 Gram's Stain of *Staphylococcus aureus*.

Source: Courtesy of Dr. Thomas F. Sellers/Emory University/CDC.

rectly toxic to host cells and induce tissue destruction. In addition, certain *S. aureus* produce *superantigens*, substances that induce an overwhelming **systemic inflammatory response syndrome (SIRS)** that can result in multiple organ failure and death without directly infecting affected tissues.[8]

Antistaphylococcal Antibiotics

Antistaphylococcal antibiotics can be broadly characterized into two groups: those that prevent bacterial replication and those that inhibit essential bacterial functions. Beta-lactams (β-lactams) such as the penicillins and cephalosporins inhibit bacterial replication by affecting bacterial cell wall formation. β-lactam antibiotics act by binding and deactivating molecules called *PBPs (penicillin binding proteins)*, which are found in the cell membrane and are critical for cell wall formation.[9] Vancomycin, a medication that is often used to treat MRSA infections, has a different mechanism from the β-lactams, but similar to them it disrupts bacterial cell wall formation (Figure 27-4).[10]

Clindamycin is an example of an antibiotic that inhibits the production of substances that are essential for bacterial function. It inhibits protein synthesis by binding to the bacterial ribosome.[11] Quinupristin-dalfopristin is a combination of two similar drugs that also act on the bacterial ribosome, resulting in decreased protein synthesis.[10] Linezolid, another antibiotic that inhibits staphylococcal protein synthesis, is useful in MRSA infections but is only available in an oral formulation.[10] Daptomycin belongs to a new class of drugs called the lipopeptides; it causes bacterial cell death by disrupting the cell membrane and is only available in an intravenous formulation.[12]

Other examples of antibiotics that inhibit bacterial protein synthesis are the macrolides (for example, erythromycin) and the fluoroquinolones (such as ciprofloxacin). Although both these classes of drugs are often well tolerated, they have been associated with high rates of staphylococcal antibiotic resistance. Mupirocin, a topical antibiotic that also inhibits protein synthesis, is useful in the treatment of superficial staphylococcal infections and to eliminate nasal carriage (colonization) by the organism.[8] Rifampin is an antibiotic that inhibits bacterial RNA formation. It is most useful for the treatment of *S. aureus* when it is used in combination with one or more other antibiotics.[8] Sulfamethoxazole, a sulfonamide, is an agent that inhibits bacterial growth by interfering with folic acid synthesis. In combination with trimethoprim, another agent that inhibits folic acid synthesis, it provides for a potent, cheap, and widely available antibiotic that has proved very useful in treating MRSA infections (Figure 27-5).[13]

Antibiotic Resistance and *S. aureus*

With so many drugs available to combat *S. aureus*, it might appear that clinicians have an adequate armamentarium with

FIGURE 27-2 Gram-positive Cell Wall.

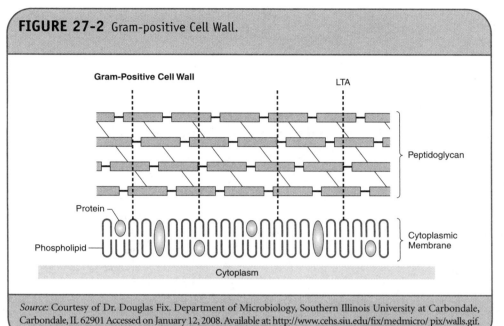

Source: Courtesy of Dr. Douglas Fix. Department of Microbiology, Southern Illinois University at Carbondale, Carbondale, IL 62901 Accessed on January 12, 2008. Available at: http://www.cehs.siu.edu/fix/medmicro/ pix/walls.gif.

FIGURE 27-3 Laboratory Diagnosis of *S. aureus*.

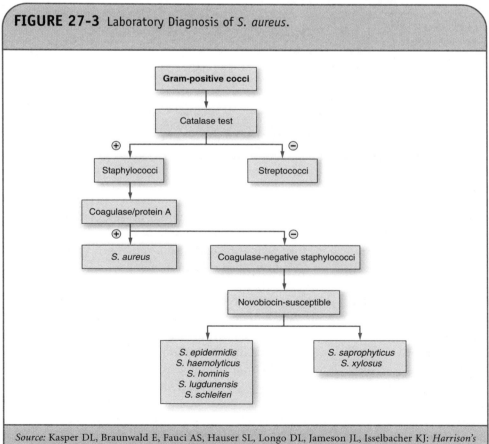

Source: Kasper DL, Braunwald E, Fauci AS, Hauser SL, Longo DL, Jameson JL, Isselbacher KJ: *Harrison's Principles of Internal Medicine*, 16th edition. Available at http://www.accessmedicine.com. © The McGraw-Hill Companies, Inc.

which to treat staphylococcal infections. Yet, efforts to treat these infections are increasingly frustrated by the bacteria's ability to develop resistance to multiple antibiotics. When penicillin was introduced in the 1940s, all *S. aureus* isolates appeared to be very sensitive to the "miracle" antibiotic. But within a few years, however, the first reports of penicillin-resistant *S. aureus* appeared and by the 1960s, 80 percent of *S. aureus* were resistant to penicillin.[4] This widespread resistance results from the ability of *S. aureus* isolates to produce **penicillinase**, an enzyme that deactivates penicillin. The genetic material that allows bacteria to produce this enzyme is easily transferred between different strains of *S. aureus* and between different types of bacteria.[4] The only way to treat infections due to organisms that produce penicillinase is to use medications that cannot be deactivated by it. In addition, one can utilize antibiotics that destroy *S. aureus* by acting on other essential cellular functions, thereby bypassing the effects of penicillinase.

The first penicillinase resistant β-lactam antibiotics were released in the 1950s. The prototype of the penicillinase-resistant semisynthetic penicillin is methicillin.[9] Other drugs in this category include nafcillin and dicloxiacillin. The cephalosporins, especially the "first generation cephalosporins" such as cefazolin, are similarly resistant to penicillinase and are widely used against penicillin-resistant *S. aureus*. Penicillinase is also inactivated by "β-lactamase inhibitors," synthetic compounds found in medications such as

FIGURE 27-4 Inhibition of Bacterial Cell Wall Synthesis.

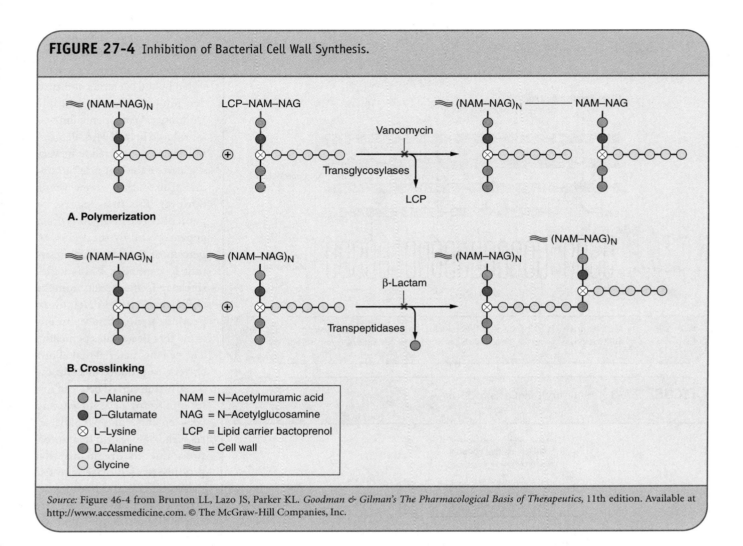

Source: Figure 46-4 from Brunton LL, Lazo JS, Parker KL. *Goodman & Gilman's The Pharmacological Basis of Therapeutics*, 11th edition. Available at http://www.accessmedicine.com. © The McGraw-Hill Companies, Inc.

clavulanic acid.[4] These medications are used in combination with drugs such as ampicillin that are useless against penicillinase-producing organisms when used alone. Methicillin resistance is mediated through bacterial expression of penicillin binding protein 2a (PBP 2a), a type of PBP that has a very low affinity for all β-lactam drugs (not just penicillin).[4] If the target bacteria are expressing PBP2a, bacterial cell wall synthesis can occur despite the presence of β-lactam antibiotics, rendering this whole class of previously potent anti-staphylococcal antibiotics useless.

Another way to bypass penicillinase resistance is to use drugs that do not act by binding to PBPs. Examples of such drugs are clindamycin, vancomycin, and the fluoroquinolones. Fluoroquinolones showed initial promise against MRSA and they were widely used for this purpose when they were first introduced. But, as expected, soon after their introduction reports of fluoroquinolone-resistant *S. aureus* began to emerge.[4] Ciprofloxacin resistance among MRSA has been attributed to

widespread use of these drugs to treat a variety of hospital and community acquired infections.[14] Because of its broad Gram-positive spectrum, clindamycin is a useful empiric drug for the treatment of cellulitis that is most likely caused by *S. aureus*. Unfortunately, resistance among *S. aureus* has been well described also and can appear among bacteria that show in vitro susceptibility to it.[14]

Vancomycin has long been considered the most useful agent against MRSA. Although it is available as an oral medication, only the intravenous formulation can be used to treat infections that involve any organs except the intestinal tract. The first reports of vancomycin intermediate-resistant *S. aureus* (VISA) were in 1997.[4] More recently, vancomycin-resistant *S. aureus* (VRSA) are being reported.[4] Some VRSA resistance appears to be mediated by a plasmid transferred from vancomycin-resistant *Enterococcus faecalis* (VRE), another "superbug" with isolates that exhibit resistance to multiple

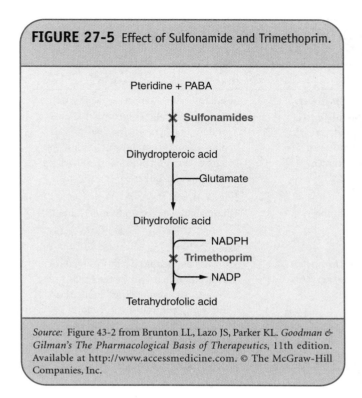

FIGURE 27-5 Effect of Sulfonamide and Trimethoprim.

Pteridine + PABA

✗ **Sulfonamides**

Dihydropteroic acid

— Glutamate

Dihydrofolic acid

— NADPH

✗ **Trimethoprim**

→ NADP

Tetrahydrofolic acid

Source: Figure 43-2 from Brunton LL, Lazo JS, Parker KL. *Goodman & Gilman's The Pharmacological Basis of Therapeutics*, 11th edition. Available at http://www.accessmedicine.com. © The McGraw-Hill Companies, Inc.

antibiotics. Because patients who are hospitalized have an increased possibility of being colonized by both VRE and MRSA, there is a genuine probability that this mechanism of transferring resistance will make VRSA more prevalent.[6]

In prescribing antibiotics, the healthcare practitioner must take several patient-specific factors into account. These include the patient's age (certain drugs such as fluoroquinolones and tetracycline cannot be prescribed to young children) and the patient's drug allergy profile. In addition, many drug-drug interactions can result in significant patient morbidity and even mortality, so the prescriber must account for the patient's prescription and nonprescription medications. Additional considerations in choosing and prescribing medications include the size of the patient and ability to metabolize and eliminate the drug. For example, a person with kidney dysfunction will need lower dosages of a medication that is cleared from the body through the urinary system. Because some medications are only available as intravenous formulations, the additional cost of hospitalization or home nursing must be added to the price of the medication to determine the true cost of the treatment.

The prescriber also must account for the cost and even the market availability of an antibiotic. An example of a situation when a medication's cost would be an important consideration is if the medication is not readily covered by a patient's insurance plan. In certain instances, a patient's insurance plan will allow for a lower patient payment for a certain drug in comparison to others that are from the same class of medication, making that medication the only one that the patient can afford. In general, antibiotics that have been in use for the longest amount of time are more cost-effective than those that have been recently introduced to the market; however, occasionally the side effect profiles and ease of administration might eclipse these benefits. Clearly, choosing the most useful antibiotic requires more than just evaluating the bacterial antibiotic sensitivity profile.

Hospital Acquired MRSA Versus Community Acquired MRSA

MRSA has long been considered a disease of the hospitalized and chronically ill patient. If MRSA is isolated from a patient 48 to 72 hours after admission, it is generally referred to as hospital acquired MRSA (HA-MRSA).[15] HA-MRSA is distinguished from community acquired (CA-MRSA) in several ways. CA-MRSA infections tend to be associated with skin and soft tissue infections in otherwise healthy hosts. In addition, CA-MRSA strains appear to be more **virulent**. This virulence is partly attributed to the increased presence of the Panton-Valentine leukocidin (PVL), a highly destructive bacterial toxin that has been associated with very aggressive staphylococcal infections.[16] Interestingly CA-MRSA are less likely than HA-MRSA to exhibit drug resistance to multiple antibiotics.[17] For example, CA-MRSA are more likely to be sensitive to the tetracyclines and to trimothoprim-sulfamethoxazole than HA-MRSA.

Other experts will classify MRSA into two broad categories: healthcare associated and community associated (Table 27-1). In the healthcare associated category, they include patients who have had hospitalization or surgery within the year before the onset of infection and refer to them as having community onset, healthcare associated MRSA infections. Persons who acquire MRSA infection over 48 hours after hospitalization are generally referred to as having hospital onset, healthcare associated MRSA.[18] As one can see, it is important to understand what classification system the author is using when trying to understand the current discourse about the rising rates of MRSA in the community.

MRSA: THE PUBLIC HEALTH PERSPECTIVE

There are many theories as to why there is a global rise in the incidence of multiresistant bacteria. What most experts do agree on is that it is unlikely that there is only one cause for the rise. Widespread use of antibiotics—often without adequate indications—in both hospital and outpatient settings is thought to have contributed to the selection of more resistant strains. In addition, the use of antibiotics in various areas

TABLE 27-1 Characteristics of CA-MRSA Versus Health Care–Associated MRSA

	CA-MRSA	Healthcare Associated MRSA
At-risk groups or conditions	Children, competitive athletes, prisoners, soldiers, selected ethnic populations (Native Americans/Alaska natives, Pacific Islanders), intravenous drug users, men who have sex with men	Residents in long-term care facility, patients with diabetes mellitus, patients undergoing hemodialysis/peritoneal dialysis, prolonged hospitalization, intensive care unit admission, indwelling intravascular catheters
SCC type	Type IV	Types I, II, and III
Antimicrobial resistance	β-Lactam resistance alone, common (Table 1)	Multidrug resistance, common (Table 1)
PVL toxin	Frequent	Rare
Associated clinical syndromes	Skin and soft tissue infections (furuncles, skin abscesses), postinfluenza, necrotizing pneumonia (see text)	Nosocomial pneumonia, nosocomial- or catheter-related urinary tract infections, intravascular-catheter or bloodstream infections, surgical-site infections

Abbreviations: CA, community acquired; MRSA, methicillin-resistant *Staphylococcus aureus*; PVL, Panton-Valentine leukocidin; SCC, staphylococcal cassette cartridge.
Source: Used with permission from the Mayo Clinic. Table 2 used with permission from Kowalski TJ, Berbari E, Osmon D. Epidemiology, treatment and prevention of community acquired methicillin-resistant *Staphylococcus aureus* infections. *Mayo Clin Proc* 2005;80:1201–1208.

of food production has been implicated. There is a growing call to both prescribing healthcare workers and infection control personnel to work together to curb the use of broad spectrum antibiotics and to limit the use of antibiotics to situations when they are clinically indicated. The judicious use of antibiotics in the treatment of infections is an essential part of controlling the rise of multidrug resistant organisms. For example, a physician might forgo antibiotics after an abscess has been adequately incised and drained. In many such instances, the host's immune system can contain the infection and antibiotics will not be needed as an adjunct. Just as important as educating the medical communities on the proper use of antibiotics, it is also important that public health officials, media personnel, and medical practitioners work together to educate the public about appropriate antibiotic use. The public needs to be aware that the unwarranted use of antibiotics is costly, results in untoward side effects, and, in a more global way, contributes to the rise of multiresistant organisms. It is imperative that research into the causes of this problem continues if we are to find a way of stemming its rise.

In addition to the judicious use of antibiotics in both the inpatient and outpatient setting, institution of infection control mechanisms are very important ways of curbing the incidence and transmission of MRSA. These include the rotation of antibiotics that are used to treat infectious diseases in hospitals and long-term care facilities.[3] Proper attention should be placed on areas in an institution where certain bacterial isolates are becoming more common. Such measures prevent the selection of bacterial isolates that are resistant to a certain class of drug. Other infection control methods are proper cleansing of furniture and equipment, frequent hand washing, and the appropriate use of barriers such as gloves and gowns.[20] If persons are identified that harbor multidrug-resistant organisms, they need to be appropriately isolated and treated to decrease transmission rates (Table 27-2).[11]

The increasingly prevalent current outbreaks of MRSA in the community have been associated with certain factors. An online CDC publication refers to these factors as the **5 C's:** "**C**rowding; frequent skin-to-skin **C**ontact; **C**ompromised skin (such as cuts or abrasions); **C**ontaminated items and surfaces; and lack of **C**leanliness. Locations where the 5 C's are common include schools, dormitories, military barracks, households, correctional facilities, and daycare centers" (available at http://www.cdc.gov/niosh/topics/mrsa/. Accessed April 22, 2008).[21] The current increase in *S. aureus* infections and

CASE STUDY

In reading about disease in textbooks, we are rarely presented with the patient's perspective of illness. One of the most moving personal accounts of how MRSA-related illness can result in significant morbidity and is that of Brandon Noble, a National Football League (NFL) player from 1997 to 2006 (Figure 27-6). A routine orthopedic operation was complicated by MRSA infection that sidelined his athletic career. His and other accounts can be found in multiple media reports and focus our attention on the very real, human toll of MRSA.[18]

IN HIS OWN WORDS: BRANDON NOBLE

Being a football player, there are certain things you can expect to deal with. From high school in Virginia Beach, Virginia, to college at Penn State, and into the NFL, I have broken bones in both hands and my leg, had concussions (probably more than I care to know about), stingers (where you go from not being able to move your arms to an incredible burning sensation), separated shoulders once or twice, torn tendons off of the end of my ring finger, torn ligaments, and dislocated my knee cap, on top of the usual wear and tear, arthritic joints, jammed fingers, bruised muscles, sprains, smashed fingers and stepped-on toes. But the worst and most unexpected thing that I have come up against in my football career (I have been playing since the age of 14 and I am 31 now) has been a tiny little thing that I cannot see. It has hurt me more than any of the others combined, and had a hand in ending my career: MRSA.

In April of 2005, I had a routine operation to clean out my right knee. The usual wear and tear of football had caused some cartilage to chip off and was floating around in my knee causing swelling and stiffness. By getting the surgery in April I felt like I would be able to be fully recovered and ready for the upcoming season. The surgery was performed and I was fine for about eight days, then the stitches were taken out. That night, a hot spot developed over the porthole used for the surgery. I began feeling sick—flu-like symptoms—and my knee hurt like someone was lighting me on fire. By the time I was put in the hospital the infection had spread from a quarter-sized red spot around the port to cover a good portion of my leg. It had taken about two days. One of the first doctors that I saw told my parents that if I had waited another 24 hours we could be talking about the loss of my leg or worse. Surgery was performed and things got better once the infection was washed out.

But now I had to deal with the rest of the treatment, which included a peripherally inserted central catheter (PICC) line for take-home IV treatment for six weeks on the drug vancomycin. A PICC line is basically a tube that is inserted into your body so you don't have a traditional needle IV in you for six weeks. This antibiotic will wear you out. Besides the fact I was told not to lift anything over 5 pounds with my arm that had the PICC line in it, the vanco exhausted me, sapping my energy and appetite. I am married with three kids (two at the time); none of them are under 5 pounds and not much else in this world is. So, that limits you in itself. Three times a day, for 1 hour and 30 minutes, I had to sit down and get my dose of vanco. Then I got redman syndrome, which happens

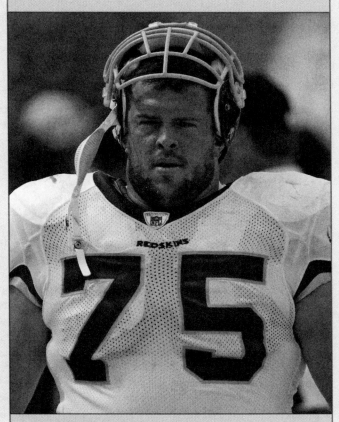

FIGURE 27-6 Brandon Noble.

Source: Infectious Disease Society of America.

when you administer the vanco too fast: a very itchy rash that will drive you crazy and turns you red. So, I was taken off of the vanco and placed on Zyvox. This is an oral med that is very strong and gives you jock itch everywhere that is dark and warm. I will leave the rest to your imagination. I completed my treatment and was given a clean bill of health.

I had at this point missed the entire off-season workout program due to the way that I felt from the antibiotics. Now I was playing catch up and tried to cram an off-season into three weeks. I was able to come back and play during preseason camp, but in compensating for a weak right leg (the one that had been infected) I hurt my left leg. I chipped off some cartilage and suffered a bone bruise requiring surgery again. I was placed on injured reserve and forced to sit out for the season.

While all this was going on we found out that my wife was pregnant with our third child. So, since I was on injured reserve I was able to stay home and help my wife out. Chasing the kids around all day I re-injured the bone bruise, which caused a gross amount of swelling in my left knee. I had the knee drained numerous times, but each time the swelling came back. In December, after draining my knee two or three times in about two weeks, I start to get sick again. Same symptoms as before—burning in the knee and the worst flu symptoms you can imagine.

I was admitted to the hospital on Dec. 15 for surgery to clean out my knee. The next day, Dec. 16th, my wife was admitted to the hospital and our third child was born. I was in the delivery room thanks to an understanding doctor. Because of my MRSA they were hesitant to let me in the delivery room (understandably so), but my wife's doctor said that as long as I wash my hands and stay clear of the actual delivery I could be there. I would not have taken it well had this not worked out. Missing the birth of a child is not acceptable to me and would have been devastating. I was scared to hold him for fear of getting him sick. It is tough not to hold your child right after he is born. I was sent home with another PICC line in my arm on the antibiotics Daptomycin and Cipro, an oral medication, because the culture was not growing. I was being treated for MRSA and whatever Cipro kills.

My PICC line is out now and I am done with the Cipro. I am taking a suppression medication called Doxycycline for at least 6 months. And then I think I will be tested to see if MRSA is still on/in me. The thing that scares me the most is I could be a carrier of this bug and have to worry about my wife and kids getting it. Knowing how painful and serious it is, that is the last thing I want to happen. I have 2 boys, the oldest is 4 and hell on wheels. If his little brother is anything like him, it will be a lifetime of cuts and scrapes. I will keep a close eye on each one because I am incredibly paranoid about them getting MRSA. Any small red bump on any of my kids and I am pestering my wife to keep an eye on it, ready to go to the doctors at the drop of a hat.

An unwelcome complication from my last surgery was developing two blood clots, one in each lung and I am now on blood thinners for at least 6 months. Because of the clots and the MRSA there is a very good chance that I will never play football again. This infection has had a huge impact on my life and will continue to impact me and my family in the near future. Hopefully, I am not a carrier and will not have to worry about this forever. Regardless, I will be vigilant in watching every cut and scrape that my kids get because I don't want them to have to suffer the way I did. To say that the last year has been difficult for me and my family would be an understatement, and we have MRSA to thank for it.

CLINICAL PERSPECTIVE

Clinical Syndromes

Although *S. aureus* have been shown to infect all human organ systems, they are recognized as the major cause of skin and soft tissue infections that can range from superficial dermatitis to deep set infection of muscle and bone. An example of a superficial infection is **impetigo**, a common skin infection characterized by vesicles or pustules that can rupture and have a characteristic "honey yellow" crust that can mimic a herpetic (cold sore) outbreak. Although impetigo rarely causes systemic symptoms, it can spread easily to other parts of the body and commonly causes disease outbreaks among persons kept in close quarters (such as daycare centers). *S. aureus* is a major cause of folliculitis, cellulitis, and soft tissue abscesses. More aggressive manifestations of staphylococcal soft tissue disease such as necrotizing fasciitis are well described and *S. aureus* is a major cause of osteomylitis and septic arthritis. Infections of other organ systems such as the cardiovascular system (for example, endocarditis) and the respiratory system (such as pneumonia) have been attributed to *S. aureus*.[2] It remains a major nosocomial (hospital-acquired) pathogen involving every organ system and it is frequently the cause of surgical site, prosthetic, and intravascular device infections.[2]

Although most of the clinical syndromes attributed to *S. aureus* are due to local tissue invasion and destruction, several well-described syndromes result directly from toxins that are elaborated by the bacteria even in the face of a small focus of infection. An example of this is toxin-associated *S. aureus* gastroenteritis. This syndrome of acute vomiting, often occurring with the clustering of cases, is related to the ingestion of pre-formed toxins. The toxins are heat-stable and although bacteria are destroyed by cooking, the toxins are not. Staphylococcal scalded skin syndrome is another illness caused by toxins elaborated by certain strains of *S. aureus* and is characterized by diffuse superficial skin peeling. Neither toxin-associated diarrheal disease nor staphylococcal scalded skin syndrome is classically life-threatening, but their occurrence should initiate an investigation to find the origin of the causative agent to prevent the emergence of new cases.

Unlike *S. aureus* toxin-associated diarrheal and scalded skin syndromes, staphylococcal **toxic shock syndrome (TSS)** is often associated with significant morbidity and mortality by inducing an overwhelming host immune response characterized by hypotension, fever, rash, and multi-organ involvement.[8] Despite the presence of this systemic inflammatory response syndrome (SIRS), bacteria are usually not isolated from blood cultures (unlike streptococcus associated TSS) and it is essential to remove the source of the offending bacteria in order to adequately treat the infection. The general public and governmental regulatory agencies became aware of the virulent nature of TSS when it was reported in 1980 with the use of super-absorbent feminine tampons.[8]

More recently, there are increasing reports in both the scientific literature and the general media of aggressive *S. aureus* in groups that are traditionally at low risk for fulminant infections with MRSA. These reports include highly publicized cases of overwhelming pneumonias in otherwise healthy children and highly destructive soft tissue infections in young athletes.

Washington Redskins defensive tackle Brandon Noble joined the team in 2003 after spending four years as a Dallas Cowboy. He has also played for the San Francisco 49ers and NFL Europe's Barcelona Dragons. He played college football at Penn State.

Source: Used with permission by the Infectious Disease Society of America, Arlington, Virginia. ©2006.

increased public awareness of the problem can help us to focus on measures that can be used to halt the spread of the bacteria. These include encouraging persons to not share towels and other such personal items, practice frequent hand washing, and to clean surfaces that could come into contact with abraded skin such as locker room benches and wrestling mats. Persons with abraded skin or open wounds should wear protective dressings to prevent infection.[21] The public also should be educated on the early recognition of *S. aureus* infection and the appropriate care of infections.

It is important that persons share "best practices" in seeking ways to contain the spread of MRSA. Many organizations ranging from physician specialty organizations (such as the Infectious Diseases Association of America) to the CDC are dedicating professional and monetary resources to this issue. Although great strides have been made toward understanding the microbiology, epidemiology, and pathophysiology of MRSA-related diseases, the consensus is that much more work has to be done toward containing these diseases. There is a multitude of ongoing efforts to improve disease **surveillance**, implement containment strategies, and educate both the general public and healthcare workers on how to prevent, diagnose, and treat staphylococcal diseases. An excellent source that is regularly updated and outlines several such efforts in the CDC's MRSA Web site.[21]

An example of an approach that has been found to be useful by some is the "search and destroy" methods used in the Netherlands that have been associated with very low rates of MRSA. This approach relies on screening patients and health-care workers for MRSA, isolation of cases, and aggressive decolonization of potential carriers.[22]

SUMMARY

If there ever was a time when human beings felt that the scourge of bacterial infections would end, our current battles against multiresistant organisms have dimmed the prospects of such a time. Rather, we seem to be entering an era of increased bacterial virulence and decreased antibiotic potency despite the great advances that have been made into the discovery and production of excellent antimicrobial medications.

CA-MRSA is a poignant example of how social, environmental, economic, and biological factors have "conspired" to lay the groundwork for an epidemic. In addition to MRSA, there are several other potent, multidrug resistant bacteria that are being encountered by medical practitioners globally. To compound this problem, there is a relative paucity of newer, more potent antibiotics on the horizon. In addressing this problem, the antimicrobial availability taskforce of the Infectious Diseases Society of America published a report in 2003 entitled, "Bad bugs, No drugs: As antibiotic R and D stagnates, a public health crisis brews."[23] Yet, it is clear that the production of new antibiotics will not be the only solution to the rise of multiresistant bacteria. Overcoming this problem will require a concerted effort by public health practitioners, governmental agencies, medical personnel, and the public at large.

TABLE 27-2 Suggested Measures to Limit the Spread of CA-MRSA

Personal and caregiver hygiene measures
    Shower daily using soap and hot water
    Wash hands frequently and/or use sanitation gels
    Cover wounds with dry, clean dressings
    Avoid contact with wound drainage (use gloves)
    Avoid sharing towels, razors, clothing, personal items
    Clean cuts and abrasions with soap and water

Enviornmental and organizational control measures
    Routinely clean shared equipment (e.g., wrestling mats, benches, athletic equipment, whirlpools)
    Clean and disinfect contaminated surfaces
    Launder contaminated clothes and/or linens in hot water with detergent or bleach
    Limit participation in contact sports unless adequate wound coverage can be obtained
    Use a barrier (e.g., clothes, towels) to bare skin when in contact with shared equipment or surfaces (e.g., sauna benches, exercise machines, massage tables)

Healthcare-initiated measures
    Use antimicrobials judiciously
    Recognize and treat CA-MRSA lesions early
    Educate and counsel patients and caregivers about appropriate wound care
    Consider decolonization strategies for recurrent disease or in localized outbreaks in consultation with infectious disease physicians

Source: Used with permission from Mayo Clinic. Table 4 used with permission from Kowalski TJ, Berbari E, Osmon D. Epidemiology, treatment and prevention of community acquired methicillin-resistant *Staphylococcus aureus* infections. *Mayo Clin Proc* 2005;80:1201–1208.

KEY TERMS

Biology/Clinical Terms

Impetigo: A common skin infection characterized by vesicles or pustules that can rupture and have a characteristic "honey yellow" crust that can mimic a herpetic outbreak.

Methicillin-Resistant Staphylococcus aureus (MRSA): Bacterial strains resistant to beta-lactam antibiotics. Benign MRSA infections typically colonize on the skin and mucous membranes but may cause severe infections.

Penicillinase: An enzyme that deactivates penicillin.

Staphylococcus aureus: Gram-positive microorganisms belonging to the genus *Staphylococcus*. It is the microorganisms involved in MRSA infections.

Systemic Inflammatory Response Syndrome (SIRS): A systemic response to a condition that forms an acute inflammatory response characterized by an occurrence of at least two symptoms.

Toxic Shock Syndrome (TSS): A condition that is often associated with significant morbidity and mortality by inducing an overwhelming host immune response characterized by hypotension, fever, rash, and multi-organ involvement.

Virulence: Capacity of a pathogen to cause an infection.

Public Health Terms

5 C's (MRSA): Certain factors that closely link an occurrence of MRSA in communities commonly known to have outbreaks. The 5 C's include: **C**rowding, **C**ontact, **C**ompromised skin, **C**ontaminated items, and **C**leanliness.

Surveillance: Continuous observation of a testing or procedure.

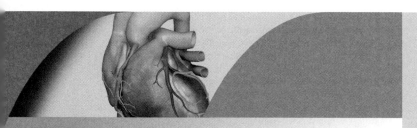

Questions for Further Research, Study, Reflection, and Discussion

For the Individual Student

In order to answer these questions, it may be necessary to research the primary literature.

1. Is there any connection between the use of antibiotics in food production and the rise of antibiotic resistant bacteria in human populations? If so, then what is the proof of this connection?

2. Your physician prescribes you a 10-day course of clindamycin at a dose of 300 mg 3 times a day for 10 days. Assuming that you are uninsured, what would the cost of the antibiotic be for you at your local pharmacy? What would the cost of a 10-day course of the following oral antistaphyloccocal antibiotics be for you at the following doses:

   Cefalexin (500 mg 4 times a day), trimethoprim-sulfamethoxazole (2 double strength tablets 2 times a day), or linezolid (600 mg 2 times a day)?

For Small Group Discussion

1. Can you define BN's risk factors for developing MRSA-related illness?

2. Could BN's illness have been prevented? If so how, if not, why not?

For Entire Class Discussion

A 7th grader at your local school returns to class after a two-day absence. He is under the care of a physician for a soft-tissue infection of his forearm.

   a. You are the principal at the school. An angry parent has come to you demanding that the affected student be removed from his son's classroom. How would you respond to the parent?

   b. The affected child is a member of the school's football team. The team's coach would like some guidance on whether the child should be allowed to participate in games and practice. He also would like to know what to tell students and parents about the risk of continuing to practice and play football this season. How would you respond to the coach?

EXERCISES/ACTIVITIES

1. Although the medical community had fully accepted the presence of MRSA in chronically ill patients, it was surprised by the sheer numbers and the widespread nature of the CA-MRSA outbreak. Do you think that anything could have been done to avert the rise of CA-MRSA? If so, then what steps should have been taken? Do you believe that we as a society are paying enough attention and putting our resources towards curbing the rise of multiply-resistant antibiotics? If so, then defend your position. If not, then propose ways in which this situation could be improved.

2. What is the STAAR Act? Would you support it? Debate the role of public advocacy and legislation in curbing multidrug-resistant organisms such as MRSA.

REFERENCES

1. Bancroft EA. Antimicrobial resistance: it's not just for hospitals. *JAMA* 2007;298:1803–1804.

2. Lowy FD. Staphylococcal infections. In: Kasper DL, Braunwald E, Hauser S, Longo D, Jameson JL, Fauci AS, eds. *Harrison's Principles of Internal Medicine*, 16th ed. Columbus, OH: McGraw-Hill; 2005.

3. Grudmann Aires-de-Sousa M, Boyce J, Tiemersma E. Emergence and resurgence of meticillin-resistant *Staphylococcus aureus* as a public-health threat. *Lancet* 2006;368:874–885.

4. Lowy FD. Antimicrobial resistance: the example of *Staphylococcus aureus*. *J Clin Invest* 2003:111:1265–1273.

5. Rice LR Antimicrobial resistance in gram-positive bacteria *Am J Infect Control* 2006;34:S11–S19.

6. Kollef MH, Micek ST. Methicillin-resistant *Staphylococcus aureus*: a new community acquired pathogen? *Curr Opin Infect Dis* 2006;19:161–168.

7. Moellering RC. The growing menace of community-acquired methicillin-resistant *Staphylococcus aureus*. *Ann Intern Med* 2006;144:368–370.

8. Moreillon P, Que YA, Glauser MP. *Staphylococcus aureus* (including staphylococcal toxic shock). In: Mandell GL, Bennett JE, Dolin R, eds. *Mandell, Bennett, & Dolin: Principles and Practice of Infectious Diseases*, 6th ed. Philadelphia: Churchill Livingstone; 2004. Available at http://www.ppidonline .com/ (subscription required). Accessed April 22, 2008.

9. Kendler JS, Hartman FJ. β-Lactam antibiotics. In: Cohen J, Powderly WD, Berkley SF, Calandra T, Clumek N, Finch RG, eds. *Cohen and Powderly: Infectious Diseases*, 2nd ed. St. Louis: Mosby; 2004.

10. Van Bambeke F, Lambert D, Mingeot-leclercq M, Tulkens P. Mechanisms of action. Ch 188. In: *Cohen and Powderly: Infectious Diseases*, 2nd ed. St. Louis: Mosby; 2004.

11. Kowalski TJ, Berbari E, Osmon D. Epidemiology, treatment and prevention of community acquired methicillin-resistant *Staphylococcus aureus* infections. *Mayo Clin Proc* 2005;80:1201–1208.

12. Hair PI, Keam SJ. Daptomycin: a review of its use in the management of complicated skin and soft-tissue infections and *Staphylococcus aureus* bacteraemia. *Drugs* 2007;67:1483–512.

13. Ellis MW, Lewis JS. Treatment approaches for community-acquired methicillin resistant *Staphylococcus aureus* infections. *Curr Opin Infect Dis* 2005;18:496–501.

14. Moran G, Krishnadasan A, Gorwitz RJ, et al., EMERGEncy ID Net Study Group. Methicillin-resistant *S. aureus* infections among patients in the emergency department. *N Engl J Med* 2006;355:666–674.

15. Vandenesch F, Naimi T, Enright MC, Lina G, Nimmo GR, Heffernan H, et al. Community-acquired methicillin-resistant *Staphylococcus aureus* carrying Panton-Valentine leukocidin genes: worldwide emergence. *Emerg Infect Dis* 2003;9:978–984.

16. Naimi TS, LeDell KH, Como-Sabetti K, Borchardt SM, Boxrud DJ, et al. Comparison of community and health care associated methicillin resistant *Staphylococcus aureus* infection. *JAMA* 2003;290:2976–2984.

17. Klevens R, Morrison MA, Nadle J, Petit S, Gershman K, et al., Active Bacterial Core Surveillance (ABCs) MRSA Investigators. Invasive methicillin-resistant *Staphylococcus aureus* infections in the United States. *JAMA* 2007;298:1763–1771.

18. Infectious Diseases Society of America. *Brandon Noble's Story*. Arlington, VA: IDSA; 2006. Available at http://www.idsociety.org/Content .aspx?id=5622. Accessed April 22, 2008.

19. Henderson DK. Managing methicillin-resistant staphylococci: a paradigm for preventing nosocomial transmission of resistant organisms. *Am J Infect Control* 2006;34(Suppl 1) S46–S54.

20. Centers for Disease Control and Prevention (CDC), National Safety Institute for Occupational Safety and Health (NIOSH). *MRSA and the Workplace* (last modified 2007). Atlanta: CDC. Available at http://www.cdc.gov/ niosh/topics/mrsa/. Accessed April 22, 2008.

21. Centers for Disease Control and Prevention (CDC). Healthcare-Associated Methicillin-Resistant *Staphylococcus aureus* (HA-MRSA). Atlanta: CDC. Available at http://www.cdc.gov/ncidod/dhqp/ar_mrsa.html. Accessed April 22, 2008.

22. Infection Prevention Working Party. Hospitals. MRSA Hospital (January 2007). Available at http://www.wip.nl/UK/free_content/Richtlijnen/ MRSA%20hospital.pdf. Accessed April 22, 2008.

23. Infectious Diseases Society of America. Bad bugs, no drugs: as antibiotic discovery stagnates a public health crisis brews. Arlington, VA: IDSA; 2004. Available at http://www.idsociety.org/badbugsnodrugs.html. Accessed April 22, 2008.

RESOURCES

Infectious Diseases Society of America (IDSA). Web site available at http://www.idsociety.org. Accessed April 22, 2008.

The Centers for Disease Control. Web site available at http://www.cdc.gov. Accessed April 22, 2008.

CROSS REFERENCES

Safe Medication Use

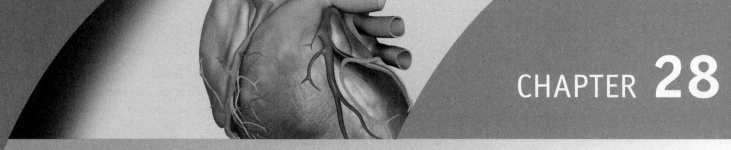

CHAPTER 28

Meningococcal Meningitis: It Strikes Without Warning

Katrina D. Hawkins
David M. Parenti

Every year, 3,000 Americans contract meningococcal disease: one out of ten will die.[1-3]

In 1996, Africa experienced the largest recorded outbreak of epidemic **meningitis** in history, with over 250,000 cases and 25,000 deaths registered.[4]

LEARNING OBJECTIVES

By the end of this chapter, the student will be able to:

- Recognize the signs and symptoms of meningococcal disease.
- Discuss the difference in the public health response for an isolated case versus an epidemic.
- Evaluate when it is appropriate to vaccinate and determine who should be vaccinated.
- Identify which groups of people are at particular risk for meningococcal disease.

HISTORY

Meningococcal meningitis was first described in Sweden in 1805 by Vieusseaux and was called episodic cerebrospinal fever. Throughout the 19th century, there were cases described of this episodic fever, mostly among children and military recruits. In 1887, the bacterium was finally isolated from the cerebrospinal fluid (CSF) of six fatal cases by Weichselbaum and was originally named *Neisseria intracellularis*. In 1893, lumbar puncture became a useful tool for collecting CSF from ill patients, making the diagnosis of meningococcal disease possible.

The first treatment for meningococcal disease came in the early 1900s when German and U.S. scientists developed anti-sera that could be injected intrathecally (directly into the cerebrospinal space) and thereby decrease the mortality rate of this disease to 25 percent. Unfortunately serum sickness and secondary meningitis limited the utility of this therapy. During World War I, there were 150 cases/100,000 troops per year with a 39 percent mortality rate. The greatest number of cases occurred during the winter months and was associated with overcrowding of military barracks. Despite efforts to control the disease with prophylactic nasal sprays, spacing between beds, and sequestering of troops, disease rates remained high. Preliminary vaccine trials began around this time and led to major vaccine trials later in the 20th century.

BASIC SCIENCE FACTS/KEY CONCEPTS REVIEW

Epidemiology

Meningococcal disease is an important cause of morbidity and mortality in the United States as well as other parts of the world. *Neisseria meningitidis* is the leading cause of bacterial meningitis in children and young adults in the United States and the second most common cause of community-acquired meningitis in adults. Each year there are 1,400 to 3,000 cases of meningococcal disease in the United States with a rate of about 0.5 to 1.1 per 100,000 persons. Unfortunately, the U.S. case rate has actually increased over the last 10 to 15 years. Most of these cases occur sporadically, with only three cases attributable to epidemics. The highest rate of disease occurs among infants less than one year of age with a rate of 9.2/100,000 (Figure 28-1).[5] In the United States, the peak season for meningococcal disease is December to January and the highest number of cases occur in the Mississippi River

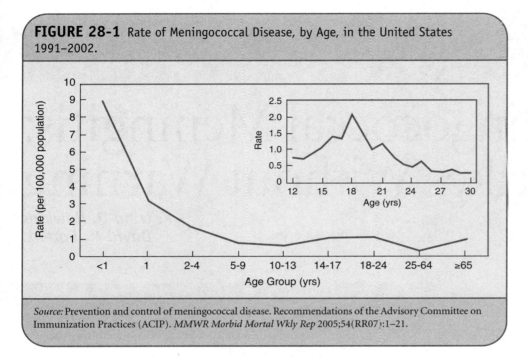

FIGURE 28-1 Rate of Meningococcal Disease, by Age, in the United States 1991–2002.

Source: Prevention and control of meningococcal disease. Recommendations of the Advisory Committee on Immunization Practices (ACIP). *MMWR Morbid Mortal Wkly Rep* 2005;54(RR07):1–21.

transmission. Prior to the advent of meningococcal vaccine, military recruits were especially high risk groups, as described above (Figure 28-3). With the introduction of the vaccine in 1972 along with other preventive measures, the rate of disease in this group has decreased to 1.4/100,000 troops (Figure 28-4 and Table 28-1).[7] College freshmen living in dorms are also at high risk due to the close living quarters, and it is now recommended that incoming freshman receive the meningococcal vaccine. Individuals who have lost their spleen due to surgery for trauma or disease as well as people with particular immunodeficiencies are vulnerable to infection with *N. meningitidis*, and should receive the vaccine as well.

Valley and the Pacific Northwest. While infants clearly have the highest rate of disease, there is another peak between the ages of 15 and 19 years, mostly due to close living quarters in college dormitories.

Worldwide, the incidence of meningitis exceeds 300,000 cases per year. Unlike the trend in the United States, the majority of cases in the rest of the world occur as **epidemic** disease, and most are found within the so called *Meningitis Belt* in sub-Saharan Africa (Figure 28-2). The rate in this Meningitis Belt approaches 20 cases per 100,000 persons, 20 to 40 times the rate in the United States. The largest outbreak of meningococcal disease occurred in sub-Saharan Africa in 1996 to 1997 with more than 300,000 cases and 30,000 deaths.[6]

Meningococcal disease is a devastating illness, with a mortality rate of 10 percent to 15 percent despite treatment with antibiotics. There are several risk factors for meningococcal disease, but the prime risk is living under crowded conditions that foster person-to-person

Microbiology

To understand the epidemiology of meningococcal disease, it is important to know a little bit about the bacteria itself. *Neisseria meningitidis* (Figure 28-5) is a Gram-negative diplococcus,

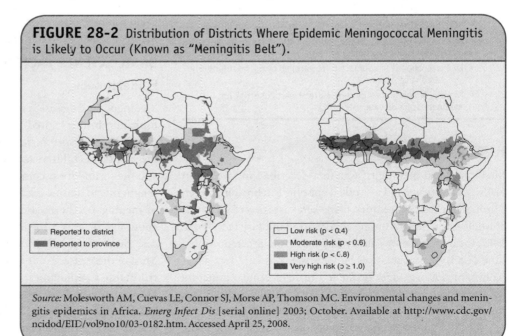

FIGURE 28-2 Distribution of Districts Where Epidemic Meningococcal Meningitis is Likely to Occur (Known as "Meningitis Belt").

Reported to district
Reported to province

Low risk (p < 0.4)
Moderate risk (p < 0.6)
High risk (p < 0.8)
Very high risk (p ≥ 1.0)

Source: Molesworth AM, Cuevas LE, Connor SJ, Morse AP, Thomson MC. Environmental changes and meningitis epidemics in Africa. *Emerg Infect Dis* [serial online] 2003; October. Available at http://www.cdc.gov/ncidod/EID/vol9no10/03-0182.htm. Accessed April 25, 2008.

FIGURE 28-3 Military Barracks.

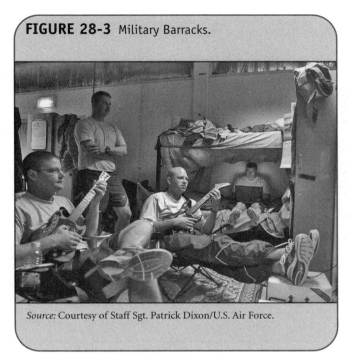

Source: Courtesy of Staff Sgt. Patrick Dixon/U.S. Air Force.

more difficult. This is particularly important as serogroup B is the most common type of disease seen in infants in the United States.

Meningococci have been shown to have *pili*, which are protein-based organelles on the outer membrane of the organism that facilitate adhesion to host cells, the first step in meningococcal host-cell interactions. Various proteins are present on the outer membrane meningococci. The first group of these proteins, called *porins*, creates channels in the cell membrane. Two major outer-membrane porins exist in meningococci, PorA and PorB. These porins allow nutrients to enter the cell and waste products to exit. Another group of outer-membrane proteins are the *opacity (Opa)* proteins. One of these proteins, Opc, is particularly important in the intimate binding of the meningococcus to the host cell. The receptor for Opc is a proteoglycan on the surface of host cells. Downregulation of capsule production allows for closer contact between Opc and the epithelial cell surface. The third group of proteins in the outer membrane is the Rmp proteins (reduction-modifiable proteins). Rmp proteins stimulate

meaning that it stains pink on routine laboratory staining and that under the microscope it looks like pairs of cocci (or berries). This bacterium has an outer capsule made of polysaccharide that contributes significantly to the pathogenicity of this organism. The **capsular polysaccharides** vary and can be used to categorize each bacterium into one of 13 possible serogroups. Serogroups that have the ability to cause clinical disease are A, B, C, W-135, and Y. In the United States, most disease is due to serogroups B, C, and Y (Figure 28-6). In Africa and Asia, however, most meningococcal disease is serogroup A or C. A successful vaccine has been developed that includes the polysaccharide of serogroups A, C, W-135, and Y, but development of a serogroup B capsular polysaccharide vaccine has proven

FIGURE 28-4 Rates of Meningococcal Disease Among Active-Duty Members of the U.S. Armed Forces in Relation to Routine Uses of Meningococcal Vaccines with Various Serogroup-Specific Components, 1964–1998. Arrows indicate dates of initiation of routine use of various vaccines.

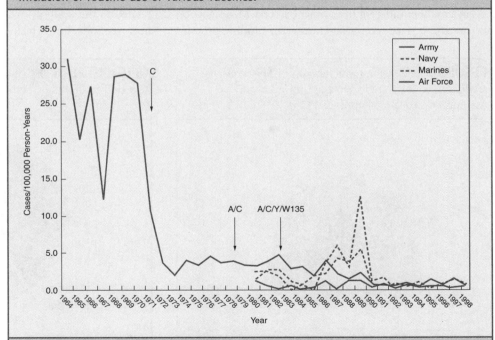

Source: Brundage JF. Meningococcal disease among United States military service members in relation to routine uses of vaccines with different serogroup-specific components, 1964–1998. *Clin Infect Dis* 2002;35:1376–1381.

TABLE 28-1 Number of Cases and Rates of Meningococcal Disease in the United States from September 1998 to August 1999*

Demographic	N cases	Population	Rate*
All persons aged 18–23 years	304	22,070,535[†]	1.4
Nonstudents aged 18–23 years	211	14,579,322[†§]	1.4
All college and university students	96	14,897,268[§]	0.6
Undergraduates	93	12,771,228[§]	0.7
Freshmen[ƒ]	44	2,285,001[§]	1.9
Dormitory residents	48	2,085,618[§**]	2.3
Freshmen[§] living in dormitories	30	591,587[§**]	5.1

Source: Bruce MG, Rosenstein NE, Capparelle JM, Shutt KA, Perkins BA, Collins M. Risk factors for meningococcal disease in college students. *JAMA* 2001;286:688–293.

Prevention and control of meningococcal disease. Recommendations of the Advisory Committee on Immunization Practices (ACIP). *MMWR Morbid Mortal Wkly Rep* 2005;54(RR07):1–21.

*Per 100,000 population.

[†]1998 census data.

[§]*Source:* National Center for Education Statistics, U.S. Department of Education, 1996–1997. Available at http://nces.ed.gov/. Accessed April 25, 2008.

[**]*Source:* National College Health Risk Behavior Survey (NCHRBS)—United States, 1995. *MMWR Morbid Mortal Wkly Rep* 1997;46(SS-6):1–54. Available at http://www.cdc.gov/mmwR/preview/mmwrhtml/ 00049859.htm. Accessed April 25, 2008.

[ƒ]Students enrolled for the first time in any postsecondary educational institution.

antibodies that block bactericidal activity against the surface antigens of meningococci. Lastly, *Neisseria* require iron for their growth and metabolism; therefore, they have developed a system that allows them to acquire iron from their human hosts in a manner different from other bacteria. Meningococci have specific surface receptors (transferrin-binding proteins and lactoferrin-binding proteins) that bind host cell transferrin and help internalize iron into the bacterium.

Approximately 50 percent of the meningococcal outer membrane is lipo-oligosaccharide (LOS). LOS is structurally related to the lipopolysaccharide expressed by many Gram-negative rods, but it lacks the repeating sugar units. Lipo-

FIGURE 28-5 A Photomicrograph of *Neisseria meningitidis* Recovered from the Urethra of an Asymptomatic Male; Magnified 1125×.

Source: From Public Health Image Library. ID # 2678. CDC and James Volk Content Providers. Available at http://phil.cdc.gov/phil/details.asp. Accessed January 8, 2008.

FIGURE 28-6 Distribution of Meningococcal Disease in United States by Serotype.

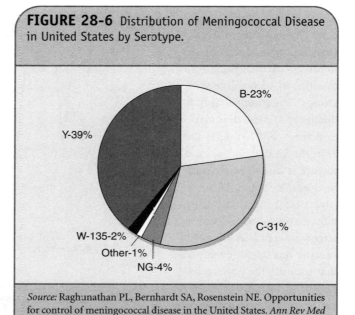

- B-23%
- Y-39%
- C-31%
- W-135-2%
- Other-1%
- NG-4%

Source: Raghunathan PL, Bernhardt SA, Rosenstein NE. Opportunities for control of meningococcal disease in the United States. *Ann Rev Med* 2004;55:333–353.

oligosaccharide is composed of lipid A and a short sugar chain of 8 to 12 saccharide units, the core oligosaccharide. The lipid A portion anchors LOS in the outer membrane and is the active moiety of endotoxin. This endotoxin induces the profound inflammatory response seen in clinical disease.

Pathogenesis and Immunity

Meningococci use pili to attach to nonciliated cells of the nasopharynx. After adhesion, colonization takes place and often patients never experience disease. In fact, 10 percent of the general population can be considered to be colonized with *N. meningitidis*. A combination of factors is probably responsible for the transition from nasopharyngeal carriage to invasive disease. Part of the process has to do with re-initiation of capsular polysaccharide production. Also, invasive meningococcal disease primarily occurs in patients who are newly infected with meningococcus. Studies have shown that epidemics occur during times of high rates of acquisition of disease, not during times of high rates of carriage.

After attachment the bacteria are internalized into phagocytic vacuoles. The re-synthesized polysaccharide capsule confers increased resistance to cationic antimicrobial peptides and helps protect the meningococci from intracellular killing. The organisms then replicate and migrate extracellularly to the submucosa where they may gain access to the bloodstream. If they replicate slowly in the bloodstream, they seed local tissues such as the meninges, joints, or pericardium. Alternatively, if they replicate rapidly, they then may cause the fulminant disease known as *meningococcemia*.

Immune protection from meningococcal disease by the host is mediated by antibodies that are directed against the capsule. Infants are provided protection by maternal antibodies; however, the protective factor of these antibodies wanes by six months of age. This is consistent with the fact that the greatest incidence of disease is in children under two years of age. Immunity also is stimulated by colonization with *N. meningitidis* or other bacteria with similar cross-reactive antigens. In addition, bacterial killing requires the terminal components of the complement system; therefore, patients with deficiencies in C5, C6, C7, or C8 are estimated to have between a 5,000- and 10,000-fold increased risk for infection with *N. meningitidis*. The complement system is made up of a group of heat-labile serum proteins that interact with antibodies and lead to the destruction of microorganisms, either through direct lysis or by enhancing phagocytosis (*opsonization*). Deficiencies in this system result in predisposition to infections with encapsulated organisms such as meningococcus. In fact, meningococcal disease is the most common infection experienced by patients with terminal complement compo-

nent deficiency, comprising up to 75 percent to 85 percent of all infections in which an etiology was identified

Clinical Features

Meningococcal disease manifests in a variety of clinical forms. The most common presentation is meningitis, which occurs in 75 percent of people who develop meningococcal disease. Of the patients with meningitis, 40 percent also have concomitant *bacteremia* (bacteria in the bloodstream). The most common initial presentation of meningococcal meningitis is the sudden onset of fever, nausea, vomiting, headache, and decreased ability to concentrate. Unfortunately, the peak season for meningococcal disease coincides with the peak season for influenza in the United States, so it is often mistaken for this viral illness. Also, most physicians see relatively few cases per year, making it difficult to identify, especially because its classic features appear somewhat late in the course of the disease. This means that healthcare professionals must have a high index of suspicion for meningococcal disease, especially during peak months. There is a narrow window of time from onset of symptoms to death in many cases, making early identification and treatment imperative.

Meningitis due to *N. meningitidis* is unique in that roughly two thirds of patients also have a petechial rash. *Petechiae* are small, nonblanching, red spots that represent minor hemorrhages of capillaries that end in the skin. The petechial rash most often appears on the trunk and lower extremities, but may also occur on the mucous membranes. Petechiae correlate with low platelet counts and therefore patients with this finding must be monitored carefully for signs of bleeding.

Purpura fulminans (Figure 28-7) is a severe complication of meningococcal disease and occurs in roughly 15 percent to 25 percent of people with meningococcemia. It is similar to septic shock from other types of bacteria, but differs by the presence of hemorrhagic skin lesions known as petechiae and purpura. These areas progress to *necrosis* (tissue death) with the formation of blisters. The necrosis can extend into deeper layers of tissue including muscle and bone if the disease goes untreated. Early and aggressive intervention with antibiotics and supportive measures are the only way to prevent these complications. If patients do not make it to the hospital in time, disfigurement, limb amputation, and often death are almost certain to occur.

Diagnosis and Treatment

Diagnosis of meningococcal disease is made by isolation of the bacteria from the cerebrospinal fluid (CSF). This is done by performing a **lumbar puncture** (also called spinal tap), where a small amount of spinal fluid is withdrawn and sent to the

FIGURE 28-7 Purpura Fulminans.

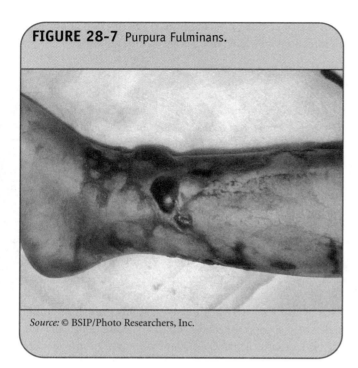

Source: © BSIP/Photo Researchers, Inc.

laboratory for analysis and culture (Figure 28-8). In bacterial meningitis, the CSF will usually show an elevated number of white blood cells, low glucose, normal to high protein, and culture will grow *N. meningitidis* within 24 to 48 hours. *N. meningitidis* is also frequently isolated from blood cultures.

FIGURE 28-8 Lumbar Puncture.

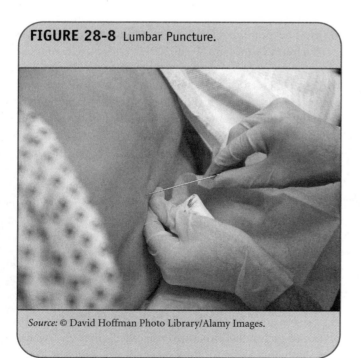

Source: © David Hoffman Photo Library/Alamy Images.

Once the idea of meningococcal disease is entertained in a patient, treatment should be initiated immediately. Penicillin is still the treatment of choice for this disease and should be administered for at least 10 to 14 days for meningitis. In patients who develop purpura fulminans and meningococcemia, there are several additional supportive measures including vascular support with fluids and possibly vasopressors, and intravenous steroids, but these measures are beyond the scope of this chapter.

PUBLIC HEALTH PERSPECTIVE FOR THE HEALTH OF THE GENERAL POPULATION AND OF HIGH RISK GROUPS

It is important to consider what public health officials should do when an isolated case of meningococcal disease is diagnosed as well as how to respond in an outbreak setting. The response to a sporadic case includes management of the case, contact identification and tracing, and maintenance of surveillance for further cases. It is important to prevent **secondary cases** and the best way of doing this is aggressive contact tracing to identify **close contacts** of the patient. The likelihood of transmission from person-to-person depends on the nature and duration of the contact. Studies performed prior to chemoprophylaxis demonstrated that household contacts were at a 500 to 1,200 times greater risk for developing meningococcal disease. Casual contacts were found to be at no increased risk and are therefore not treated in the case of sporadic disease. All close contacts should receive chemoprophylaxis with antibiotics if they have been in contact with the patient within seven days of the onset of symptoms. They should receive antibiotics regardless of whether they have been vaccinated in the past. Close contacts should also be alerted to the symptoms of meningococcal disease and advised to seek medical attention if they experience any febrile illness or other symptoms consistent with the disease.

What about the case of an infected air traveler? The CDC recommends that contact tracing be initiated if the infected person traveled within seven days of the onset of symptoms and the total time on the aircraft was at least eight hours.[8] Passengers on either side of the infected person or passengers/staff that were in direct contact with respiratory secretions should be contacted and receive prophylaxis.

In either an **organization-based** or **community-based outbreak** contract tracing, identification of close contacts and distribution of chemoprophylaxis to close contacts should be performed as described above for sporadic cases. Widespread chemoprophylaxis for people who are not close contacts is not performed as this is impractical and ineffective.[8] Vaccination of the population at risk should be performed if the attack rate

CASE STUDY
A CASE OF THE OMINOUS SPOTS
Scenario

A 19-year-old otherwise healthy college freshman presents to the Emergency Room complaining of headache, body aches, and fever since she woke up. She is seen by the ER physician and found to have a temperature of 102.4°F, a pulse of 112, and a blood pressure of 102/65 mm Hg. She appears lethargic and is perspiring but appears to have chills; her heart is beating fast but with a regular rhythm. Her neck is slightly stiff and she says that the light is bothering her eyes. She has no rash and the rest of her exam is normal. She reports that the only shot she received prior to entering college was a tetanus booster. The physician asks the nurse to place an intravenous line and administer intravenous fluids while she prepares to do a lumbar puncture. She returns to the patient's room 45 minutes later to find the patient barely arousable with a diffuse petechial rash, blood pressure is now 63/39 and her pulses are weak. She rapidly decompensates and has to be resuscitated with chest compressions, intravenous medications to support her blood pressure, and defibrillation.

The resuscitation effort is successful, but the patient remains on a ventilator for several days while she is stabilized. She undergoes amputation of two toes due to necrosis but after an extensive rehabilitation period she fully recovers her mental status. After six weeks of hospitalization and rehab her parents take her home.

Defining the Issues

1. The patient is presenting with headache, neck stiffness, and sensitivity to light, which should prompt a rapid workup for meningitis.
2. The patient needs standard workup for meningitis, which involves performing a lumbar puncture, and antibiotics should be initiated immediately. The patient should not be left alone without antibiotics if the physician is suspicious of meningococcal disease.
3. The patient is a college student living in a dorm, placing the patient in the group most at risk for meningitis. Because college freshmen living in dorms have higher incidence of meningococcal disease, this population should be vaccinated prior to entering college.

Patient's and Family's Understanding

In addition to the tremendous impact this disease has on the patient, it also has a profound effect on the patient's families and friends. The patient described above is a college student and this situation undoubtedly affects her roommates. They have the fear of losing a roommate to a potentially fatal disease coupled with learning that it is highly infectious and the risks that imparts to them. The patient's family is also hugely impacted by this situation. It is stressful for a family as they watch their loved one struggle through weeks in the hospital followed by a long rehabilitation period. For most patients, the experience does not end once they go home. The psychological and physical effects of this illness last long beyond the days after rehabilitation; depending on the physical consequences of their disease, the effects may last throughout their lifetime.

CLINICAL PERSPECTIVE FOR THE INDIVIDUAL PATIENT

Endemic meningococcal infection occurs primarily during the late winter when concurrent influenza virus is in the community; therefore, many cases of meningococcal disease are mistaken initially for severe influenza. However, patients with meningococcal meningitis either present with, or soon develop, a degree of illness that is much too severe to warrant these diagnoses. The patient will frequently tell the physician that this is the sickest they have ever felt; many express feelings of impending death. With infants, the parents are frequently more worried than the early symptoms may warrant. The clinical expression of this infection varies widely, and thus, a high index of suspicion and a careful search for clues of the disease are required to make a diagnosis, particularly in the absence of an epidemic. The difficulty in identifying meningococcal disease is due in part to the fact that clinicians in the community see so few cases in their lifetime and because the classic clinical features of meningococcal disease (that is, hemorrhagic rash, stiff neck, and impaired consciousness) appear late in the course of the illness. The narrow time window between progression from initial symptoms to death underscores the need for early recognition and treatment. If patients are fortunate enough to receive the immediate attention necessary to survive this disease, they must then often endure an extensive rehabilitation period. The patient described above lost two toes, but many patients lose entire limbs and undergo therapy aimed at teaching them to perform the typical activities of daily living.

is greater than 10 cases/100,000 persons.[3] In cases that occur on college campuses, records of immunization should be available to confirm the adequacy of immunization in that population. While treatment should not be delayed, genotyping of the cases of meningococcal disease should be performed to identify the outbreak strain and to ensure that individual cases are in fact related. Lastly, community education on early recognition of symptoms and where to seek treatment is extremely important in preventing the fatal consequences of meningococcal disease.

Due to the risk of meningococcal disease among dormitory occupants, many colleges have recommended (and some require) that their students receive the meningococcal vaccine prior to entry (Figure 28-9). Requirement by law is established on a state-by-state basis. Presently, 34 out of 51 states (if you include the District of Columbia) have some sort of requirement for the meningococcal vaccine. Of these, 34 states with laws requiring vaccination, four only require vaccination for public institutions, and eight require it only in universities with on-campus housing.[9]

In most countries outside of Africa, serogroup B infection comprises a significant proportion of cases of meningococcal disease and development of an effective vaccine to date has been difficult. There are many reasons for the difficulty in creating an effective serogroup B vaccine. Firstly, the serogroup B capsular polysaccharide is weakly immunogenic and there-

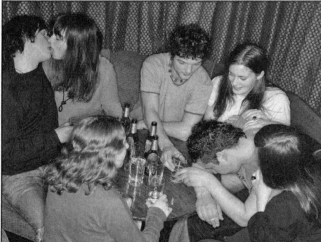

FIGURE 28-9 Party in a College Dormitory.

Source: © www.imagesource.com/Jupiterimages

fore a poor vaccine candidate. Another potential vaccine candidate is composed of "outer membrane proteins" of the meningococcus. These are certain proteins that are components of the cell membrane that lies just below the capsule. There is significant heterogeneity among the outer membrane proteins with multiple subtypes that vary by geographic location and by genetic adaptability of the organism, again making it a difficult target for a vaccine.

New Zealand is one country that has attempted to solve this problem when they experienced an epidemic of group B disease between 1991 and 2003. Eighty-five percent of these cases happened to be due to a clone with a single *PorA* gene coding for a specific outer membrane protein. This made creating a vaccine somewhat easier than it has been in the United States. They have created a vaccine called MeNZB that in studies has shown an immune response in 87 percent to 100 percent of vaccines. In 2004, universal immunization was implemented for individuals between the ages of 6 weeks to 19 years.[10] Evaluation of its overall efficacy is still in progress.

KEY TERMS

Biology and Clinical Terms

Capsular Polysaccharide: Water soluble, acidic, thick layer of carbohydrate produced by certain bacteria to prevent the host from being able to destroy it. They are linear and consist of regularly repeating subunits of one to six monosaccharides. The capsular polysaccharides displayed on the capsular surface allow for subtyping or grouping of bacteria. *Neisseria meningitidis* has 13 serogroups based on capsular antigens displayed on the surface of the bacterium.

Lumbar Puncture (also, **spinal tap**): A procedure in which a needle is inserted through an area in the lower back and into the spinal canal to obtain spinal fluid. The fluid is then sent for analysis to help make the diagnosis of meningitis.

Meningitis: An infection of the lining of the brain and or spinal cord that can be caused by bacteria or viruses.

Purpura Fulminans: A life-threatening condition involving cutaneous hemorrhage and necrosis, bacteremia, low blood pressure, and abnormalities of the blood clotting system.

Public Health Terms

Close Contacts: Close contacts of a patient who has meningococcal disease include: 1) household members; 2) childcare center contacts; and 3) persons directly exposed to the patient's oral secretions (such as by kissing, mouth-to-mouth resuscitation, endotracheal intubation, or endotracheal tube management).

Community-Based Outbreak: The occurrence of three or more confirmed or likely cases of meningococcal disease within three months among persons who are not in close contact, but reside in the same area, who do not share a common affiliation, with a primary disease attack rate of ≥10 cases/100,000 persons.

Endemic: A disease that is constantly present to a greater or lesser degree in a particular group of people or in a particular location.

Epidemic: Widespread outbreak of a disease, or a rapidly expanding cluster of cases of a disease in a single community or relatively small area.

Organization-Based Outbreak: The occurrence of three or more confirmed or likely cases of meningococcal disease of the same serogroup within three months among persons with a common affiliation but without close contact, resulting in primary disease attack rate of ≥10 cases/100,000 persons.

Secondary Case: A secondary case of meningococcal disease is one that occurs among close contacts of a primary patient ≥24 hours after onset of illness in the primary patient.

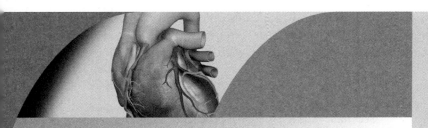

Questions for Further Research, Study, Reflection, and Discussion

For the Individual Student

In order to answer these questions, it may be necessary to research the primary literature.

- What is the role of surveillance in public health programs, and how is it performed?
- How effective is the meningicoccal vaccine? Are booster doses necessary?
- What progress is being made in the development of serogroup B vaccines?

For Small Group Discussion

- What types of contact are important in determining exposure risk?
- What public health entities are responsible for contact tracing and treatment of significant contacts?
- What determines who will develop meningitis after exposure?

For Entire Class Discussion

- What public health education tools or programs might be helpful to reduce the risk of meningococcal infection? What populations would you target?
- How will universal immunization impact on *Neisseria meningitidis* serogroup distribution?
- How well do insurance companies reimburse for meningococcal immunization?

EXERCISE/ACTIVITY

Divide the class into two groups and assign half to each of the following scenarios:

- Your are the resident advisor in a college dormitory. One of the dormitory residents shows up on Friday afternoon to say that Alice is sick and in the hospital with meningitis. What do you do?
- Your are the public health officer at the local health department. A nurse from an area boarding high school calls to inform you that one of the students is sick and in the hospital with meningitis. Outline what steps you would take in this situation.

Ask each group to present its recommendations and to outline steps to be taken. Ask both groups to engage in a two-way discussion about possible interaction between college dormitory administrative staff and health department staff.

Healthy People 2010

Indicators: Immunization

Focus Area: Immunization and Infectious Diseases

Goal: Prevent disease, disability, and death from infectious diseases, including vaccine-preventable diseases.

Objectives:

14-4. Reduce bacterial meningitis in young children.

14-7. Reduce meningococcal disease.

REFERENCES

1. Centers for Disease Control and Prevention. Summary of Notifiable Disease, United States 1996. *MMWR Morbid Mortal Wkly Rep* 1997;45:1–14.

2. Centers for Disease Control and Prevention. Summary of Notifiable Disease, United States 2002. *MMWR Morbid Mortal Wkly Rep.* 2004;51:1–34.

3. Granoff DM, Feavers IM, Borrow R. Meningococcal vaccines. In: Plotkin SA, ed. *Vaccines,* 4th ed. Philadelphia: WB Saunders Co.; 2004:959–987.

4. Lemon SM, Hamburg MA, Sparling PF, Choffnes ER, and Mack A. Ethical and Legal Considerations in Mitigating Pandemic Disease: Workshop Summary. Washington, DC: The National Academy Press; 2007:37.

5. Prevention and Control of Meningococcal Disease: Recommendations of the Advisory Committee on Immunization Practices (ACIP). *MMWR Morbid Mortal Wkly Rep* 2005;54(RR07)1–21.

6. Stephens DS, Munford RS, Wetzler LM. Meningococcal Infections. In: Weiner MW, Kasper DL, Braunwald E, et al., eds. *Harrison's Principles of Internal Medicine,* 16th ed. McGraw Hill; 2005:849–855.

7. Brundage JF. Meningococcal disease among United States military service members in relation to routine uses of vaccines with different serogroup-specific components, 1964–1998. *Clin Infect Dis* 2002;35:1376–1381.

8. Centers for Disease Control. Summary of notifiable diseases —United States, 2005. *MMWR Morbid Mortal Wkly Rep* 2007;54:2–92.

9. Meningococcal Prevention Mandates for Colleges and Universities. October 16, 2006. Available at http://www.immunize.org/laws/menin.htm Accessed April 25, 2008.

10. Thornton V, Lenon D, Rasanathan K, O'Hallahan J, Oster P, Stewart J, et al. Safety and immunogenicity of New Zealand strain meningococcal serogroup B OMV vaccine in healthy adults: beginning of epidemic control. *Vaccine* 2006;24:1395–1400.

RESOURCES

Active Bacterial Core Surveillance (ABCs) Report. Emerging Infections Program Network, *Neisseria meningitidis,* 2006. Available at http://www.cdc.gov/ncidod/DBMD/abcs/survreports/mening06.pdf. Accessed April 25, 2008.

Centers for Disease Control and Prevention. Exposure to patients with meningococcal disease on aircrafts—United States 1999–2001. *MMWR Morbid Mortal Wkly Rep* 2001;50:485–489.

Raghunathan PL, Bernhardt SA, Rosenstein NE. Opportunities for control of meningococcal disease in the United States. *Ann Rev Med* 2004;55:333–353.

Steffen R, DuPont H. Manual of Travel Medicine and Health. Hamilton, Ontario, Canada: B.C. Decker; 1999:267–273.

Tondella ML, Popovic T, Rosenstein NE. Distribution of *Neisseria meningitidis* serogroup B serosubtypes and serotypes circulating in the United States. *J Clin Microbiol* 2000;38:3323–3328.

CROSS REFERENCES

Communicating Health Information
HPV
MRSA
Research Methods for Health Information

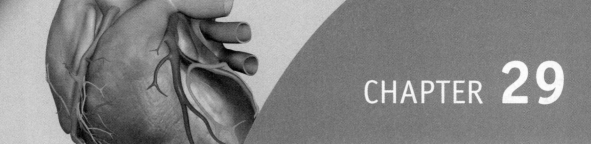

CHAPTER 29

Human Papillomavirus (HPV) Infection and Immunization

James F. Cawley
Lawrence D'Angelo

The human papillomavirus (HPV) is the most common sexually transmitted infection (STI) in the United States, with about 6.2 million cases diagnosed annually.[1]

LEARNING OBJECTIVES

By the end of this chapter, the student will be able to:

- Explain the major epidemiologic features of HPV infection.
- Describe the progression of HPV infection to cervical cancer.
- Describe the clinical features of HPV infections.
- Discuss the concept of **immune evasion** as it applies to HPV infection.
- Identify the groups who are candidates for the HPV vaccine.
- List the strengths and limitations of the HPV vaccine.

HISTORY

A vaccine to prevent cancer has long been considered akin to the holy grail of public health and preventive medicine. The development of a vaccine to prevent cervical cancer through the use of the cervical cytology (Papanicolaou [Pap] smear) has reduced the incidence of cervical cancer by 70 percent. However, cervical cancer remains a leading cause of death in countries without screening programs. Vaccines that prevent these persistent HPV infections have the potential to reduce the burden of disease.

BASIC SCIENCE FACTS/KEY CONCEPTS REVIEW

Human papillomaviruses (HPV) are highly prevalent, tissue-specific DNA viruses that infect epithelial cells.[2] **Persistent** viral **infections** with **oncogenic** types of HPV lead to cancer of the cervix, anus, vagina, vulva, penis, mouth, and sinus.[3] Cervical cancer is the second most common malignant disease in women worldwide and has a bimodal onset in the third and sixth decades of life. There are more than 100 strains of HPV, more than 30 of which can infect the genitals. Although most HPV infections are benign, HPV has been found to be associated with cervical cancer and genital warts.

Immune Evasion

What happens when HPV infects human tissue? The virus initially infects the basal stem cell of the mucosal epithelium, the lining cells of tissues like the human cervix. HPV is able to continually infect new layers of mucosal cells even as these short-lived cells desquamate. There are several mechanisms by which HPV infection evades the immune system. HPV infection leads to downregulation of interferon expression and regulatory pathways, which subsequently prohibits the activation of **cytotoxic T cells**.[4] No associated cytolysis or release of proinflammatory cytokines occurs as a result of basal cell infection. In the absence of the usual signals that identify a virally infected cell, the cellular immune system is not activated and HPV infection persists. The importance of cellular immunity is clinically apparent in HIV-infected patients and in renal transplant patients who have a higher incidence of HPV-related disease.

Approximately 75 percent to 90 percent of HPV infections will clear within a year of infection. Clearance is mediated mostly by the natural desquamation of epithelial cells and in part by low levels of neutralizing antibody responses to the specific HPV L1 **epitope**. There is a limited antibody response from natural infection and a significant loss of detectable antibodies within three years.

In one large study of data pooled from 11 case-controlled studies, HPV type 16 was detected in nearly 60 percent of cervical cancer cases, and HPV type 18 was implicated in an additional 15 percent.[5]

> **THE SCIENCE: KEY POINTS**
> - HPV infection is a prevalent viral STI worldwide.
> - Nearly all cases of cervical cancer are linked to HPV infection.
> - Most HPV infections will clear by themselves.

CLINICAL PERSPECTIVE FOR THE HEALTHCARE PROVIDER

Genital HPV infection is an STD that is caused by HPV. Human papillomavirus is the name of a group of viruses that includes more than 100 different strains or types and has DNA as their genetic material. More than 30 of these viruses are sexually transmitted, and they can infect the genital area of men and women including the skin of the penis, vulva (area outside the vagina), or anus, and the linings of the vagina, cervix, or rectum. Most people who become infected with HPV will not have any symptoms and will clear the infection on their own.

Only certain of these viruses are "high-risk" types, that is, capable of inducing cytologic changes believed to be the precursor to the development of cervical cancer. The most common of these are types 16 and 18, which account for 70 percent of all cases of cancer of the cervix.[11] Infection with these subtypes also may lead to cancer of the vulva, vagina, anus, or penis. Other viral subtypes are known as "low-risk" types, and they may cause mild Pap test abnormalities or genital warts (for instance, types 6 and 11). Genital warts are single or multiple growths or bumps that appear in the genital area, and sometimes are cauliflower shaped.

Most people who have a genital HPV infection do not know they are infected. The virus lives in the skin or mucous membranes and usually causes no symptoms. Only a small percentage of infected individuals will get visible genital warts or have precancerous changes in the cervix, vulva, anus, or penis.

Genital warts usually appear as soft, moist, pink, or flesh-colored swellings, usually in the genital area. They can be raised or flat, single or multiple, small or large, and sometimes cauliflower shaped. They can appear on the vulva, in or around the vagina or anus, on the cervix, and on the penis, scrotum, groin, or thigh. After sexual contact with an infected person, warts may appear within weeks or months, or not at all.

Genital warts are diagnosed by visual inspection. Visible genital warts can be removed by medications the patient applies, or by treatments performed by a healthcare provider. Some individuals choose to forego treatment to see if the warts will disappear on their own. No treatment regimen for genital warts is better than another, and no one treatment regimen is ideal for all cases.

Regular PAP smears are still the "gold standard" for making the diagnosis of chronic HPV infection. The American College of Obstetrics and Gynecology currently recommends that sexually active women receive a PAP smear at age 21 or within three years of the initiation of sexual intercourse, whichever comes first, and annually thereafter until age 30. Luckily, most adolescent women with abnormal PAP smears will experience spontaneous regression, so initial abnormal changes may not necessitate anything more than careful follow-up.

Healthcare providers have been caught squarely in the middle of the controversy over the HPV vaccine. On the one hand, the possibility that an effective vaccine with few if any significant side effects can prevent cancer is exciting. On the other hand, most practitioners did not appreciate the aggressive direct-to-consumer marketing plan that was launched as soon as the vaccine became available, particularly because it was accompanied by a far less extensive educational campaign for providers. Moreover, most providers have respect for the strong family values that serve as the focus of many of the objections to the routine use of HPV vaccine. Finally, the considerable expense of the vaccine ($120–$150/dose) has put the provider in a difficult position because the reimbursement offered by many insurance companies is not sufficient to offset the expense of the vaccine, its storage, and its administration.[12]

PUBLIC HEALTH PERSPECTIVE FOR THE HEALTH OF THE GENERAL POPULATION AND OF HIGH RISK GROUPS

In 2005, there were 500,000 new cases of cervical cancer worldwide, and 260,000 women died of cervical cancer. The overwhelming majority of these women were in developing countries, where cervical cancer screening programs and infrastructures for prevention and diagnoses are weak.

In the United States, the cervical cancer incidence rate is much lower. It is estimated that there will be 9,710 cases of invasive cervical cancer and approximately 3,700 deaths from cervical cancer in the United States in 2006. This lower rate is attributable to the success of the widespread use of the **Papanicolaou (Pap) test**, which detects changes in cervical tissue, and is a major tool in screening for early identification of cervical cancer.[13]

CASE STUDY
Scenario

Jessica is a 14-year-old African-American female who comes to her primary care provider's office for a routine physical examination. She is accompanied by her mother. The provider interviews both Jessica and her mother together, and then requests time to speak to and examine Jessica alone. Jessica's mother initially objects, but relents when Jessica looks at her and says, "Oh Mom, I'm not a baby."

Jessica confides to the provider that she has a boyfriend but has not had sexual intercourse and doesn't plan to have intercourse in the near future. The provider completes her examination, which is completely normal, reviews with her the findings of the exam, and then invites her mother back for final recommendations.

DEFINING THE ISSUES

One of the recommendations the clinician makes is for Jessica to initiate the HPV vaccine series. The provider emphasizes the fact that this is a "cancer prevention vaccine" and shares with mother and Jessica some of the data on cervical cancer and of the importance of a vaccine to prevent HPV infection. Jessica seems interested, asks some appropriate questions about the vaccine series, and indicates that she would like to receive the vaccine. At this point, her mother, who has been quiet during the previous discussion speaks up. "Isn't this an experimental vaccine that is being tried out on women of color? And why do you think my daughter needs this vaccine, anyway? Do you think that all young women of color are sexually active?"

Patient's Understanding

In this case study, the patient appears to understand what the vaccine is and how it is supposed to work. Jessica also understands that her mother appears to be opposed to her receiving the vaccine, despite the fact that her care provider believes strongly that this is an important clinical and public health intervention. Her mother understands her role as her minor adolescent's healthcare agent who is intent on protecting her from harm.

CLINICAL PERSPECTIVE FOR THE INDIVIDUAL PATIENT

HPV infection is an STI that can be transmitted—albeit rarely—through genital contact without intercourse. Most HPV infections are asymptomatic and will typically resolve themselves. Certain strains, however, can have serious clinical consequences, including genital warts and cervical cancer. HPV infection is associated with the vast majority of cases of cervical cancer.[6] If detected early, cervical cancer is highly treatable. In the United States, it is recommended that women receive Pap tests at least once every three years. However, many women still do not receive Pap tests at the recommended frequency. In particular, Asian/Pacific Islander women have significantly lower rates of Pap tests than women of other races.[7] Cervical cancer incidence and mortality are approximately 1.5 times higher among African American and Latina women, compared to white women.[8] Researchers have postulated several reasons for these disparities, including fear, cost, lack of physician referral, and cultural issues.[9]

Most women are diagnosed with chronic HPV on the basis of abnormal Pap tests. A Pap test is the primary cancer-screening tool for cervical cancer or precancerous changes in the cervix, many of which are related to HPV. Also, a specific test is available to detect HPV DNA in women. The test may be used in women with mild Pap test abnormalities, or in women older than 30 years at the time of Pap testing. The results of HPV DNA testing can help healthcare providers decide if further tests or treatment are necessary.

There is no "cure" for HPV infection, although in most women the infection goes away on its own. The treatments provided are directed to the changes in the skin or mucous membrane caused by HPV infection, such as warts and pre-cancerous changes in the cervix.

Recently, a new vaccine against four of the most common subtypes of HPV has been approved by the Food and Drug Administration (FDA) and has begun to be marketed for young women between the ages of 9 and 26. The vaccine is administered in three separate shots over the course of six months (months 0, 2, and 6). The vaccine has shown a high degree of efficacy with little serious side effects or consequences.[10] A number of jurisdictions have begun to debate the wisdom of requiring the vaccine for school entry. Unfortunately, the vaccine has been very controversial with a vocal minority of detractors attempting to prevent widescale use of the vaccine.

Approximately 20 million people are currently infected with HPV. At least 50 percent of sexually active men and women acquire genital HPV infection at some point in their lives. By age 50, at least 80 percent of women will have acquired genital HPV infection. About 6.2 million Americans get a new genital HPV infection each year. Each year about 15,000 women in the United States learn that they have cervical cancer; an estimated 4,100 women will die of the disease this year. Worldwide, about 500,000 new cases of cervical cancer are diagnosed each year, resulting in 250,000 deaths. The disease is the second or third most common cancer among women (cervical cancer and colorectal cancer are virtually tied for second place after breast cancer).

Primary Prevention: The HPV Vaccine

The new **quadrivalent** (directed against four viral strains) HPV vaccine was approved for use in June 2006. This new vaccine is produced by Merck and Company and is called Gardasil®. Proteins from the capsule of the virus are incorporated into the vaccine. The four strains included in this vaccine are types 6, 11, 16, and 18. The former two types are the cause of 90 percent of genital warts while the later two are responsible for 70 percent of all cases of cervical cancer. In extensive clinical trials, the vaccine has been shown to be between 90 percent and 95 percent effective in protecting those immunized against cancer or precancerous changes. It is currently approved for use in girls and women ages 9 to 26. A second bivalent vaccine (directed against cancer-causing types 16 and 18) is expected to be available sometime in the near future.[14]

While this advance has the potential to improve the health and longevity of millions of women, policymakers and health professionals are being forced to address many issues to assure the large scale administration of this new vaccine. These include: public and provider education, healthcare financing, parental consent and confidentiality, and access to care.

Following the FDA approval of the Gardasil vaccine, the federal Advisory Committee on Immunization Practices (ACIP), a committee of the Centers for Disease Control and Prevention (CDC) that establishes guidelines for the use of approved vaccines, recommended the new vaccine be administered routinely to girls 11 to 12 years of age. Use at a health provider's discretion was also recommended for girls and women between the ages of 9 to 26. These recommendations were designed to encourage vaccination before initiation of sexual activity and were based on data from clinical trials demonstrating a greater immune response in girls ages 10 to 15 compared to young women ages 16 to 25.[15]

As good as the vaccine is, it still does not protect against all types of cervical cancer–causing HPV. Therefore, regular Pap tests remain a critical tool for early detection of precancerous cells. The vaccine should be administered in three doses over six months. Presently, there is only enough research to show vaccine effectiveness for five years. Further research will determine whether booster shots are needed. Furthermore, clinical trials were conducted in 9- to 26-year-old females, so effectiveness is only known for this age group and not for older women or males.

Vaccine Implementation and Costs

It is usual that ACIP recommendations are followed closely by healthcare professionals.[16] Healthcare professional associations often base their own policies on these recommendations. After ACIP makes its recommendations, each state decides whether the vaccine should be required for entry into childcare or school. There are no federal laws that mandate vaccination; thus, mandatory vaccination laws will vary from state to state. Currently, legal exemptions to vaccination on the basis of medical, religious, or philosophical grounds also vary from state to state. Some groups have already expressed opposition to mandatory vaccination for entry into school. In addition, to date any vaccine administered to an individual under the age of 18 requires parental consent. It is not yet clear how states and providers will handle consent issues, particularly with women ages 18 and under who do not need consent for STD preventive services or treatment.

Another major hurdle will be the price of the vaccine. Merck has said that the list price of the vaccine will be $360 for the three doses, making it one of the costliest vaccines on the market. Private insurance companies usually cover ACIP recommended vaccines, so most insured individuals will likely have coverage, although it is still too soon to tell. The Vaccines for Children (VFC) program, a federal entitlement program, covers the cost for children under age 19 who are uninsured, on Medicaid, Alaska Natives, or American Indians.[17]

Public Acceptability

Numerous studies have evaluated acceptability and attitudes regarding the use of the HPV vaccine.[11] Acceptability among gynecologists and physicians is generally high, depending on factors such as a patient's gender, age, and sexual history as well as efficacy of the vaccine.[18] A review of research regarding STI and HPV vaccine acceptability also indicates that healthcare providers and professional health organizations play a large part in a parent's decision to vaccinate his or her child.[19] Parents are more likely to follow the recommendations and information put forth by healthcare providers, and healthcare providers are more apt to follow a professional health organization's endorsement of a vaccine.[20] Thus, healthcare providers will likely play a pivotal role in relaying information about HPV and HPV immunization in order to ensure the targeted population is vaccinated.

Approval of this new vaccine holds great promise for millions of women. Not only can it greatly reduce deaths attributable to cervical cancer, but it also has the potential to reduce the economic and emotional burdens that women experience when they are faced with an abnormal Pap smear that requires further testing and treatment. The key to the success of this new vaccine will be in how policymakers, healthcare providers, parents, women, and girls respond to make sure that all those who can benefit from this new technology have access to it.[21]

Limitations

The vaccine tested in this study has several limitations. First of all, the vaccine offers no protection against other types of HPV that also can cause cervical cancer. In addition, it is unknown whether the vaccine's protection against HPV-16 is long-lasting. Finally, it does not prevent HPV-16/18 infections already present at the time of vaccination from progressing to cancer.

The HPV vaccine was initially approved for administration to women ages 9 to 26. It is generally accepted that it is best to administer the vaccine to young women before they initiate sexual intercourse, because once they are sexually active, they have a significant chance of being infected with HPV, even if they have only a single sexual partner with no past history of HPV infection. The vaccine is highly efficacious, providing virtually 100 percent protection against long-term consequences of HPV infection. Numerous clinical trials in diverse populations have substantiated these recommendations.

Because of numerous abuses and discrepancies in involving women and men of color in ethical research studies, many communities have long and deeply established suspicions of being "experimented on" by healthcare providers. Unfortunately, many of these suspicions originated for very valid reasons. When the vaccine first became available, these suspicions were exacerbated by the aggressive marketing campaign of direct–to-consumer advertising that saturated print and electronic media as soon as the vaccine became available. This marketing campaign was accompanied by an equally aggressive campaign for the establishment of state and local requirements of proof of immunization for entry into schools.[22]

The issues for the individual providers are compounded by the issues for public health professionals. This is an excellent vaccine that is highly protective. However, in addition to being controversial for the reasons cited above, the vaccine is very expensive, with pricing of the vaccine being in the range of $120 to $150 per dose. As a vaccine approved by the ACIP, jurisdictions are responsible for providing it for children and adolescents covered under government insurance programs such as Medicaid and the Children's Health Insurance Program (CHIPS). Public health authorities not only face the community concerns about how and for whom the vaccine should be utilized, they also have to cope with the significant cost issues the vaccine raises.[23]

Secondary Prevention: Pap Tests Still Needed

Most cervical cancers develop slowly through a series of abnormal changes in the cells of the cervix, changes most often related to an HPV virus. Regular Pap tests can detect these changes and the abnormal tissue can be removed. Pap tests would still be needed even if the experimental vaccine used in this study proves widely effective because the vaccine only works against one kind of HPV.

Pap tests are not 100 percent accurate, however, and many women do not have the tests regularly. In one national health survey, a fifth of women aged 18 to 64 had not had a Pap test in the past three years. A vaccine that prevented the HPV infections known to be behind most cervical cancers would be a powerful addition to disease prevention strategies.

KEY TERMS

Clinical Terms

Cytotoxic T Cells: Cell capable of destruction of other immune and non-immune cells.

Epitope: An antigenic determinant, in simplest form, of a complex antigenic molecule.

Immune Evasion: Capability of invading microorganisms to avoid detection and/or destruction by the immune system.

Oncogenic: Leading to the development of cancer.

Papanicolaou (Pap) Test: Laboratory identification of HPV infected cervical tissues that may be in neoplastic transformation.

Persistent Infections: Infection not cleared by the immune system.

Quadrivalent: A vaccine directed against four viral strains.

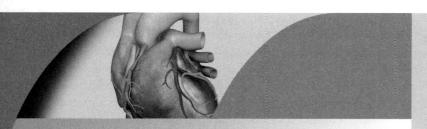

Questions for Further Research, Study, Reflection, and Discussion

For the Individual Student

In order to answer these questions, it may be necessary to research the primary literature.

- List the major advantages and limitations of the HPV vaccine.
- What has been the overall outcome of the use of the Pap smear?
- Summarize the arguments against the routine use of HPV vaccine.

For Small Group Discussion

- What arguments can be used for the routine use of HPV vaccine in young women?
- Should state legislatures mandate the vaccine for young women? Defend your position.
- What regulations and policies are needed to allow low-income and underinsured individuals to gain greater access to vaccinations at both the state and federal level?
- There are good lessons in vaccine public health policy that can be observed in case of the introduction of the HPV vaccine. Identify the major aspects of this policy discussion.

For Entire Class Discussion

- What are the barriers to making this vaccine mandatory? How could these barriers be addressed?
- What options would be needed to improve access for uninsured women ages 19 to 26?
- Should young men be vaccinated against HPV? Why or why not?

EXERCISES/ACTIVITIES

- Present testimony to the FDA for the approval of HPV for men. Assume that the vaccine is as efficacious for young men as it is for young women.
- A prominent African-American columnist for the *Washington Post* has written an Op/Ed piece decrying the use of HPV in African-American young women. His argument is that this is an experimental vaccine being tested on young women of color. Write a letter to the editor either supporting or disagreeing with the columnist.
- Present testimony to the Senate Committee on Children and Families in support of federal subsidies for any state mandating the use of HPV vaccine for school entry. Present a rebuttal to this argument.

Healthy People 2010

Indicator: Responsible Sexual Behavior

Focus Area: Sexually Transmitted Diseases

Goal: Promote responsible behaviors, strengthen community capacity, and increase access to quality services to prevent sexually transmitted disease (STDs) and their complications.

Objectives:

25-5. Reduce the proportion of persons with human papillomavirus (HPV) infection.

REFERENCES

1. Centers for Disease Control and Prevention. *HPV and HPV Vaccine—Information for Healthcare Providers*, August 2006. Available at http://www.cdc.gov/std/hpv/STDFact-HPV-vaccine-hcp.htm. Accessed April 27, 2008.

2. Dunne EF, Markowitz LE. Genital human papillomavirus infection. *Clin Infect Dis* 2006;43:624–629.

3. American Cancer Society. *Detailed Guide: Cervical Cancer*. Available at http://www.cancer.org/docroot/CRI/CRI_2_3x.asp?dt=8. Accessed April 27, 2008.

4. Steinbrook R. The potential of human papillomavirus vaccines. *N Engl J Med* 2006;354:4–12.

5. Munoz N, Bosch FX, de Sanjose S, et.al. International Agency for Research on Cancer Multicenter Cevical Cancer Study Group. Epidemiologic classification of human papillomavirus types associated with cervical cancer. *N Engl J Med* 2003;348:518–527.

6. Cox JT. Introduction. *Curr Opin Obstet Gynecol* 2006;18(Suppl 1):s3.

7. World Health Organization. *Comprehensive Cervical Cancer Control: A Guide to Essential Practice*, 2006. Available at http://www.who.int/reproductive-health/publications/cervical_cancer_gep/index.htm. Accessed April 27, 2008.

8. The Office of Minority Health. Eliminate Disparities in Cancer Screening & Management, June 30, 2006.

9. Centers for Disease Control and Prevention. *CDC Press Briefing: ACIP Recommends HPV Vaccination*, June 29, 2006. Available at http://www.cdc.gov/od/oc/media/transcripts/t060629.htm. Accessed April 27, 2008.

10. U.S. Food and Drug Administration, Center for Biologics Evaluation and Research (CBER). *Product Approval Information—Licensing Action*, June 2006. Available at http://www.fda.gov/cber/products/hpvmer060806qa.htm. Accessed April 27, 2008.

11. Centers for Disease Control and Prevention. *HPV Vaccine Questions and Answers*, June 2006. Available at http://www.cdc.gov/std/Hpv/STDFact-HPV-vaccine.htm. Accessed April 27, 2008.

12. Sanders GD, Taira AV. Cost-effectiveness of a potential vaccine for human papillomavirus. *Emerg Infect Dis* 2003;9:37–48.

13. Centers for Disease Control and Prevention. *United States Cancer Statistics: 2002 Incidence and Mortality*, 2005. Available at http://www.cdc.gov/cancer/NPCR/uscs/2002/download_data.htm. Accessed April 27, 2008.

14. Goldie, SJ, Kohli, M, Grima, D. et.al. Potential health and economic impact of adding human papillomavirus 16/18 vaccine. *J Nat Cancer Inst* 2004;96:604.

15. Koutsky LA, Ault KA, Wheeler CM, et al. A controlled trial of a human papillomavirus type 16 vaccine. *N Engl J Med* 2002;347:1645–1651.

16. Centers for Disease Control and Prevention. *Advisory Committee on Immunization Practices (ACIP)*, June 2006. Available at http://www.cdc.gov/od/oc/media/pressrel/r060629.htm. Accessed April 27, 2008.

17. Centers for Disease Control and Prevention. *Vaccines for Children (VFC) Program*, July 19, 2006. Available at http://www.cha.state.md.us/edcp/html/vfchmpg.html. Accessed April 27, 2008.

18. Raley JC, Followwill KA, Zimet GD, Ault KA. Gynecologists' attitudes regarding human papilloma virus vaccination: a survey of fellows of the American College of Obstetricians and Gynecologists. *Infect Dis Obstet Gynecol* 2004;12:127–133.

19. Riedesel JM, Rosenthal SL, Zimet GD, Bernstein DI, Huang B, Lan D, Kahn JA. Attitudes about human papillomavirus vaccine among family physicians. *J Pediatr Adolesc Gynecol* 2005;18:391–398.

20. Zimet GD. Improving adolescent health: focus on HPV vaccine acceptance. *J Adolesc Health* 2005;37:S17–S23.

21. Sprigg P. "Pro-Family, Pro-Vaccine—But Keep It Voluntary," editorial. *The Washington Post* July 15, 2006;A21.

22. Allen A. "Don't Rush to Mandate HPV Vaccine." *The Baltimore Sun* February 8, 2007.

23. Allen A. *Vaccine: The Controversial Story of Medicine's Greatest Lifesaver*. New York: W.W. Norton, 2006.

RESOURCES

Fishbein DB, Broder KR, Markowitz L, Messonnier N. New, and some not-so-new, vaccines for adolescents and diseases they prevent. *Pediatrics* 2008;121(Suppl 1):S5–S14.

McCauley MM, Fishbein DB, Santoli JM. Introduction: strengthening the delivery of new vaccines for adolescents. *Pediatrics* 2008;121(Suppl 1):S1–S4.

CROSS REFERENCES

Immunization
Meningococcal Meningitis
MRSA

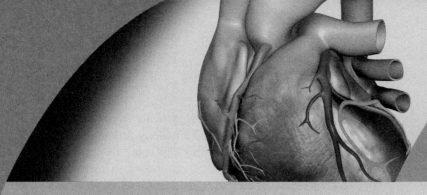

CHAPTER 30

Helicobacter Infection and Peptic Ulcer

James F. Cawley

As many as two thirds of the world's population is infected with *Helicobacter pylori*.[1]

LEARNING OBJECTIVES

By the end of this chapter, the student will be able to:

- Discuss the basic process of infection with *Helicobacter pylori*.
- Describe peptic ulcer disease and how it occurs.
- Explain the relationship between infection, peptic ulcer, and gastric cancer.
- Indicate the commonly used diagnostic and therapeutic approaches to treating *H. pylori* infection.
- Analyze the economic aspects of eradicating *H. pylori* infection.
- Discuss the worldwide epidemiology of *H. pylori* infection and gastric cancer.

HISTORY

In the 1980s, scientists began to notice the presence of curved bacteria, which later became known as *Helicobacter pylori* (*H. pylori*), in tissue samples taken from patients with **ulcers** of the stomach and upper small intestine. Believing that no bacterium could survive the harsh stomach environment, most scientists thought these mysterious bacteria were either due to contamination of tissue samples or just another harmless species of bacteria like many found in the gut. Australian researchers Barry J. Marshall and J. Robin Warren believed that the bacteria were actually the cause of ulcers. Marshall, frustrated with the lack of a good animal model of infection, infected himself with the curved bacteria. He became ill,

developed inflammation of the stomach, and was able to culture the bacterium from his own ulcers, thereby proving the microbe to be the cause of stomach ulcers. For their discovery of *H. pylori* and its role in gastric ulcer formation, Marshall and Warren were awarded the 2005 Nobel Prize in Medicine.

Helicobacter pylori is a bacterium responsible for most ulcers and many cases of chronic gastritis (inflammation of the stomach). This organism can weaken the protective coating of the stomach and duodenum (first part of the small intestines), allowing the damaging digestive juices to irritate the sensitive lining of these body parts.

Those living in developing countries or crowded, unsanitary conditions are most likely to contract the bacteria, which is passed from person to person. *H. pylori* only grows in the intestines and is usually contracted during childhood.

Helicobacter pylori is a small, highly motile, gram-negative bacillus (Figure 30-1) that is one of the most common bacterial pathogens in humans. At least half of the world's populations are infected by *H. pylori*. Most of the infected persons (>70 percent), however, are asymptomatic, whereas only fewer than 30 percent are symptomatic. Half of the symptomatic patients develop peptic ulcer diseases, lymphoproliferative disorders, or gastric cancer. Again, some infected individuals develop duodenal ulcer whereas others develop gastric ulcer. Prevalence of infection is different between developing and developed nations. It is not known how *H. pylori* is transmitted or why some patients become symptomatic while others do not. The bacteria most likely are spread from person to person through fecal-oral or oral-oral routes, but possible environmental reservoirs include contaminated water sources. **Iatrogenic** spread through contaminated endoscopes

FIGURE 30-1 *Helicobacter pylori* and Peptic Ulcer.

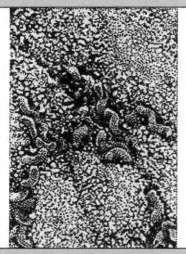

Source: National Digestive Diseases Information Clearinghouse (NDDIC), NIDDK, NIH. Publication No. 07–4225 10/1/2004. Available at http://digestive.niddk.nih.gov/ddiseases/pubs/hpylori/. Accessed April 28, 2008.

Helicobacter pylori is almost always acquired in childhood and, if untreated, infection is usually life-long. Although prevalence of *H. pylori* infection is very high, only 15 percent of infected persons develop peptic ulcer disease. Factors determining the subset of infected individuals developing disease compared with those remaining as *H. pylori* carriers remain unclear. Both host and bacterial factors contribute to differences in *H. pylori* pathogenicity.

Before 1982, when this bacterium was discovered, spicy food, acid, stress, and lifestyle were considered the major causes of ulcers. The majority of patients were given long-term medications, such as histamine-2 (H2) blockers, and more recently, proton pump inhibitors, without a chance for permanent cure. These medications relieve ulcer-related symptoms, heal gastric mucosal inflammation, and may heal the ulcer, but they do NOT treat the infection. When acid suppression is removed, the majority of ulcers, particularly those caused by *H. pylori*, recur. Because we now know that most ulcers are caused by *H. pylori*, appropriate antibiotic regimens can successfully eradicate the infection in most patients, with complete resolution of mucosal inflammation and a minimal chance for recurrence of ulcers.[2]

THE SCIENCE: KEY POINTS

- *H. pylori* causes more than 90 percent of duodenal ulcers and up to 80 percent of gastric ulcers.
- *H. pylori* is a spiral-shaped bacterium found in the gastric mucous layer or adherent to the epithelial lining of the stomach.
- The bacteria are most likely spread from person to person through fecal-oral or oral-oral routes. Possible environmental reservoirs include contaminated water sources.

has been documented but can be prevented by proper cleaning of equipment.

BASIC SCIENCE FACTS/KEY CONCEPTS REVIEW

Helicobacter pylori is a spiral-shaped bacterium found in the gastric mucous layer or adherent to the epithelial lining of the stomach. *H. pylori* causes more than 90 percent of duodenal ulcers and up to 80 percent of gastric ulcers.

CASE STUDY
A Case of Secondary Peptic Ulcer

Scenario

A 56-year-old male presented to the emergency department with the sudden onset of severe, sharp mid-epigastric pain approximately. He began having episodes of nausea and vomiting starting the day before, especially after trying to eat or drink. He had no hematemesis, diarrhea, melena, or hematochezia; he denied any dizziness or fainting. On close questioning, he reported taking ibuprofen three to four times per week for five months for joint aches after beginning a cardio-theraputic walking program. He often would take as much as 800 milligrams each day. He had last taken ibuprofen the day before the pain began. He denied having taken steroids, and there was no personal or family history of peptic ulcer disease or endocrine problems.

Physicial examination revealed a slighty obese man in some distress with a temperature of 101.6°F, a pulse of 120, and a blood pressure of 130/74. He was sitting up in bed with knees flexed and clutching his abdomen. His abdomen was soft without rigidity but with considerable tenderness in the mid-epigastric region; the bowel sounds were diminished. There was also tenderness in the right lower quadrant. He had negative Rovsing's and obturator signs but a positive heel drop. Rectal exam was normal without blood in the stool.

With a pre-operative diagnosis of perforated gastric ulcer, the patient underwent a laparoscopy, which confirmed the diagnosis of perforated gastric ulcer. There was a dime-sized perforation through the anterior portion of the pre-pyloric region of the stomach. No other ulcers or perforations were noted. There was no frank pus in the peritoneum, but some of the gastric contents had tracked down into the right lower quadrant.

The postoperative course was uncomplicated and there was no postoperative infection at the wound site. A serum gastrin level was normal. He was discharged on hospital day seven and instructed to avoid all nonsteroidal anti-inflammatory agents. Follow-up gastroduodenoscopy two months later demonstrated healing of the mucosa with no signs of gastritis and a negative rapid urease test. Antral and fundal biopsies were consistent with normal mucosa.

Defining the Issues

About one in five patients, especially patients taking non-steroidal anti-inflammatory drugs have no antecedent symptoms of pain. Secondary ulcers generally present more acutely than primary ulcers (the majority of which are now known to be due to *H. pylori*). Secondary ulcers often do not present until a complication such as hemorrhage or perforation develops, as in this case (Figure 30-2). Hence, they have a higher need for surgery and a higher morbidity and mortality rate.

A patient with a perforated ulcer will present with a history of epigastric abdominal pain that suddenly became diffuse. There may be pain in the right lower quadrant as enteral contents track down the right gutter. This may mimic an appendicitis. On exam, the patient is often febrile with tachycardia and hypotension, and lies still to avoid exacerbating the pain. The knees may be flexed. Bowel sounds are typically diminished to absent. The abdomen is very tender and is often described as boardlike, though not so in this case. Laboratory tests reveal an elevated white cell count, and an upright abdominal Roentgenogram may reveal free air under the diaphragm.[3]

CLINICAL PERSPECTIVE FOR THE HEALTHCARE PROVIDER

Signs and Symptoms

Most persons who are infected with *H. pylori* never suffer any symptoms related to the infection; however, it causes chronic active, chronic persistent, and atrophic **gastritis** in adults and children. Infection with *H. pylori* also causes duodenal and gastric ulcers. Infected persons have a 2- to 6-fold increased risk of developing gastric cancer and **mucosal-associated lymphoid-type (MALT) lymphoma** compared with their uninfected counterparts. The role of *H. pylori* in non-ulcer dyspepsia remains unclear.

Peptic ulcers are holes in the lining of the stomach or upper small intestine (duodenum) that extend deep into the muscular layers of these organs. An ulcer forms when surface cells become inflamed, die, and are shed (Figure 30-3). Damage can be caused by mechanical abrasion, infection, or inflammation, which results from an overreaction of immune cells. The most common ulcer symptom is gnawing or burning pain in the **epigastrium**.

This pain typically occurs when the stomach is empty, between meals, and in the early morning hours, but it can also occur at other times. It may last from minutes to hours and may be relieved by eating or by taking antacids. Less common ulcer symptoms include nausea, vomiting, and loss of appetite. Bleeding can also occur; prolonged bleeding may cause anemia, leading to weakness and fatigue. If bleeding is heavy, **hematemesis, hematochezia**, or **melena** may occur.

Signs and symptoms of peptic ulcer may also include:

- burning or gnawing pain in the epigastric region
- loss of appetite

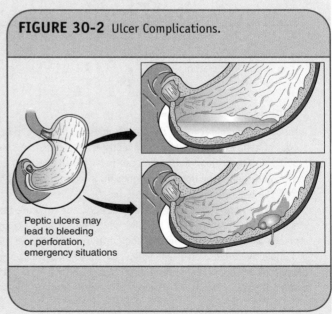

FIGURE 30-2 Ulcer Complications.

Peptic ulcers may lead to bleeding or perforation, emergency situations

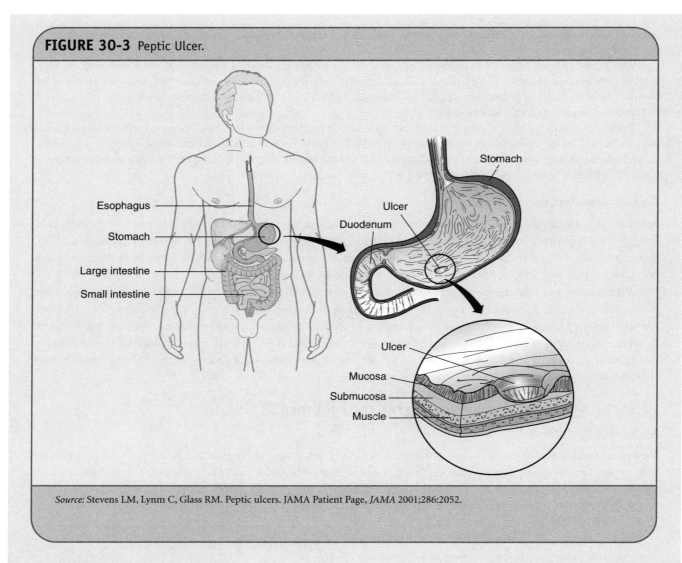

FIGURE 30-3 Peptic Ulcer.

Esophagus
Stomach
Large intestine
Small intestine

Stomach
Ulcer
Duodenum

Ulcer
Mucosa
Submucosa
Muscle

Source: Stevens LM, Lynm C, Glass RM. Peptic ulcers. JAMA Patient Page, *JAMA* 2001;286:2052.

- vomiting
- blood in the stool
- anemia

Diagnosis

Accurate and simple tests for the detection of *H. pylori* infection are available. They include blood antibody tests, urea breath tests, stool antigen tests, and endoscopic biopsies. Blood tests for the presence of antibodies to *H. pylori* can be performed easily and rapidly. However, blood antibodies can persist for years after complete eradication of *H. pylori* with antibiotics. Therefore, blood antibody tests may be good for diagnosing infection, but they are not good for determining if antibiotics have successfully eradicated the bacterium.

The urea breath test (UBT) is a safe, easy, and accurate test for the presence of *H. pylori* in the stomach. The breath test relies on the ability of *H. pylori* to break down the naturally occurring chemical, urea, into carbon dioxide that is absorbed from the stomach and eliminated from the body in the breath. Ten to 20 minutes after swallowing a capsule containing a minute amount of radioactive urea, a breath sample is collected and analyzed for radioactive carbon dioxide. The presence of radioactive carbon dioxide in the breath (a positive test) means that there is active infection. The test becomes negative (there is no radioactive carbon dioxide in the breath) shortly after eradication of the bacterium from the stomach with antibiotics. Despite the fact that individuals having the breath test are exposed to a minute amount of radioactivity, the breath test has been modified so that it also may be performed with urea that is not radioactive.

Endoscopy is an accurate test for diagnosing *H. pylori* as well as the inflammation and ulcers that it causes. To perform the text, the clinician inserts a flexible viewing tube (endoscope) through the mouth, down the esophagus, and into the stomach and duodenum. During endoscopy, small tissue samples (biopsies) from the stomach lining can be removed and the biopsy specimen placed on a special slide containing urea (for example, CLO test slides). If the urea is broken down by *H. pylori* in the biopsy, there is a change in color around the biopsy on the slide. This means that there is an infection with *H. pylori* in the stomach.

The most recently developed test for *H. pylori* can detect the presence of the bacterium with a sample of stool. The test uses an antibody to *H. pylori* to determine if the bacterium is present in the stool. A positive test means that *H. pylori* is infecting the stomach. Like the UBT, in addition to diagnosing infection with *H. pylori*, the stool test can be used to determine if eradication has been effective shortly after treatment.

Persons with active gastric or duodenal ulcers or documented history of ulcers should be tested for *H. pylori*, and if found to be infected, they should be treated. To date, there has been no conclusive evidence that treatment of *H. pylori* infection in patients with non-ulcer dyspepsia is warranted. Testing for and treatment of *H. pylori* infection are recommended following resection of early gastric cancer and for low-grade gastric MALT lymphoma.

Treatment

Therapy for *H. pylori* infection consists of ten days to two weeks of one or two effective antibiotics, such as amoxicillin, tetracycline (not to be used for children < 12 years), metronidazole, or clarithromycin, plus either ranitidine bismuth citrate, bismuth subsalicylate, or a proton pump inhibitor. Acid suppression by the H2 blocker or proton pump inhibitor in conjunction with the antibiotics helps alleviate ulcer-related symptoms (that is, abdominal pain, nausea), helps to heal gastric mucosal inflammation, and may enhance efficacy of the antibiotics against *H. pylori* at the gastric mucosal surface. Currently, eight *H. pylori* treatment regimens are approved by the Food and Drug Administration (FDA); however, several other combinations have been used successfully also. Antibiotic resistance and patient noncompliance are the two major reasons for treatment failure. Eradication rates of the eight FDA-approved regimens range from 61 percent to 94 percent depending on the regimen used. Overall, triple therapy regimens have shown better eradication rates than dual therapy. Longer length of treatment (14 days versus 10 days) results in better eradication rates.

PUBLIC HEALTH PERSPECTIVE FOR THE HEALTH OF THE GENERAL POPULATION AND OF HIGH RISK GROUPS

Approximately 25 million Americans suffer from peptic ulcer disease at some point in their lifetime. Each year there are 500,000 to 850,000 new cases of peptic ulcer disease and more than one million ulcer-related hospitalizations.

Peptic ulcer disease (PUD) is responsible for over three million visits to the doctor per year in the United States.[2] Stomach pain similar to heartburn or indigestion is the most prevalent symptom of a stomach ulcer.

Risk of Gastric Cancer

Gastric cancer, or cancer of the stomach, was once considered a single entity, but now epidemiologists divide this cancer into two main classes: gastric cardia cancer (which is cancer of the top inch of the stomach, where it meets the esophagus) and non-cardia gastric cancer (cancer in all other areas of the stomach). This classification was adopted because these two types of stomach cancer have different risk factors and different patterns of occurrence. For example, *H. pylori* has been established as a strong risk factor for non-cardia gastric cancer, whereas its association with gastric cardia cancer is controversial.

In 2006, there will be an estimated 22,280 new cases of gastric cancer and approximately 11,430 deaths due to the disease in the United States. Gastric cancer is the second most common cause of cancer-related deaths in the world, killing approximately 700,000 people in 2002. Gastric cancer is more common in developing countries than in the United States.

Overall gastric cancer incidence rates are decreasing. However, this decline is mainly in non-cardia gastric cancer rates. In contrast, gastric cardia cancer rates are increasing, particularly in Western countries, such as the United States and many parts of Europe. Gastric cardia cancer, which was once very uncommon, now constitutes nearly half of all stomach cancers in white males in the United States.

Infection with *H. pylori* is the most important risk factor for gastric cancer. Other risk factors include chronic gastritis (inflammation of the stomach); older age; being male; a diet high in salted, smoked, or poorly preserved foods and low in fruits and vegetables; certain types of anemia; smoking cigarettes; and a family history of stomach cancers.

Recent studies have shown an association between long-term infection with *H. pylori* and the development of gastric cancer. Gastric cancer is the second most common cancer worldwide; it is most common in countries such as Colombia and China, where *H. pylori* infects over half the population in early childhood. In the United States, where *H. pylori* is less common in young people, gastric cancer rates have decreased since the 1930s.

Economic Impact

One out of ten Americans suffers from peptic ulcer disease during their lifetime. Ulcers cause an estimated 1 million hospitalizations and 6,500 deaths per year. In the United States, annual healthcare costs of peptic ulcer disease have been estimated at nearly $6 billion: $3 billion in hospitalization costs, $2 billion in physician office visits, and $1 billion in decreased productivity and days lost from work.[4]

We now know that nine out of ten peptic ulcers are caused by an infection with the bacterium *Helicobacter pylori* and not by stress or spicy foods as previously thought. Curing the infection with antibiotics shortens ulcer healing time and significantly reduces the ulcer recurrence rate compared with traditional ulcer therapies such as acid-reducing medications. *H. pylori* infection can usually be cured with a two-week regimen of antibiotics. In more than 80 percent of patients, the ulcer is cured and does not recur.[5]

Studies indicate that curing an ulcer with antibiotics takes less time and costs less than one-tenth the amount of treating ulcer symptoms over a lifetime. Maintenance therapy with acid-reducing medications costs approximately $11,000 and requires 187 days of treatment over 15 years. **Vagotomy**, a more extreme treatment, is also quite costly at $17,000 and requires 307 days of treatment over a 15-year period. Conversely, antibiotic therapy takes 17 days and costs less than $1,000 over the same period of time.[6]

Recent cost analyses, economic decision models, and a randomized controlled trial have all shown that eradicating *H. pylori* from patients with peptic ulcer disease results in decreased healthcare costs. In a study at a large health maintenance organization, *H. pylori* eradication in peptic ulcer disease patients resulted in a decreased use of outpatient services and, thus, a decreased cost of follow-up care.[7]

KEY TERMS
Clinical Terms

Epigastrium: Area of the abdomen located between the costal margins and the subcostal plane.

Endoscopy: Visual examination of the inner surface of the esophagus, stomach, and/or small bowel performed using a lighted scope passed into the body under sedation.

Gastritis: Inflammation of the lining of the stomach.

Hematemesis: Vomiting of blood.

Hematochezia: Passage of bloody stools.

Iatrogenic: Disease or disorder attributed to medical therapy or intervention.

Mucosal-Associated Lymphoid-Type (MALT) Lymphoma: Rare form of lymphoid cancer.

Melena: Tarry stool.

Ulcer: A lesion on the skin or mucosal surface caused by loss of tissue, usually with necrosis and inflammation.

Vagotomy: Surgical division of the vagus nerve designed to reduce stomach acid secretion.

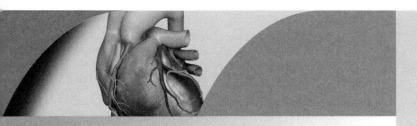

Questions for Further Research, Study, Reflection, and Discussion

For the Individual Student

In order to answer these questions, it may be necessary to research the primary literature.

- Why is MALT lymphoma relevant in the discussion of *H. pylori* and peptic ulcer?
- Indicate the possible mechanisms of transmission of *H. plylori.*
- Discuss the various options for the treatment of *H. pylori* infection.

For Small Group Discussion

- Discuss the factors that may contribute to the differing prevalence of *H. pylori* infection between developed and developing countries.
- What public health measures could be taken to reduce the prevalence of peptic ulcer?

- Discuss the linkages and hypothesized pathways of progression from *H. pylori* infection to peptic ulcer to gastric cancer.
- Because the prevalence of peptic ulcer is common and many public health students choose this career path due to personal experience, ask for volunteers in the class who have had family members with the disease to describe their feelings.

For Entire Class Discussion

- Ask class members how many have a friend or relative who has had peptic ulcer. If they have had surgery or antibiotic treatment for the disease ask if they would describe their experience.
- Ask students in the class what they think should be public health measures that would reduce the occurrence of *H. pylori* infection.
- Develop a time line of the history of gastric cancer, peptic ulcer, and the discovery of the bacterium that causes both of these diseases.

EXERCISES/ACTIVITIES

- Visit a gastroenterology practice or department and ask to see an endoscope. Ask the clinicians to describe the process of sedation, patient preparation, and procedure of viewing the upper gastrointestinal tract.
- Ask individuals who have had an endoscopic procedure to describe their experiences.

Healthy People 2010

Focus Area: Immunization and Infectious Disease

Goal: To prevent disease, disability, and death from infectious diseases, including vaccine-preventable diseases.

Objectives:

14-17. Reduce hospitalizations caused by peptic ulcer disease in the United States

REFERENCES

1. Centers for Disease Control and Prevention. *Helicobacter pylori and Peptic Ulcer Disease: The Key to Cure.* Atlanta: CDC. Available at http://www.cdc.gov/ulcer/keytocure.htm#howcommon. Accessed April 28, 2008.

2. NIH Consensus Development Conference. *Helicobacter pylori* in peptic ulcer disease. *JAMA* 1994;272:65–69.

3. Viera AJ, Cubano M. *Resident Clinical Case Report Perforated Gastric Ulcer in an Eleven Year Old.* Jacksonville, FL: Jacksonville Medicine. Available at http://www.dcmsonline.org/jax-medicine/1998journals/september98/casereport.htm. Accessed April 28, 2008.

4. Sonnenberg A, Everhart JE. Health impact of peptic ulcer in the United States. *Am J Gastroenterol* 1997;92:614–620.

5. Graham DY, Lew GM, Klein PD, Evans DG, Evans DJ Jr, et al. Effect of treatment of *Helicobacter pylori* infection on the long term recurrence of gastric or duodenal ulcer: a randomized controlled study. *Ann Intern Med* 1992;116:705–708.

6. Sonnenberg A, Townsend WF. Costs of duodenal ulcer therapy with antibiotics. *Arch Intern Med* 1995;155:922–928.

7. Levin TR, Schmittdiel JA, Henning JM, Kunz K, Henke CJ, et al. A cost analysis of a *Helicobacter pylori* eradication strategy in a large health maintenance organization. *Am J Gastroenterol* 1998;93:743–747.

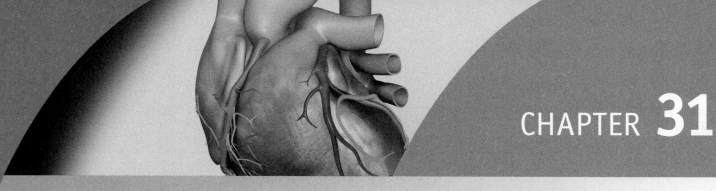

Avian and Seasonal Influenza

John M.P. Cmar
Gary L. Simon

CHAPTER 31

The first pandemic clearly consistent with influenza occurred in 1580, which spread from Asia to Europe via North Africa, resulting in over 8,000 dead in Rome and near-total mortality in several Spanish cities.[1]

LEARNING OBJECTIVES

By the end of this chapter, the student will be able to:

- Understand the basic science topics relevant to the public health ramifications of a possible influenza pandemic, especially:
  - The role of antigenic drift and shift in pandemic influenza.
  - The use of antiviral medications for treatment and prophylaxis of influenza.
  - The role of vaccines in the prevention of influenza infection.
- Define key terms necessary to discuss influenza and public health.
- Identify both important clinical features and public health concerns in a real-world case involving a possible influenza outbreak.

HISTORY

As illustrated by the above fact, influenza has been a persistent global threat to human life and health for nearly 500 years. The 1918 **influenza** pandemic killed 50 to 100 million people worldwide and over 549,000 in the United States alone. This is at least five times as many people who died in World War I, and at least as many people who died in World War II. While the 1957 and 1968 **pandemic influenza** viruses resulted from genetic reassortment between a human and avian virus (Figure 31-1), the 1918 pandemic was the result of an avian virus di-

rectly jumping to humans. Understanding the science and circumstances of past influenza outbreaks is crucial in order to formulate plans for prevention, surveillance, and treatment of a possible pandemic.

BASIC SCIENCE FACTS/KEY CONCEPTS REVIEW

Influenza has long been associated with issues of public health. Indeed, in many ways it represents the prototypical public health concern. Seasonal influenza, an illness associated with substantial morbidity and significant mortality, is a predictable and persistent threat to both individual well-being and societal resources. As a result of its prevalence and its potential severity, an infrastructure has been established to promote prevention through education and yearly vaccination. **Avian influenza,** that is, infection with the H5N1 strain of influenza, for which there is an as-yet undefined potential for sustained human-to-human transmission, represents a possible pandemic illness for which our current public health organization is inadequately prepared.

Nomenclature

The colloquialism *influenza* is often used by the public to denote any significant respiratory illness associated with systemic symptoms, such as myalgias or fever. While numerous viruses are associated with respiratory illnesses, only a few are actual influenza viruses. The influenza virus family consists of three species (A, B, and C) classified by their core proteins, which vary in terms of the severity of disease that they cause and the hosts that they can infect. The most significant of these is influenza A, which has the capacity to be highly pathogenic in humans, causes seasonal outbreaks peaking during the winter

FIGURE 31-1 Generation of a Potentially Pandemic Strain of Influenza Through Reassortment.

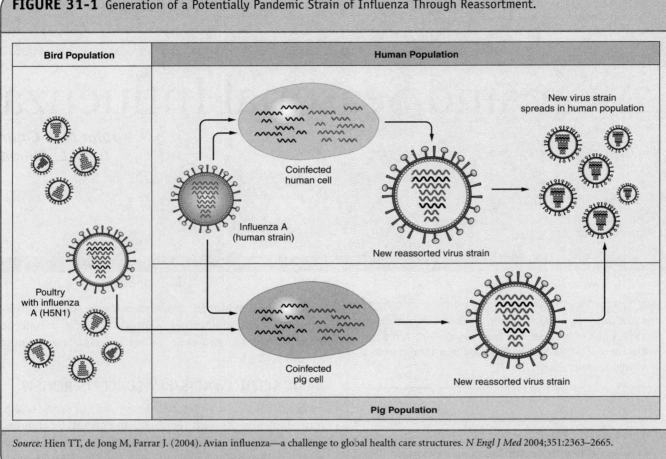

Source: Hien TT, de Jong M, Farrar J. (2004). Avian influenza—a challenge to global health care structures. *N Engl J Med* 2004;351:2363–2665.

months in both hemispheres. Influenza A, of which H5N1 avian influenza is an example, infects a wide variety of mammals and birds. The H5N1 classification of avian influenza represents two major surface molecules, a **hemagglutinin** and a **neuraminidase**, which contribute to the pathogenic potential of influenza. Influenza B, although less common and generally less pathogenic, is still a significant cause of human illness. It also manifests as seasonal outbreaks, although its host spectrum is limited to humans and seals. Influenza C is a relatively minor pathogen, causing mild disease without seasonal variation, and is confined to humans and pigs as hosts.

The nomenclature for the influenza viruses is based on the specific influenza type, the site of isolation, the strain designation and the year of isolation. For influenza A isolates, the hemagglutinin and neuraminidase activity are also specified to further characterize the specific strain of virus. For example, one of the viral strains included in the 2006–07 vaccine was Influenza A/Wisconsin/67/2005(H3N2); this was an isolate of

influenza A obtained from a patient in Wisconsin in 2005. It was strain number 67 and contained an H3 hemagglutinin and an N2 **neuraminidase**.

Seasonality

Influenza A and B viruses exhibit a seasonal pattern of outbreaks, peaking during the winter months in both the northern and southern hemispheres, respectively (Figure 31-2). In avian influenza, this seasonality appears to be tied to bird migration patterns and social behavior. It is poorly understood why this seasonal variation is observed in humans, or how the virus persists during the summer months between outbreaks. Certainly small sporadic outbreaks can occur year round. Contributing to the seasonal variation of influenza is the tendency of people to congregate indoors during the winter. The virus may survive longer on exposed surfaces in colder temperatures favoring fomite transmission. An additional theory espouses the role of vitamin D in the immune response, and

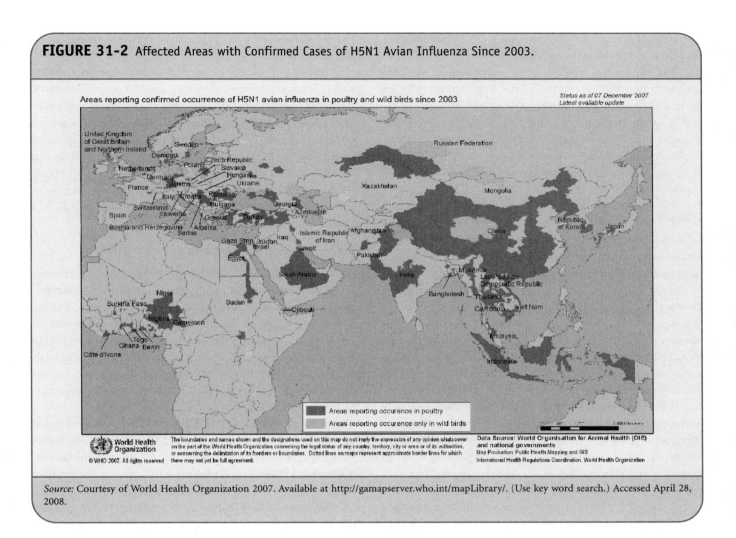

FIGURE 31-2 Affected Areas with Confirmed Cases of H5N1 Avian Influenza Since 2003.

Source: Courtesy of World Health Organization 2007. Available at http://gamapserver.who.int/mapLibrary/. (Use key word search.) Accessed April 28, 2008.

suggests that a decrease in vitamin D metabolism due to reduced periods of sunlight in the winter may contribute as well.

Antigenic Variation

The hemagglutinin and neuraminidase proteins play important roles in disease caused by influenza, including pathogenicity, recognition by the host's immune system, and targets for medical therapy. Hemagglutinins bind to surface molecules on epithelial cells lining the respiratory tract and other mucous membranes, allowing the virus to invade and infect the cells. Fifteen different hemagglutinin subtypes have been described, all of which can infect birds. Among mammals there is a wide variation in hemagglutinin specificity. In humans, six subtypes contribute to disease, including H5, although H1, H2, and H3 are the most common. Neuraminidases function to liberate progeny viruses from host cells. All nine described neuraminidases affect birds, while only three affect humans, but N1 and N2 are the most common.

The two central concepts that underlie the potential for influenza to impact public health are antigenic drift and antigenic shift. Antigenic drift occurs when, as a particular strain of influenza virus is circulating through a community, minor genetic changes occur to the hemagglutinin and neuraminidase molecules during replication and transmission. The result is a virus that is less well recognized by the host immune system of the at-risk population. These minor shifts in hemagglutinin and neuraminidase result in the nearly annual influenza epidemic and necessitate updating the influenza vaccine on a yearly basis. Antigenic drift occurs with all three influenza subtypes. Antigenic shift, on the other hand, occurs only with influenza A and refers to a more dramatic change in antigenicity. When two influenza A viruses with different subtypes of hemagglutinin and neuraminidase infect the same animal host, there can be exchange of genetic components during replication such that the resultant virus has a new combination of surface molecules. This "new" virus is poorly recognized by the circulating immunity of the population. When antigenic shift occurs, a pandemic may result.

The avian influenza virus H5N1 represents an antigenic shift such that there is relatively little host immunity to this particular strain of virus. Fortunately, at least at this time, the ability of this virus to spread via human-to-human transmission appears to be quite limited. Additional mutations could alter this, however, such that this particular strain of virus would become highly contagious and lead to worldwide pandemic.

Transmission, Symptoms, and Complications

Influenza viruses are spread primarily through inhalation of **aerosolized** viral particles expelled via coughing from an infected subject. Respiratory **droplets** can contaminate surfaces, on which the virus can survive for a period of hours. **Contacting** a contaminated surface followed by direct inoculation of mucous membranes represents a secondary form of transmission. Other routes more specific to avian influenza include exposure to contaminated water via ingestion or direct intranasal or conjunctival inoculation, and contamination of hands through handling of bird feces.

Influenza can cause a wide range of symptoms. Typically, both systemic (fever, headache, myalgia, malaise) and respiratory tract (cough, sore throat) symptoms can occur, although one or the other may predominate. Most patients with influenza have inflammation of the upper airways; laryngitis, tracheitis, and bronchitis. Pneumonia is relatively uncommon and can be quite severe. Pregnant women are at especially high-risk for primary influenza pneumonia as are patients with mitral stenosis. In these patients bronchiolitis and alveolitis are seen. Alveolar involvement appears to be considerably more common among patients with influenza due to H5N1, contributing to the reported mortality of approximately 50 percent for patients with infection with this strain of virus.

Bacterial superinfection, that is, secondary bacterial pneumonia, is a more common complication of influenza than primary viral pneumonia. In patients with influenza, secondary bacterial pneumonia can be severe and contributes to the morbidity and mortality associated with annual influenza epidemics. Infection with *Streptococcus pneumoniae* is the most frequently encountered infecting organism, but there is a marked increase in pneumonia caused by *Staphylococcus aureus*. Recently, a particular strain of *S. aureus*, methicillin-resistant *S. aureus* (MRSA) has become more prevalent in the community (see Chapter 27). Post-influenza pneumonia caused by this community-acquired MRSA is of particular concern. Isolates of this organism frequently contain the Panton-Valentine leukocidin, which can cause a severe necrotizing infection with tissue necrosis, abscess formation, and increased mortality.

Traditionally, the populations with the greatest morbidity and mortality were the very young and the elderly. However, during the avian influenza epidemic of 1918 there was a substantial mortality among young, healthy adults. This has been attributed to an overexuberant immune response—a cytokine storm—which led to severe tissue damage in the host. In this case, the more robust immune response of young adults resulted in a greater mortality in that group. There is some speculation that the severity of H5N1 infection is related to a cytokine storm.

Treatment and Prophylaxis

Antiviral medications have two roles in managing an influenza outbreak: treatment and prophylaxis. Treatment with currently available agents is only beneficial if initiated within 24 hours of onset of symptoms. The effect of therapy in patients with influenza is a decrease in the duration of symptoms by two to three days at most, with no impact demonstrated on mortality. Prophylaxis is useful if started prior to symptoms in the setting of an active outbreak, although it is not 100 percent effective in preventing the acquisition of influenza.

There are two classes of drugs that have activity directed against the influenza virus: the **M2 ion channel inhibitors** (amantadine and rimantadine) and the **neuraminidase inhibitors** (oseltamivir and zanamivir). Currently, greater than 90 percent of seasonal influenza isolates are resistant to the M2 inhibitors, leading to the recommendation that they not be used for either prophylaxis or treatment. Similarly, most isolates of H5N1 avian influenza are resistant to the M2 inhibitors. To date, resistance to neuraminidase inhibitors has been rarely reported among circulating seasonal influenza isolates. The use of neuraminidase inhibitors has been recommended for patients with H5N1 avian influenza, but there are few clinical data demonstrating efficacy. Indeed, there is some concern that the dose of oseltamivir that is used for the treatment of seasonal influenza is not adequate for the treatment of H5N1 isolates. It has been observed that some H5N1 strains require higher doses to be effective. This has raised the concern that administration of the standard dose of oseltamivir during a pandemic could promote the development of high-level resistance.

Several additional potential problems exist with reliance on neuraminidase inhibitors for the treatment of H5N1 avian influenza. The manufacturing process for oseltamivir is complex, and the parent compound, shikimic acid, is efficiently isolated only from the Chinese star anise. This plant grows only in four provinces of China and is available for harvest only from March through May. Given these caveats, there is concern that in the event of a pandemic, supplies could quickly become depleted. Many governments and corporations have been stockpiling oseltamivir for prophylaxis in the event of an outbreak, but these supplies are far from adequate should a worldwide pandemic occur.

Prevention

The primary mode of prevention for influenza infection has been the use of vaccines. There is both a killed virus vaccine that is administered parenterally as well as the live attenuated virus vaccine that can be given intranasally. Seasonal influenza vaccines are prepared annually, based on the most recent circulating influenza A and B strains. In the event of an avian influenza pandemic, seasonal influenza vaccine would still be recommended in order to prevent co-infection with multiple types of virus as well as to gain possible benefits from cross-immunity between the two strains. Vaccines for H5N1 are under development, and the first license for such a vaccine was granted by the FDA in April of 2007 for high risk groups, such

as healthcare professionals and laboratory workers. These vaccines are considered to be "pre-pandemic," in that they would have reduced efficacy for a pandemic strain of H5N1 due to intercurrent antigenic drift and shift. In the event of a pandemic, it would take at least six months with current vaccine production technology to develop and produce a vaccine targeted against the pandemic strain.

There is some controversy regarding the population that should receive vaccination. Current Centers for Disease Control Guidelines stress the need for immunizing elderly individuals and high-risk subjects such as immunosuppressed individuals and pregnant women. Children and young adults are not routinely targeted. However, many individuals within the targeted groups, such as elderly subjects, do not manifest a robust immune response. Studies from Japan have shown that immunizing children produces a herd immunity and reduces infections in adults. This is an important consideration in the event that a pandemic occurs.

CASE STUDY
Scenario

Mr. A is a 35-year-old man of Vietnamese descent who presented to his outpatient physician with a three day history of cough, fever, and myalgias. He is physically fit, with no past medical history, and currently takes no medications or supplements. He "doesn't like doctors" and avoids receiving routine medical care for this reason, including never having received an influenza vaccination. He lives in an apartment with his female partner and three children, all younger than 10 years of age. Mr. A is employed as a security guard at a local college dormitory and is the only source of income for his family. He smokes two packs per day of cigarettes and denies any regular alcohol or illicit drug use.

Just over two weeks ago, in February, he took a vacation to visit extended family in Vietnam. Although he spent most of his time in downtown Hanoi, he did visit his cousins in the outlying country for three days just prior to returning to the United States. His cousins were chicken farmers, and while staying with them he helped out with daily chores, including tending to the flock. He noticed that many of the chickens seemed "ill," and was told that this had been observed for several days. The cousins had not reported the sick poultry due to fear that they would be forced to cull their flocks out of concern for avian influenza, which would be financially devastating to their already meager subsistence. Due to limited space, Mr. A had been unable to stay in the main house, so he slept in a shack near where the chickens were penned. One of his cousins did have a "severe cold" at the time of his visit.

On the day of his return to the United States, Mr. A noted the acute onset of fever, myalgias, and cough. He had no further available leave from his job and did not want to risk termination, so he reported for work despite his illness. Over the next two days, Mr. A felt progressively more ill with profound fatigue and noticeable shortness of breath with exertion. During those two days, he went about his usual activities in the dormitory, which included the breakup of two large parties on the dormitory floors and supervising a crowded Family Day activity in a common room in that building. On the third day of his illness, Mr. A found it difficult to accomplish his usual morning activities due to his worsening symptoms. He still insisted on reporting for work, and asked his girlfriend to drive him there, but she brought him to his outpatient physician instead. Mr. A believed that he picked up "a bad cold" from one of the students in the dormitory. He heard of avian influenza in the news a couple of years ago, but expressed to his physician that he is unconcerned, as clearly a pandemic has not occurred. He was initially unwilling to provide details of his trip to Vietnam to his physician, but did so only after insistent prompting from his girlfriend.

Defining the Issues

There are several issues presented in this scenario. Mr. A was unwilling to engage in routine health care, and so neither received a seasonal influenza vaccination, nor sought medical advice prior to travel back to Vietnam. When confronted with illness, he believed himself unable to take leave due to the risk of losing his job because he was the only source of income for his family. Unfortunately, his employer contributed to the problem by having an inadequate sick leave policy, especially in the face of a possibly communicable disease. When ill, Mr. A did not seek prompt medical attention, but continued to work in a situation where he exposed numerous people in close conditions to a potentially easily transmissible disease in addition to the potential for exposure of his family, including his young children. In terms of Mr. A's relatives in Vietnam, their living conditions and means of subsistence put them at the highest risk for contracting avian influenza from infected birds. Furthermore, their unwillingness to consider the need to cull their flock due to livelihood considerations is at odds with a major public health initiative to control the spread of known avian influenza from infected birds.

Patient's Understanding

Mr. A's understanding of the medical issues involved in this case is quite poor. He is concerned with supporting his family over his own personal health, and appears to have little insight into the fact that he may be infected with a communicable disease that he could easily transmit to both his family and to the students with whom he works. He appears to have little insight into avian influenza and how it is spread among people. Alternatively, his reluctance to provide information about his trip to Vietnam suggests that he might be attempting to avoid laying blame on his family in Vietnam, either for his own illness or for not reporting sick poultry to the government.

CLINICAL PERSPECTIVE FOR THE INDIVIDUAL PATIENT

Level of Intervention Now

Mr. A has an illness that is clinically consistent with influenza. Excluding other possible infectious etiologies, two options that might be considered relative to this episode are seasonal influenza or avian influenza. Mr. A may have contracted seasonal influenza from an exposure in Hanoi or from his ill cousin, who could have acquired seasonal influenza from a non-family human exposure. Alternatively, Mr. A may have acquired avian influenza either from close contact with chickens or, more disturbingly, as a result of human-to-human transmission from his ill cousin, who could have contracted it from the poultry.

A nasal swab for rapid influenza would be the easiest test to establish the diagnosis. If positive, it would confirm the presence of an influenza A or B virus, but would not distinguish between seasonal influenza A and avian influenza. Given the history in this case, tests that specifically identify for H5N1, such as a nasal or throat swab for viral culture and/or PCR, would be appropriate. These samples should be processed with appropriate biosafety precautions and sent to the CDC for confirmatory testing.

Potential Level Earlier

Mr. A has had symptoms for three days. Therapy should be simply supportive because he is well beyond the 24-hour window in which antiviral therapy with oseltamivir could alter the course of his disease. However, treatment with oseltamivir might be considered with the intention of quantitatively reducing the amount of virus shed by Mr. A in his respiratory secretions. Potentially, this would reduce infectivity and lower the risk of transmitting virus to others. This could be an even more important consideration if his infection was due to a strain of avian influenza that had developed efficient human-to-human transmission.

Clearly, opportunities for primary preventative measures were missed in this case. An influenza vaccination would have significantly decreased the risk of acquiring seasonal influenza and possibly allowed for some cross-immunity to avian influenza. A pre-travel visit with a physician would have allowed Mr. A to be more educated as to the threat of exposure to avian influenza, especially if his specific destinations were reviewed. Specific recommendations could have included avoidance of live poultry in general, such as in markets or his cousin's flock, safe handling and thorough cooking of food, and practicing meticulous hand hygiene with, preferably, an alcohol-based hand sanitizer. When visiting his rural cousins in Vietnam, Mr. A should have been counseled to avoid ill chickens or related products. Alternative sleeping arrangements in which he was removed from the area where the flock was penned could have been more vigorously sought as well. If Mr. A insisted on working with the animals despite being informed of the risks associated with avian influenza and knew that the flock contained ill animals prior to his arrival, he should have utilized an N95-rated mask and **barrier precautions** to reduce the likelihood of exposure.

Secondary prevention of clinical influenza in this scenario would have hinged on Mr. A seeking medical evaluation within 24 hours of the onset of his symptoms. Given the burden of suspicion for influenza, seasonal or avian, a rapid influenza swab could have been performed and, if positive, oseltamivir could have been started in order to reduce the duration of Mr. A's symptoms.

PUBLIC HEALTH PERSPECTIVE FOR THE HEALTH OF THE GENERAL POPULATIONS AND OF HIGH RISK GROUPS

Mr. A's cousin, immediate family, and the students and their family members who were potentially exposed during the dormitory event constitute high-risk groups in this scenario. If human-to-human transmission were to occur, infection among these individuals who have the capacity to disseminate it widely could portend the start of a pandemic. Appropriate interventions at this stage would include identification of all potentially exposed persons and subsequent medical evaluation. Prophylactic therapy with oseltamivir could be initiated in order to prevent or reduce disease in affected persons as well as to decrease viral shedding and thereby reduce the likelihood of transmission. **Social distancing**, along with close monitoring for symptoms, should also be stressed.

Mr. A's cousins and infected chicken stock represent a potential source for an avian influenza pandemic. Despite their understandable reluctance to do so, **culling** of the entire ill poultry population is appropriate, along with improvements in sanitation and removal of wild birds that could transmit the virus to domesticated populations. Vaccination of the healthy poultry population is a consideration but should be done with strict oversight, as subpotent dosing could lead to partial immunity that could accelerate viral antigenic mutation and result in a more pathogenic virus.

The potential for the events outlined in this case to herald a widespread pandemic raises significant issues for control and prevention. General vaccine development, as previously noted, would not be a "first line" response. With current technology, it takes at least six months to produce an effective vaccine for the pandemic viral strain. In addition, current vaccine manufacturing processes utilize chicken egg–based technology originally developed in the 1950s. Besides its inefficiency, the possibility for this influenza strain to infect the chicken population that generates the needed eggs must be considered. Efforts are under way to develop cell culture-based vaccine development technology for quicker and more efficient vaccine turnaround.

Thus, antiviral agents would be the "first line" of response in a pandemic situation. While there would only be enough oseltamivir to treat or prophylax a small proportion of the at-risk population, one strategy that has been suggested would be to treat front-line healthcare workers until an effective vaccine could be distributed. To this end, many governments and organizations have been stockpiling the drug. This has raised some concerns on the part of individuals or groups who lack the resources to acquire oseltamivir in any quantity, as to the equality of the distribution of these stockpiles.

In the event of a pandemic, antivirals and vaccine coverage need to be combined with social distancing. On the basis of patterns observed in the 1918 influenza pandemic, transmission occurs in roughly even distributions among the general community, workplaces and schools, and individual households. Targeted school and business closings would be part of a **containment strategy**, and employer liberalization of illness-related leave is an important policy consideration. Travel and trade with an infected region or country may have to be severely curtailed.

A final consideration in the management of an outbreak of pandemic influenza would be the logistics of healthcare delivery to a large numbers of ill persons. Most hospitals and healthcare sites have poor **surge capacity**, both in terms of available space as well as technology (such as ventilators) and supplies. Temporary or mobile health centers would need to be established, and it may be necessary for these temporary facilities to remain active for prolonged periods, perhaps as long as one to two years. Healthcare workers, because of their close contact with ill individuals, would be at especially high risk of becoming infected if an effective vaccine was not readily available. Besides the strain on facilities, the impact of infection among the already limited number of healthcare workers would add to the logistical nightmare. Additional pragmatic issues that would need to be addressed include the handling and disposal of a large number of corpses, increasing production of masks and barrier equipment, and establishing fair and clear guidelines for overriding confidentiality and consent procedures in the interest of public health. Finally, establishing appropriate infrastructure, reliable communication, and recognized leadership at both local and national levels would be imperative to successfully coordinate a public health response.

KEY TERMS

Biology Terms

Aerosol Spread: Dissemination of virus in airborne particles less than five micrometers in size that can be carried in the air over long distances, filtered only by a N95 rated mask.

Antigenic Drift: Minor genetic changes to circulating influenza viruses that occur seasonally and cause small, localized outbreaks of varying severity and extent.

Antigenic Shift: Major genetic reassortment between two different influenza A viruses resulting in a pandemic strain (see Pandemic Influenza).

Avian Influenza: A strain of influenza A that infects birds and may cause severe disease in humans; potentially could cause a pandemic if the virus were to undergo antigenic shift and become easily transmissible from human-to-human.

Barrier Precautions: Use of gloves, gowns, and hand washing to prevent contact spread of infections (see Contact Spread).

Contact Spread: Dissemination of virus via touching a contaminated surface and self-inoculation of mucous membranes.

Hemagglutinin: Surface protein on influenza A that attaches to respiratory tract cells to cause infection; the abbreviation of it and its numbered type is used as a component of the virus name (for example, H5).

Influenza: Illness caused by any of several types (A, B, and C) of influenza virus, spread by airborne and tactile routes, and causing both upper and lower respiratory disease of varying degrees of severity.

M2 Ion Channel Inhibitors: Class of antiviral medications including amantadine and rimantadine, to which greater than 90 percent of circulating seasonal influenza is resistant.

Neuraminidase: Surface protein that releases new viruses from infected cells; the abbreviation of it and its numbered type is used as a component of the virus name (for example, N1).

Neuraminidase Inhibitors: Class of antiviral medications including oseltamivir and zanamivir.

Public Health Terms

Containment Strategy: Multifaceted plan to control an outbreak of influenza and prevent its further spread.

Culling: Depopulation of infected birds from a localized area to prevent spread of illness (such as avian influenza), which lessens the chance of human disease involvement.

Droplet Spread: Dissemination of virus in airborne particles greater than five micrometers in size that travel only several feet in the air.

Pandemic Influenza: Influenza virus that has spread to cause epidemic disease on a continental or worldwide level, regardless of source (such as avian).

Social Distancing: Removal of someone with an easily transmissible infection from normal situations in which they would potentially expose a large number of people, such as a job site or school.

Surge Capacity: The amount of patients a given medical facility can accommodate in an emergency situation beyond its standard maximum amount, such as in a pandemic.

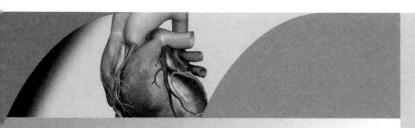

Questions for Further Research, Study, Reflection, and Discussion

For the Individual Student

In order to answer these questions, it may be necessary to research the primary literature.

- What are other described varieties of avian influenza beyond H5N1 that have caused outbreaks in humans, and what have been the impacts of those outbreaks?
- What are the different clades or strains of H5N1 in circulation among birds currently, and how do they differ in terms of geographic distribution, ability to cause disease, and sensitivity to antiviral medications?
- What is the difference in between oseltamivir and zanamivir, and how does that impact their use in preventing and treating influenza?

For Small Group Discussion

- Discuss practical ways for public institutions to encourage someone in Mr. A's situation to practice meticulous hand hygiene, and to appropriately cover coughs/wear a mask to prevent transmission of influenza to others.
- What roles could student health play in the given scenario at the college, assuming that some of the students and family members begin to develop symptoms after the Family Day event?
- Assume Mr. A's children are all in varying grades of school and have started to exhibit symptoms. From the standpoint of Mr. A's girlfriend, what are the potential social and financial ramifications of their situation, if (a) Mr. A continues to insist on reporting for work, or (b) if Mr. A chooses to stay home and convalesce?

For Entire Class Discussion

- Discuss options for companies, both in terms of sick leave policy and providing barrier precautions (masks, gloves, etc.) to employees, in order to responsibly prevent transmission of influenza in an outbreak or pandemic setting among its employees, without penalizing said employees through compulsory leave without pay or possible termination of employment.
- Assume that you are on the medical staff of a hospital with a total of 25 ventilators, all of which are being utilized at the start of a pandemic. Over the course of a day, 5 more patients, varying in range from 2 to 84 years of age, present in pulmonary failure due to influenza and meet necessary criteria for mechanical ventilation. Additionally, several of the respiratory therapists and staff are ill, but have continued to report to work, and two have a worsening respiratory status necessitating cessation of their clinical duties and use of supplemental oxygen. What factors are important in rationing the limited resources of the hospital to meet patient and staff needs? Would there be other creative ways of increasing mechanical ventillation capacity?
- Consider the population and economic distribution of the United States by geography and location of resources. In the event of an influenza pandemic, what areas and industries are most likely to be severely affected? The least likely? Are there any basic changes in population or industrial infrastructure that could lessen such a pandemic-related impact?

EXERCISE/ACTIVITY

Each class member should assume the role of one of the people involved in the case study above, from the following list: Mr. A, Mr. A's girlfriend, the physician, a college student, a parent of one of the students, and Mr. A's cousin. Assume the following: some of the students in the dormitory are becoming ill with similar symptoms the day after Mr. A presented to his physician; someone in the student body has made a connection between Mr. A's recent trip and illness with the current illness; one of

Mr. A's children has also become significantly ill; and both Mr. A's cousin and physician have been made aware of these further illnesses through him. From an individual standpoint, consider the following from the perspective of the role chosen:

- How did each person contribute to the development of the outbreak, both through specific actions and inaction?
- What factors unique to each person's situation motivated them to do so?

- What steps can they take now to prevent further spread of the disease for themselves, or those around them?
- Do you personally agree with your assigned role's motivations in the case? After addressing these questions, gather as a group and compare/discuss responses. In particular, examine differences between the responses of your classmates who shared the same assigned role.

Healthy People 2010

Indicator: Immunization

Focus Area: Immunization and Infectious Diseases

Goal: Prevent disease, disability, and death from infectious diseases, including vaccine-preventable diseases.

Objectives:

14-1. Reduce or eliminate indigenous cases of vaccine-preventable diseases

14-29. Increase the proportion of adults who are vaccinated annually against influenza and ever vaccinated against pneumococcal disease

REFERENCE

1. Potter C. W. (2001). A History of Influenza. *The Journal of Applied Microbiology 91*, 572–579.

RESOURCES

Belshe RB. The origins of pandemic influenza—lessons from the 1918 virus. *N Engl J Med* 2005;353:2209–2211.

Centers for Disease Control. *Avian Influenza (Bird Flu)*, 2007. Available at http://www.cdc.gov/flu/avian/. Accessed April 28, 2008.

Hien TT, de Jong M, Farrar J. Avian influenza—a challenge to global health care structures. *N Engl J Med* 2004;351: 2363–2365.

Kaye D, Pringle CR. Avian influenza viruses and their implication for human health. *Clin Infect Dis* 2004;40:108–112.

Osterholm MT. Preparing for the next pandemic. *N Engl J Med* 2005:352:1839–1842.

Treanor JJ. Influenza virus. In: Mandell GL, Bennett JE, Dolin R, eds. *Principles and Practice of Infectious Diseases*. Philadelphia: Elsevier; 2005:2060–2085.

World Health Organization. *Avian influenza*, 2007. Epidemic and Pandemic Alert and Response (EPR). Geneva: WHO. Available at http://www.who.int/csr/disease/avian_influenza/en/index.html. Accessed April 29, 2008.

World Health Organization. Avian influenza A (H5N1) infection in humans. *N Engl J Med* 2005;353:1374–1385.

CROSS REFERENCES

Behavioral Determinants of Health
Information-Seeking Strategies in Public Health
The Public Health Triad

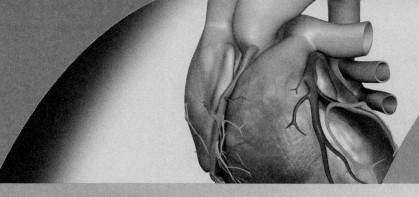

CHAPTER 32

Bioterrorism: Medical and Public Health Implications

Christina L. Catlett
Christopher Scott

> "Although we all hope that events such as the anthrax attacks of 2001 will never occur again and that our efforts to prepare and protect ourselves will be successful, the challenge of bioterrorism will be with us indefinitely. It is difficult to assess the probability of future deliberate releases of microbes or their products, but the potential consequences of such attacks are enormous."[1]

LEARNING OBJECTIVES

By the end of this chapter, the student will be able to:

- Discuss the history of bioterrorism.
- List characteristics that make "Category A" biological agents a threat to our national security.
- Discuss the basic clinical presentation and management of anthrax, smallpox, plague, botulism, tularemia, and viral hemorrhagic fevers.
- Describe key public health strategies used to respond to an attack with a biological agent.

HISTORY

September 11, 2001, and the subsequent anthrax attacks ushered in a new age of awareness for most Americans on the threat of terrorism; therefore, some may be surprised to learn that bioterrorism has been around for centuries. In the 6th century bc, Assyrians used rye ergot to poison the wells of its enemies. In the 400 BC, Scythian archers dipped arrows in decomposing bodies or manure to cause wound infections.

During the 15th to 18th centuries, smallpox-laden clothing and blankets were given to enemies to induce outbreaks.

The 20th century brought industrialism and mass production to the concept of bioterrorism. By World Wars I and II, several countries had well-developed biological weapons programs, including Japan, Russia, United Kingdom, and the United States. President Nixon put an end to offensive research and production of biological weapons in the United States in 1969. In 1972, a treaty known as the Biological Weapons Convention was developed by the international community that prevented the stockpiling of biological agents and research into offensive biological weapons. Despite being signatories of the treaty, several countries, particularly Iraq and the Soviet Union, continued active biological weapons production.

For experts in homeland security, a series of events and discoveries in the 1990s led to growing concern over the possibility of an attack on the United States with a biological agent:

- The dissolution of the former Soviet Union in 1991 led to a mass exodus of scientists to other countries, bringing with them expertise in bioterrorism and possibly samples or caches of bioweapons.
- In 1995, Iraq revealed to United Nations inspectors its extensive bioweapons research and production capabilities during the Persian Gulf War. Thousands of liters of concentrated botulinum toxin, anthrax, and aflatoxin were produced and loaded into munitions.
- Also in 1995, a Russian defector disclosed details of the former Soviet Union's bioweapons program, including

extensive production capabilities and genetic engineering of more virulent and resistant biological organisms.[2]

- After its successful attack on Tokyo with sarin (chemical agent), an investigation into the Japanese cult Aum Shinrikyo in 1995 revealed that the terrorist group had attempted to obtain and deploy botulinum toxin and anthrax on several occasions.

In the wake of the terrorist attacks in New York, Pennsylvania, and Washington, D.C. on September 11, 2001, many federal, state, and local initiatives began to address bioterrorism preparedness and response. Response to an act of biological terrorism presents many challenges to the medical and public health communities. Unlike an attack with an explosive or a chemical agent where the effects are immediate and dramatic, an attack with a biological agent is likely to be covert. Because of the delay in onset of illness (**incubation period**), people can travel over long distances after exposure, making identification of the release site and other exposed individuals difficult. Many biological agents cause non-specific, flu-like illnesses initially, which can delay diagnosis of the disease. Also, most clinicians are unfamiliar with diseases related to biological terrorism due to the rarity of naturally occurring cases. Finally, because we live in a very mobile society, contagious disease outbreaks have the potential to spread rapidly across borders.

While certainly many viruses and bacteria could be used as terrorist weapons, the Centers for Disease Control and Prevention (CDC) have designated three categories to classify different bioterrorism agents, dubbed A, B, and C. The six agents discussed in this chapter are classified as Category A Agents. In addition to the high risk they pose as weapons of bioterrorism, these six share the following characteristics:

- Easily disseminated within a population including person to person transmission;
- Potential to cause high severity of illness with extraordinary death rates;
- Ability to incite public panic and chaos; and
- The requirement of special resources or procedures to prepare for and combat.

Source: These criteria for Category A Agent status were adapted from the CDC's Web site at http://www.bt.cdc.gov/bioterrorism/overview.asp. Accessed April 28, 2008.

While certainly any bioterrorism agent would fulfill some of the above criteria and some may fulfill all the above criteria, knowledge preparation for the six Category A Agents will better enable us to respond to all agents, regardless of their classification.

ANTHRAX

CASE STUDY

The morning of October 16, 2001, was miserable for Joseph Curseen, a 47-year-old United States Postal Service employee at the Brentwood processing facility in Washington, D.C. He woke up feeling fatigued with little desire to spend his day sorting mail. Throughout the day, Mr. Curseen got progressively more nauseated, and by that night he began vomiting and had diarrhea.

After five days of what he thought would be a quick stomach bug, he went to the emergency room. He had a chest x-ray and received intravenous fluids, then was sent home to rest and recover from presumed viral illness. Twenty-six hours later, when he passed out for the second time, Mr. Curseen returned to the same emergency room. He continued to have the same flu-like complaints but now looked much sicker. Mr. Curseen was drenched in sweat and was having difficulty breathing. A second chest x-ray and computerized axial tomography (CAT) scan revealed a widened mediastinum (swollen lymph nodes between the lungs) and bilateral pulmonary effusions, abnormal and concerning findings. By this time, concerns over an anthrax attack were well publicized, and the physician recognized Mr. Curseen's case as pulmonary anthrax, the same thing his co-worker had been hospitalized with three days earlier. He was admitted to the intensive care unit (ICU), but on October 22, Joseph Curseen became the third person to die as a result of a biological attack on the United States.

An extensive investigation revealed that *B. anthracis* spores had been delivered through the mail to several media outlets and Senator Daschle's office. Once it was over, 22 people had developed anthrax and 5 had died. To date, the perpetrator remains at large.

Historical Perspective

Anthrax is a **zoonotic disease** of grazing animals that has been around for centuries. The skin or **cutaneous** form occurs in people working with infected animal and hides; *woolsorter's disease* refers to the inhalation form. The incidence of naturally occurring anthrax is low in the United States. In the 50 years between 1944 and 1994, there were only 224 cases of naturally occurring cutaneous anthrax.

Anthrax was identified as a potential bioweapon in the 20th century. The United States weaponized spores until the termination of its offensive program, as did the Soviet Union. An accident in the Sverdlovsk region of the former Soviet Union in 1979 demonstrated the lethality of aerosolized anthrax. A military microbial facility accidentally released approximately 1 milligram of anthrax spores into the air outside of the facility. Ninety-six individuals up to 4 kilometers downwind developed the disease and at least 68 people died.

In 1995, Iraq admitted to producing mass quantities of anthrax and loading it onto ballistics; that same year, a defector from the former Soviet Union's bioweapons program revealed the production of large quantities of anthrax for use as a weapon by the Soviets. Anthrax was deployed successfully against the United States by an unknown perpetrator in 2001 (Exhibit 32-1).

Clinical Perspective

Anthrax is caused by *Bacillus anthracis*, a Gram-positive, rod-shaped, aerobic bacteria that can form a protective spore coat in the proper environment. *B. anthracis* spores are engineered to withstand hostile environments including exposure to heat, cold, radiation, desiccation, disinfectants, and anaerobic conditions. Spores can last up to 40 years in the environment and remain infective.

Anthrax typically presents in people in three forms: cutaneous and inhalational (seen in the 2001 anthrax attacks), and gastrointestinal (rare in humans).

In cutaneous (or skin) anthrax, inoculation occurs through a break in the skin in an area exposed to the environment, like the hand, arm, or neck. A small itchy bump (papule) develops one to seven days later that may be mistaken for an insect bite. The papule evolves into the characteristic ulcer, usually 1 to 3 centimeters in diameter with a red, raised border around a coal-black scab, called an *eschar* (Figure 32-1). The patient may develop systemic signs of illness, including fever, malaise, swollen lymph nodes, and headache. Cutaneous anthrax is fatal in 20 percent of cases when left untreated.

Inhalational (lung) anthrax occurs after inhalation of spores into the lungs (Figure 32-2). The incubation period is typically one to six days, but can last up to six weeks. Initial symptoms resemble the flu, including fever, malaise, non-productive cough, and chest discomfort. Following a brief period of improvement, the patient develops severe respiratory distress; death occurs 24 to 36 hours later. Inhalational anthrax is 89 percent to 96 percent fatal if left untreated.

Anthrax is not contagious, so **standard precautions** can be utilized by healthcare workers. Fortunately, *B. anthracis* is susceptible to many common antibiotics including penicillin,

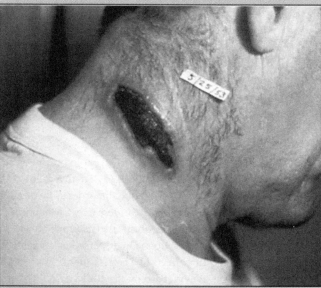

FIGURE 32-1 Cutaneous Anthrax Lesion on the Neck.

Source: From Public Health Image Library. ID # 1934. CDC Content Provider. Available at http://phil.cdc.gov/phil/details.asp. Accessed August 14, 2007.

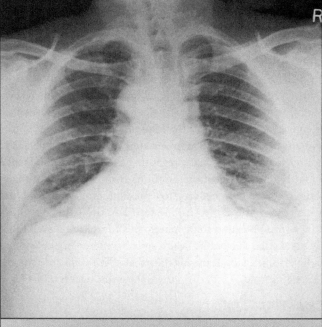

FIGURE 32-2 Chest X-ray of Patient with Pulmonary Anthrax.

Source: From Public Health Image Library. ID # 5146. CDC and Arthur E. Kaye Content Providers. Available at http://phil.cdc.gov/phil/details.asp. Accessed August 14, 2007.

clindamycin, and ciprofloxacin. Because anthrax is not contagious, contacts of victims do not need to receive antibiotics; however, victims of the attack itself must. For **prophylaxis** of exposures, guidelines state that 60 days of antibiotics is needed to prevent any long-lasting spores in the lungs from germinating and infecting the individual. There is a vaccine that appears to be 93 percent effective at preventing anthrax. It is currently only recommended for laboratory personnel working with anthrax, persons handling potentially infected animal hides or carcasses, and deployed military.

Public Health Perspective

Anthrax has been described as the perfect biological weapon. *Bacillus anthracis* is found naturally in the environment and, until the events of the fall of 2001, could be ordered from multiple biological supply houses for use in research. Production of anthrax spores does not require sophisticated machinery or techniques. Anthrax spores could be easily dispersed as an aerosol. Finally, the socioeconomic effects of a large-scale anthrax attack would be devastating, as evidenced by the 2001 attack.

A mass prophylaxis campaign was initiated as a countermeasure to the 2001 anthrax attacks, which proved to be a significant challenge. The logistics of distribution of medication to a large population were complex. Many people believed that they were receiving substandard care when their treatment regimens changed or were different from others. People began demanding screening tests and moved from hospital to hospital to get them when they were refused. The public and physicians began to hoard antibiotics, which could have led to a shortage of vital therapies. Adherence to 60 days of therapy with antibiotics was difficult to maintain in the face of declining infections and medication side effects.

There were many other important lessons learned from the 2001 anthrax attacks about the public health response to a biological attack. Post-event analysis demonstrated that information management was one of the biggest challenges. The rapidly evolving situation resulted in disparate information and lack of consensus decision-making regarding exposure risks and treatment regimens. Recommendations from the CDC changed daily. Coordination between federal, state, and local health departments was lacking, leading to frustration and confusion. Risk communication to the public was complicated even more by the media. The public health system suffered organizational and personnel fatigue during the exhaustive response to the anthrax attacks, particularly in the wake of the events of 9/11.

SMALLPOX

Historical Perspective

Prior to its eradication, smallpox ravaged the world for centuries. The first smallpox outbreaks occurred in 10,000 BC in the Nile Valley and Mesopotamia. The mummy of the Egyptian Pharaoh Ramses V, who died in 1157 BC, bears the characteristic pustules of smallpox. One of the first uses of smallpox as a biological weapon was at Fort Pitt (Pittsburg) during the French and Indian War in 1754 when the English distributed blankets from smallpox patients to Native Americans in an effort to decimate the tribes.

In 1796, Edward Jenner demonstrated that cowpox inoculation protected against smallpox, initiating the practice of smallpox vaccination worldwide. Yet smallpox continued to wreak havoc on the world, causing nearly 100 million deaths during the 20th century alone. As the result of an aggressive worldwide immunization program during the 1960s and 1970s, the last case of naturally occurring smallpox was in Somalia in 1977. The disease was declared eradicated by the World Health Organization in 1980.

Currently, there are only two official repositories of smallpox virus in the world, The Centers for Disease Control and Prevention (CDC) in Atlanta and the Russian State Research Center of Virology and Biotechnology in Koltsovo, Novosibirsk region of Russia, but it is suspected that other countries have clandestine stockpiles that may be used in a biological attack.

Clinical Perspective

Smallpox, also known as *variola*, is caused by a DNA virus. Before it was eradicated, there were two forms of the disease: variola major, which was more common and had a case fatality rate of 30 percent in the unvaccinated, and variola minor, a much milder form with a 1 percent mortality rate.

A smallpox attack is likely to occur through aerosolization of the virus. Exposure is followed by an incubation period, during which the patient is asymptomatic. Twelve to 14 days later, the patient develops a flu-like illness, with high fever, malaise, headache, and back pain. The characteristic rash begins in the mouth and on the face and arms, before spreading to the trunk and legs. This rash may resemble chickenpox at first glance; however, unlike chickenpox, smallpox lesions are all in the same stage of development and tend to be focused on the face and extremities (Figure 32-3). The lesions turn to blisters that fill with pus, leaving significant scars if the patient recovers.

The patient is most contagious during the first seven to ten days of the rash. Smallpox is easily spread through the air by droplets from coughing or sneezing, or through direct contact with an infected person, contaminated bedding, or clothing. Hospitalized patients require specialized rooms with negative air pressure and air-handling filtration. Hospital employees must take special precautions and wear protective gear to protect themselves from becoming infected with smallpox.

Currently there is no proven effective treatment for smallpox. The patient is given supportive therapy, which may include antibiotics to prevent secondary bacterial infection.

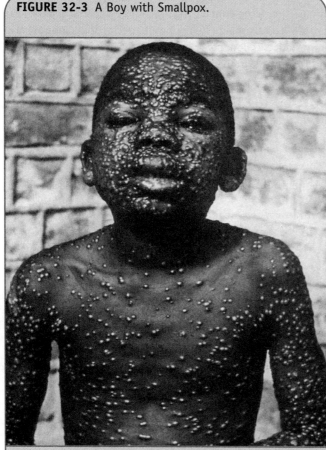

FIGURE 32-3 A Boy with Smallpox.

Source: From Public Health Image Library. ID # 3268. CDC Content Provider. Available at http://phil.cdc.gov/phil/details.asp. Accessed August 14, 2007.

Public Health Perspective

Smallpox is perhaps the most feared of the biological agents. Renowned bioterror expert D.A. Henderson stated that, "the deliberate reintroduction of smallpox as an epidemic disease would be an international crime of unprecedented proportions." A single case of smallpox in the world would be an international health emergency.

Because routine vaccination against smallpox ended in the early 1980s, the United States population is susceptible to smallpox. In December of 2002, President Bush released his plan to begin vaccinating "smallpox response teams" that could provide initial care for victims in the event of a smallpox attack. In 2003, nearly 40,000 civilian medical and public health workers were vaccinated. However, the controversial program was discontinued due to adverse reactions to the vaccine. Now the vaccine is approved for post-exposure prophylaxis.

Response to a smallpox attack must be rapid and aggressive. Infected persons need to be identified quickly through intensive surveillance and isolated to prevent further transmission. If administered in the first four days after exposure, smallpox vaccine may prevent or lessen the severity of the disease; therefore, an exhaustive **epidemiologic investigation** would ensue. All household members and primary contacts of cases would be immunized; then, close contacts of the primary contacts would be immunized in growing concentric circles. In addition to this "ring vaccination" strategy, key populations would be targeted for immunization, including healthcare workers, first responders, public health staff, and transit workers. The United States currently has sufficient vaccine to immunize everyone in the country if needed. The CDC's *Smallpox Plan and Response Guide* (available on the Internet) describes the vaccination plan and other important smallpox public health strategies such as surveillance, case reporting, contact tracing, laboratory confirmation, and **quarantine**.

PLAGUE

Historical Perspective

The first known plague pandemic occurred from 542 to 767 AD, killing an estimated 40 million people from Africa to the Mediterranean. The earliest recorded use of plague as a biological weapon occurred in the 14th century. During its attack on Kaffa, the Tartar army experienced a plague outbreak. Soldiers hurled the corpses of plague victims over the city walls in an attempt to induce an epidemic in its enemies. This tactic may have led to the most devastating pandemic in history, known as the *Black Death*. Experts estimate that the plague pandemic killed one third to two thirds of the population of Europe and 75 million people worldwide. The resulting depopulation and devastating socioeconomic, cultural, and religious effects has earned plague a remarkable place in history.

There is evidence that the Japanese investigated the use of plague-infested fleas as a biological weapon during World War II. The United States also experimented with *Yersinia pestis* in the 1950s and 1960s before termination of its offensive biological weapons program.

The WHO reports 1,000 to 3,000 cases of plague worldwide every year. The United States has between 5 and 15 naturally occurring bubonic plague cases each year, usually in the West where plague is considered endemic in 17 states.

Clinical Perspective

Plague is caused by a Gram-negative bacterium called *Yersinia pestis*. The bubonic form of plague is usually transmitted to humans through the bite of an infected flea from a rodent. The typical case presentation of a patient with bubonic plague is swollen lymph nodes under the arms or in the groin (called buboes) and high fever (Figure 32-4). Bubonic plague is not contagious.

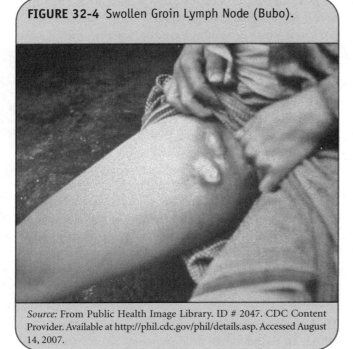

FIGURE 32-4 Swollen Groin Lymph Node (Bubo).

Source: From Public Health Image Library. ID # 2047. CDC Content Provider. Available at http://phil.cdc.gov/phil/details.asp. Accessed August 14, 2007.

Terrorists are more likely to disseminate the organism in an aerosolized form, leading to **pneumonic** (lung) plague. Following inhalation of the bacteria and an average incubation period of one to six days, the patient develops a flu-like **prodrome** and a cough with watery and then bloody sputum. A chest x-ray reveals evidence of pneumonia. If untreated, the patient rapidly develops severe respiratory distress, shock, and death.

Pneumonic plague can be treated with antibiotics, which must be started within 24 hours of the onset of illness to be effective. Pneumonic plague has a 100 percent mortality rate if left untreated. Pneumonic plague is very contagious through respiratory droplets from coughing or sneezing; therefore, hospitalized patients with confirmed or suspected plague should be isolated and placed on respiratory precautions.

Public Health Perspective

Syndromic surveillance is an important strategy to mitigate the impact of a biological attack with plague. Fortunately, most physicians have been trained to send a sputum (phlegm) sample to the lab in patients with bloody sputum to rule out tuberculosis, but it is important that clinicians are trained to consider the diagnosis of plague as well. Furthermore, laboratory technicians must be trained to identify the characteristic strain of the plague organism under the microscope so they can notify the appropriate public health officials.

People who have been exposed to plague from a face-to-face contact or a known biological attack can receive prophy-

lactic antibiotics. Therefore, a coordinated public health response including contact tracing and an aggressive antibiotic prophylaxis campaign following an attack with plague are also important components of mitigation. Currently there is no vaccine for plague in the United States, but research is under way.

BOTULINUM TOXIN

Historical Perspective

Botulism comes from the Latin word *botulus*, meaning sausage. When naturally occurring botulism was first recognized in Europe in the 18th century, many cases were due to homemade blood sausage. The Japanese were the first to use botulinum toxin as a weapon in the 1930s when they fed cultures of the bacteria to their prisoners during the occupation of Manchuria. The toxin was weaponized by the United States during World War II, and more recently by Russia, Iraq, Iran, North Korea, and Syria. Following the Persian Gulf War, Iraq admitted to United Nations inspectors that it had produced 19,000 L of botulinum toxin, loading 10,000 L into weapons. In the 1990s, the Japanese cult Aum Shinrikyo attempted numerous times to deploy botulinum toxin before its successful attack in a Tokyo subway station with sarin in 1995.

Although terrorists could use botulinum toxin to contaminate food or a water source, it is likely to be aerosolized as a weapon. It is extremely potent: experts estimate that if deployed effectively, a single gram of botulinum toxin could kill more than a million people.

In the United States, there is an average of 110 naturally occurring cases of botulism each year; approximately 72 percent are infantile botulism (from ingestion of the bacteria and production of toxin in the intestine) and 25 percent are foodborne (from improperly prepared or canned food). Wound infections in injection drug users are a rising cause of botulism.

Clinical Perspective

Botulism is caused by exposure to one or more of the seven neurotoxins produced by *Clostridium botulinum*, a spore-forming bacterium that is found naturally in soil.

Whether ingested or inhaled, the clinical syndrome of botulism poisoning is the same (Figure 32-5). After an incubation period of six hours to two weeks (often 12–36 hours), the victim begins experiencing paralysis in a descending pattern. Symptoms include double vision, difficulty swallowing and talking, and then descending weakness and difficulty breathing as the respiratory muscles become paralyzed. Botulism does not affect the mental status, and the patient does not develop a fever.

Because most clinicians have never seen a case of botulism, victims initially may be misdiagnosed with another neurolog-

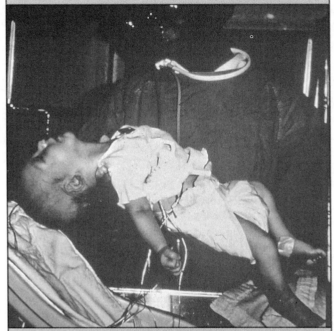

FIGURE 32-5 Six-Week-Old Infant with Botulism.

Source: From Public Health Image Library. ID # 1935. CDC Content Provider. Available at http://phil.cdc.gov/phil/details.asp. Accessed August 14, 2007.

ical process, such as stroke. Diagnosis is made based on symptoms; laboratory testing is not generally helpful. Botulism is not contagious; therefore, patients do not need to be isolated, and healthcare providers may use standard precautions. The mainstay of treatment in botulism poisoning is ventilatory support, and recovery can take weeks to months. A botulinum *antitoxin* is available in limited quantities from the CDC and from some state health departments. It can prevent progression of the disease but is not a cure. There is no vaccine against botulism.

Public Health Perspective

Botulinum toxin is considered a major biological threat due to its ease of production, extreme potency, and need for prolonged intensive care of victims. This presents a challenge for the healthcare system, as there is a limit to intensive care unit (ICU) capacity. **Surge capacity** planning is a major component of healthcare system emergency preparedness, and one of the focuses of federal funding in the last five years has been increasing ICU bed spaces. Extra ventilators are an important component of the CDC's Strategic National Stockpile.

Surveillance is a key public health strategy against botulism in the United States. Botulism is a reportable disease, and every suspected case is treated as a public health emergency and must be investigated immediately to determine the source.

TULAREMIA

Historical Perspective

In the early 1900s, the investigation of a suspected plague outbreak in San Francisco turned up a new organism dubbed *Bacterium tularense*. A United States Public Health Service physician, Dr. Edward Francis, devoted his life to researching this new disease and as such the organism was renamed *Francisella tularensis* in his honor. The organism was weaponized in the 1950s by the United States, and probably other countries, but U.S. stockpiles were destroyed when its program was abolished.

Tularemia occurs naturally in the United States with about 150 cases per year, mostly in Arkansas. In 1995, the CDC removed tularemia from the list of reportable diseases but reversed that decision in 2000 due to the threat of bioterrorism.

Clinical Perspective

Tularemia, also known as *rabbit fever* and *deer fly fever*, is caused by a small Gram-negative coccobacillus. While the most common natural route of exposure is via a bite from an infected arthropod, infection can also occur by direct contact with infected animal tissue, ingestion of contaminated food and inhalation. *F. tularensis* is a highly virulent organism when inhaled, requiring only 10 to 50 organisms to infect an individual.

The clinical presentation depends on the location of inoculation with the bacteria (Figure 32-6). Up to six different forms of infection have been documented including: typhoidal,

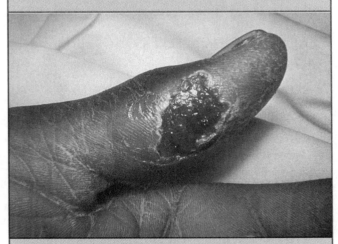

FIGURE 32-6 Skin Ulcer of Ulceroglandular Tularemia.

Source: From Public Health Image Library. ID # 1344. Emory U. and Dr. Sellers Content Providers. Available at http://phil.cdc.gov/phil/details.asp. Accessed August 14, 2007.

ulceroglandular, glandular, oculoglandular, oropharyngeal, and pneumonic. As with all other Category A agents, terrorists are likely to disseminate tularemia as an aerosol, leading to the typhoidal form of illness. The average incubation period is three to five days. Patients present with fever, prostration, cough, chest pain, and weight loss in addition to pneumonia, which may be severe.

No person-to-person spread of tularemia has been reported; therefore, standard precautions should be followed for those treating suspected tularemia patients. Untreated tularemia results in approximately 35 percent mortality, but with antibiotics that rate can drop to 1 percent to 3 percent. Fortunately tularemia responds well to common antibiotics including streptomycin, gentamicin, and ciprofloxacin.

Public Health Perspective

In the 1970s, the World Health Organization published a report stating that 50 kg of aerosolized tularemia dispersed in a metropolitan area with 5 million inhabitants would cause 250,000 disabling illnesses and 19,000 deaths. Tularemia is an attractive weapon of terrorism due to its high virulence, nonspecific symptomatology, and high mortality rate. Fortunately, the high mortality rate can be mitigated with treatment.

In the event of an attack with tularemia, a mass prophylaxis campaign will be an important strategy. As very few organisms are needed to cause the typhoidal or pneumonic form of the disease, a successful aerosol attack could lead to a frightening number of victims. Ciprofloxacin or doxycycline for two weeks provides adequate prophylactic protection to exposed individuals. An investigational live attenuated vaccine is being studied; however, a post-exposure vaccination program with an unapproved vaccine might be difficult to institute within the short incubation period.

VIRAL HEMORRHAGIC FEVERS

Historical Perspective

Viral hemorrhagic fevers (VHFs) are popular with Western media for their grotesque and dramatic symptomatology including extensive bruising, bleeding from mucous membranes, and high mortality rates. The 1995 movie *Outbreak* features an Ebola-like illness from Zaire with 100 percent mortality. Popular nonfiction and fiction books on Ebola include Richard Preston's *The Hot Zone* and Tom Clancy's *Executive Orders*. Ebola-like illnesses also have been featured on television shows like *CSI* and *24*.

VHFs were weaponized by the former Soviet Union and by the United States up until the end of its biological weapons program in 1969. Some terrorist organizations, most notably the Aum Shinrikyo cult in Japan, have tried unsuccessfully to weaponize the viruses. In his book *Biohazard*, defector Ken Alibek describes the former Soviet Union's bioweapons program in which Ebola was genetically engineered and combined with smallpox to increase transmissibility and lethality. To date there are no known instances of VHFs being used as biological weapons.

Clinical Perspective

The viral hemorrhagic fevers are a diverse group of illnesses caused by at least 15 RNA viruses, of which 7 are classified as Category A biological agents by the CDC. While each of the viruses has specific symptoms and a predilection for certain organs, they all eventually result in a common end: uncontrollable bleeding.

VHF should be suspected in any patient who presents with severe flu-like illness, high fever, and evidence of involvement of the vascular system including: low blood pressure, flushing of the face and chest, and bruising of the skin. Approximately 70 percent of Ebola patients will experience the cardinal sign of bleeding mucous membranes including gums, nose, gastrointestinal tract, and eyes. During the second week of the infection, the patient either recovers or quickly deteriorates and succumbs to the disease. The mortality rate for VHFs ranges from 23 percent to 90 percent. There is no specific treatment recognized to decrease mortality, so supportive therapy is all healthcare professionals can provide.

Public Health Perspective

A terrorist attack with a viral hemorrhagic fever is a frightening prospect for many reasons. The potential for dissemination via an aerosolized particle and ease of spread is worrisome, as is the potentially long incubation period that could make identifying a source of release difficult. Diagnosis of VHF is uncommon in the United States, with very few physicians ever seeing a case. This rarity can lead to missed or delayed diagnoses allowing the patient to continue infecting those around him or her.

Fortunately, the weaponization of VHFs is relatively difficult. Without proper equipment and protection, as can be found in a highly specialized laboratory at the CDC, exposure to and infection by a VHF is exceedingly possible for those attempting to develop the agent as a weapon.

CONCLUSION

Biological weapons continue to pose a significant threat to our nation (Table 32-1). United States countermeasures include the development of vaccines, implementation of early warning surveillance systems, and stockpiling of medications, equipment, and supplies to care for potential victims. These efforts do not take place in a vacuum, however; they are integrated

TABLE 32-1 Category A Biological Agents

Disease	Transmission	Treatment	Special Precautions	Potential Threat
Smallpox	Contact with infected materials including cadavers, droplet and airborne	Supportive care once infected, vaccine available for prophylaxis	Gown, gloves, HEPA mask, and negative pressure room. Isolation of patient.	High: Over half the U.S. population is not vaccinated. High mortality rate.
Plague	Inoculation by flea, inhalation of aerosolized bacteria	Antibiotics	Gown, gloves, HEPA mask, and negative pressure room. Isolation of patient.	High: Relatively ubiquitous in nature. Dissemination via rodents and fleas possible.
Tularemia	Environmental exposures, animal bites, inhalation. No person-to-person transmission	Antibiotics	Gown and gloves	High: Initial cases may mimic natural occurrences. Low inoculation size for infection.
Anthrax	Inhalation or contact with spores, or infected tissue. No person-to-person transmission	Antibiotics, vaccine available to select populations	Gown and gloves, decontaminate infected person if spores remain on skin.	High: Easily disseminated via aerosolized spores. High mortality rate.
Botulinum Toxin	Must be ingested, inhaled, or injected	Supportive care including ventilation until toxin is metabolized	None.	High: Most potent toxin known to man.
Viral Hemorrhagic Fevers	Contact with infected materials including cadavers, droplet and possibly airborne	Supportive care	Gown, gloves, HEPA mask, and negative pressure room. Isolation of patient.	High: Naturally occurring in epidemics, may not be recognized early on.

into the wider context of public health as a whole. Monies invested in bioterrorism preparedness have the dual benefit of enhancing preparedness for epidemics and pandemics of naturally occurring diseases, such as influenza, and emerging infectious diseases, such as severe acute respiratory syndrome (SARS).

The public health arena plays a vital role in preparation for, and response to, a biological weapons attack. Only through a strong public health infrastructure and a coordinated medical response will we be ready to face the threat of bioterrorism.

KEY TERMS

Biology Terms

Cutaneous: Relating to the skin (for example, cutaneous anthrax is infection of the skin resulting from direct contact with the bacteria *Bacillus anthracis*).

Incubation Period: Time lapse between exposure to a biological agent (infection) and the onset of clinical symptoms, usually several days to several weeks.

Pneumonic or **Pulmonary:** Relating to the lung, from inhalation of the biological agent (for example, pneumonic plague results from inhalation of *Yersinia pestis*).

Prodrome: Early symptoms indicating development of a disease; in biological terrorism, the most common prodrome is a flu-like illness, with fever, muscle pain, headache, and profound weakness.

Standard Precautions: Measures that healthcare personnel take to reduce the risk of transmission of infection, including the donning of gown, gloves, mask, and eye protection during patient care involving bodily fluids.

Zoonotic Disease: Infectious disease that can be transmitted from animals to humans (for example, anthrax, plague, and tularemia).

Public Health Terms

Epidemiologic Investigation: Process that determines the presence of an outbreak or biological attack, confirms the diagnosis, establishes the case definition, traces exposures and contacts, and characterizes the outbreak or attack (where, when, how, etc.).

Isolation: Separation of patients with a communicable disease from noninfected individuals, preventing transmission of infection to others, and allowing focused care.

Prophylaxis: Medical intervention to prevent disease. Antibiotics and antivirals are chemoprophylactics (medications); vaccines are referred to as immunoprophylactics.

Quarantine: Enforced isolation of the sick or exposed from healthy people to contain the spread of disease.

Surge Capacity: Ability to expand healthcare during periods of excessive and/or prolonged demand.

Syndromic Surveillance: Use of certain symptom complexes and other health-related data to detect a potential outbreak or biological attack in its early phases so that public health measures may be rapidly mobilized to decrease morbidity and mortality. Examples of surrogate data sources include school absenteeism, sale of over-the-counter medications, and Emergency Department presenting complaints.

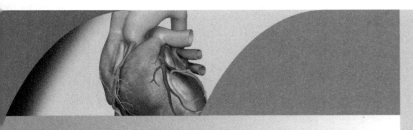

Questions for Further Research, Study, Reflection, and Discussion

In order to answer these questions, it may be necessary to research the primary literature.

- Why is a biological attack so difficult to detect initially? What are some epidemiological clues that a biologic attack has occurred?
- What is the Centers for Disease Control and Prevention's *Strategic National Stockpile*? What preparations has the CDC made for deployment and how would it be implemented?
- Community containment strategies are fundamental public health measures used to control the spread of disease. What is "social distancing"? What are the challenges to enforced quarantine?
- How might preparedness for bioterrorism improve preparedness for pandemic influenza?

EXERCISES/ACTIVITIES

- You are the Emergency Preparedness Coordinator for a 300-bed hospital in an urban area on the East Coast. What kinds of equipment, supplies, and medications would you purchase to create a bioterrorism stockpile? Describe one source of federal funding that is being used by the healthcare system to improve bioterrorism preparedness.
- Read Chapter One ("Filth and Decay") of Laurie Garrett's *Betrayal of Trust: The Collapse of Global Public Health*.[3] Discuss the confluence and cascade of events that culminated in the plague epidemic and societal panic in India in 1994. Do you think the public's response to a biological attack with plague in a major U.S. city would be similar or different?

REFERENCES

1. Hirschberg R, La Montagne J, Fauci AS. Biomedical research—an integral component of national security. *N Engl J Med* 2004;350:2119–2121.

2. Alibek K, Handelman S. *Biohazard: The Chilling True Story of the Largest Covert Biological Weapons Program in the World—Told from the Inside by the Man Who Ran It.* New York: Delta (Random House); 2000: 319 pp.

3. Garrett L. *Betrayal of Trust: The Collapse of Global Public Health.* New York: Hyperion; 2000.

RESOURCES

Centers for Disease Control and Prevention. Update: investigation of bioterrorism-related anthrax and interim guidelines for exposure management and antimicrobial therapy, October 2001. *MMWR Morbid Mortal Wkly Rep* 2001;50: 909–919 (see Erratum).

Centers for Disease Control and Prevention. Smallpox response plan and guidelines. Version 3.0. Atlanta: CDC; 2002. Available at http://www.bt.cdc.gov/agent/smallpox/response-plan/. Accessed April 29, 2008.

Arnon SS, Schechter R, Inglesby TV, et al., for the Working Group on Civilian Biodefense. Botulinum toxin as a biological weapon: medical and public health management. *JAMA* 2001;285:1059–1070.

Borio L, Inglesby TV, Peters CJ, et al., for the Working Group on Civilian Biodefense. The hemorrhagic fever viruses as biological weapons: medical and public health management. *JAMA* 2002;287:2391–2405.

Darling RG, Catlett CL, Huebner KD, et al. Threats in bioterrorism I: CDC category A agents. *Emerg Med Clin N Am* 2002;20:273–309.

Dennis DT, Inglesby TV, Henderson DA, et al. Tularemia as a biological weapon: medical and public health management. *JAMA* 2001;285:2763–2773.

Gursky E, Inglesby TV, O'Toole T. Anthrax 2001: observations on the medical and public health response. *Biosecurity Bioterrorism* 2003;1:97–110.

Henderson DA, Inglesby TV, Bartlett JG, et al., for the Working Group on Civilian Defense. Smallpox as a biological weapon: medical and public health management. *JAMA* 1999;281:2127–2137.

Inglesby TV, Dennis DT, Henderson DA, et al., for the Working Group on Civilian Biodefense. Plague as a biological weapon: medical and public health management. *JAMA* 2000;283:2281–2290.

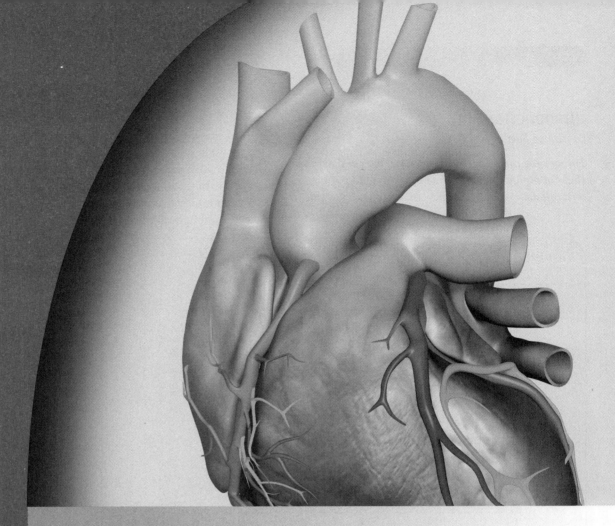

PART V

The Public Health Burden of Chronic Disease

INTRODUCTION

Constance Battle

Hungry Joe collected lists of fatal diseases and arranged them in alphabetical order so that he could put his finger without delay on any one he wanted to worry about.[1]

—Heller J. *Catch 22*

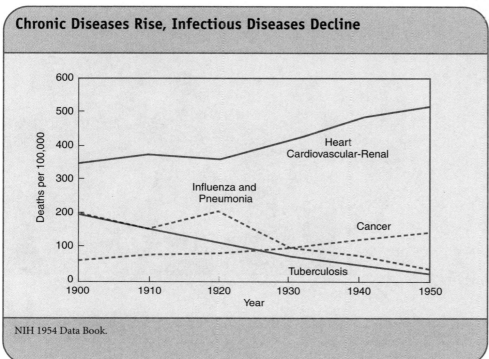

Chronic Diseases Rise, Infectious Diseases Decline

NIH 1954 Data Book.

The above graph, recreated from a dramatic page in the 1954 NIH data book, reveals one of the many extraordinary transitions in the history of public health.[2] This illustration appeared among a group used to buttress NIH's budget presentation to Congress. It clearly demonstrates the acknowledged highest place award to heart disease as the greatest killer as far back as the graph goes, 1900, reflecting perhaps the seemingly inevitability of heart disease and stroke in old age. Medicine did not make a major inroad against these diseases until the blood pressure–lowering drugs became available in the 1950s and the ACE inhibitors in the 1980s and until the National Heart and Lung blood pressure education program was started in 1972. The rising trend for cancer deaths parallels the rise of public concern with cancer as a major problem and the establishment of the National Cancer Institute at the NIH in 1937. Cancer deaths surpassed infectious disease deaths in the 1930s, and by 1937 sulfa drugs had been introduced. The message of this graph is that both cancer and heart disease rose annually after World War II while tuberculosis, flu, and pneumonia decreased as causes of death.

This historical snapshot captures the dramatic change during the last century in the profile of diseases contributing most heavily to deaths among Americans. As a result, the field of public health shifted and expanded its past primary focus on infectious disease to embrace a focus on major non-communicable diseases (NCDs). In summary, the rise of the public health burden of chronic disease has not simply replaced the burden of infectious disease but rather contributed to a double burden of disease globally today.[3]

At the beginning of the 21st century, chronic diseases such as those covered in this part (hypertension, heart disease, diabetes, asthma, stroke, kidney disease, arthritis, osteoporosis, Alzheimer disease, and depression) are the leading causes of death and disability in the United States and account for the vast majority of the health care spending.[4] These diseases are responsible for 7 out of every 10 deaths in the United States per year and when they do not kill, they profoundly affect the quality of life for 133 million Americans.[4,5]

The chapter on depression addresses patterned maladaptation encompassing problems in three domains: biological, physiological, and behavioral adjustment. The chapter on sleep addresses the important biochemical and physiological processes which occur during sleep. The importance of sleep loss has been documented repeatedly to impact negatively on metabolic and hormonal physiology, diabetes and obesity, immune system function, and cardiac disease. Society faces numerous problems due to poor sleep, which have major public health consequences across the lifespan.

REFERENCES

1. Heller J. (1955). *Catch 22* New York: Simon and Schuster.
2. National Institutes of Health. *1954 NIH Data Book* Bethesda, MD p. 3.
3. Yach D, Hawkes C, Gould CL, Hofman KJ. The global burden of chronic diseases overcoming impediments to prevention and control. JAMA 2004;291(21):2616–2622.
4. Centers for Disease Control and Prevention National Center for Chronic Disease Prevention and health Promotion. Chronic disease overview. Available at: http://www.cdc.gov/nccdphp/overview.htm Accessed January 19, 2008.
5. Wu S, Green A. Projection of chronic illness prevalence and cost inflation. RAND Corporation, October 2000.

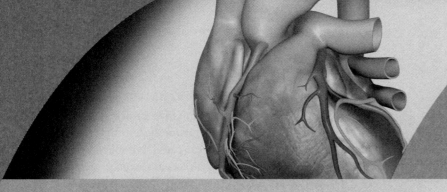

CHAPTER 33

Hypertension and the Kidney

Randall Packer
Richard Billingsley
Daniel Webb

According to the American Heart Association (2007) one in three U.S. adults has high blood pressure, but because there are no symptoms, nearly one third of these people don't know they have it. In fact, many people have high blood pressure for years without knowing it. Uncontrolled high blood pressure can lead to stroke, heart attack, heart failure, or kidney failure. This is the reason why high blood pressure is often called the "silent killer."

LEARNING OBJECTIVES

By the end of this chapter, the student will be able to:

- Discuss the factors that contribute to high blood pressure.
- Explain the functional anatomy of the kidneys.
- Outline the body physiological responses to changes in extracellular fluid volume (ECFV).
- Explain the complex relationship between kidney disease and hypertension.
- Discuss diet-related and pharmaceutical-based clinical interventions to control hypertension.
- Analyze the public health burden of hypertension and discuss which populations face the highest risk.

INTRODUCTION

In the United States approximately 60 million people suffer from **hypertension**. Around 90 percent of those are said to have primary hypertension, that is, no specific cause of hypertension can be identified. The remaining 10 percent suffer from secondary hypertension, which can be caused by a number of different conditions. Most of us are aware that high blood pressure contributes to cardiovascular disease such as strokes and heart attacks, but it is also true that hypertension is often associated with chronic kidney disease (CKD). It is well established that treatment of hypertension in people with CKD slows further deterioration of renal function. However, the complex relationships between hypertension and kidney disease are incompletely understood. CKD in hypertensive patients often progresses to end-stage renal disease (ESRD). In the United States in 2004 over 300,000 individuals were being treated for ESRD. Of that number, about 100,000 were new patients and the number of new patients treated each year is increasing. ESRD is treatable by dialysis or transplant but treatment is very expensive. ESRD contributes significantly to morbidity and mortality, especially in the oldest quartile of the population. The dramatic increases in the incidence of hypertension and kidney disease are associated with the well publicized increase in obesity in many developed nations, including the United States.

When we speak of blood pressure what we are really discussing is systemic arterial pressure, which in a healthy adult is about 120/80 mm Hg. **Systolic pressure** refers to the level of blood pressure while the heart is contracting and is represented by the top number (120 mm Hg). **Diastolic pressure**, the level of blood pressure in between heart contractions, is represented by the bottom number (80 mm Hg). Hypertension is clinically defined as pressures greater than 140/90 mm Hg.

OVERVIEW

What Causes High Blood Pressure?

In the most immediate terms, blood pressure is determined directly by two factors: cardiac output, the volume of blood pumped by the heart each minute, and the resistance to blood flow in the vessels, primarily the arterioles. Vascular resistance is a result of friction as blood flows through the vessels and the smaller the diameter of the vessels the higher the resistance. The relationships among pressure, flow, and resistance are quite simple:

$$Pressure = Flow \times Resistance$$

An increase in the volume of blood the heart is pumping per minute or a decrease in the diameter of vessels (an increase in resistance) will increase blood pressure.

A number of neural and hormonal pathways act on the cardiovascular system to regulate blood pressure. The most important neural regulation is via the autonomic nervous system. Sympathetic stimulation increases both the rate and force of contraction of the heart to increase cardiac output. In many blood vessels, sympathetic stimulation causes contraction of vascular smooth muscle. That contraction increases resistance due to the decreased arteriolar diameter. Somewhat counterintuitively, contraction of vascular smooth muscle in veins has little effect on systemic resistance. Instead, the effect is to increase venous return and thus cardiac output (flow). Hormones, including epinephrine from the adrenal medulla, act directly on the cardiovascular system to affect blood pressure. Abnormal function of any of the pathways that regulate cardiovascular function or pathological changes in the heart or vessels can cause hypertension.

What Does Kidney Function Have to Do with Blood Pressure?

In addition to excreting wastes, the kidneys help regulate blood pressure through regulation of extracellular fluid volume (ECFV). If, for example, a person eats a salty meal and drinks a large amount of water, ECFV increases. In a healthy person the kidneys act quickly to excrete the excess salt and water, returning ECFV to normal. If, on the other hand, some of the excess salt and water is retained rather than excreted, ECFV may be maintained above normal causing a long-term increase in blood pressure. Hypertension can be caused by pathological changes in kidney tissue or in the associated nervous or hormonal regulatory systems.

In the medical literature, there is an ongoing discussion of the complex relationship between hypertension and renal disease. It is well known that hypertensive individuals are at risk of developing kidney disease. Similarly, abnormal activation of the renin-angiotensin-**aldosterone** system that regulates several aspects of renal function can cause secondary hypertension, hypertension for which a direct cause can be identified.

Drugs that are used to treat blood pressure include pharmacological agents that directly target the circulatory system and reduce both flow and resistance, including the so-called beta-blockers (atenolol, propranalol) and calcium channel blockers (lacidipine, nicardipine). They decrease cardiac output by decreasing the force and rate of ventricular contraction, thus lowering cardiac output. They also cause arterioles to dilate, lowering resistance.

BASIC SCIENCE FACTS/KEY CONCEPTS REVIEW

Functional Anatomy of the Kidneys

To understand more completely how kidney function and hypertension are related, we first summarize several basic aspects of kidney function as they relate to control of blood pressure. We do that by looking at the anatomy of the kidneys and relating structure at the tissue and cellular levels to regulation of sodium and water balance.

As can be seen in Figure 33-1, the kidneys are paired organs that lie against the dorsal body wall in the abdominal cavity. Each kidney is a bean-shaped organ about the size of your fist. Two large vessels, the renal artery and the renal vein, enter and exit each kidney along with a thin-walled duct, the ureter, which carries urine to the urinary bladder where it is stored, awaiting periodic urination (Figure 33-2).

If you were to cut a section through a freshly dissected kidney, you could observe that there are two distinct tissue layers: the outer cortex and a number of pyramidal-shaped structures underneath that comprise the renal medulla (Figure 33-2). Each medullary pyramid is attached at the bottom to one of the branches of the ureter. Those branches form the renal pelvis; urine flows from small openings in the tip of each medullary pyramid into the renal pelvis and then into the ureter.

What the gross anatomy of the kidney does not reveal is the orderly arrangement of blood vessels and small tubules called **nephrons** that are the functional units of the kidney. Each human kidney contains about one million nephrons. The parts of the nephron are shown in Figure 33-3. In fact, there are two types of nephron, cortical nephrons (the larger number) that have short loops of Henle and juxtamedullary nephrons that have long loops of Henle, descending deep into the medulla.

Both types of nephrons filter plasma across the glomerular capillaries, delivering fluid very much like plasma, less blood cells and proteins, into the first part of the proximal tubule.

FIGURE 33-1 Drawing of Torso Showing the Location of the Kidneys and the Urinary System.

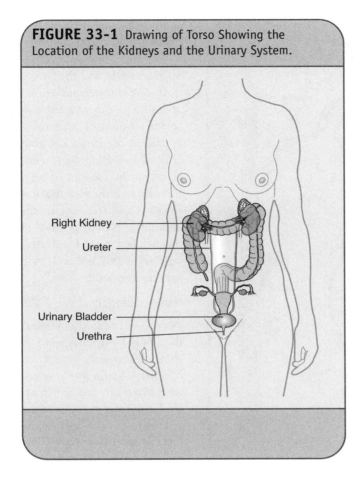

Right Kidney

Ureter

Urinary Bladder

Urethra

FIGURE 33-2 A Sagittal Section of the Kidney.

Adrenal Gland

Renal Artery

Renal Vein

Renal Pelvis

Ureter

Cortex

Medulla

About 120 mL/min of filtrate (the **glomerular filtration rate** [GFR]) is produced in an adult. In contrast, only about 1 mL/min of urine is delivered to the ureters. This means that more than 99 percent of the fluid filtered in the glomeruli is reabsorbed back into the peritubular capillaries that adjoin all the various segments of the nephron. Maintenance of normal ECFV requires precise regulation of **reabsorption** of both sodium and water.

As mentioned earlier, kidney function affects blood pressure primarily by regulating sodium and water excretion, thereby controlling ECFV. An important aspect of that regulation is that the kidneys are able to vary water and solute excretion somewhat independently of one another. For example, if a person eats a diet containing a moderate amount of salt and drinks a large volume of water, urine volume is high and the salt concentration is moderate. On the other hand, if the same diet is eaten but water intake is limited, the urine volume will be lower but salt concentration will be higher. In both examples, the amount of sodium excreted in urine is the same but water excretion is different.

The ability to vary the amount of water excreted in urine depends on water and solute transports in the loops of Henle and in collecting ducts. Those transports, especially in juxtamedullary nephrons, can establish an axial gradient of osmotic concentration that increases reabsorption of water from the urine in the collecting ducts back into blood capillaries when a person is dehydrated. Under those conditions, the osmotic concentration of the interstitial fluid increases from 300 mOsm in the cortex, the osmotic concentration of extracellular fluid throughout the body, to as high as 1,200 mOsm in the inner medulla. That osmotic gradient can extract water from collecting duct fluid, decreasing urine volume and conserving water when water intake is low.

Sodium Ion and Water Transports

Sodium Balance

To a large degree, the sodium content of the body determines ECFV and thus blood volume and blood pressure. To maintain constant body sodium and extracellular fluid sodium ion (Na+) concentration, urinary Na+ output must be adjusted in response to differing amounts of Na+ in the diet. The rate of glomerular filtration is held nearly constant over the long term in a healthy kidney so the amount of Na+ delivered to the

FIGURE 33-3 Nephron Structure.

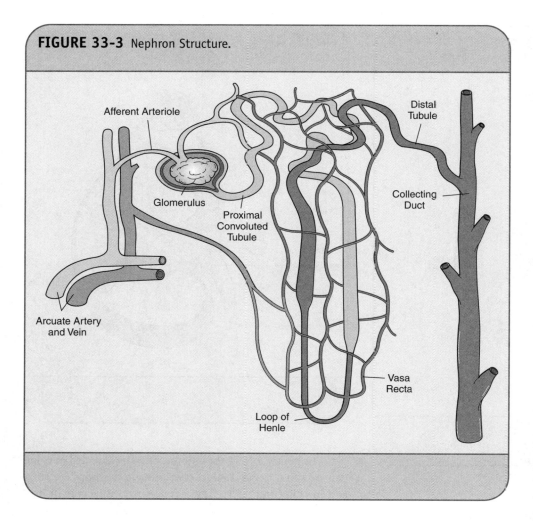

- Afferent Arteriole
- Glomerulus
- Proximal Convoluted Tubule
- Arcuate Artery and Vein
- Loop of Henle
- Distal Tubule
- Collecting Duct
- Vasa Recta

sodium channel (ENaC). Several hormones, including atrial natriuretic peptide (ANP), angiotensin II, and the steroid hormone aldosterone, are responsible for precise regulation of the amount of Na+ reabsorbed in the distal nephron and the collecting duct to ensure that the amount of Na+ excreted in urine plus that lost in sweat and feces equals the amount of Na+ consumed in the diet, helping to keep extracellular fluid volume and blood pressure constant.

Water Balance

Water is added to the extracellular fluid by drinking and by oxidative metabolic production of water. Water is lost in sweat, in expired air, and in urine. Under normal conditions the amount of water lost in the feces is relatively small. The kidneys adjust the amount of water lost in urine in response to changes in ECFV and composition.

first part of the proximal tubule is also more or less constant. Since there is a relatively high Na+ concentration in plasma, a large and precisely regulated quantity of Na+ must be reabsorbed back into the blood from the fluid in the nephrons.

About 70 percent of filtered Na+ is reabsorbed in the proximal tubule where Na+ reabsorption is linked to reabsorption of filtered metabolites such as glucose and amino acids and transport of wastes such as protons and ammonium ions. Some of the transporters involved in Na+ reabsorption are illustrated in Figure 33-4. Although the bulk of the filtered Na+ is reabsorbed here, the linkage of Na+ reabsorption to transport of other molecules means that Na+ transport here is not regulated in a way that optimizes Na+ balance. That role is played by more distal parts of the nephron.

Fine adjustments of Na+ reabsorption, and thus Na+ balance, begin in the distal tubule where Na+ and Cl– are reabsorbed via the Na-Cl cotransporter (NCC). In the principle cells of the collecting duct, final adjustments to the balance between Na+ reabsorption and excretion are made by regulation of the amount of Na+ reabsorbed through the epithelial

The amount of water lost in urine is regulated by the antidiuretic peptide hormone vasopressin, released from the posterior pituitary. Vasopressin has three major effects:

1. It increases NaCl reabsorption in the thick ascending limb of nephrons. A countercurrent mechanism establishes a gradient of NaCl concentration in medullary interstitial fluid.
2. Water channels (aquaporin 2) are recruited to the apical membrane of collecting duct cells, increasing water permeability.
3. The urea permeability of the terminal segment of the collecting duct increases dramatically by stimulating the urea transporter (UT1). Urea exits the collecting duct at the end before it drains urine into the renal pelvis, establishing a high urea concentration in the interstitial fluid of the inner medulla.

Together, the high concentrations of NaCl and urea in medullary interstitial fluid draw water out of the collecting duct by osmosis through water channels, decreasing urine vol-

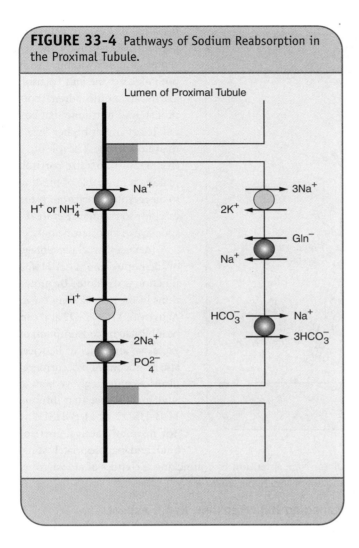

FIGURE 33-4 Pathways of Sodium Reabsorption in the Proximal Tubule.

Lumen of Proximal Tubule

response to low blood pressure and to decreases in the amount of Na+ in glomerular filtrate. Acting as an enzyme, renin converts the plasma protein angiotensinogen to angiotensin I. As blood passes through the lungs and kidneys angiotensin I is converted to angiotensin II by angiotensin-converting enzyme (ACE). Angiotensin II acts in several ways to increase blood pressure:

1. The hypothalamus–pituitary axis is activated by angiotensin II to increase thirst as well as increase the release of vasopressin. Drinking and decreased urine output increase and maintain ECFV.
2. Angiotensin II is a vasoconstrictor that increases arteriolar resistance and blood pressure.
3. In the proximal and distal tubules as well as the collecting duct, angiotensin II directly increases Na+ reabsorption aiding in maintenance of ECFV.
4. The adrenal cortex releases aldosterone in response to angiotensin II. In the distal tubule NCC is upregulated by aldosterone and ENaC activity is enhanced in the principle cells of the collecting duct, increasing Na+ reabsorption.

Increased ECFV

If extracellular fluid volume increases, blood pressure goes up and the volume of blood returning to the heart increases, stretching the walls of the atria more than normal. In response, atrial cells release the hormone ANP. ANP decreases thirst as well as reabsorption of Na+ in the collecting duct. It also suppresses the release of renin and vasopressin. The overall effect is increased NaCl and water excretion, increased urine volume, and decreased ECFV. Stretching of the atria also activates neural sensory pathways from the heart back to the brain to decrease vasopressin release. Pressure receptors in the carotid arteries and in the aorta signal neural regulatory centers in the brainstem to decrease sympathetic stimulation of the cardiovascular system, lowering blood pressure. Decreased sympathetic stimulation of the renal vasculature increases glomerular filtration. Activity the RAAS is downregulated by decreased sympathetic stimulation as well as by blood pressure sensing within the kidney itself, reducing Na+ reabsorption and thus increasing urinary Na+ excretion and urine volume.

Kidney Disease and Hypertension

As mentioned earlier, the relationships between kidney disease and hypertension are complex. Epidemiological studies show that hypertension predisposes people to chronic kidney disease, as does diabetes. In both cases, the specific causes of renal failure are incompletely known but are the subject of intensive clinical and basic science research.

ume. The recovered water is returned to capillaries in the renal medulla, minimizing water loss but allowing excretion of wastes and excess ions.

Responses to Changes in Extracellular Fluid Volume

Decreased ECFV

Substantial decreases in ECFV and low blood pressure can result from dehydration, Na+ loss, or blood loss. Both the cardiovascular system and the kidneys respond. In response to low blood pressure, there is a rapid increase in sympathetic activity that stimulates cardiac output and increases arteriolar resistance, raising blood pressure. Sympathetic stimulation also increases the release of the enzyme renin from the juxtaglomerular cells of the juxtaglomerular apparatus (Figure 33-5). The release of renin activates the renin-angiotensin-aldosterone pathway (RAAS) (Figure 33-6). Renin is also released from juxtaglomerular cells in direct

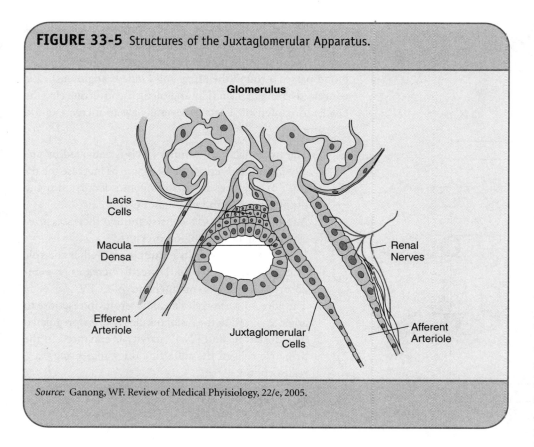

FIGURE 33-5 Structures of the Juxtaglomerular Apparatus.

Glomerulus

Lacis Cells

Macula Densa

Renal Nerves

Efferent Arteriole

Juxtaglomerular Cells

Afferent Arteriole

Source: Ganong, WF. Review of Medical Phyisiology, 22/e, 2005.

In the small fraction of patients with secondary hypertension, specific mechanisms are clear. There are several genetic mutations identified in human populations that cause hypertension due to abnormal kidney function. They mainly affect NCC in the distal tubule and ENaC in the collecting duct.

For example, in Liddle syndrome ENaC activity is abnormally high, causing excess Na+ reabsorption, increased ECFV, and hypertension.

Excess secretion of aldosterone, primary aldosteronism, can be caused by aldosterone-secreting tumor cells or other factors. Excessive amounts of circulating aldosterone lead to increases in Na+ reabsorption in nephrons so that total body sodium increases, ECVF increases, and hypertension develops.

As mentioned earlier, obesity is correlated with high blood pressure. Abnormally high levels of aldosterone are associated with abdominal obesity. No matter what the source, excess aldosterone can contribute to hypertension. Also, obese individuals often have high insulin levels due to type 2 diabetes and insulin increases Na+ retention.

A rare but interesting cause of kidney-associated hypertension results from dysregulation of the enzyme 11β-hydroxysteroid dehydrogenase (11 β-HSD2). In target cells, aldosterone binds to an intracellular receptor complex that migrates to the nucleus, modifying gene expression. Surprisingly, the receptor complex will bind with both aldosterone and cortisol. Cortisol is another adrenal cortical steroid hormone that circulates at much higher levels than aldosterone. The role of 11 β-HSD2 is to oxidize cortisol, making it incapable of binding to the receptor. This protects the receptor so that the cells are responsive to aldosterone only.

In a very small percentage of the population, 11 β-HSD2 function is disrupted by mutations in the gene coding for it. Activity of 11 β-HSD2 also can be inhibited by consumption of excessive amounts of licorice, also an uncommon occurrence. Licorice contains glycyrrhetinic acid, a substance that inhibits 11 β-HSD2. If 11 β-HSD2 is not normally active, cortisol binds and inappropriately stimulates Na+ retention by mimicking the effect of aldosterone, causing severe hypertension.

Managing Hypertension: Renal Aspects

Diet

People in the general population can be divided into non–salt-sensitive and salt-sensitive groups. In salt-sensitive people, ingestion of NaCl increases ECFV and blood pressure, at least transiently. Despite the fact that there is considerable disagreement in the scientific literature concerning the link between dietary salt intake and hypertension, physicians recommend that all hypertensive patients reduce salt intake. Because of the links between obesity, type 2 diabetes, hypertension, and kidney disease, increased exercise and weight loss are recommended also for overweight people with high blood pressure.

Drugs

A number of drugs that target kidney functions are commonly used to help manage hypertension. For many years, **diuretics** have been used to decrease blood pressure by increasing urine volume. Lasix is an example. It blocks the reabsorption of Na+ in the loop of Henle, reduces the medullary interstitial Na+ concentration gradient, and increases Na+ excretion.

FIGURE 33-6 Renin-Angiotensin-Aldosterone System.

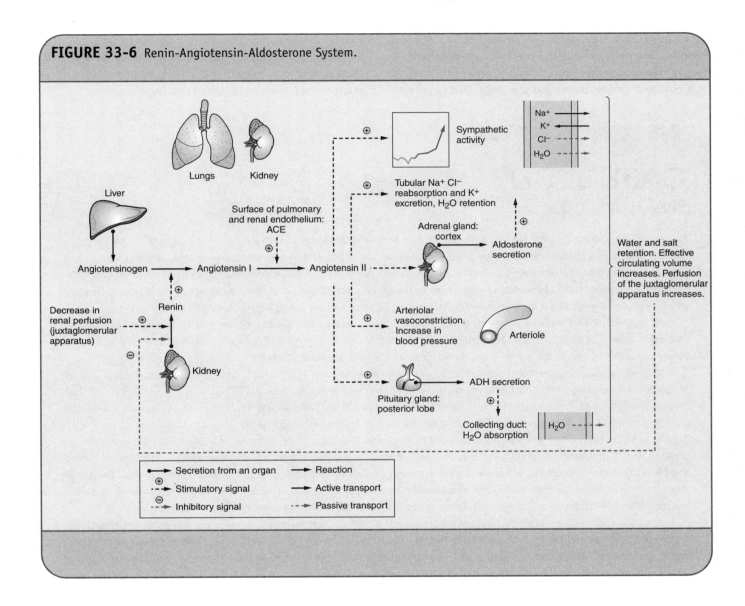

Both factors contribute to the resulting increased urine volume, decreased ECFV, and reduced blood pressure. Other diuretics such as thiazides inhibit reabsorption of NaCl by suppressing activity of NCC in the distal tubule.

Increasingly, pharmacological management of hypertension includes drugs that target the hormones and paracrine secretions of the RAAS. Spironolactone and eplerenone block the action of aldosterone. ACE inhibitors such as lisinopril and enalapril block the conversion of angiotensin I to angiotensin II, thereby attenuating all the pathways by which angiotensin II increases blood pressure (Figure 33-6). Finally, the cellular effects of angiotensin II are also blunted by drugs like losartan that block the binding of angiotensin II to its cellular receptors.

SUMMARY

Precise regulation of body Na+ content and extracellular fluid volume by the kidneys is necessary to maintain blood pressure within the normal range. Despite the elegant, interacting renal and cardiovascular control systems, problems develop. Hypertension and chronic kidney disease, especially as they are associated with obesity, are increasingly important public health problems. All the inter-relationships between hypertension and the development and progression of renal disease are not understood. In a relatively small proportion of people with secondary hypertension, renal defects like those outlined above cause hypertension. It is not so clear that hypertension in and of itself causes chronic kidney disease, but hypertension and kidney disease often develop together. It is also well documented that lowering the blood pressure of people with hypertension slows the progression of kidney disease and that drugs that target renal function, such as ACE inhibitors and angiotensin II blockers, are useful in lowering blood pressure. Future epidemiological, clinical, and basic science research undoubtedly will answer many of the intriguing questions that are unresolved.

CASE STUDY
Scenario

Mr. Samuel Johnson is a 52-year-old African-American man who was initially seen in the emergency department complaining of a two-day history of a severe headache with slight dizziness. He has noticed these headaches with related dizziness for the past two years, but admits that these symptoms are occurring more frequently. Mr. Johnson denies any chest pain, shortness of breath, radiating pain, or pain when he walks. He hasn't been to the doctor since he got out of the army at age 24 because he is "healthy as a horse," and doesn't like to go to the doctor ("they always find something wrong when you go").

Mr. Johnson started smoking cigarettes at age 16 and is a two pack-per-day smoker. He admits that he drinks beer, but denies other alcohol or illicit drug use. His history is not remarkable, with many years of apparent good health. His only reported illness was a broken arm at age 8 from a bicycle accident, which healed without problem.

His social history includes being married for 33 years with three children (ages 22, 24, and 28, all in good health). Both of his parents are deceased (father died from unknown causes at age 44 when Mr. Johnson was just a young boy, and his mother just recently died at age 69 from complications of diabetes). He has two siblings, ages 40 and 47. Both of his siblings are female; the younger one is healthy, the older one is a breast cancer survivor of 4 years, otherwise healthy.

On physical examination at admission, his blood pressure was 190/110 mm Hg, pulse 98, respiration rate 18, and oral temperature 98.6°F. His height is 66 inches and he weighs 250 pounds, giving him a body mass index of 40.3. Although he denied any chest discomfort or shortness of breath, a chest x-ray and an electrocardiograph were performed and were normal. The physician also ordered laboratory tests to determine routine blood counts, blood glucose, cholesterol and lipid measurement, and electrolytes. After two follow-up evaluations, Mr. Johnson was diagnosed as having hypertension.

As part of the treatment plan, Mr. Johnson was counseled on the medical dangers of tobacco use and about smoking cessation methods. He was scheduled to speak with a dietician about dietary issues such as weight loss, sodium intake, saturated fat intake, and portion control, and he was also counseled about eating more fruits and vegetables and about avoiding red meat and excess alcohol consumption. Finally, Mr. Johnson was started on an exercise plan that included walking every day for one hour, taking breaks as needed.

Defining the Issues

Left untreated, hypertension is a major **risk factor** for coronary heart disease (CHD), stroke, and kidney damage. It is categorized into three different groups depending upon blood pressure readings:

- **Prehypertension** is defined as systolic if the blood pressure is between 120 and 139 mm Hg and/or diastolic if the blood pressure is between 80 and 89 mm Hg in adults, and if the blood pressure is between the 90th and the 95th percentile values in children.
- **Stage 1 hypertension** is defined as a systolic blood pressure of 140 to 159 mm Hg and a diastolic blood pressure of 90 to 99 mm Hg.
- **Stage 2 hypertension** is defined as a systolic blood pressure greater than or equal to 160 mm Hg, or a diastolic blood pressure greater than or equal to 100 mm Hg

Blood pressure varies naturally and is also sensitive to short-term stress, such as the nervousness a patient may experience when visiting a doctor's office. Hypertension refers to consistently elevated blood pressure over a period of time and can therefore only be diagnosed after measuring a patient's blood pressure twice per visit for a minimum of three visits (a baseline visit with two follow ups). A patient with hypertension will only require hospitalization if he is also suffering from acute target-organ damage such as a stroke or heart attack. If his blood pressure is drastically higher than stage 2 levels, the patient will need to start drug therapy immediately. Otherwise, hypertension is a long-term concern, and treatment should start within several weeks of diagnosis.

Mr. Johnson is suffering from stage 2 hypertension. He will need to take steps to lower his blood pressure, or he will face increased risks of CHD, stroke, heart failure, and kidney disease.

Patient's Understanding

Mr. Johnson's serves as testimony to the fact that hypertension is a silent killer. In fact, over 30 percent of people suffering from hypertension are not aware of their condition. By eschewing regular medical check ups for nearly 30 years, Mr. Johnson had allowed his hypertension to remain undiagnosed, meaning he was likely unaware of how his lifestyle choices were contributing to his illness. Although it is widely advertised that family history of hypertension is an important risk factor for contracting the disease, Mr. Johnson does not know what factors contributed to his parents' deaths and is therefore unlikely to pay attention to warnings targeted at people with a family history of the disease.

To address his lack of understanding, he needs to be educated about all facets of hypertension, including the cause of the disease, its long-term and short-term impact on his health, and about potential behavior changes that can improve his prognosis.

CLINICAL PERSPECTIVE FOR THE INDIVIDUAL PATIENT

Level of Intervention Now

When treating hypertension, the main aim of treatment is to reduce the risk of clinically overt cardiovascular disease. To reduce risk, blood pressure should be reduced to less than 140/90 mm Hg (and ideally to 120/80 mm Hg). For patients like Mr. Johnson who are experiencing elevated stage 2 hypertension, the best level of intervention is combining pharmaceutical treatments with changes in lifestyle, including diet, exercise, smoking, and other relevant behaviors. For patients with less severe hypertension, changes in lifestyle may be sufficient to lower their blood pressure, and those patients will not need to be treated with pharmaceuticals.

The main factor to remember when treating hypertension is that blood pressure should not be viewed in isolation. The whole cardiovascular risk profile of the patient (including smoking, dyslipidemia, obesity, and diabetes) should be taken into account to design a personalized intervention.

Potential Level Earlier

Patients do not develop stage 2 hypertension overnight; rather their blood pressure slowly increases over time. Normal blood pressure slowly gives way to **prehypertension**, which in turn develops into stage 1 hypertension. Mr. Johnson's case illustrates this point. Presumably, he has maintained behaviors putting him at risk for hypertension for quite some time. He has been a smoker for over 35 years and does not seem to adhere to a healthy diet and exercise regimen. Screening is the best early intervention for hypertension because catching the disease before it has progressed beyond prehypertensive levels has implications for both the patient's health and for overall economic costs associated with treating the disease. Prehypertension is easily treated with lifestyle modifications and does not require drug therapy, thereby reducing the overall costs per incident. Had Mr. Johnson had his blood pressure measured earlier and more consistently, he would have been aware of the importance of adopting a healthy lifestyle and would have had the opportunity to prevent his blood pressure from progressing to stage two. Because he was not diagnosed earlier, he must now take a pill every day and is also at much greater risk for acute target organ damage.

Other early interventions, such as encouraging the public to inquire about their family history, can bolster screening efforts. If those individuals with a family history are made aware of their increased risk, they are more likely to be screened. Similarly, if more people are targeted by preventative programs emphasizing the importance of diet, exercise, and other healthy lifestyle habits, many case of hypertension could be prevented. Empowering people to adopt healthier lifestyles is a formidable challenge, however, and education alone is unlikely to make a strong impact on reducing hypertension rates. A more thorough discussion on behavior change is in Chapter 8.

PUBLIC HEALTH PERSPECTIVE FOR THE HEALTH OF THE GENERAL POPULATION AND OF HIGH RISK GROUPS

Hypertension is a major medical and public health issue in the 21st century. The prevalence of hypertension has shown a marked increase with age; as many as 50 percent of all individuals over the age of 60 are affected. The major risk factor is old age, and older women are especially vulnerable. The prevalence is also higher among African Americans.

As discussed in the Case Study section, uncontrolled hypertension is a major risk factor of stroke, myocardial infarction, renal failure, congestive health failure, progressive atherosclerosis, and other chronic diseases. Hypertension also shares many common risk factors with other diseases. Risk factors such as obesity, family history, diets high in salt, and lack of exercise can combine with other widespread health risks, such as hyperlipidemia (high lipid levels in the blood), tobacco smoking, diabetes, and a sedimentary lifestyle to contribute to decreased quality of life. The negative synergy between risk factors also can lead to hypertension-related complications such as chest pain, shortness of breath, headaches, and an overall decreased life expectancy. With persistently high levels of obesity, diabetes, and cardiovascular disease, the interaction of multiple risk factors is of growing concern. The high comorbidity of hypertension with other diseases complicates treatment. Hypertension must therefore be considered as a piece of a larger public health puzzle.

The good news is that hypertension is both highly treatable and preventable and therefore is an appropriate candidate for public health interventions. Because hypertension tends to be asymptomatic until major damage is detectable, regular blood pressure monitoring should be performed to determine a patient's normal range. Early and frequent screening can detect hypertension before it becomes a problem. When caught early, changes in diet, activity levels, and the use of lipid-lowering medicatins can be utilized to prevent continual and further damage.

Not surprisingly, one of the most successful hypertension-related public health efforts to date focused on expanding early and frequent screening to detect cases before they caused major traumatic events. The National High Blood Pressure Education Program (NHBPEP), started in 1972, sought to educate patients and providers about the importance of controlling hypertension. At the time of its launch, only 16 percent of patients with hypertension were successfully controlling their high blood pressure with healthy behaviors and antihypertensive drugs. As a direct result of NHBPEP outreach activities, however, hypertension captured the nation's attention. Patients became aware of the need to know and monitor their blood pressure, and more clinicians learned how to properly treat the disease. As a result, after 20 years of program activities, the number of patients successfully controlling their hypertension stood at 65 percent, an increase of nearly 50 percentage points. Nationwide, average blood pressure levels have fallen by 10 to 12 mm Hg as a direct result of the NHBPEP. The program also has resulted in significant declines in age-adjusted mortality rates for stroke and coronary heart disease. After 30 years of successful operations, the NHBPEP proves not only the importance of monitoring for and detecting hypertension early, but it also illustrates the huge impact a simple, well-designed public health program can have on an entire population.

Looking Ahead

Historically, hypertension has been of primary concern as a health risk to the middle-aged and elderly. Although old age remains the number one risk factor, the pandemic of childhood obesity, along with the development of new clinical knowledge, is fueling new concern about hypertension among the young. Due to changes in diet and activity levels, children are exposed to many more risk factors for hypertension than they were in the past. Furthermore, new epidemiological and clinical evidence has strengthened clinicians' abilities to associate childhood hypertension with progressive target organ damage occurring later in life. Both rising rates of childhood obesity and hypertension and new predictive capacities make a compelling case for dedicating more resources to prevent childhood hypertension and ultimately preventing sequelae in adulthood.

Monitoring children's risk factors for hypertension has proved to be somewhat of a challenge. A lack of resolution of the basic science surrounding childhood hypertension serves as a roadblock to developing comprehensive policies. Furthermore, treatment and prevention efforts geared towards children face unique hurdles not accounted for in existing protocols for adults. Although establishing effective education and behavior change campaigns has successfully impacted the health of certain adult populations, such techniques cannot be readily transferred to children. Children are limited not only by their understanding but also by their lack of autonomy. Very few children shop for their own groceries, cook their own meals, or purchase gym memberships. One of the great public health challenges down the road, therefore, will be to develop effective treatment and prevention efforts for children, especially in situations where a child's family fails to encourage the development of healthy behavior.

KEY TERMS

Biology Terms

Aldosterone: A steroid hormone released from the adrenal cortex. It acts in the distal tubule and the collecting duct.

Diuretic: A drug that increases urine flow, usually by inhibiting sodium reabsorption.

Glomerular Filtration Rate (GFR): The volume of filtrate formed in both kidneys and passing into the proximal tubule. In adults it averages about 120 mL/min.

Hypertension: Blood pressure exceeding 140/90 mm Hg.

Nephron: The functional unit of the kidney. Each human kidney has about one million of these tiny tubular structures.

Reabsorption: In the kidney, reabsorbed solutes are transported out of the fluid in the lumen of the nephron and returned to the blood.

Public Health Terms

Diastolic Blood Pressure: The bottom number is the diastolic blood pressure reading. It represents the pressure in the arteries when the heart is at rest.

Systolic Blood Pressure: The top number is the systolic blood pressure reading. It represents the maximum pressure exerted when the heart contracts.

Prehypertension: Systolic if the blood pressure is between 120 and 139 mm Hg and/or diastolic if the blood pressure is between 80 and 89 mm Hg in adults.

Risk Factor: A behavior or predicament that places an individual in harm's way; the probability that an untoward event will occur.

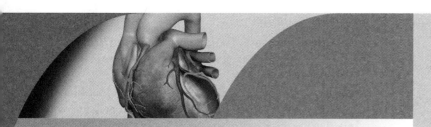

Questions for Further Research, Study, Reflection, and Discussion

In order to answer these questions, it may be necessary to research the primary literature.

For the Individual Student

- Describe two different cellular signaling pathways by which aldosterone increases sodium reabsorption in target cells.
- Outline the cellular mechanisms by which angiotensin II increases sodium reabsorption in the proximal and distal tubule as well as in the collecting duct.
- The rate of filtration of blood in the glomerulus (GFR) is driven by arterial blood pressure. Surprisingly, changes in mean blood pressure over the range of 60 to 140 mm Hg result in only very modest changes in GFR. Describe a mechanism that limits increases in GFR as mean arterial pressure increases.
- Make a detailed drawing of the structures in the glomerulus and describe how the filtration process works.
- If a person eats a very low protein diet, they are unable to produce urine that is as osmotically concentrated as a person eating a high protein diet. Explain why.

For Small Group Discussion

- What are the consequences of unregulated hypertension?

- Are there any risk factors in Mr. Johnson's family history that make him more at risk for hypertension?
- What lifestyle behaviors might have led to Mr. Johnson's hypertension?
- Identify some barriers to hypertension prevention, and identify ways to overcome these barriers with education, screening, routine checkups, and medical intervention.
- Discuss how the community can serve as an interventional point for the prevention, early diagnosis, and management of hypertension.

For Entire Class Discussion

- Discuss what steps would be necessary to plan a public blood screening program in your community.
  (a) Identify your target audience.
  (b) How and where would you publicize the event?
  (c) What materials and supplies would be necessary?
  (d) Identify numbers and type of staff you would need.
  (e) Determine what statistics you would collect.
  (f) Where you would refer those that need immediate medical attention and follow-up monitoring?
  (g) Identify factors you would use to evaluate effectiveness of the program.

EXERCISE/ACTIVITY

- Identify a specific population in your city, gather health statistics about that population, and, using the statistics that you gathered, identify one health intervention to screen for or prevent hypertension in that specific population. Develop an outreach plan. How would you evaluate if your plan was successful?

HEALTHY PEOPLE 2010

Indicator: Physical Activity

Focus Area: Heart Disease and Stroke

Goal: Improve cardiovascular health and quality of life through the prevention, detection, and treatment of risk factors; early identification and treatment of heart attacks and strokes; and prevention of recurrent cardiovascular events.

Objectives:

12-9. Reduce the proportion of adults with high blood pressure.

12-10. Increase the proportion of adults with high blood pressure whose blood pressure is under control.

12-11. Increase the proportion of adults with high blood pressure who are taking action (for example, losing weight, increasing physical activity, or reducing sodium intake) to help control their blood pressure.

12-12. Increase the proportion of adults who have had their blood pressure measured within the preceding two years and can state whether their blood pressure was normal or high.

RESOURCES

Beutler KT, Masilamini S, Turban S, Nielsen J, Brooks HL, Ageloff S, Fenton R, Packer RK, Knepper MA. Long-term regulation of ENaC expression in kidney by angiotensin II. *Hypertension* 2003;41:1143–1150.

Campese VM, Park J. The kidney and hypertension: over 70 years of research. *J Nephrol* 2006;19:691–698.

Centers for Disease Control and Prevention (2004). State-specific trends in chronic kidney failure—United States, 1990–2001. *MMWR Morbid Mortal WklyRep* 2004; 53:918–920.

Chobanian AV, Bakris GL, Black HR, et al., for the National High Blood Pressure Education Program Coordinating Committee. Seventh report of the Joint National Committee on Prevention, Detection, Evaluation, and Treatment of High Blood Pressure. *Hypertension* 2003;42:1206–1252.

Hajjar I, Kotchen TA. Trends in prevalence, awareness, treatment, and control of hypertension in the United States, 1988–2000. *JAMA* 2003;290:199–206.

Silverthorn DU. *Human Physiology: An Integrated Approach*, 4th ed. San Francisco: Pearson/Benjamin Cummings; 2007.

Jones DW, Hall JE. The National High Blood Pressure Education Program: thirty years and counting. *Hypertension* 2002;39:941–942.

Locatelli F, Pozzoni P, Del Vecchio L. Renal manifestations in the metabolic syndrome. *J Am Soc Nephrol* 2006;17(Suppl 2): S81–S85.

Boron WF, Boulpaep EL. *Medical Physiology: A Cellular and Molecular Approach*. Philadelphia: Saunders; 2003.

Mullins LJ, Bailey MA, Mullins JJ. Hypertension, kidney, and transgenics: a fresh perspective. *Physiol Rev* 2006;86: 709–746.

Department of Health and Human Services, National Institutes of Health, National Heart, Lung, and Blood Institute. *Prevention, Detection, Evaluation, and Treatment of High Blood Pressure*, December 2003. Available at http://www.nhlbi.nih.gov/guidelines/hypertension/. Accessed April 30, 2008.

Wexler R, Aukerman G. Nonpharmacologic strategies for managing hypertension. *Am Fam Physician,* 2006;73:1953–1956.

CROSS REFERENCES

Atherosclerosis

Behavioral Determinants

Stroke

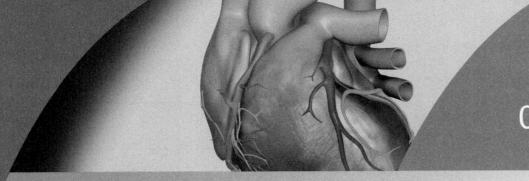

CHAPTER **34**

Epidemiology of Atherosclerosis

Cynthia M. Tracy
Richard V. Milani

During the next 40 minutes that it will take you to read this chapter, 75 people will die suddenly as a result of cardiovascular disease in this country.

LEARNING OBJECTIVES

By the end of this chapter, the student will be able to:

- Recognize the national health importance of cardiovascular disease.
- Describe the role of atherothrombosis in the development of vascular disease.
- Discuss the importance of risk factors and risk factor modification.
- Recognize the interplay of science and public health initiatives.
- Define key terms necessary to discuss cardiovascular disease.
- Identify important clinical features and public health concerns in a case involving a deadly manifestation of cardiovascular disease.

HISTORY

Atherosclerosis is a generalized and progressive disease that affects the arterial circulation. There are five recognized stages to atherosclerosis that generally progress over a period of decades (Figure 34-1) leading to clinical manifestations usually in middle-age to older adults.[1,2] The impact of this disease has reached epidemic proportions such that the most recent World Health Report documents that **atherothrombosis** has overtaken infectious disease as the leading cause of death worldwide, representing 23 percent of all deaths. Currently in the United States, cardiovascular disease—the major result of ath-

erosclerosis leading to heart attack and stroke—affects over 71 million individuals with an annual mortality exceeding 900,000 per year.[3] The impact of this disease costs U.S. taxpayers approximately 400 billion dollars per year and represents over 6 million hospital discharges, accounting for 37 percent of all deaths (1 out of 2.7 deaths).

BASIC SCIENCE FACTS/KEY CONCEPTS REVIEW

Risk Factors

Shortly after World War II, the **National Institutes of Health** (NIH) funded the Framingham Heart Study to describe any relationship between unhealthy behaviors or traits and the subsequent development of heart attack and stroke. These unhealthy characteristics have since been called *risk factors* for heart attack and stroke. Today several additional important risk factors have been identified (Table 34-1).

Risk factors can behave synergistically to promote the onset and progression of atherothrombosis and increase the risk of heart attack and death.[4] More recently, one can calculate any individual's 10-year risk for the development of heart attack (also known as *myocardial infraction*) and death due to heart disease by using an online calculator provided by the Framingham Heart Study if one knows his or her risk factors (http://hp2010.nhlbihin.net/atpiii/calculator.asp?user type=prof).

Among the known risk factors for the development of coronary heart disease, some are more easily controlled than others. For example, it is possible to avoid or to stop smoking and to pursue a healthy lifestyle but it is not possible to alter ones family history. Similarly, some risk factors are more

FIGURE 34-1 Initiation, Progression, and Complication of Human Atherosclerotic Plaque.

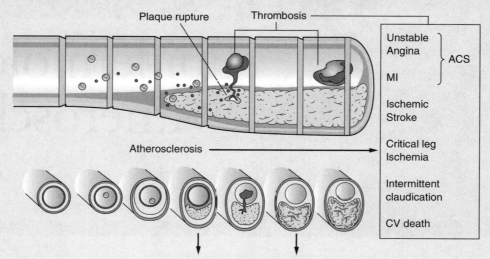

ACS = acute coronary syndrome, CV = cardiovascular, MI = myocardial infarction
Initiation, progression, and complication of human atherosclerotic plaque. Top: Longitudinal section of artery depicting "time line" of human atherogenesis from normal artery to atheroma that caused clinical manifestations by thrombosis or stenosis. Bottom: Cross sections of artery during various stages of atheroma evolution.

Source: Adapted from Libby P. Current concepts of the pathogenesis of the acute coronary syndromes. *Circulation* 2001;104:365–372.

TABLE 34-1 Risk Factors and Coronary Heart Disease

AHA Scientific Position

What are the major risk factors that can't be changed?
- Increasing age
- Male sex (gender)
- Heredity (including race)

What are the major risk factors you can modify, treat, or control by changing your lifestyle or taking medicine?
- Tobacco smoke
- High blood cholesterol
- High blood pressure
- Physical inactivity
- Obesity and overweight
- Diabetes mellitus

What other factors contribute to heart disease risk?
- Individual response to stress may be a contributing factor
- Drinking too much alcohol

Source: Adapted from American Heart Association. AHA Scientific Position. Risk Factors and Coronary Heart Disease. Dallas: AHA; 2008. Available at http://www.americanheart.org/presenter.jhtml?identifier=4726. Accessed April 30, 2008.

powerful than others and their impact is different among men and women. Having an unfavorable lipid profile, elevated low-density lipoprotein (LDL) **cholesterol**, and reduced high-density lipoprotein (HDL) cholesterol quadruples the risk of developing coronary artery disease. It has been demonstrated over time that there is a linear relationship between LDL level and the development of coronary artery disease (Figure 34-2).[4]

Therapeutic lifestyle changes including obtaining and maintaining ideal body weight, reducing fats in the diet, and exercise are important tools for managing risk factors. A healthy diet may decrease the risk of coronary artery disease by nearly 30 percent. It has been demonstrated that maximal dietary therapy can result in LDL-C reductions of up to 25 percent to 30 percent.[5] Much more emphasis is needed to target much younger aged people on the importance of a healthy lifestyle.

Today very powerful drugs are available for modifying cholesterol levels. The statins are a group of drugs that lower the total cholesterol and LDL by inhibiting an important step in the production of cholesterol that requires an enzyme called HMG-CoA reductase. Statin drugs inhibit this enzyme and are thus called HMG-CoA reductase inhibitors. Other drugs such as ezetimibe block cholesterol absorption in the gut. Increasing the level of HDL (so-called "good") cholesterol would seem to be desirable, but unfortunately this often proves difficult. One class of drugs that can increase the HDL to a modest degree is the fibrates, which act by modulating fat metabolism. Niacin, also known as nicotinic acid or vitamin B3, can also increase HDL by 7 percent to 30 percent as well as lower LDL and total cholesterol. When taken in large doses niacin blocks the breakdown of fats in adipose tissue.

Diabetes, another important risk factor for coronary disease, has been increasing at an alarming rate in the United States and has doubled over the past three decades (Figure 34-3), probably owing to sedentary lifestyles and poor dietary habits. The importance of diabetes as a risk factor for coronary artery disease differs in men and women. Having diabetes quadruples the risk for coronary artery disease in women and doubles it in men. The prevalence of diabetes is particularly high among African Americans (Figure 34-4).

Hypertension, an important risk factor for coronary disease, is highly prevalent in the United States; an estimated 72,000,000 people have blood pressures of ≥140 mm Hg systolic and/or diastolic of ≥90 mm Hg; are taking antihypertensive medication; or have been told at least twice by a health professional that they have high blood pressure.[1,6] Similar to diabetes, hypertension is particularly prevalent among African Americans (Figure 34-5). In men, hypertension nearly triples the risk for developing coronary artery disease and in women it nearly doubles the risk.

A more recently recognized risk for coronary disease is the metabolic syndrome. In 2004, the American Heart Association and the National Heart Lung and Blood Institutes published an updated definition of the metabolic syndrome (Table 34-2).[6] While the cause of the metabolic syndrome is unknown, several predisposing factors have been identified including advancing age, genetics, sedentary lifestyle, and excess caloric intake. It is not

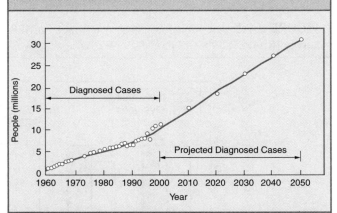

FIGURE 34-3 Prevalence of Diagnosed Diabetes in the United States.

Source: Diabetes: a national plan for action. Steps to a healthier US. U.S. Department of Health and Human Services. December 2004. Data for 1960–1998 from the National Health Interview Survey, National Center for Health Statistics (NCHS). Centers for Disease Control and Prevention (CDC) projected data for 2000–2050 from the Behavioral Risk Factor Surveillance System, Division of Diabetes Translation, CDC. Available at aspe.hhs.gov/health/blueprint/images/figure3.gif. Accessed May 1, 2008.

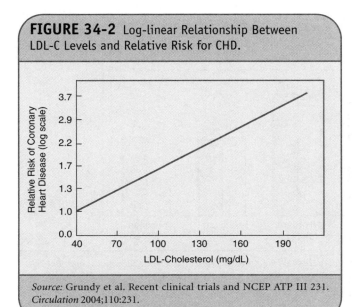

FIGURE 34-2 Log-linear Relationship Between LDL-C Levels and Relative Risk for CHD.

Source: Grundy et al. Recent clinical trials and NCEP ATP III 231. *Circulation* 2004;110:231.

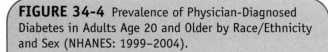

FIGURE 34-4 Prevalence of Physician-Diagnosed Diabetes in Adults Age 20 and Older by Race/Ethnicity and Sex (NHANES: 1999–2004).

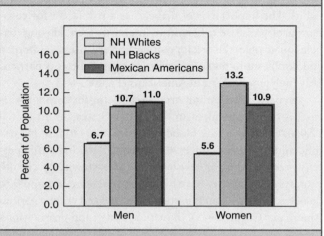

Source: Rosamond W, et al. Heart disease and stroke statistics—2007 update. A report from the American Heart Association Statistics Committee and Stroke Statistics Subcommittee Circulation. 2007;115:e69–e171. Chart 13-1. Source: NCHS and NHLBI. Available at http://www.circ.ahajournals.org. Accessed May 1, 2008.

TABLE 34-2 American Heart Association/Updated NCEP Definition of the Metabolic Syndrome

- Elevated waist circumference
  - Men: Equal to or greater than 40 inches (102 cm)
  - Women: Equal to or greater than 35 inches (88 cm)
- Elevated triglycerides: Equal to or greater than 150 mg/dL
- Reduced HDL ("good") cholesterol
  - Men: Less than 40 mg/dL
  - Women: Less than 50 mg/dL
- Elevated blood pressure: Equal to or greater than 130/85 mm Hg or use of medication for hypertension
- Elevated fasting glucose: Equal to or greater than 100 mg/dL (5.6 mmol/L) or use of medication for hyperglycemia

Source: From Centers for Disease Control: Diabetes. National Diabetes Fact Sheet: United States, 2008. Accessed March 2007 at http://www.cdc.gov/diabetes/pubs/pdf/ndfs_2005.pdf

clear whether obesity or insulin resistance is the cause of the metabolic syndrome or whether it is part of a broader metabolic derangement. The insulin resistance of the metabolic syndromes results in a cascade of events that promotes the development of atherosclerosis. Increased fasting insulin levels and increased fasting glucose levels lead to arterial stiffness, which promotes hypertension. Insulin resistance results in low HDL-C as well as increased levels of LDL and triglycerides. An increased risk of clotting and a decreased ability to break down clots can occur. Abdominal fat is particularly rich in insulin-resistant adipose cells that result in increased free fatty acids and deposition of lipid in arterial walls. Vascular inflammation results along with evidence for systemic inflammation as shown by increased levels of inflammatory markers like C-reactive protein, fibrinogen, interleukin 6 (IL-6), and tumor necrosis factor-alpha (TNFα).[7,8] Abdominal obesity more than doubles the risk of developing coronary artery disease.

FIGURE 34-5 Age-Adjusted Prevalence Trends for HBP in Adults Age 20 and Older by Race/Ethnicity, Sex, and Survey (NHANES: 1988–1994 and 1999–2004).

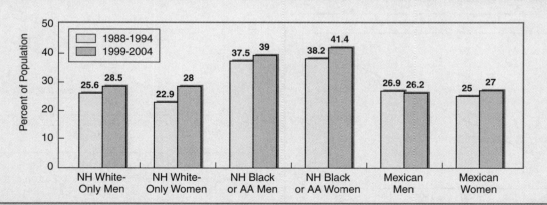

Source: Rosamond W, et al. Heart disease and stroke statistics—2007 update. A report from the American Heart Association Statistics Committee and Stroke Statistics Subcommittee. *Circulation* 2007;115:e69–e171. Chart 5-2. Source: NCHS and NHLBI. NH indicates non-Hispanic; AA, African American. Available at http://www.circ.ahajournals.org. Accessed May 1, 2008.

Cigarette smoking is an independent risk factor for the development of coronary artery disease and can also work with other risk factors to accelerate the disease process. Smokers are at two to four times the risk of developing coronary disease than are nonsmokers. Chemicals in tobacco smoke accelerate the development of atherosclerosis. Smoking contributes to arterial stiffening and hastens the breakdown, or oxidation, of certain fats resulting in increased LDL. Secondhand smoke has much the same effects.

While several risk factors can be eliminated or modified, basic genetic makeup cannot. It has long been recognized that family history plays an important role in the development of coronary artery disease. Part of this may be shared environment and habits, but new genetic testing has allowed for the identification of several genetic loci that affect the risk of development of coronary artery disease.[9] To date genetic modification is not possible, but understanding one's risk can help enforce engaging in risk factor modification and allow for earlier detection and treatment.

Pathology

A series of seminal pathologic studies were conducted over 50 years ago using autopsy examinations of young soldiers killed in combat during the Korean War.[10,11] During the1950s, early atherosclerosis was documented in these young men (typically aged 18–25 years) by demonstration of fatty streaks (types II lesions). Today in the United States atherosclerosis has been shown to develop at much younger ages, with fatty streaks now revealed in childhood suggesting that poor lifestyle habits are being acquired earlier in life.[12,13] Recently conducted autopsy studies in the United States have described more pronounced lesions (> 40 percent blockages in major coronary arteries) occurring in approximately one out of five men by the time they reach ages 30 to 40 and in 8 percent of women that age. As a result of this earlier development, clinical events including heart attack and stroke are being documented at younger and younger ages.[14] The National Health Nutrition Examination Survey (NHANES) report from 1988–1994 and the follow-up survey from 1999–2002 demonstrate a 32 percent increase in the prevalence of cardiovascular disease in young men and a 23 percent increase in the prevalence of cardiovascular disease in young women over just a decade of time. It is also noteworthy that the first clinical episode related to atherosclerosis can be cardiac death.[15]

Development of atherosclerosis is a lifelong process that begins with the fatty streaks seen in the artery walls. This slow progression of atherosclerotic lesions and the close connection with thrombotic complications are known as atherothrombosis.

The process of atherothrombosis has five phases (Figure 34-1).[16] In the first phase, LDL deposits into the cells of the inner wall of the artery. During the second and third phases, inflammatory cells move into the vessel wall and the **plaque** continues to grow. Smooth muscle cells move into the damaged area and replicate. Cholesterol (LDL)-filled foam cells begin to accumulate. As the plaque matures, its surface calcifies and forms a fibrous cap. In the fourth stage of atherothrombosis, the smooth muscle cell proliferation changes and begins to break down. The fibrous cap ruptures, or the LDL-filled plaque erodes to the inner surface of the vessel and is exposed to the bloodstream. The contents of the plaque contain materials that encourage clot formation (prothrombotic). In the fifth stage, platelets are attracted to this prothrombotic material and a clot forms in the vessel. If the clot is large enough to interrupt blood flow beyond its location, damage occurs to the tissue that would normally be supplied by the blood vessel beyond the clot.

Because of the widespread nature of atherosclerosis, if it is detected in any of the arteries of the body (that is, arteries supplying the limbs or the brain), then it is very likely to also be present in the arteries supplying the heart muscle (coronary arteries). In 2001, the Expert Panel on the Detection, Evaluation, and Treatment of High Blood Cholesterol in Adults (Adult Treatment Panel III) recommended that all forms of atherosclerosis disease be considered the equivalent as having coronary heart disease, or atherosclerosis of the heart arteries, recognizing that patients with atherosclerosis in any of these non-heart arteries were also dying of heart disease with the same prevalence as those individuals with documented coronary artery disease.[5] Additionally, if atherosclerosis affects the arteries supplying the brain, then those individuals are at increased risk for stroke or other clinical events that are similar to strokes except they resolve (called *transient ischemic attack [TIA]*).

Heart Circulation

By virtue of the dramatic nature with which heart events (also called *coronary events*) occur, the heart circulation (also known as the *coronary circulation*) is certainly the most "newsworthy" territory that atherosclerosis affects. The major events that occur from coronary disease include acute coronary syndromes, which comprise myocardial infarctions (heart attacks) and episodes of unstable angina. Currently in the United States, approximately 1.7 million acute coronary syndromes occur per year.[3] As described earlier in the stages of atherothrombosis, we now have a much better understanding of how this process occurs. Plaque growth and rupture with release of thrombogenic material and subsequent clot formation and interruption of blood flow are the core of the process. Two factors that lead to plaque rupture are inflammation within plaques that can lead to weakening of the fibrous cap and high shear stress within the blood vessel.[17,18] The occluding clots can be opened emergently by using either clot-busting drugs (that is, tissue plasminogen activator [tPA]) or coronary angioplasty with or without placing a small expandable stent in the opened blood vessel. Time is of the essence in opening closed arteries, and major healthcare initiatives are under way to promote a "door to balloon time" of 90 minutes or less. In other words, from the time a patient arrives at the emergency room, is triaged, diagnosed, transported to a cardiac catheterization laboratory, has catheters inserted into the body, and the culprit blood vessel is opened should take 90 minutes or less. This requires tremendous coordination of care.

Peripheral Circulation

Peripheral arterial disease is defined as the presence of a stenosis or an occlusion in the aorta or the arteries of the limbs. This is almost exclusively caused by atherothrombosis and represents to the individual a dramatic increase risk of cardiovascular and cerebrovascular events including death, myocardial infraction, and stroke (Figure 34-6). Currently, peripheral arterial disease affects 8 to 12 million Americans a prevalence second only to coronary heart disease.[3] It is estimated by the year 2050, the prevalence of peripheral arterial disease will reach 19 million Americans. Peripheral arterial disease increases in the population with age and is likely to be present in approximately 29 percent of individuals over age 70, or between ages 50 and 69 with a history of either diabetes or cigarette smoking.[19] Although the risk factors for peripheral arterial disease are similar to the risk factors for coronary heart disease, some risk factors take on greater importance in peripheral arterial disease.[20] The most potent risk factors for the development of peripheral arterial disease impacts individuals in two ways. First, because of the widespread nature of atherosclerosis, individuals with peripheral arterial disease are at very high risk for heart attack, stroke, and death due to heart disease. Second, peripheral arterial disease affects the limb arteries, leading to leg pain, and, in some cases, ulcers and amputation.

Polyvascular Disease

It is important to understand that atherosclerosis is nondiscriminating and typically does not limit itself to a single circulation. Atherosclerosis represents a widespread disorder impacting many "territories" of the arterial circulation including coronary, peripheral, and cerebrovascular (the arteries feeding the brain). As an example, in patients over age 60 who present with peripheral arterial disease, roughly 68 percent also will demonstrate coronary artery disease and another 42 percent will further demonstrate cerebrovascular disease.[21] When atherosclerosis is documented in more than one circulation, we label the individual as having *polyvascular disease* (mean ing many vascular bed effects). Of all the risk groups known, those with the highest risk for subsequent myocardial infarction, stroke, or death due to heart disease is the polyvascular patient. In a recent worldwide study, individuals with polyvascular disease carry a 20 percent to 25 percent annual risk of heart attack, stroke, death, or hospitalization due to complications of atherosclerosis.[22]

PUBLIC HEALTH PERSPECTIVE FOR THE HEALTH OF THE GENERAL POPULATION AND OF HIGH RISK GROUPS

Many think that heart disease is a man's disease. In fact, heart disease is the number one killer in women (Figure 34-8 and Figure 34-9). Women tend to develop heart disease about ten years later than men. Many public health initiatives have relied on studies where the study group was comprised disproportionately of men. To address this inequity of evidence-based knowledge, in 1991 the National Institutes of Health launched the **Women's Health Initiative (WHI)**. The WHI consisted of a set of clinical trials and an observational study

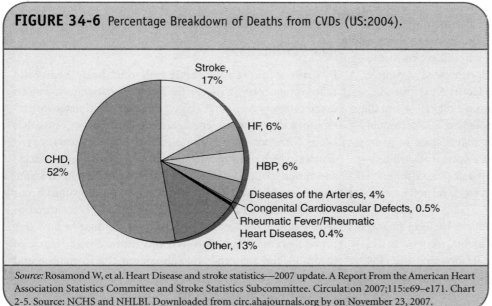

FIGURE 34-6 Percentage Breakdown of Deaths from CVDs (US:2004).

Stroke, 17%
HF, 6%
CHD, 52%
HBP, 6%
Diseases of the Arteries, 4%
Congenital Cardiovascular Defects, 0.5%
Rheumatic Fever/Rheumatic Heart Diseases, 0.4%
Other, 13%

Source: Rosamond W, et al. Heart Disease and stroke statistics—2007 update. A Report From the American Heart Association Statistics Committee and Stroke Statistics Subcommittee. Circulation 2007;115:e69–e171. Chart 2-5. Source: NCHS and NHLBI. Downloaded from circ.ahajournals.org by on November 23, 2007.

CASE STUDY

ACUTE MYOCARDIAL INFARCTION AND SUDDEN CARDIAC ARREST

Scenario

DT is a 49-year-old woman of African-American descent who works as a paralegal in a high pressure multi-partner law office in Washington, DC. She and her husband of 23 years recently divorced largely over differences in how to raise their three teenage sons, one of whom recently has been in trouble at his high school. Her oldest son is a sophomore in college. Her ex-husband has left the United States and as a result, she is solely responsible for raising her sons. Her 70-year-old mother recently experienced a stroke that left her unable to care for herself on her own. Her mother has moved in with DT and her sons. DT's only brother, three years her elder, died last year of a heart attack. Although DT's salary is quite good, being a single parent and the primary care provider for her mother has left her financially strapped.

DT has generally been healthy but underwent a hysterectomy along with removal of both ovaries after the birth of her youngest son because of complications at his birth. She has been on hormone replacement therapy since that time.

Personnel turnover in her office is large and, although she genuinely likes the lawyer for whom she typically works, her new immediate supervisor is fifteen years her junior and in DT's opinion is out to make a name for herself regardless the cost to others. DT has recently resumed smoking and has gained approximately 25 pounds since her divorce. She frequently takes on additional cases to get overtime pay in an attempt to cope with her additional financial burden. Her late work hours and financial status have completely eliminated her trips to the gym.

The heath insurance offered through her employer covers major medical illnesses but does not cover medications. DT typically gets her prescriptions at a discount pharmacy located 15 miles from her home. She still finds the cost of her three prescription blood pressure medications prohibitive and will often miss taking them for days at a time.

DT has been feeling exhausted and experiences shortness of breath when she walks to and from her metro stop. She has been experiencing episodes of dizziness as well, all of which she attributes to her return to smoking and hectic work and home schedules. She keeps meaning to call her physician whom she hasn't seen in two years.

On a Monday morning, DT reported to work having been unable to complete a project over the weekend as she had meant to do. Her supervisor chastised her in front of several other people in the office. DT appeared to drop her head to her chest. The staff initially though she was overcome by emotions until DT fell from her chair to the floor. The supervisor immediately recognized that DT was in trouble and instructed one of the staff to call 9-1-1 and began cardiopulmonary resuscitation (CPR). A colleague rushed to the elevator where the **automated external defibrillator (AED)** was stored and applied the device. DT received two shocks before paramedics arrived to initiate advanced life support. DT was transported to the nearby George Washington University Hospital where she underwent emergency heart catheterization.

Defining the Issues

There are several issues involved in DT's case. At age 49, she is surgically postmenopausal. She has multiple risk factors for developing atherosclerosis such as hypertension, overweight, sedentary lifestyle, cigarette smoking, and stress. She also has been on an estrogen-progesterone combination for several years, placing her at higher risk for heart attack and stroke. In addition, DT has a family history both of coronary disease and hypertension. Her personal support system is weak, as is often the case in the "Sandwich Generation," a generation of people who care for their aging parents while supporting their own children. To keep down costs, DT's employers offer reasonable healthcare benefits but these do not extend to prescription coverage and DT is too young to benefit from Medicare.

DT has experienced one of the most deadly first manifestations of coronary artery disease—**sudden cardiac arrest**—in the setting of a heart attack. The emergency catheterization showed that a major blood vessel traveling down along the bottom surface of the heart called the *right coronary artery* was completely occluded by clot. The doctors were able to open the blood vessel and placed a stent. The findings at the catheterization procedure and subsequent blood tests confirmed that she had undergone a myocardial infarction (heart attack). The catheterization procedure showed that she had some minor plaque buildup in the other two major blood vessels that supply the heart with blood, but the amount was not severe. Fortunately, tests days later showed that her overall heart function remained normal despite the heart attack. Additional tests showed that she had elevated cholesterol and a high LDL level.

Like many women, DT's symptoms of coronary artery disease were somewhat cryptic. For both men and women, the most common heart attack symptom is chest pain or discomfort. However, women with coronary disease are somewhat more likely to experience other symptoms such as fatigue, dizziness and shortness of breath, nausea/vomiting, and back or jaw pain.

DT's first clinical presentation with heart disease was with a cardiac arrest or aborted sudden cardiac arrest. As the blood vessel supplying the bottom surface of her heart closed, the area beyond the blockage suffered from a lack of blood supply (ischemia) and some of it ultimately died (infarct) despite the early catheterization. During the ischemic phase, the cells of the heart muscle became electrically unstable and this led to the potentially fatal abnormal heart rhythm ventricular fibrillation. When in ventricular fibrillation the heart is not effectively pumping blood and the person collapses; if quick intervention is not given, the person dies within minutes. In the United States approximately 325,000 sudden cardiac arrests occur out-of-hospital or in hospital emergency departments annually.[23] This equates to about 890 people per day or roughly one person every minute and a half. DT was fortunate to have a witnessed cardiac arrest, especially because only around 6.4 percent of those who experience a cardiac arrest will survive to make it out of the hospital.[24] Fifty percent of men and 64 percent of women who die suddenly as a result of heart disease had no previous symptoms.[3]

Patient's Understanding

Like many women, DT was not aware of the significance of heart disease. Surveys conducted by the American Heart Association in 2003 showed that only 46 percent of respondents were aware that heart disease is the number one killer in women. This lack of awareness is worse among African Americans and Hispanics. Responders in these categories showed awareness in 30 percent and 27 percent of the women, respectively. Among white women, 50 percent were aware of the significance of heart disease.[3] An even more interesting survey conducted in 1997 showed that only 8 percent of women respondents identified heart disease as their greatest health concern.[3]

DT was unaware that her symptoms of fatigue, shortness of breath, and dizziness might reflect more than being out of shape but could actually be signs of a serious heart condition. DT had no awareness of the difference between a heart attack and a cardiac arrest. Like many women, she was using her obstetrician/gynecologist as her primary care physician and had not received the proper evaluations or treatments that might have prevented her heart attack and cardiac arrest.

DT was not aware of resources in her community that could have helped relieve the amount of stress she had and she had no awareness that stress could contribute to a heart attack. She did acknowledge her weight, sedentary lifestyle, and cigarette smoking as unhealthy behaviors.

CLINICAL PERSPECTIVE FOR THE INDIVIDUAL PATIENT

Level of Intervention Now

The critical care needed at the time of the cardiac arrest was prompt resuscitation with quick correction of the abnormal heart rhythm and good quality CPR. Survival after a cardiac arrest falls off dramatically for every minute delay in restoring the heart to its normal rhythm: seven to ten percent for each minute delay.[25]

Then next critical phase is prompt restoration of blood flow. The critical window of 90 minutes has been shown to be important in preserving as well as possible the heart function. The more damage the heart sustains with a heart attack, the worse the long-term prognosis. After these steps were achieved, protecting DTs health in the future is of the utmost importance. Testing has shown that her heart function overall remains reasonably well preserved but that she does have other vascular disease. The strictest levels of cholesterol control will need to be put in place combining diet, exercise, and drugs to lower her cholesterol. A careful history and physical will show whether additional tests of other vascular beds such as the carotid arteries are needed.

DT's blood pressure will need better regulation. Unfortunately, the price of prescription drugs and the lack of a prescription plan for many make this difficult. Fortunately, many generic drugs exist which can be prescribed for less cost than brand name pharmaceuticals. DT's hormone replacement therapy was immediately discontinued on admission to the hospital. Testing for other risk factors such as diabetes were undertaken and found to be negative. She showed little or no damage to sensitive organs such as the eyes and kidneys from her poorly treated hypertension.

DT received diet and smoking cessation counseling. A case manager and a social worker saw her while she was in the hospital. They discussed the role of stress in her health crisis and identified that DT's mother under her Medicare benefits qualified for long-term home health care. DT was also given a list of clinical social workers covered by her insurance plan with whom she could establish a therapeutic relationship as an outpatient. DT liked and trusted the cardiologist who cared for her in the hospital, and made arrangements to see her as an outpatient to continue monitoring and treating her heart-related issues. The cardiologist was able to refer her to a good primary care physician who would assume her general medical care.

Potential Level Earlier

The Framingham Study was invaluable at showing the relationship between behaviors and the development of heart disease years later. This awareness needs to translate into early primary prevention strategies as shown by the earlier ages at which fatty streaks are identified in arteries. The time to begin preventing heart disease is during childhood and teenage years. Public awareness campaigns are critical to raise awareness that risk factors often begin their insidious process to heart attack or stroke at a very young age. Children and teens need to be assessed for high blood pressure and elevated cholesterol. Smoking prevention campaigns must seriously address prevention of smoking at an early age. The incidence of obesity in childhood is alarming in this country and is coupled with inactivity. The American Academy of Child and Adolescent Psychiatry estimates that between 16 percent and 33 percent of children and teenagers are obese (Figure 34-7). Obese children are more likely to become obese adults. Along with the rise in obesity, in children and teenagers, there has been a rise in the type of diabetes normally seen only in adults.[26]

Primary prevention generally refers to efforts at modifying risk factors and the earlier these efforts are undertaken the better. DT missed primary prevention strategies and so is now a candidate for secondary prevention. Secondary prevention includes therapy to decrease recurrent events and decrease coronary mortality once the patient already has established heart disease. This includes many of the steps that would be included in a primary prevention strategy such as therapeutic lifestyle changes. In addition, secondary prevention involves introduction of medication to modify risk factors to prevent further plaque formation and atherothrombosis (same as above).

Tertiary prevention refers to the rehabilitative efforts after the event has occurred. DT has already received many of these interventions including revascularization and establishment of a better support system to allow her to reenter her daily life more effectively.

FIGURE 34-7 Trends in the Prevalence of Overweight Among US Children and Adolescents by Age and Survey (NHANES: 1971–1974, 1976–1980, 1988–1994, and 2001–2004).

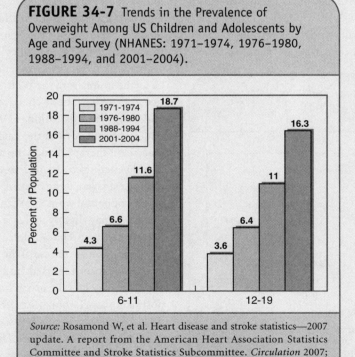

Source: Rosamond W, et al. Heart disease and stroke statistics—2007 update. A report from the American Heart Association Statistics Committee and Stroke Statistics Subcommittee. *Circulation* 2007; 115:e69–e171. Chart 2-17. Source: Annual Final Mortality. NCHS and NHLBI. Note: The overall comparability for CVD between the ICD-9 (1979–1998 and ICD-10 (1999–2004) is 0.9962. No comparability ratios were applied. Download from circ.ahajournals.org by on November 23, 2007.

and involved 161,808 generally healthy postmenopausal women.

Clinical trials were designed to test the effects of different treatments (hormone therapy), dietary modifications, and supplements such as calcium and vitamin D. The effects of the modifications on heart disease, bone fractures, and breast and colorectal cancer were studied over time.[27] The menopausal hormone therapy clinical trial had two parts. The first involved 16,608 postmenopausal who took either estrogen plus progestin therapy or a placebo. The second study involved 10,739 women who had had a hysterectomy and took estrogen alone or a placebo. Both of these studies were important and sought to address the widespread belief that using hormone replacement therapy after menopause might protect women from developing heart disease and strokes because at earlier ages, when hormone levels are higher, women are at less risk than are men.

Women were enrolled into these studies between 1993 and 1998. Their enrolling physicians monitored the women closely and an independent Data and Safety Monitoring Board (DSMB) reviewed events. The studies were planned to continue until 2005 but both were stopped early. The estrogen plus-progestin study was stopped in July 2002, and the estrogen-alone study in February 2004. Women continued to be followed and monitored closely until 2007.

The estrogen plus progestin study was stopped because of an increased risk of breast cancer and it was determined

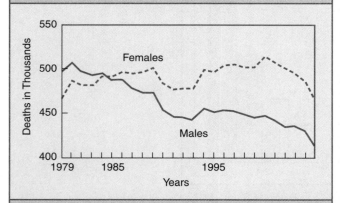

FIGURE 34-8 CVD Mortality Trends for Males and Females (United States; 1979–2004).

Source: Rosamond W, et al. Heart disease and stroke statistics—2007 update. A report from the American Heart Association Statistics Committee and Stroke Statistics Subcommittee. *Circulation* 2007; 115:e69–e171. Chart 2-17. Source: Annual Final Mortality. NCHS and NHLBI. Note: The overall comparability for CVD between the ICD-9 (1979–1998 and ICD-10 (1999–2004) is 0.9962. No comparability ratios were applied. Download from circ.ahajournals.org by on November 23, 2007.

that the risk from taking the combination hormone therapy outweighed any potential gain. The combination therapy increased the risk for heart attack, stroke, and blood clots. Although the risk of heart attack was particularly high in the first year of hormone, it continued for several years.

The estrogen-alone study was stopped after around seven years when it was determined that the hormone therapy increased the risk of stroke and did not reduce the risk of coronary heart disease. Estrogen-alone therapy was associated with a statistically significant increased risk for venous **thrombosis** and a trend towards increased risk for pulmonary embolism (blood clots in the lungs) that was not statistically significant. The therapy had no significant effect on the risk of colorectal cancer. Estrogen alone reduced the risk for hip fractures and there was a trend towards a decrease in breast cancer but this was not statistically significant. Importantly, neither the estrogen plus progestin nor estrogen alone affected the risk of death.

The Women's Health Initiative is an excellent example of a public health initiative that had enormous impact on medical care. Prior to the WHI, most clinical trials had not included enough women to truly gage the effects of different interventions. Medical guidelines that are used by clinicians to guide therapy based on evidence-based medicine did not take into account gender differences. Aside from dispelling medical myths about the benefits of hormone replacement therapy, the WHI provided evidence upon which clinical decisions can be rationally based. While more information will be forthcoming from the WHI, several changes in clinical practice already have been changed. For example, the U.S. **Food and Drug Administration** (FDA) reviewed data from the WHI and as a result revised the package labeling for hormone replacement therapy. Following publication of the data in 2002, the FDA required changes to the labels of all products containing estrogen alone or combined with progestin for use by postmenopausal women. Warnings were included stating that the drugs may slightly increase the risk of heart attack, stroke, breast cancer, and blood clots.

Following the release of the data regarding an increased risk of breast cancer reported from the WHI study, there was an abrupt decrease in the use of hormone replacement therapy in postmenopausal woman. Researches noted a concomitant sharp decline in the rate of new breast cancer cases in 2003 that may be related to a decline in the use of hormone replacement therapy.[28] The report used data from the Surveillance, Epidemiology and End Results (SEER) program of the National Cancer Institute (NCI), part of the National Institutes of Health (NIH).

The outcomes exemplify the impact of powerful, population-based studies. Not only were erroneous assumptions about the benefit of hormone replacement therapy

FIGURE 34-9 Dangerous Ruptures.

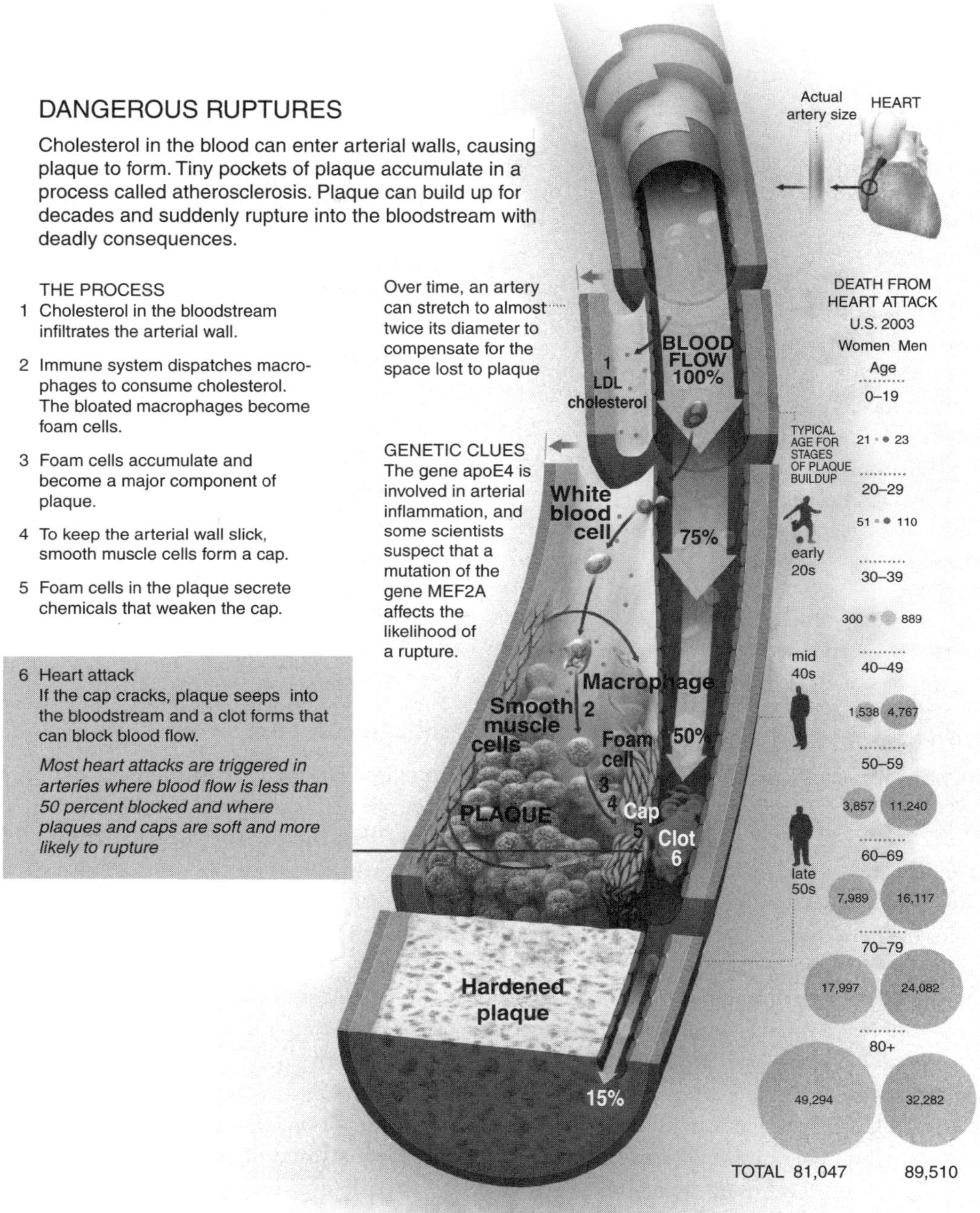

DANGEROUS RUPTURES

Cholesterol in the blood can enter arterial walls, causing plaque to form. Tiny pockets of plaque accumulate in a process called atherosclerosis. Plaque can build up for decades and suddenly rupture into the bloodstream with deadly consequences.

THE PROCESS

1 Cholesterol in the bloodstream infiltrates the arterial wall.

2 Immune system dispatches macrophages to consume cholesterol. The bloated macrophages become foam cells.

3 Foam cells accumulate and become a major component of plaque.

4 To keep the arterial wall slick, smooth muscle cells form a cap.

5 Foam cells in the plaque secrete chemicals that weaken the cap.

6 Heart attack
If the cap cracks, plaque seeps into the bloodstream and a clot forms that can block blood flow.

Most heart attacks are triggered in arteries where blood flow is less than 50 percent blocked and where plaques and caps are soft and more likely to rupture

Over time, an artery can stretch to almost twice its diameter to compensate for the space lost to plaque

GENETIC CLUES

The gene apoE4 is involved in arterial inflammation, and some scientists suspect that a mutation of the gene MEF2A affects the likelihood of a rupture.

Actual artery size   HEART

BLOOD FLOW 100%

1 LDL cholesterol

White blood cell

75%

Macrophage

Smooth muscle cells   2

Foam cell   50%

3
PLAQUE   4 Cap
5   Clot 6

Hardened plaque

15%

DEATH FROM HEART ATTACK

U.S. 2003

Age	Women	Men
0–19	21	23
20–29	51	110
30–39	300	889
40–49	1,538	4,767
50–59	3,857	11,240
60–69	7,989	16,117
70–79	17,997	24,082
80+	49,294	32,282
TOTAL	**81,047**	**89,510**

TYPICAL AGE FOR STAGES OF PLAQUE BUILDUP

early 20s

mid 40s

late 50s

Source: National Geographic Magazine, February 2007, pg. 54.

Healthy People 2010

Focus Area: Heart Disease and Stroke

Goal: Improve cardiovascular health and quality of life through the prevention, detection, and treatment of risk factors; early identification and treatment of heart attacks and strokes; and prevention of recurrent cardiovascular events.

Objectives:

12-1. Reduce coronary heart disease deaths.

12-13. Reduce the mean total blood cholesterol levels among adults.

12-14. Reduce the proportion of adults with high total blood cholesterol levels.

12-16. Increase the proportion of persons with coronary heart disease who have their LDL-cholesterol level treated to a goal of less than or equal to 100 mg/dL.

debunked, saving countless women from harm, governmental agencies such as the FDA responded with changes in drug labeling. Healthcare professionals worldwide rely on drug labeling for proper use of medications. Furthermore, much of the data from the WHI were incorporated in the Cardiovascular Disease Prevention in Women: Evidence-Based Guidelines.[29]

CONCLUSION

Atherosclerosis and its manifestations represent the leading cause of death in United States as well as worldwide. There are clear risk factors for the development of atherosclerosis, most of which are modifiable. These risk factors, which are often related to unhealthy lifestyle, often begin in childhood, leading to adverse events developing in younger adults. Atherosclerosis disorders are uncommon in a single arterial bed and represent a generalized disorder affecting multiple arterial beds. Clinical risk for heart attack, stroke, and death due to heart disease, increase dramatically based on the number of arterial beds affected. The economic costs of all forms of vascular disease are difficult to calculate, as many people have more subtle limitations related to their vascular disease other than the dramatic presentations of sudden cardiac arrest, heart attack, amputation, or stroke. The estimated annual cost is 400 billion dollars. The other societal costs related to the premature loss of loved ones cannot be estimated.

KEY TERMS

Clinical Terms

Atherosclerosis: Process through which deposits of fatty materials build up in the inner lining of an artery causing plaque buildup.

Atherothrombosis: A sclerotic plaque disruption in the arteries with a superimposed blood clot (see *Thrombosis, Plaque*).

Cholesterol: A soft, fat-like, waxy substance found in the blood and in all body cells. Cholesterol cannot be dissolved and has to be transported to and from the cells by carriers called lipoproteins. Low-density lipoprotein (LDL) is known as "bad" cholesterol. High-density lipoprotein (HDL) is known as "good" cholesterol. LDL plus HDL along with triglycerides and Lp(a) cholesterol comprise the total cholesterol count, which is measured through blood testing.

Plaque: Built up material on the inner lining of an artery made up of cholesterol and fatty substances. Plaque build-up results in narrowing of the blood vessel.

Sudden Cardiac Arrest: Unexpected death occurring less than an hour from the onset of a cardiac event; usually caused by an abnormal heart rhythm that develops during a heart attack; often is referred to as *sudden death*.

Thrombosis: Formation or presence of a blood clot inside a blood vessel.

Public Health Terms

Automated External Defibrillator (AED): A small, portable device that is attached to a person's chest with wires; used to check the person's heart rhythm; if that rhythm is abnormal, it gives the heart an electric shock (called a *defibrillating shock*) if needed to restores the heart's rhythm to normal.

Food and Drug Administration: Agency of the U.S. Department of Health and Human Services responsible for protecting public health by assuring safety, efficacy, and security of human and veterinary drugs, biological products, and medical devices. The FDA is also responsible for advancing the public's health.

National Institutes of Health: A federal entity that is made up of 27 institutes and centers; one of eight health agencies of the Public Health Service, which is part of the U.S. Department of Health and Human Services.

Women's Health Initiative (WHI): A 15-year national health study that involved over 161,000 women aged 50 to 79 that focused on preventing heart disease, breast and colorectal cancer, and bone fractures.

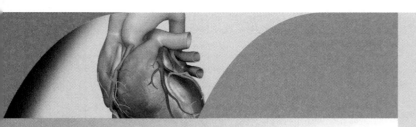

Questions for Further Research Study, Reflection, and Discussion

For the Individual Student

In order to answer these questions, it may be necessary to research the primary literature.

- In the United States, which groups of people are at greatest risk for developing atherothrombosis?
- How does atherothrombosis differ in other countries? What factors might account for the differences?
- What other patient populations are at risk for sudden cardiac arrest? What can be done to help them prevent sudden cardiac arrest?

For Small Group Discussion

- Discuss ways that corporations, such as the law firm where DT works, can promote prevention of atherothrombosis.
- What are the expected impacts of DT's cardiac arrest and heart attack on her family?
- What steps can DT take to promote the health and well-being of her family?

For Entire Class Discussion

- Discuss how the Food and Drug Administration can meet its goal of advancing public health.
- With the aging of the baby boomers, what can be anticipated in terms of future access to care for people with cardiovascular disease? What steps might prevent or relieve any foreseeable problems?
- What evidence is there for the effectiveness of public education campaigns and what steps might improve their efficacy?

EXERCISE/ACTIVITY

Knowledge of risk factors and their "ownership" on an individual basis is critical to preventing heart disease and stroke. Organize a group activity that measures a modifiable risk factor in the general public. An example would be to organize a blood pressure screening clinic at local churches or health clubs.

1. What equipment would be needed?
2. What skill sets are needed to perform a blood pressure screening clinic?
3. What educational materials would be useful to have at the clinic?
4. Who should be targeted for screening?
5. What supervision would be required?
6. What might be the projected costs of your program? Identify a funding source(s).

REFERENCES

1. Stary HC, Chandler B, Dinsmore RE, Fuster V, Glagov S, et al. A definition of advanced types of atherosclerotic lesions and a histological classification of atherosclerosis. A report from the Committee on Vascular Lesions of the Council on Arteriosclerosis, American Heart Association. *Circulation* 1995;92:1355–1374.

2. Libby P. Current concepts of the pathogenesis of the acute coronary syndromes. *Circulation* 2001;104:365–372.

3. Rosamond W, Flegel K, Friday G, Furie K, Go A, et al. Heart disease and stroke statistics—2007 update: a report from the American Heart Association Statistics Committee and Stroke Statistics Subcommittee. *Circulation* 2007;115:e69–171.

4. Yusuf S, Hawken S, Ounpuu S, Dans T, Avezum A, et al., INTERHART Study Investigators. Effect of potentially modifiable risk factors associated with myocardial infarction in 52 countries (the INTERHEART study): case-control study. *Lancet* 2004;364:937–952.

5. Jenkins DJ, Kendall CWC, Marchie A, Faulkner DA, Wong JMW, et al. Effects of a dietary portfolio of cholesterol lowering foods vs lovastatin on serum lipids and C-reactive protein. *JAMA* 2003;290:502–510.

6. Grundy SM, Brewer HB, Cleeman JI, Smith SC, Lenfant D, for the Conference Participants. Definition of metabolic syndrome: report of the National, Heart, Lung, and Blood Institute/American Heart Association conference on scientific issues related to definition. *Circulation* 2004;109:433–438.

7. McFarlane SI, Banerji M, Sowers JR. Insulin resistance and cardiovascular disease. *J Clin Endocrinol Metab* 2001;86:713–718.

8. Reusch JEB. Current concepts in insulin resistance, type 2 diabetes mellitus, and the metabolic syndrome. *Am J Cardiol* 2002;90:19G–26G.

9. Samani NJ, Erdmann J, Hall AS, Hengstenberg C, Mangino M, et al., WTCCC and the Cardiogenics Corporation. Genomewide association analysis of coronary artery disease. *N Engl J Med* 2007;357:443–453.

10. Enos WF, Holmes RH, Beyer J. Coronary disease among United States soldiers killed in action in Korea; preliminary report. *JAMA* 1963;152:1090–1093.

11. Enos WF, Beyer JC, Holmes RH. Pathogenesis of coronary disease in American soldiers killed in Korea. *JAMA* 1955;158:912–914.

12. Berenson GS, Srinivasan SR, Nicklas TA. Atherosclerosis: a nutritional disease of childhood. *Am J Cardiol* 1998;82:22T–29T.

13. Berenson GS, Srinivasan SR, Bao W, Newman WP, 3rd, Tracy RE, Wattigney WA. Association between multiple cardiovascular risk factors and atherosclerosis in children and young adults. The Bogalusa Heart Study. *N Engl J Med* 1998;338:1650–1656.

14. McGill HC Jr, McMahan A, Zieske AW, Tracy RE, Malcolm GT, et al. Association of coronary heart disease risk factors with microscopic qualities of coronary atherosclerosis in youth. *Circulation* 2000;102:374–379.

15. Kaikkonen KS, Kortelainen ML, Linna E, Huikuri HV. Family history and the risk of sudden cardiac death as a manifestation of an acute coronary event. *Circulation* 2006;114:1462–1467.

16. Fuster V, Lewis A. Conner Memorial Lecture: mechanisms leading to myocardial infarction: insights from studies of vascular biology. *Circulation* 1994;90:2126–2146. [erratum 1995;91:256].

17. Davies MJ, Richardson PD, Woolf N, Katz DR, Mann J. Risk of thrombosis in human atherosclerotic plaques: role of extracellular lipid, macrophage, and smooth muscle cell content. *Br Heart J* 1993;69:377–381.

18. Loree HM, Kamm RD, Stringfellow RG, Lee RT. Effects of fibrous cap thickness on peak circumferential stress in model atherosclerotic vessels. *Circ Res* 1992;71:850–858.

19. Hirsch AT, Criqui MH, Treat-Jacobson D, Regensteiner JG, Creager MA, et al. Peripheral arterial disease detection, awareness, and treatment in primary care. *JAMA* 2001;286:1317–1324.

20. Smith SC Jr, Milani RV, Arnett DK, Crouse JR III, McDermott MM, et al. Atherosclerotic Vascular Disease Conference: Writing Group II: risk factors. *Circulation* 2004;109:2613–2616.

21. Ness J, Aronow WS. Prevalence of coexistence of coronary artery disease, ischemic stroke, and peripheral arterial disease in older persons, mean age 80 years, in an academic hospital-based geriatrics practice. *J Am Geriatr Soc* 1999;47:1255–1256.

22. Bhatt DL, Steg PG, Ohman EM, Hirsch AT, Ikeda Y, et al., REACH Registry Investigators. International prevalence, recognition, and treatment of cardiovascular risk factors in outpatients with atherothrombosis. *JAMA* 2006;295:180–189.

23. American Heart Association. Heart Disease and Stroke Statistics—2007 Update At-a-Glance. Dallas: American Heart Association; 2007. Available at http://www.americanheart.org/downloadable/heart/1166711577754HS_Stats InsideText.pdf Accessed May 1, 2008.

24. American Heart Association. Statistical Fact Sheet—Miscellaneous. 2007 Update. Out-of-Hospital Cardiac Arrest—Statistics. Dallas: AHS; 2007. Available at: http://www.americanheart.org/downloadable/heart/116863 9579314OUTOFHOSP07.pdf Accessed May 1, 2008.

25. Cummins RO. From concept to standard-of-care? Review of the clinical experience with automated external defibrillators. *Annals Emerg Med* 1989;18:1269–1275.

26. Scott M, Balady GJ, Criqui MH, Fletcher G, Greenland P, et al. Primary prevention of coronary heart disease: guidance from Framingham. A statement for healthcare professionals from the AHA Task Force on Risk Reduction. *Circulation* 1998;97:1876–1887.

27. Department of Health and Human Services, National Institutes of Health, National Heart, Lung, and Blood Institute. *Women's Health Initiative.* Available at http://www.nhlbi.nih.gov/whi/index.html. Accessed May 1, 2008.

28. Ravdin PM, Cronin KA, Howlader N, Berg CD, Chlebowski RT, et al. The decrease in breast-cancer incidence in 2003 in the United States. *N Engl J Med* 2007;356:1670–1674.

29. Mosca L, Banka CL, Benjamin EJ, Berra K, Bushnell C, et al. Evidence-based guidelines for cardiovascular disease prevention in women: 2007 update. *Circulation* 2007;115:1481–501.

CROSS REFERENCES

Atherosclerosis

Communicating Health Information

Diabetes

Inflammation

Smoking or Health

Stroke

The Nutrition Transition

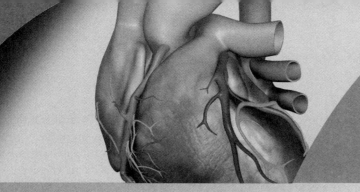

CHAPTER 35

Stroke: A Guide for Prevention for Patients and Families*

Ronald Riechers
Geoffrey S. F. Ling

> Stroke is the third leading cause of death and the leading cause of disability in the United States. Every 45 seconds, someone will suffer a new or recurrent stroke. Every 3.1 minutes, someone will die from a stroke.[1]

LEARNING OBJECTIVES

By the end of this chapter, the student will be able to:

- Discuss the public health impact of stroke.
- Distinguish between hemorrhagic and ischemic stroke.
- Recognize the common signs and symptoms of stroke.
- List the risk factors for stroke.
- Discuss the treatment and prevention of ischemic stroke.

INTRODUCTION

Stroke is a disease that both kills and maims. It attacks suddenly and usually without any warning. Patients are typically devastated: paralyzed, unable to communicate, yet awake and fully comprehending the awful nature of what has happened. This is terrifying to both patient and family. It is life altering for both. Who will care for this terribly injured person? Will there be recovery or instead worsening? Alarmingly, this disease can and often does return to strike the victim yet again.

However, there are steps one can take to avoid suffering a stroke. It begins by paying proper attention to one's own health. A lot has been learned about stroke and the health conditions that lead to it. As a result, leading health organizations such as the American Heart Association (AHA), the American Stroke Association (ASA), the National Institutes of Health (NIH), and others have recommended health-related guidelines that medical care providers can use to help their patients avoid stroke and its close relatives, heart attack and peripheral vascular disease.

HISTORY

Stroke has plagued humankind for eons. Early works from ancient Egypt, China, Rome, and Greece record stroke. Even the father of medicine, Hippocrates, wrote about stroke in his ancient texts. More recent historical medical texts from the 1700s and 1800s give detailed descriptions of the deadly disease they termed *apoplexy*.

Even today, stroke is a common disorder. It is estimated that in the United States, there are approximately 700,000 new strokes per year and 500,000 new **transient ischemic attacks** (**TIAs**). This statistic leads to an estimate of one stroke occurring every 46 seconds. Of the 700,000 strokes, 500,000 were first time occurrences and the remaining 200,000 were recurrent strokes. Each year 150,000 people die as a result of stroke, which is one death every three to four minutes, making stroke

---

*(Editor's note: In choosing to present their chapter as a guide for patients and families, Riechers and Ling demonstrate how to present and explain complex diseases to patients and families.)

the third leading killer in the United States. Given that approximately 80 percent of individuals with stroke survive, there are an estimated 5.7 million stroke survivors in the United States, of this group, nearly 60 percent are women. In addition to being the third leading cause of death in the United States, it is the leading cause of disability. Of stroke survivors over the age of 65, approximately one fourth are dependent on others for assistance or institutionalized in a nursing home within six months of their stroke. Because of this very high morbidity and mortality, stroke will cost the United States an estimated $62.7 billion dollars in 2007. This, of course, does not include the incalculable cost in human suffering.[1]

BASIC SCIENCE FACTS/KEY CONCEPTS REVIEW
Pathophysiology

Simply defined, **stroke** is the sudden onset of loss of function (movement, feeling, speaking, etc.) because of an interruption of blood flow to the portion of the brain responsible for controlling that function. The brain is a very active organ and uses prodigious amounts of oxygen and glucose, its primary metabolic fuels. Thus, it depends on a continuous blood flow to deliver more oxygen (O_2) and glucose as well as remove metabolic waste products, such as carbon dioxide (CO_2). In fact, about 25 percent of the heart's output of blood goes to supply the brain. Once that blood flow is interrupted, within a few minutes *neurons* (brain gray matter cells) lose their ability to function and rapidly die. As the flow of oxygen and glucose to the neuron stops, the basic energy-generating processes within the cell become dysfunctional. The mitochondria rely on O_2 to produce adenosine 5β-triphosphate (ATP), the basic currency of cellular energy, and the cells require glucose to create substrate for the mitochondria. Cellular energy production in neurons functions primarily to maintain the electrical state of the neuron as well as its ability to signal other neurons. When cellular energy stores are depleted, the electrical state of the neuron changes and communication with other neurons ceases. This change in electrical state also sets into motion the programmed cell death (*apoptosis*) of the neuron. Without the neurons, the body functions that are controlled by that portion of the brain will cease. Clinically, this results in the symptoms and signs of stroke.[2,3]

Stroke's Two Killer Faces: Ischemic and Hemorrhagic

There are two major types of strokes. They are ischemic stroke and hemorrhagic stroke. *Ischemic stroke* is when the blood flow to the brain region is interrupted because of a blockage in the artery. *Hemorrhagic stroke* is due to a rupture of the blood vessel. The end result for both types of strokes is that blood flow is interrupted and downstream neurons die.

Ischemic stroke accounts for the majority of strokes, approximately 80 percent to 85 percent. The decrease in blood flow is due to blockage of a blood vessel supplying the brain. Blood vessels become occluded either from disease affecting the blood vessel directly or from clots traveling up the blood vessel from a more central source, otherwise known as an *embolus*. Narrowing and hardening of the arteries, also known as **atherosclerosis**, cause stroke via *thrombosis* (direct occlusion of blood vessel) or *embolism* (clot breaking off of the narrowing and traveling down to a smaller blood vessel). In Caucasian populations, the common site of atherosclerosis leading to stroke is the carotid artery in the neck. In African-American and Asian populations, the arteries more commonly involved are the blood vessels within the skull, known as the *intracranial arteries*. Another common source of embolism is the heart. Within the heart, diseases such as atrial fibrillation, patent foramen ovale, cardiomyopathy, valvular disease, or large *myocardial infarction* ([*MI*] heart attack) can lead to areas of decreased blood flow or turbulent blood flow in the heart, which would allow formation of large clots. From these large clots, smaller pieces can break off and travel down the course of arteries leading to the brain. Other causes of ischemic stroke include small vessel or lacunar disease, paradoxical embolism, and dissection, among others.[2,3]

There are two types of hemorrhagic strokes. *Intracerebral hemorrhage (ICH)* is when there is bleeding into the brain itself. If bleeding occurs around the surface of the brain, it is known as *subarachnoid hemorrhage (SAH)*. Both conditions are very dangerous as persistent bleeding can compress the brain itself.

Strokes that result in hemorrhage in the brain occur for different reasons than ischemic stroke. Intracerebral hemorrhage occurs as the result of hypertension, *amyloid vascular disease* (protein deposits within the walls of blood vessels), blood vessel anomalies such as arteriovenous malformation (AVM), bleeding disorders, or tumors. Hemorrhage around the surface of the brain, subarachnoid hemorrhage (SAH), occurs most often as a result of a ruptured aneurysm, which is a weakness in the wall of the blood vessel such that it pouches out like a balloon which then bursts.[2,3]

CLINICAL PERSPECTIVE FOR THE INDIVIDUAL PATIENT
Signs and Symptoms of Stroke

Symptoms of a stroke depend on several factors including the region of the brain involved as well as hemorrhage versus ischemia.

CASE STUDY
Scenario

Charles is a 73-year-old man with several chronic medical problems who experienced a life-changing event while eating dinner with his wife. He was eating his normal dinner consisting of meatloaf, au gratin potatoes, and canned green beans when he lost control of his fork. He was holding his fork in the right hand and while bringing it to his mouth, it fell from his hand. Within seconds of this, he noted a sensation of heaviness in the upper arm and leg, causing his arm to fall at his side and his body to lean to the right. His wife noticed some drooping of the right side of his face and asked him what just happened. He was able to respond only with a brief grunt. As his wife attempted to ask him more questions, he became visibly frustrated but continued to only grunt in reply. He attempted to rise from his chair and fell to the ground. His wife screamed, got up from her chair and called 9-1-1. Emergency Medical Service (EMS) technicians arrived in seven minutes and took Charles to the nearest emergency room.

While in the emergency room (ER), his symptoms remained the same. He was rapidly seen by an ER provider who reviewed his past medical history with the wife. Charles was being treated for high blood pressure and high cholesterol. He smoked for 40 years ranging from one to three packs of cigarettes per day. He lived a sedentary lifestyle following retirement from a local factory. His wife admitted that he was poorly compliant with his prescribed blood pressure medications and cholesterol medication due to side effects. After the brief history and examination, Charles was taken to the computed tomography (CT) scanner and a head CT was obtained, which was normal. Charles presented to the ER within three hours of the onset of his symptoms and was found to be a good candidate for tissue plasminogen activator (tPA), the clot-busting drug. tPA was administered and over the subsequent days, his speech improved as did his weakness. Following a short hospitalization, Charles was transferred to a rehabilitation unit where he remained for several weeks. Following his discharge from the rehabilitation unit, he returned home but required a walker for ambulation and had significant impairments in his ability to speak in full sentences.

Defining the Issues

Charles' case demonstrates several important issues regarding stroke. First, based on the history and the evaluation, he has suffered an ischemic stroke. He has many risk factors for ischemic stroke including his age, high blood pressure, high cholesterol, and cigarette smoking. These risk factors have led to the development of atherosclerosis that affects not only the blood vessels supplying his brain but also those supplying the heart and the extremities. As an individual, his risk of stroke could have been potentially decreased by alterations in his lifestyle including smoking cessation, exercise, and changes in his diet. Additionally, the medical system could have lessened his risk of stroke by encouraging these lifestyle changes as well as emphasizing the importance of medication compliance. Ultimately, while he did not die from his stroke, he has suffered significant disability that will impact his day-to-day life as well as incur significant healthcare costs for the rest of his life.

Patient's Understanding

Charles showed poor understanding of the importance of treatment of systemic disorders that predispose to the development of atherosclerosis. He was noncompliant with his medications to treat high blood pressure and high cholesterol. Unfortunately, this is common as there are no symptoms of these conditions. They are simply detected with vital sign checks or a blood draw, otherwise the patient is unaware of their presence. Additionally, he neglected to change his behavior at the time these disorders were identified. His current diet remained high in fat and sodium after his initial diagnosis, both which can increase his chances of developing atherosclerosis. Additionally, smoking cessation and increasing his activity level may have modified these risks. In the acute setting however, he and his wife demonstrated good judgment in activating EMS immediately after the onset of his symptoms. This likely improved his ultimate outcome by making him eligible for tPA treatment.

Stroke symptoms generally occur with a sudden onset or reach maximal intensity within a matter of a few minutes. Transient ischemic attack (TIA) is a subset of stroke. A TIA, as implied by its name, is the sudden onset of stroke-like symptoms but, unlike stroke, the symptoms go away within a certain period of time. Thus, within 24 hours, the afflicted patient is back to where he/she was prior to the event. However, it must be emphasized that the TIA is a significant warning that an individual patient is at a more imminent risk of developing a completed stroke.

Common symptoms of stroke or TIA include inability to move or feel parts of the body (face, arm, hand, or leg) on one side, inability to speak or understand speech, any loss of vision (in one eye or to one side), double vision, dizziness/vertigo, confusion, or sudden severe headache. Severe headache is more frequent in patients who have bleeding into or around the brain.[2,3]

Treating an Acute Stroke: Time Is Tissue

A stroke is remarkably similar to a heart attack. In both diseases, symptoms can be rapid onset or can slowly develop over time, and immediate medical treatment is critical to ensure the best possible recovery. When deprived of oxygen and nutrients, brain tissue begins to die almost instantly. By quickly recognizing symptoms and seeking treatment, patients can drastically improve their long-term health outcomes. In fact, due to the time-sensitive demands of treating a stroke, strokes are now commonly referred to as *brain attacks*.

As was mentioned in the case study, although Charles did a poor job taking preventative steps before his stroke, immediately calling EMS may have saved his life. If a patient suffering a stroke presents early (within 3–6 hours) after the onset of symptoms, they may be a candidate for treatment with the clot-dissolving medication tPA. This drug works by increasing the amount and activity of the body's natural clot breakdown system. It can be administered into a peripheral vein if the patient presents within the first three hours of stroke and can be administered directly into the blocked artery if a patient presents within the first six hours. Unfortunately, many patients do not present within the necessary timeframe or have other medical conditions that prevent the use of tPA. At present, only about 5 percent to 10 percent of acute stroke patients will receive tPA therapy. Only by increased public awareness about stroke and, specifically, the signs of acute stroke will this improve.[4]

Even though tPA may not be administered to many patients, the antiplatelet medications can be given. Although these will not lead to reversal of stroke symptoms as tPA can, they will improve outcome, mainly by preventing recurrent strokes.

Prevention by Controlling Risk Factors

In the 1960s, a remarkable thing happened: the stroke rate began to decline. This was because of the tremendous advances in understanding about another disease, heart attack. During this period, a large epidemiological study was conducted to find out what causes heart attacks. It was called the *Framingham Study* because it was conducted in Framingham, Massachusetts. This study identified a number of health conditions associated with developing MI or heart attack. These health conditions, such as high blood pressure or **hypertension**, high blood sugar or diabetes, and others, became known as risk factors as their presence increased the risk of having an MI. It was subsequently found that by treating these risk factors, MIs decreased. A fortunate consequence of this was that the number of strokes also decreased.

There are two major categories of risk factors (Table 35-1). The first are **non-modifiable risk factors**, that is, ones you cannot do anything about. They are advancing age, male predilection, ethnicity, and family history.

Advancing age is a major non-modifiable risk factor for developing stroke. As patients grow older, the risk of stroke increases dramatically such that the incidence of stroke doubles for each decade over 60 years old.

There are significant racial and gender differences in the incidence of stroke in the United States. In the United States, African Americans have a nearly two times higher occurrence of first time stroke than Caucasians and have 1.5 times greater death rates from stroke than Caucasians. When comparing men and women, men have higher incidence of stroke from ages 55 to 74, while women have a higher incidence of stroke at older ages. Women account for 61 percent of all stroke deaths, likely related to their increased longevity compared to men.[1]

There are certain genes that are associated with increased stroke risk such as *APO-E*.

TABLE 35-1 Stroke Risk Factors

Non-Modifiable	Modifiable
Age	Hypertension
Gender	Cigarette Smoking
Race	Hyperlipidemia
Geographic Location	Diabetes Mellitus
Genetics	Obesity
	Alcohol Consumption

The second category of risk factors is modifiable, that is, ones you can do something about. There are multiple, well-identified **modifiable risk factors** for stroke. The most important are hypertension, diabetes mellitus, obesity, tobacco use, and elevated cholesterol or **hyperlipidemia**. Hypertension is likely the most important modifiable risk factor for stroke. These are all risk factors for development of coronary artery disease leading to MI as well as peripheral vascular disease (blocked arteries in the legs) leading to critical limb ischemia (poor circulation) and thus amputation.

Levels of Prevention

Identification of risk factors in an individual patient is critically important for stroke prevention. Prevention of a medical condition can be primary or secondary (Table 35-2). **Primary prevention** refers to preventing the stroke before it occurs, whereas **secondary prevention** refers to prevention of a repeat stroke.

Primary prevention of stroke is accomplished via treatment of modifiable risk factors. Hypertension is perhaps the most important modifiable risk factor for stroke. Hypertension is a factor in approximately 70 percent of all strokes. The treatment of hypertension leads to an estimated reduction of stroke risk by 40 percent to 45 percent. As such, identification and treatment of hypertension is critical for prevention of stroke. Patients should be screened every two years for blood pressure elevation. When hypertension is diagnosed, treatment includes lifestyle and dietary changes as well as medications. Increasing physical activity and initiating a low sodium diet are important non-pharmacologic (medication) interventions. Many medications are available for the treatment of hypertension; the selection of a particular drug is made on a case-by-case basis because no single class of blood pressure–lowering medication has been shown to be significantly superior to another for reducing stroke risk. Typically, patients are started on a diuretic such as thiazide or angiotensin-converting enzyme inhibitor (ACEI). However, often the decision on which medication to use is predicated on other disease conditions a patient might have, such as an ACEI because the patient has diabetes mellitus. The reduction in blood pressure associated with benefit for stroke risk reduction is 10 mm Hg systolic and 5 mm Hg diastolic. The guidelines goal for optimal blood pressure control is < 140/90 mm Hg.[5,6]

Cigarette smoking is a significant risk factor which is imminently modifiable. Smokers have up to a six times higher risk of stroke than nonsmokers. Cessation of smoking has a tremendous impact on decreasing stroke risk. In fact, in the first year after quitting cigarette smoking, the risk of stroke is reduced by 50 percent and after five years the risk of stroke returns to that of a nonsmoker.[6]

Diabetes mellitus increases risk of stroke occurrence especially when combined with other disorders including hypertension and hyperlipidemia. The prevention of stroke in diabetic patients focuses on management of these conditions because strict control of blood sugar alone has not been found to impact primary prevention. More stringent blood pressure goals are recommended and are less than 130/80 mm Hg. The goal of blood glucose control is a hemoglobin A1C < 7 percent.[5,6]

Treatment of high cholesterol or hyperlipidemia leads to approximately a 30 percent stroke risk reduction in primary prevention. Thus, patients who have experienced a stroke should be tested for elevations in fasting cholesterol. In patients with elevated LDL ("bad cholesterol") treatment with cholesterol-lowering agents should begin. The first-line agents for this should be statin drugs. Other options include niacin, oatmeal, and diet modification. The goal for reduction in LDL should be to levels less than 100 mg/dL, unless the patient is considered high risk, where the goal LDL should be less than 70 mg/dL. In a patient who had a stroke but has normal cholesterol levels, statin therapy should still be initiated; however, it is not necessary to target a specific level. Statin medications probably have some benefit for reducing stroke risk outside of their impact on cholesterol levels.[5,6]

Alcohol consumption at heavy levels increases the risk of stroke and as such, patients who have had a stroke should stop or significantly reduce consumption. Some studies have suggested however that light daily consumption (1–2 beverages per day) may reduce the risk of vascular events.

Obesity is an additional modifiable risk factor. Patients who have suffered a stroke should begin a weight reduction program to bring their weight down to a body mass index of under 25 kg/m² and reduce waist circumference to under 35 inches in females and under 40 inches in males.[5,6]

TABLE 35-2 Risk Factor Modification Goals

Hypertension	<140/90 mm Hg
Cigarette Smoking	Total cessation
Diabetes Mellitus	Hgb A1C < 7
Hyperlipidemia	LDL < 100
Alcohol Consumption	< 2 beverages per day
Obesity	BMI < 25
Exercise	30 min of moderate exercise 3 times per week

Increasing physical activity is a behavioral modification that can have a variety of benefits for prevention of stroke. Patients who have had a stroke and are capable of exercise are recommended to get 30 minutes of moderate intensity exercise at least three times per week. This exercise can help in weight reduction as well as improve control of blood pressure and diabetes.[5]

Treatment with Medications: Antiplatelets and Anticoagulants

Aspirin has routinely been used for the prevention of first myocardial infarct (MI or heart attack). There is very good scientific evidence to support this use. A recent study has shown that aspirin may have a benefit in preventing the first stroke in women who have reached menopause. Preventing the first event is known as *primary prevention*. There is no such evidence supporting aspirin in a role for stroke primary prevention in men as of yet. Of note, aspirin is the only medication that has evidence showing benefit for primary prevention of either first heart attack or first stroke.[6]

Other antiplatelet medications can be used for secondary prevention of stroke. There are four drugs currently available for preventing subsequent stroke: aspirin, aspirin-dipyridamole ER (extended release), clopidogrel, and ticlopidine. Aspirin remains the most commonly used medication as it is inexpensive, only has to be taken once per day, is generally well tolerated by patients, and, most importantly, it is effective. The optimal dose to use is a subject of debate and there is evidence supporting doses as low as 50 mg/day to as much as 325 mg/day. Neurologists typically use 325 mg/day, which is a single adult size table. Clopidogrel and aspirin-dipyridamole ER have demonstrated efficacy and can be used as well. The medication that is being used less often is ticlopidine, because it has the most severe side effects of this group of drugs.[4,5]

Conditions such as atrial fibrillation require the use of an anticoagulation medication, coumadin, which interrupts the normal clotting cascade. This drug has been shown to reduce the risk of stroke 60 percent to 70 percent in atrial fibrillation patients. For patients who are over age 65 and/or have risk factors, coumadin is used. The dose used is that which leads to a blood INR (international normalization rate) of 2.0 to 3.0. The low risk patient may be treated with aspirin instead of coumadin. If a patient who suffers atrial fibrillation is younger than 65 years old and does not have any risk factors, then he/she may be treated with aspirin (325 mg) alone.[4,5]

Non-Pharmaceutical Treatments: Stents and Carotid Endarterectomy

Placement of a stent will re-open the blood vessel but it does not remove the plaque causing the narrowing. Scientific data are less robust for treatment of narrowing of the vertebral arteries in the neck, but this can be considered when repeated strokes have occurred in the posterior portions of the brain despite maximum medical therapy. Angioplasty and stenting of the arteries within the brain has uncertain benefit and is considered investigational at this time.

With coronary artery disease and MI, invasive treatments such as angioplasty, stenting, or surgical bypass are a mainstay of treatment in the acute phase and for primary and secondary prevention. In stroke, there are very limited situations where invasive treatment is indicated. Conditions in which invasive treatment is useful include carotid artery and vertebral artery narrowing. When carotid artery narrowing in the neck is detected in the evaluation of a stroke patient, surgical intervention should be considered. Several factors are important in determining the safety and benefit of surgery. First, the stroke should have occurred on the same side of the brain as the narrowed carotid artery. Secondly, the narrowing in the artery should be greater than 70 percent. Finally, the surgical complication rate for the performing surgeon should be less than 6 percent. The surgical procedure generally performed is a carotid endarterectomy. This procedure involves removing the atherosclerotic plaque from within the vessel. When there are medical conditions that make surgery too risky, insertion of a stent into the narrowed blood vessel can also be considered. The role of stents is not as well established as surgical carotid endarterectomy. However, as stenting is less invasive, a number of studies are under way to determine its effectiveness, especially as compared to carotid endarterectomy.[4,5]

After carotid endarterectomy, risk factor reduction is necessary and vitally important. It must be recognized that the surgery improved just the lesion; it did not "cure." Thus, subsequent strokes can be avoided mainly through risk factor reduction. Aspirin (325 mg/day) use should be continued also.

If a stent is placed, risk factor reduction must be aggressively accomplished. Typically, a patient will be prescribed a combination of aspirin and clopidogrel for one year after the procedure. Thereafter, aspirin alone will be continued.

STROKE AS A RISK FACTOR FOR MYOCARDIAL INFARCTION

The risk of heart attack after stroke is three to four times higher than patients who have not had a stroke. Among stroke survivors, the highest risk of death is due largely to recurrent stroke and heart attack. In some studies of stroke patients, heart attack outnumbers stroke as the cause of death by as much as two to one. For this reason, medical providers should determine whether or not the stroke victim is also at risk of heart attack. This means obtaining a detailed medical history on the patient as well as an appropriate physical exam. It might also mean an electrocardiogram (ECG), cardiac ultrasound or echo, stress test, and possibly cardiac angiography. Possibly, an ankle-brachial index will be needed as well to identify peripheral vascular disease. If unrecognized cardiac and peripheral vascular disease exists, then risk factor reduction becomes even more critical. Of the antiplatelet medications, only aspirin and clopidogrel are U.S. Food and Drug Administration (FDA) indicated for stroke and heart attack, and only clopidogrel is FDA indicated for peripheral vascular disease.[5]

PUBLIC HEALTH PERSPECTIVE FOR THE HEALTH OF THE GENERAL POPULATION AND OF HIGH RISK GROUPS

Although the mortality rates from strokes and other cardiovascular disease have been in decline since the 1970s, the overall number of deaths attributable to stroke increases each year. The increase in deaths is fueled primarily by the aging of the baby boomers and also by the obesity epidemic. Despite declines in the overall mortality rate, stroke persists as the third largest killer of Americans. Internationally, stroke is also on the rise, accounting for 5 million deaths worldwide and 5 million more cases of disability each year. By 2020, stroke is estimated to account for the 4th largest share of Disability Life Year (DALY) statistics, up from its current position as 7th.

Despite its prominence as a major killer, programs to prevent stroke and heart disease account for less than 3 percent of the budgets of U.S. state public health agencies. Unlike many diseases, the causes and risk factors for stroke are quite well known and modifying several risky behaviors can greatly reduce risks, making it an ideal target for public health prevention programs.

Current public health efforts to address stroke include a National Public Health Action Plan, which was developed by the U.S. Department of Health and Human Services in conjunction with other national partners from both the public and private sectors. The five essential components of the plan are:

1. *Taking Action.* Develop new policies in accordance with advances in science and implement new intervention programs in a timely manner in multiple settings, for all age groups, for whole populations, and especially for high-risk groups, on a scale sufficient to have measurable impacts.
2. *Strengthening Capacity.* Strengthen public health agencies and create training opportunities, model standards, and resources for continuous technical support for these agencies and their partners.

3. *Evaluating Impact.* Enhance data sources and systems to monitor key indicators relevant to heart disease and stroke prevention, and to systematically evaluate policy and program interventions.
4. *Advancing Policy.* Foster research on policies and public health programs aimed at preventing atherosclerosis and high blood pressure, especially at the community level. Continue to evaluate the public health role of genetic and other biomarkers of risk. Develop innovative ways to evaluate public health interventions, particularly those related to policy and environmental change and population-wide health promotion.
5. *Engaging in Regional and Global Partnerships.* Work with regional and global partners to reap the full benefit of sharing knowledge and experience in heart disease and stroke prevention with these partners.

Special At-Risk Populations

Certain populations are disproportionately affected by stroke, and African Americans are particularly vulnerable. Their increased risk relative to other populations results from a complex set of factors. African Americans suffer from higher rates of hypertension, obesity, diabetes, and have high rates of alcohol and tobacco usage. Adding to their high prevalence of risk factors, African Americans also have less access to health services compared to other cohorts. As a result of these factors, blacks have almost twice the risk of first-ever strokes compared with whites, and after suffering a stroke, they are less likely to survive. The disproportionate burden of stroke born by African Americans continues to be of great public health concern.[7]

CONCLUSION

Stroke is a devastating medical condition, which has major medical morbidity for sufferers and a significant societal cost. The prevention of stroke can occur both before and after the stroke has occurred. Before the stroke or TIA has occurred, the prevention should center on management of systemic diseases and behaviors that are vascular risk factors. After the stroke, management of these conditions should come under further scrutiny. Additionally, secondary stroke prevention will include medications that can affect the platelets or clotting system to decrease the chances of recurrent occlusion of blood vessels within the brain. Stroke or TIA is reflective of cerebrovascular (brain's blood vessels) disease, which highly correlates with vascular disease in other areas of the body including the heart and legs. Thus, the interventions taken to prevent stroke will likely also modify the risk for coronary artery and peripheral vascular disease.

KEY TERMS

Biology Terms

Athersclerosis: Narrowing of arteries characterized by deposition of lipid, inflammation, and calcification.

Hyperlipidemia: Elevations of lipids (cholesterol, triglycerides) in the plasma.

Hypertension: Transitory or sustained elevation of systolic and diastolic blood pressure.

Stroke: Sudden onset of persistent neurologic deficits resulting from vascular causes.

Transient Ischemic Attack (TIA): Sudden onset of neurological deficits resulting from cessation of blood flow, which recovers in less than 24 hours.

Public Health Terms

Modifiable Risk Factor: Condition present within an individual that increases the risk of disease occurrence that can be changed to alter subsequent risk of disease occurrence.

Non-Modifiable Risk Factor: Condition present within an individual that increases the risk of disease occurrence but cannot be changed.

Primary Prevention: Intervention to prevent a disease before it has occurred.

Secondary Prevention: Intervention to prevent a recurrence of a disease after its initial occurrence.

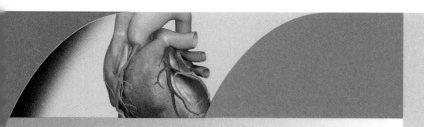

Questions for Further Research, Study, Reflection, and Discussion

For the Individual Student

In order to answer these questions, it may be necessary to research the primary literature.

- Define the term *ischemic penumbra* and describe its relevance to treatment of stroke.
- Describe how an atherosclerotic plaque leads to occlusion of a blood vessel.

For Small Group Discussion

- What steps would you recommend for Charles to change his long-term risk of stroke? Discuss med-ical and non-medical interventions and how you also help to ensure that he accomplishes them.
- How would your approach to question 1 change if Charles was 53 instead of 73?
- Are there other problems/conditions that must be considered?

For Entire Class Discussion

- Given the limited resources to begin a stroke pre-vention campaign, how would you prioritize which risk factors to address?
- If you were to design a stroke assessment team, what specialists would you include? What labs, tests, or assessments should be standard?

EXERCISES/ACTIVITIES

- Design an educational program for the lay popu-lation discussing common signs and symptoms of stroke as well as risk factors for stroke.
- Review and critique the NIH Guidelines for Stroke Centers of Excellence as it pertains to secondary prevention.

DISCLAIMER

The views and opinions expressed in this work belong solely to the authors. They do not and should not be interpreted as those of or endorsed by the Uniformed Services University of the Health Sciences, Walter Reed Army Medical Center, Department of the Army, Department of Defense, or the federal government.

Healthy People 2010

Indicator: Overweight and Obesity

Focus Area: Heart Disease and Stroke

Goal: Improve cardiovascular health and quality of life through the prevention, detection, and treatment of risk factors; early identification and treatment of heart attacks and strokes; and prevention of recurrent cardiovascular events.

Objectives:

12-7. Reduce stroke deaths.

12-8. Increase the proportion of adults who are aware of the early warning symptoms and signs of a stroke.

12-11. Increase the proportion of adults with high blood pressure who are taking action (for example, losing weight, increasing physical activity, or reducing sodium intake) to help control their blood pressure.

12-15. Increase the proportion of adults who have had their blood cholesterol checked within the preceding 5 years.

REFERENCES

1. American Heart Association. *Heart Disease and Stroke Statistics: 2007 Update At-A-Glance*. Dallas: American Heart Association; 2007. Available at http://www.americanheart.org/downloadable/heart/1166712318459HS_Stats InsideText.pdf. Accessed May 2, 2008.

2. Biller J, Love BB. Ischemic Cerebrovascular Disease. In: Bradley WG, Daroff RB, Fenichel G, Jankovic J. *Neurology in Clinical Practice*. Philadelphia: Butterworth Heinemann; 2004:1197–1250.

3. Kasner SE, Gorelick PB. *Prevention and Treatment of Ischemic Stroke*. Philadelphia: Butterworth Heinemann; 2004.

4. Van der Worp HB, van Gijn J. Clinical practice: acute ischemic stroke. *N Engl J Med* 2007;357:572–579.

5. Sacco RL, Adams R, Albers G, Alberts MJ, Benevente O, et al. Guidelines for prevention of stroke in patients who have had an ischemic stroke or transient ischemic attack. *Circulation* 2006;113:e409–e449.

6. Goldstein LB, Adams R, Alberts MJ, Appel LJ, Brass LM, et al. Primary prevention of ischemic stroke: a guideline from the American Heart Association/American Stroke Association Stroke Council. *Stroke* 2006; 37:1583–1633.

7. American Stroke Association. *Know the Facts*. Available at: http://www.strokeassociation.org/presenter.jhtml?identifier=3035006 Accessed May 2, 2008.

CROSS REFERENCES

Atherosclerosis

Communicating Health Information

Diabetes

Inflammation

Smoking or Health

The Nutrition Transition

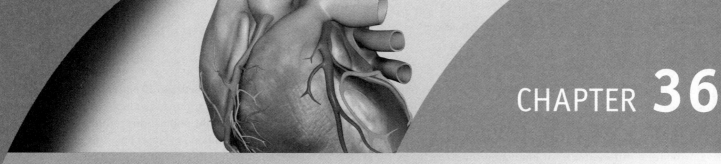

CHAPTER 36

Diabetes: A Public Health Pandemic

Mary Beth Bigley

Every 24 hours:[1]
- 4,100 new cases
- 810 deaths
- 230 amputations
- 120 kidney failures
- 55 blindness

LEARNING OBJECTIVES

By the end of this chapter, the student will be able to:

- Understand the basic science and pathophysiology of diabetes types 1 and 2.
- Summarize the United States and global **epidemiology** of diabetes.
- Describe characteristics of an individual at risk for diabetes.
- Discuss public health preventive measure related to diabetes.

INTRODUCTION

Diabetes is a major public health problem affecting the United States population in epidemic proportions. The prevalence has doubled since 1991 from 7.0 million to 14.6 million in 2005. In addition, 6.2 million people are unaware that they have the disease.[1] Diabetes is a serious chronic disease that is costly. It causes significant **morbidity** and **mortality** ranking as the sixth leading cause of death in the United States. Globally, in 2006, diabetes affected approximately 246 million people and is expected to affect 380 million by 2025. Acute and chronic complications from diabetes lead to damage, dysfunction and failure of several vital organs.

Diabetes is a group of metabolic disorders marked by inappropriate **hyperglycemia** due to a deficiency in **insulin** secretion, insulin action, or a combination of **insulin resistance** (action) and inadequate insulin secretion. *Type 1 diabetes*, previously called insulin-dependent diabetes mellitus (IDDM) or juvenile-onset diabetes, accounts for less than 10 percent of the cases. It is primarily due to pancreatic islet B cell destruction and affects children and young adults. Currently there is no way to prevent type 1 diabetes. Type 2 diabetes, previously called non-insulin dependent diabetes mellitus (NIDDM) or adult onset diabetes, results from insulin resistance with a defect in compensatory insulin secretion. The terms IDDM and NIDDM are no longer being used.

Diabetes type 1 disease used to be primarily a childhood disease almost always resulting in premature death. However, we are now seeing well-controlled type 1 diabetics living with similar life expectancies as normal adults. Type 2 diabetes was thought to be mostly an adult disease, but very recently, with the prevalence of obesity in adolescence and even childhood, type 2 diabetes has become a pediatric chronic disease.

Important advances in prevention, detection, and treatment of diabetes provide evidence that the consequences of diabetes can be altered. Much of the information regarding diabetes—current medical treatment, healthcare delivery system, and cost—frames the issue from an illness or medical prospective. However, prevailing causes of type 2 diabetes are physical inactivity, obesity, and poor nutrition. Theses are public health problems that require an individual and population approach to resolve. Primary and secondary prevention that promotes exercise and nutrition has been and will continue to be challenging.

Framing the issue from a public health wellness prospective provides a different way of analyzing the diabetes as chronic disease. Evidence-based healthcare, implementation of community programs, and evaluations of lifestyle intervention impact on the incidence of diabetes. There is an immediate need to maximize the use of primary and secondary preventive measures and a population approach to avert the projected morbidity and mortality.

HISTORY

The earliest known record of diabetes was in 1552 BC by a physician named Hesy-Ra, who mentioned polyuria as a symptom in a journal written on 3rd Dynasty Egyptian papyrus. Up until the 11th century, diabetes was commonly diagnosed by the "water taster," who drank urine to determine if it was sweet-tasting. The Latin word for honey (sweetness), *mellitus*, was attached to diabetes, thus the term *diabetes mellitus*. Insulin was discovered in 1922 at the University of Toronto by Dr. Fredrick Banting, Dr. Charles Best, Professor J.J.R. Macleod, and Dr. James Collip. The first successful insulin treatment was on January 23, 1922 on a 14-year-old boy, Leonard Thompson. The link between diabetes and the complications related to diabetes was established in the 1940s; however, the distinction between type 1 and type 2 diabetes was determined later in 1959. Blood glucose meters and insulin pumps were developed in 1970.

Mapping of the human genome has advanced the treatment of diabetes. Understanding the molecular genetics of diabetes has begun to inform researchers on variation in gene mutations. Different mutations respond to different treatment. Although the science is incomplete, there is promise that by understanding gene mutation and developing therapies that respond to the specific gene mutation, individual treatment plans will be enhanced. The research and development in understanding the disease process and the burden of suffering as well as maximizing prevention strategies and treatment plans, is just starting.

EPIDEMIOLOGY

In 2005, 14.6 million Americans had been diagnosed with diabetes with another 6.2 million with the disease who had not yet been diagnosed. The total number, 20.8 million people, accounts for 7 percent of the U.S. population. Of those cases diagnosed, 5 to 10 percent have type 1 diabetes while the remaining cases are individuals with type 2 diabetes.[2] Almost 10 percent of the population aged 20 years or older has diabetes, with 1.5 million new cases being diagnosed in 2005. Moreover, several minority populations are at increased risk of diabetes, resulting in more deaths (Table 36-1).[3]

With the combination of growth and aging of the U.S. population, it is projected that the prevalence of diabetes will exceed 29 million in the year 2050. The largest percent increase will be seen in individuals older than 75 years along with a significant percent increase seen among black males.[4] These statistics will directly impact resources and the current healthcare delivery model.

Direct medical and indirect expenditures attributable to diabetes in 2002 were estimated at $132 billion. These expenditures have increased as the number of type 2 diabetes patients has risen. A diabetic person spends twice as much on medical care compared to a person without diabetes. In 2002, direct medical expenditures alone totaled $91.8 billion, which was comprised of $23.2 billion for diabetes care, $24.5 billion for chronic complications attributable to diabetes, and $44.1 billion general medical conditions.[5,6] The indirect cost, including disability, work loss, and premature mortality is estimated to be $40 billion annually.[6] This cost is likely to increase as the prevalence increases.

Global concerns of diabetes have labeled this disease as a pandemic with diabetes affecting 246 million people, estimated to be 7.3 percent of adults aged 20 to 79. Similar to the projections in the United States, this number is expected to reach 380 million by 2025. According to the International Diabetes Federation, an organization that collects data from most countries, in 2007 diabetes is expected to cause 3.8 million deaths, which is equivalent to 6 percent of global mortality, approaching the same rate as HIV/AIDS. The five countries with the highest diabetes prevalence in their adult population are Nauru (30.7%), United Arab Emirates (19.5%), Saudi Arabia (16.7%), Bahrain (15.2%), and Kuwait (14.4%).[7,8]

TABLE 36-1 Relative Risk of Diabetes for Race/Ethnicity Population as Compared to Non-Hispanic Whites Among People Age 20 Years or Older in the United States, 2005

Population	Relative Risk
Non-Hispanic white	1.0
American Indians and Alaska Native	2.2
African Americans	1.9
Mexican Americans	1.7
Asians, native Hawaiians and Pacific Islanders in Hawaii	2.0
California Asians	1.5

Source: Centers for Disease Control: Diabetes. *National Diabetes Fact Sheet: United States, 2005.* Available at http://www.cdc.gov/diabetes/pubs/pdf/ndfs_2005.pdf. Accessed May 5, 2008.

BASIC SCIENCE FACTS/KEY CONCEPTS REVIEW

Diabetes mellitus is a common endocrine disorder in which the body cannot metabolize carbohydrates, fats, and proteins due to a lack of or ineffective use of insulin.

The pancreas is an elongated organ next to the first portion of the small intestine. The endocrine pancreas refers to the cells within the pancreas that synthesize and secrete hormones. The endocrine portion of the pancreas takes the form of many small clusters of cells called **islets of Langerhans**. The islets house three major cell types: **alpha** cells, **beta** cells, and **delta** cells. The physiologic effect of insulin comes from the beta cells, the main endocrine component of the islet of Langerhans in the pancreas. Alpha cells make and release a hormone called **glucagon**. When blood glucose is high or low, after eating or fasting, the body's normal physiological response is to regulate glucose.

The complete science and mechanisms of insulin secretion are not fully understood. Still, some features of the physiology and pathophysiology have been confirmed. After eating, your blood sugar rises; then glucose, proteins, and fatty acids from the intestines are distributed in the bloodstream. Insulin, made and secreted by beta cells, is released into the bloodstream to open up cells throughout the body. Insulin stimulates the absorption of glucose in the liver and muscle cells. As the body maintains a constant state of glucose, excess glucose, proteins, and fatty acids are absorbed by the liver and muscles and stored as **glycogen**. The result of decreased blood glucose in the bloodstream is that insulin production ceases.

In a fasting state, glucagon secretes from alpha cells into the bloodstream. This stimulates the release of glycogen stored in the muscle as well as fat stored in adipose tissue for energy. The brain is also affected by the level of glucose in the blood with a low glucose level resulting in symptoms of **hypoglycemia** and a high glucose level resulting in symptoms of ketoacidosis. The balance of the release of insulin and glucagon throughout the day keeps the body's blood glucose levels constant (Figure 36-1).

Type 1 Diabetes

Type 1 diabetes results from B-cell destruction, usually leading to absolute insulin deficiency.[9] The typical onset is during childhood with signs and symptoms of hyperglycemia: increased thirst and hunger, frequent urination, weight loss, and fatigue. It is due to the destruction of pancreatic beta cells (which is most likely caused by an environmental or autoimmune reaction), a genetic predisposition, or an environmental exposure to a virus, toxin, or stress. Due to the lack of insulin, the body is unable to utilize glucose for energy and begins to metabolize free fatty acids instead, which can result in coma and even death. The incomplete metabolism of fatty acids results in an accumulation of substances and a state termed **diabetic ketoacidosis**. Individuals

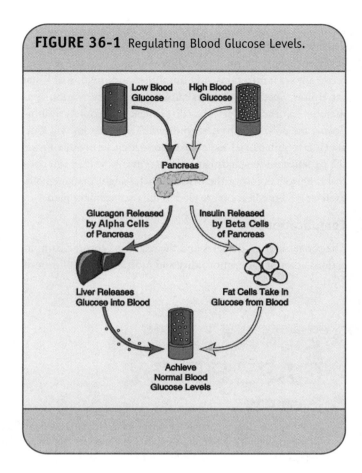

FIGURE 36-1 Regulating Blood Glucose Levels.

with type 1 diabetes control glucose levels with insulin as well as diet and exercise. Education and monitoring of theses activities as well as blood glucose level are paramount to controlling the signs and symptoms of diabetes and the results of fluctuating blood glucose levels that leads to organ system complications.

Type 2 Diabetes

Type 2 diabetes results from a progressive insulin secretory defect in the background of insulin resistance.[9] For mechanisms unclear, but possibly due to excess oxidized free fatty acids from abdominal fat, the peripheral tissues in type 2 diabetics become insensitive to insulin. Initially, the pancreas tries to compensate by producing excess amounts of insulin. Eventually, however, the pancreas is not able to keep up, and the beta cells begin to atrophy. The resultant beta cell dysfunction ultimately leads to insulin deficiency. Decreased insulin secretion occurs when the pancreas does not secrete enough insulin in response to glucose levels. Insulin resistance is the body's inability to utilize insulin that it makes because of a cell receptor defect or an absorption defect; absorption of glucose into the cells. There is an increased prevalence of type 2 diabetes in people with a genetic predisposition and a sedentary lifestyle as well as in obese children, adolescents, and adults. Like type 1 diabetes, signs and symptoms include hyperglycemia, increased thirst and hunger, frequent urination, weight loss, and fatigue. Additionally, individuals may experience extreme tiredness, blurred vision, delayed healing, recurrent yeast infections, and numbness and tingling of distal extremities. Specific to diabetes caused by insulin resistance, signs include acanthosis nigricans (dirty-neck syndrome), dyslipidemia, and polycystic ovarian syndrome. Treatment for type 2 diabetes is multifactorial. Essential to good long-term outcomes is the patient's understanding of diabetes and how they can control the progression of the disease. Diet, weight management, exercise, and medication are vital to the management plan.

Complications

The progression of diabetes and the results of chronic complications account for its morbidity and mortality. Complications are classified as macrovascular or microvascular and infectious. Macrovascular complications such as coronary artery disease, stroke, and peripheral vascular disease, are the main cause of death. Diabetics are two to five times more likely to have myocardial infarction. They are at increased risk for diffuse atherosclerosis thus prone to cerebrovascular and peripheral vascular disease. Secondary prevention of hypertension, dyslipidemia, and hypercoagulability is routine care for an individual with diabetes.

Microvascular complications such as retinopathy, nephropathy, and neuropathy are the main cause of decreased quality of life, disability, and morbidity. Diabetic retinopathy is the most common cause of blindness in adults, while nephropathy leads to kidney failure. Neuropathy results in loss of peripheral sensation, gastroparesis, orthostatic hypotension,

CASE STUDY
Scenario

James has been your patient for many years. Five years ago, at age 40, he was diagnosed with hypertension. For the first two years after his diagnosis he kept all of his appointments. He lost seven pounds and started to learn more about living a healthy life. Today you are seeing him for a physical examination. He is now 45 years old (born in 1962) and much heavier than the last time you saw him.

James has an African-American father and Native American mother. You start your visit asking him about his family, children, and job. You find out that three years ago, he changed jobs and now is much busier and travels more often. His children are grown and his wife has started working full time. You ask him why he did not continue with the routine care appointments to monitor his hypertension. He responded that he felt fine and that he was just too busy. What brought him in today was that a very good friend of his suddenly died from a "heart attack." Other information you learn is that he restarted smoking about one year ago (he had quit shortly after being diagnosed with hypertension), he does not have a regular physical fitness program, and he has been having headaches as well as blurred vision. Recently, his father had a kidney transplant due to uncontrolled diabetes leading to end organ kidney failure.

On physical exam he is calm with a **body mass index (BMI)** of 29.5, with excess weight notably in his abdominal area. Blood pressure is elevated 182/96 mm Hg. The exam was unremarkable except for the funduscopic exam notable for hard exudates and the foot exam notes fungus between his toes. A urine dipstick shows +2 glucose and +1 protein. A fasting finger stick glucose is 182 mg/dL. Fasting is defined as no caloric intake for at least eight hours.

Categories of the Basal Metabolic Index (BMI):

- Underweight = <18.5
- Normal weight = 18.5–24.9
- Overweight = 25–29.9
- Obesity = BMI of 30 or greater[10]

You continue to talk with James during and after the exam to find out more about his daily routine, diet, and extended family. You tell him that his blood pressure is too high and based on the information collected, it is likely he has diabetes. You order additional blood work, provide him medication for his elevated blood pressure, and schedule him to come back next week. But before he leaves, you ask James what he wants to do to get healthy. He says he will quit smoking today and start eating better. You encourage him and suggest that he should keep a diary of what he eats as well as to check his blood pressure three or four times before the next visit. The additional tests confirm a diagnosis of type 2 diabetes.

Defining the Issues

As noted, James at age 40 had several risk factors for diabetes: first degree relative with diabetes, hypertension, a current smoker, and from a high risk ethnic population (African American and Native American). By stopping his routine follow-up care for his hypertension, he was not screened for diabetes or provided with education that may have delayed the onset of the diagnosis of type 2 diabetes.

Another notable aspect of this case is that James made an appointment after he had heard about his friend's heart attack. The case informs us of his father's long-standing history of diabetes and subsequent kidney failure. If James had understood the relationship between his medical history and his father's medical history, then he may have made the appointment years earlier. James's delay in receiving medical care to diagnose his type 2 diabetes as well as helping him to control his hypertension increases his risk of co-morbidities.

Patient's Understanding

James' lack of knowledge regarding routine healthcare and chronic illness care clouded his judgment to continue with his appointments and commitment to a proactive, healthy lifestyle. This is not an isolated occurrence. Many individuals with chronic health conditions are not regularly followed by a healthcare provider. They do not understand the progression of a disease, especially when they are asymptomatic. Communication to the general public that provides information stressing the importance of regular healthcare, along with healthcare providers assuming the role as educator, may help to improve an individual's understanding of this chronic disease.

Many of the issues in this case have to do with health communication: first the communication between the provider and patient, and second the communication of health information from other sources about hypertension, diabetes, and healthy lifestyle behaviors. Although we do not have the benefit of knowing the conversation between James and the provider, based on the information communicated to James initially regarding his hypertension as well as information about his risk factors for diabetes given his family history, James did not understand the importance of the information and failed to make appropriate health decisions. This case points out the value of health literacy, defined as "the degree to which individuals have the capacity to obtain, process, and understand basic health information and services needed to make appropriate health decisions."[11] Schillinger et al.'s studies with type 2 diabetics found that inadequate health literacy is independently associated with worse glycemic control and higher rates of retinopathy. Inadequate health literacy may contribute to the disproportionate burden of diabetes-related problems among disadvantaged populations.[12]

CLINICAL PERSPECTIVE FOR THE INDIVIDUAL PATIENT

Screening for diabetes is not recommended for the general population by any of the associations or task forces that publish guidelines. The American Diabetes Association (ADA) recommends screening for individuals 45 years old or older with a BMI greater than or equal to 25, and screening for those less than 45 years old who are overweight and have additional risk factors.

Managing diabetes requires an understanding of the disease and its co-morbidities. The most effective approaches to achieving glycemic control are patient education, lifestyle modification, and appropriate medical therapy. Secondary prevention includes maintaining a healthy weight, following a balanced diet, being physically active, taking medication as prescribed, and managing stress. Additionally, checking your glucose levels and blood pressure regularly and keeping them in your target range, along with routine medical visits, are vital. The National Standards for diabetes self-management education provides a robust framework to develop an individualized plan of care. The multidisciplinary team approach considers individual aspects such as setting for obtaining healthcare, work schedule, eating patterns, cultural factors, and other medical conditions.

In general, people with diabetes are medically managed and monitored for the end organ damage that occurs. Routine care consists of lifestyle modification, glycemic control, and nutrition therapy that primarily focuses on balancing carbohydrate and fat intake. Several major studies have shown that individuals with an intensive treatment plan were found to have prevented or slowed the progression of diabetic complications as compared to individuals who received standard care. Prognosis can be positive if the individual is well cared for and conversely cares for themselves.

Family health history information can serve as a tool to estimate an individual's risk of diabetes. Evidence suggests that having one or both biological parents with diabetes increases the risk of diabetes.[13] Because population screenings for diabetes are not indicated, using information entered into a pedigree chart can generate one's risk for diabetes. Preventive measures such as exercise, diet, and eliminating smoking can be offered to those identified as high risk for developing diabetes. Additional public health methods to inform and educate family members about diabetes and their risk of developing diabetes further the utility of gathering a family health history to reduce the incidence of diabetes.

and erectile dysfunction. Patients with diabetes have a higher rate of infection, especially if they experience frequent hyperglycemic periods. It is the primary and secondary prevention of these chronic conditions, as well as blood sugar control, which limits the progress of these complications.

PUBLIC HEALTH PERSPECTIVE FOR THE HEALTH OF THE GENERAL POPULATION AND OF HIGH RISK GROUPS

National efforts to understand and provide guidance to individuals, communities, businesses, organizations, and providers are ongoing. Former Secretary of Health and Human Services (2004–2005) Tommy Thompson identified diabetes as central to his health agenda. Documents such as *Steps to a Healthier US: Putting Prevention First, the Diabetes Detection Initiative, and the Small Steps, Big Rewards, Prevent Type 2 Diabetes* campaign were released. The Diabetes Detection Initiative provides resources for providers and the public to identify new cases of diabetes. The "Steps" programs provide funding to communities to implement prevention and health promotion programs. The Medicare Prescription Drug Improvement and Modernization Act of 2004 established coverage for annual diabetes screen for individuals with two diabetes risk factors. In late 2004, *Diabetes: A National Plan for Action* was released to mobilize the nation to address the rising rates of diabetes. The document provides prevention, detection, and treatment information with simple steps for all segments of the population to utilize as a comprehensive action-oriented approach to diabetes. For example, local communities can take steps to prevention of diabetes by promoting walking trails that are safe or promoting sponsored "cook offs" that create healthy meal options that are culturally appropriate. Business can join with communities to promote these activities as well as offer worksite health promotion and disease prevention programs. Studies have shown that there is a cost benefit to healthy employees, noting the return on investment for worksite programs. This cost benefit to cost ratio ranges from $1.49 to $4.91 in benefits per dollar spent on the program.[14]

Over the years there has been an increased focus on gathering data and setting up surveillance systems related to diabetes, evident in the increase of Healthy People (HP) objectives from five objectives for HP 2000 to 17 objectives for HP 2010. This has led to a better understanding of the condition and its health disparities. A midcourse review of the HP 2010 diabetes objectives noted that the nation has exceeded target for diabetes-related death in persons with diabetes (5–6) as well as cardiovascular deaths in persons with diabetes (5–7). Several objectives, however, have moved away from the target goal:

new cases, for example, of diabetes in persons aged 18 to 84 years and overall diagnosis of diabetes.[15]

One social challenge to implementing lifestyle interventions is targeting the populations that would benefit the most. Over the next 50 years the increase in diabetes will be in African Americans, American Indians, Alaska Natives, Asian, and Hispanic/Latino persons.[16] These populations are medically underserved and lack the means to search out appropriate information and resources. The lack of culturally appropriate care and language barriers further puts these populations at a disadvantage. New models of care that link community resources with the population's unique culture and values are needed to ensure access and evidence-based care. These new models are innovative ways to achieve change. Healthcare providers working in a team each contribute their own unique knowledge and skills in the treatment of diabetes. Teams should include the patient, family members, and community resources to maximize individualized care and targeted lifestyle interventions.

Delivery of evidence-based diabetic care is essential to all individuals with diabetes. This includes providing clear and individualized lifestyle interventions. However, the current healthcare system does not encourage healthcare providers to counsel patients. Counseling is not a billable service and clinicians working in a traditional clinic setting do not have time to offer behavior change information. Few practices utilize a team approach having health educators, nurses, and nutritionist in their practices to provide individual and group education. This in part is due to the limited research that endorses a team approach supporting the initial education and clinical oversight by trained staff.

The economic impact of delivering lifestyle interventions as an integral part of the evidence-based care model is not fully understood. Examining the cost and value of lifestyle interventions is complex. The current evidence-based care included interventions such as regular follow-up, periodic foot exam, annually eye exams, and hemoglobin A1c testing. Providers have not yet incorporated these elements of care into the routine diabetes care. For example, in 2002 the CDC found that only 63.3% of persons with diabetes had an eye exam within the last year. It may be difficult in the current healthcare delivery system to require providers to offer lifestyle modification education.

The ideal model to address the medical, nursing, behavior, and social factors of diabetic care is the team approach. The Chronic Care Model (CCM) by Wagner and colleagues[17] has shown to be successful in providing a team approach to diabetic care. The model is designed so that the care targets the

Diabetic Quality Improvement Project performance indicators; those factors that parallel evidence-based diabetes care. Another unique aspect of the CCM is that it emphasizes partnering with the community. The next step to ensure optimal care is to demonstrate both to purchases and payer that prevention and lifestyle interventions minimize complication in diabetics. This will be a challenging but necessary step.

CONCLUSION

Scientific evidence suggests that the trajectory of diabetes can be altered. As we learn more about the impact of primary and secondary lifestyle intervention, the messages of early lifestyle interventions that promote exercise and nutrition must be clear, consistent, and practical. Additionally, emerging scientific information and a better understanding of a diabetic's genetic profile can lead to individualized pharmacogenetic therapy. The public health of the world is in danger if we cannot avert the projected mortality and morbidity related to diabetes.

KEY TERMS

Biology Terms

Alpha Cell: A type of cell in the pancreas in areas called the islets of Langerhans; alpha cells make and release a hormone called glucagon, which raises the level of glucose (sugar) in the blood.

Beta Cell: A type of cell in the pancreas in areas called the islets of Langerhans; beta cells make and release insulin, a hormone that controls the level of glucose (sugar) in the blood.

Body Mass Index (BMI): A measure to gauge total body fat that takes into account a person's weight and height. For adults, a BMI of 30 or more is considered obese. For children, proper determination of BMI depends on additional factors. The higher the BMI, the greater the risk of developing additional health problems.

Delta Cell: A type of cell in the pancreas in areas called the islets of Langerhans; delta cells make somatostatin, a hormone that is believed to control how the beta cells make and release insulin and how the alpha cells make and release glucagon.

Diabetic Ketoacidosis (DKA): Severe, out-of-control diabetes (high blood sugar) that needs emergency treatment. DKA is caused by a profound lack of circulating insulin. This may happen because of illness, taking too little insulin, or getting too little exercise. The body starts using stored fat for energy, and ketone bodies (acids) build up in the blood. Ketoacidosis starts slowly and builds up. Signs include nausea and vomiting, which can lead to loss of water from the body, stomach pain, and deep and rapid breathing. Other signs are a flushed face, dry skin and mouth, a fruity breath odor, a rapid and weak pulse, and low blood pressure. If the person is not given fluids and insulin right away, ketoacidosis can lead to coma and even death.

Glucagon: A hormone that raises the level of glucose (sugar) in the blood. The alpha cells of the pancreas, in areas called the islets of Langerhans, make glucagon when the body needs to put more sugar into the blood.

Glycogen: A substance made up of sugars. It is stored in the liver and muscles and releases glucose (sugar) into the blood when needed by cells. Glycogen is the chief source of stored fuel in the body.

Hyperglycemia: Too high a level of glucose (sugar) in the blood; a sign that diabetes is out of control. Many things can cause hyperglycemia. It occurs when the body does not have enough insulin or cannot use the insulin it does have to turn glucose into energy. Signs of hyperglycemia are a great thirst, a dry mouth, and a need to urinate often. For people with type 1 diabetes, hyperglycemia may lead to diabetic ketoacidosis.

Hypoglycemia: Too low a level of glucose (sugar) in the blood. This occurs when a person with diabetes has injected too much insulin, eaten too little food, or has exercised without extra food. A person with hypoglycemia may feel nervous, shaky, weak, or sweaty and have a headache, blurred vision, and hunger. Taking small amounts of sugar, sweet juice, or food with sugar will usually help the person feel better within 10 to 15 minutes.

Insulin: A hormone that helps the body use glucose (sugar) for energy. The beta cells of the pancreas (in areas called the islets of Langerhans) make the insulin. When the body cannot make enough insulin on its own, a person with diabetes must inject insulin made from other sources, such as beef, pork, human insulin (recombinant DNA origin), or human insulin (pork-derived, semisynthetic).

Insulin Resistance: The body's inability to respond to and use the insulin it produces; insulin resistance may be linked to obesity.

Islets of Langerhans (pronunciation: EYE-let): Clumps of cells within the pancreas that include those that make insulin and other hormones. The cells include several subvarieties including: alpha cells (which make glucagon); beta cells (which make insulin); delta cells (which make somatostatin); and PP cells and D1 cells (about which little is known). Islet cells appear under low-power magnification to be islands (islets) within the pancreas. First described by Dr. Paul Langerhans in 1869, whose name is now associated with these islands.[18]

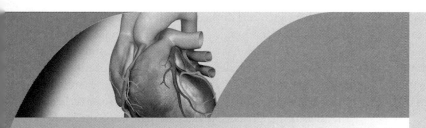

Questions for Further Research, Study, Reflection, and Discussion

For the Individual Student

In order to answer these questions, it may be necessary to research the primary literature.

- Explain the pathophysiology of type 2 diabetes.
- List the microvascular changes that occur due to diabetes and their associated symptoms and describe the pathophysiology.

For Small Group Discussion

- As James's provider, you give him two behavior changes to make to his lifestyle. What two changes will you recommend, and discuss your rationale for suggesting these two specific recommendations?
- You are a member of the team who is responsible for keeping an individual with diabetes healthy. Roles include the patient, his family members, the provider, the community, or the government. Take a role and discuss your plan, rationale, and action items. How does your plan interrelate with the other members of the team and what they are recommending?
- Keep a 24-hour journal to record what you eat, drink, and the type of exercise (from casual walking to organized aerobic and weight lifting). If you have access to a pedometer, count your steps. Also note your sleep pattern, stress, and medications (prescribed and over-the-counter) taken.

After reviewing this information, reflect on the positive and negative activities as if you were a type 2 diabetic. Discuss in your small group your reflections of this exercise.

For Entire Class Discussion

- The global impact of diabetes affects economic stability of countries. Using Internet resources, research the global economic impact of diabetes. What statistics are available, and what countries report high rates? Compare U.S. prevention programs to those in other countries. What lessons can be learned?
- Design a marketable "Diabetes Fact Sheet" that you would provide to a unique population. For example, what facts would you like the immigrant Asian-American population to know about diabetes? Include statistical data and lifestyle information with the resource.

EXERCISES/ACTIVITIES

- Complete the *My Family Health Portrait Tool* (U.S. Surgeon General, U.S. Public Health Service. Available at https://familyhistory.hhs.gov. Accessed May 5, 2008). Identify patterns of health conditions such as diabetes or cancers that may exist in your family and discuss generally.
- Using Internet resources, research several different community programs that have been implemented with outcomes that have impacted the incidence of diabetes. What are the target populations? Describe how the different programs are implemented. What are the strengths and limitations to these programs? Three or four groups in the class should compare and contrast the information they found about different community programs. If possible, one or two members of each group should visit the programs personally to learn more about them in advance of the discussions.

Healthy People 2010

Indicator: Overweight and Obesity

Focus Area: Diabetes

Goal: Through prevention programs, reduce the disease and economic burden of diabetes, and improve the quality of life for all persons who have or are at risk for diabetes.

Objectives:

5-1. Increase the proportion of persons with diabetes who receive formal diabetes education.

5-2. Prevent diabetes

5-3. Reduce the overall rate of diabetes that is clinically diagnosed.

5-4. Increase the proportion of adults with diabetes whose condition has been diagnosed.

5-5. Reduce the diabetes death rate.

5-6. Reduce diabetes-related deaths among persons with diabetes.

Public Health Terms*

Epidemiology: The study of the distribution and determinates of health-related states or events in specified populations, and the application of this study to control the health problems.

Morbidity: Any departure, subjective or objective, from a state of physiological or psychological well-being.

Mortality: Death; number of deaths in a given time or place.

Relative Risk: Ratio of the risk of disease or death among the exposed to the risk among the unexposed.

ACKNOWLEDGMENT

Special acknowledgements to Daniel Adam Lyons for his contributions to the Chapter Questions and Exercises/Activities.

REFERENCES

1. American Diabetes Association (ADA). *Diabetes Statistics*, 2006. Available at: http://www.diabetes.org/diabetes-statistics.jsp. Accessed May 5, 2008.

2. National Intitutes of Health. National Institute of Diabetes and Digestive and Kidney Diseases. National Diabetes Information Clearinghouse. National Diabetes Statistics fact sheet: general information and national estimates on diabetes in the United States. Bethesda: NIH; 2005. Available at http://diabetes.niddk.nih.gov/dm/pubs/statistics/. Accessed May 5, 2008.

3. Centers for Disease Control and Prevention (CDC). *National Diabetes Fact Sheet. United States, 2005.* Available at: http://www.cdc.gov/diabetes/pubs/pdf/ndfs_2005.pdf. Accessed May 5, 2008.

4. Boyle JP, Honeycutt AA, Narayan KM, Hoerger TJ, Geiss LS, Chen H, et al. Projection of diabetes burden through 2050: impact of changing demography and disease prevalence in the U.S. *Diabetes Care* 2001;24:1936–1940.

5. Hogan P, Dall T, Nikolov P. Economic costs of diabetes in the US in 2002. *Diabetes Care* 2003;26:917–932.

6. Lewin Group, Inc. Estimating Diabetes Cost in the United States in 2002. In: *Diabetes Care* 2003;26: 917–932.

7. International Diabetes Foundation (IDF). *Diabetes Atlas*, 3rd ed. Brussels, Belgium: IDF; 2006.

8. World Health Organization (WHO). *Diabetes Programme.* Available at http://www.who.int/diabetes/en/. Accessed May 5, 2008.

9. American Diabetes Association (ADA). Standards of Medical Care in Diabetes-2007, Position Paper. *Diabetes Care* 2007;30(Suppl 1):S4–S41.

10. National Health Lung and Blood Institute. Body mass calculator. Available at http://www.nhlbisupport.com/bmi/. Accessed May 5, 2008.

11. Institute of Medicine (IOM) of the National Academies. *Health Literacy.* Available at http://www.iom.edu/?id=31489.Accessed May 5, 2008.

12. Schillinger D, Grumbach K, Piette J, Wang F, Osmond D, Daher C, et al. Association of health literacy with diabetes outcomes. *JAMA* 2002;288: 475–482.

13. Harrison TA, Hindorff LA, Kim H, Wines RC, Bowen DJ, McGrath BB, et al. Family history of diabetes as a potential public health tool. *Am J Prevent Med* 2003;24:152–159.

14. U.S. Department of Health and Human Services (DHHS). *Prevention makes "cents."* Available at http://www.aspe.hhs.gov/health/prevention. Accessed May 5, 2008.

15. U.S. Department of Health and Human Services (DHHS). Healthy People 2010 Midcourse Review. Available at www.healthypeople.gov/data/midcourse. Accessed on May 5, 2008.

16. Schillinger D, Grumbach K, Piette J, Wang F, Osmond D, Daher C, et al. Association of health literacy with diabetes outcomes. *JAMA* 2002;288: 475–482.

17. Wagner, E, Austin, B, Davis, C, Hindmarsh, M, Schaefer, J, & Bonomi, A. Improving Chronic Illness Care: Translating Evidence Into Action. *Health Aff (Millwood)* Nov 01, 2001;20:64–78.

18. Diabetes123. *Diabetes Dictionary.* Available at http://www.diabetes123.com/dictionary/a.htm. Accessed May 5, 2008.

CROSS REFERENCES

Atherosclerosis

Chronic Kidney Disease

Communicating Health Information

Inflammation

Stroke

The Nutrition Transition

Source: Last JM. *A Dictionary of Epidemiology*, 4th ed. Oxford; New York: Oxford University Press; 2001.

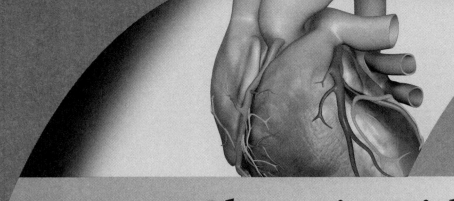

CHAPTER 37

Chronic Kidney Disease: The New Epidemic

Sudhindra Pudur
Paul L. Kimmel

Twenty million adults in the United States adults are estimated to have chronic kidney disease. Chronic kidney disease is an independent risk factor for death from cardiovascular disease.[1-5]

LEARNING OBJECTIVES

By the end of this chapter, students will be able to:

- Recognize chronic kidney disease as a major public health problem.
- Identify the major causes of chronic kidney disease and be aware of initial treatment approaches.
- Discuss the morbidity and mortality attributed to chronic kidney disease.
- List preventive strategies for chronic kidney disease.

HISTORY

Chronic kidney disease (CKD) is a worldwide health problem. In the United States, the National Kidney Foundation (NKF) estimates that twenty million Americans (1 in 9 adults) suffer from CKD, an increase of more than fivefold since 1980, with 20 million more at risk.[5] Undiagnosed and untreated CKD may lead to **end-stage renal disease** (ESRD), requiring treatment with **dialysis** or renal transplantation. As of 2006 more than 470,000 Americans are being treated for ESRD. Of these, more than 330,000 patients are treated with dialysis, and more than 130,000 have a functioning kidney transplant. CKD is now one of the major health problems in the United States, and the **prevalence** of ESRD patients is expected to rise exponentially in concurrence with the ongoing epidemic of hypertension and diabetes (Figure 37-1).

BASIC SCIENCE FACTS/KEY CONCEPTS REVIEW

Normal Kidneys and Their Function

The kidneys are a pair of bean-shaped organs that lie on either side of the spine in the lower middle of the back. Each kidney weighs about 150 grams and contains approximately one million filtering units called nephrons. Each nephron is composed of a glomerulus and a tubule. The glomerulus is a filtering or sieving device while the tubule is a tiny tubelike structure attached to the glomerulus. The kidneys are connected to the urinary bladder by tubes called *ureters*. The bladder is connected to the outside of the body by another tubelike structure called the *urethra* (Figure 37-2).

The main functions of the kidneys are listed below.

1. *Maintenance of body composition:* The kidney regulates the volume of fluid in the body, as well as its osmolarity, electrolyte content, and the concentration of many of the ionic constituents of plasma. In addition, the kidney plays a major role in regulating the acidity of the blood. The kidneys achieve these functions by variation of the amounts of water and ions excreted in the urine.

2. *Excretion of metabolic end products and foreign substances:* The kidneys are responsible for removal of

FIGURE 37-1 Incidence and Prevalence of End-stage Renal Disease in the United States.

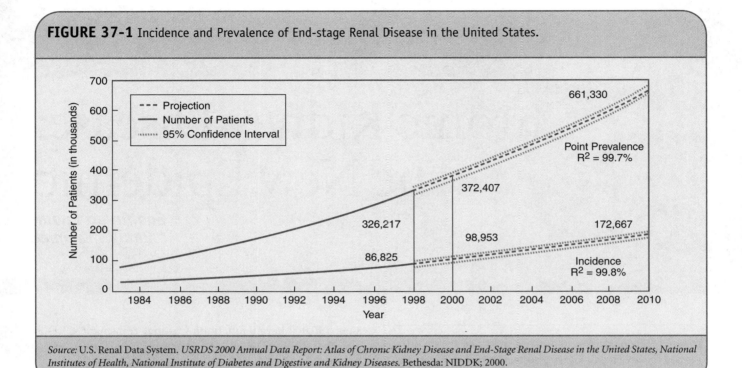

Source: U.S. Renal Data System. *USRDS 2000 Annual Data Report: Atlas of Chronic Kidney Disease and End-Stage Renal Disease in the United States, National Institutes of Health, National Institute of Diabetes and Digestive and Kidney Diseases.* Bethesda: NIDDK; 2000.

FIGURE 37-2 Anatomy of Normal Kidneys.

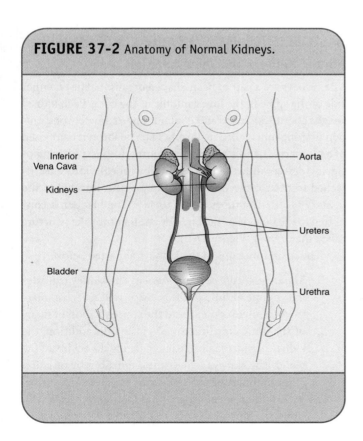

metabolic end products such as urea as well as drugs and toxins.

3. *Hormone synthesis:* Hormones produced and secreted by the kidneys include:
   a) Renin, produced by the juxtaglomerular apparatus, catalyzes the formation of angiotensin from angiotensinogen. Angiotensin is a potent vasoconstrictor and is involved in the balance of the salt content of the body as well as the regulation of blood pressure.
   b) Erythropoietin, which stimulates the maturation (and production) of red blood cells (erythrocytes) in the bone marrow.
   c) Vitamin D_3, the most active form of vitamin D. Vitamin D_3 is a steroid hormone that plays an important role in the regulation of body calcium and phosphate balance.

Pathophysiology

Gradual and permanent loss of kidney function over time leads to CKD. Typically, the development of kidney disease takes place over months to years, although in some cases such disease can progress very rapidly. Table 37-1 lists the risk factors for development of CKD. CKD is classified into five stages

TABLE 37-1 Risk Factors for Chronic Kidney Disease

Clinical Factors	Sociodemographic Factors
Hypertension	Older age
Diabetes	Ethnicity: African Americans,
Autoimmune diseases	Native Americans, and
Low birth weight	Hispanics
Exposure to certain drugs like NSAIDs	Low income/education
Family history of kidney disease	

based on level of renal function, using the glomerular filtration rate (GFR). CKD Stage 5 includes patients who require treatment for end-stage renal disease (ESRD), with dialysis or transplantation. Major causes of ESRD include diabetes mellitus (40 percent), hypertension (27 percent), glomerulonephritis (12 percent), and cystic kidney diseases (11 percent). Other diseases comprise about 10 percent of the ESRD population.

Signs and Symptoms of CKD

CKD is often silent until late in the course of disease, when the GFR is diminished below 10 percent to 15 percent of normal. Numerous clinical abnormalities are associated with advanced CKD. Some important clinical problems are listed below.

1. Fluid and electrolyte abnormalities, such as hyperkalemia, metabolic acidosis, and volume overload.
2. Cardiovascular abnormalities, such as hypertension, congestive heart failure, pericarditis, and cardiac rhythm disturbances.
3. Gastrointestinal abnormalities, such as nausea, lack of appetite, and vomiting.
4. Hematologic abnormalities, such as anemia, or bleeding.
5. Neurologic system disturbances, such as irritability, sleep disorders, muscle cramps, seizures, and in advanced stages, coma and death.
6. Endocrine system abnormalities, such as carbohydrate intolerance, bone disorders, and secondary hyperparathyroidism.
7. Dermatologic symptoms, such as itching, pallor, and bruising.

PUBLIC HEALTH PERSPECTIVE FOR THE HEALTH OF THE GENERAL POPULATION AND OF HIGH RISK GROUPS

CKD is now a major public health problem.[3] CKD meets all the criteria for a major public health issue, including the presence of a high disease burden, higher **incidence** in certain ethnic groups such as African Americans[6] and Native Americans, increased prevalence in underprivileged and low socioeconomic groups,[7] and availability of preventive measures that can be implemented at the community level to decrease the disease burden. Screening tests for kidney disease include measurement of blood pressure and checking for level of urine protein excretion as well as assessment of GFR using serum creatinine concentration levels and patient demographic factors. These are relatively inexpensive and easy to perform. The National Kidney Foundation is implementing a similar screening program, the Kidney Early Evaluation Program (KEEP) in high-risk groups. GFR can be easily calculated using a formula that requires the serum creatinine concentration, age, race, and gender. GFR and the level of urinary protein excretion are commonly used to estimate renal function and detect CKD. Several studies have shown that early detection and treatment of patients with microalbuminuria prevents development of CKD in people with diabetes mellitus. Use of medications like ACEIs (angiotensin converting enzyme inhibitors) or ARBs (angiotensin receptor blockers) has been shown to delay progression of diabetic and non-diabetic nephropathies, in addition to reducing proteinuria. Recent studies have also shown that reduction of proteinuria may be associated with reduced cardiovascular morbidity.[8]

Unfortunately, CKD is often diagnosed late in the course of illness. Lack of awareness among patients, the often asymptomatic nature of early stage CKD, and the insidious onset of the disease are likely contributory factors. An elevated serum creatinine concentration is often the first sign of kidney disease detected by health care providers, although estimated GFR rather than serum creatinine concentration provides a better marker of renal function. Serum creatinine is a product of muscle breakdown, and therefore at any level of renal function the serum concentration directly correlates with patients' muscle mass. So a patient with diminished muscle mass (such as an elderly nursing home patient) with significant renal dysfunction can have a misleadingly "normal" serum creatinine concentration. Reliance only on the level of serum creatinine in absence of consideration of other patient factors used to estimate the GFR may lead to delay in referral to a nephrologist until an advanced stage of the kidney disease is present.

CASE STUDY

Scenario

Ms. Smith is a 45-year-old African-American woman referred to the renal clinic by her primary care physician for evaluation of renal insufficiency. She was diagnosed with hypertension and diabetes mellitus five years ago. She reports taking all her blood pressure and diabetes medications consistently. Two years ago, she lost her health insurance when she was laid off at work. Her blood pressure and diabetes were under excellent control at that time, and she thought she no longer needed to take medications. She subsequently found a new job but did not have time to see her new primary care physician until recently because of a busy work schedule.

DEFINING THE ISSUES

1. What is chronic kidney disease?
2. What are the risk factors for development of chronic kidney disease?

Ms. Smith was shocked to find out from her primary care physician that she had kidney insufficiency. She was concerned that she will need dialysis like her father and is willing to do anything to prevent it. Her physician in the renal clinic performed some simple blood and urine tests. He told her that the cause of her renal insufficiency was likely secondary to uncontrolled diabetes and hypertension.

Patient's Understanding

She remarked, "I never knew that high blood pressure and diabetes can lead to kidney disease." She promised to start taking all her medications conscientiously and follow up regularly with her primary care physician as well as the renal clinic physicians.

CLINICAL PERSPECTIVE FOR THE INDIVIDUAL PATIENT

The patient is a 45-year-old African-American woman with diabetes and hypertension. Risk factors for development of CKD in the patient include hypertension, diabetes, and African-American ethnicity as well as a family history of kidney disease. Diabetes (followed by hypertension) is the most common etiology for development of CKD in the United States. African-American race, low socioeconomic status, and low income are the other risk factors associated with the development of CKD. The patient therefore had multiple risk factors for the development of CKD. Lack of awareness of risk factors that lead to the development of CKD has been cited as one of the reasons for the increasing prevalence of ESRD in the United States. It is common to see family members of patients on dialysis (like this patient) who are unaware of kidney disease. Figure 37-3 shows the stages in initiation and progression of CKD.

Potential Level of Intervention Earlier

Primary prevention would include early detection and aggressive treatment of risk factors (hypertension, diabetes) prior to the development of CKD. Increasing awareness of CKD and the potential benefits of treatment of multiple risk factors might have improved compliance in following with primary care physician recommendations and in taking medications. Close monitoring of renal function in high-risk populations is necessary for early detection of kidney disease.

Level of Intervention Now

Unfortunately, Ms. Smith's kidneys had already been damaged. Diagnoses can be confirmed by the finding of abnormalities on urinalyses (microalbuminuria or proteinuria), by assessing markers of GFR such as the serum creatinine concentration, or using imaging studies (such as an ultrasound examination of the kidneys) to determine if the size of the kidneys is normal. Focus now should be placed on delaying the progression of established CKD. **Secondary prevention** measures can be implemented to reduce the extent of disease and disease burden. These include optimizing hypertension management to a goal blood pressure of less than 130/90 mm Hg or less than 125/75 mm Hg if the patient has already developed proteinuria. Drugs belonging to the class of angiotensin converting enzyme inhibitors (ACE inhibitors) and angiotensin receptor blockers (ARBs) delay the progression of CKD to ESRD. Tight control of blood sugar and lipid levels are also recommended for patients with diabetes mellitus or chronic kidney disease and lipid disorders. Patients need to be followed closely to monitor for progression of CKD. In addition, depression, pain, and sleep disturbances may be common problems for patients with chronic illness. Attention to these symptoms might improve well-being and compliance with the treatment regimen.

Tertiary prevention measures include careful monitoring for and treatment of complications arising out of CKD including anemia, secondary hyperparathyroidism, and volume overload. As patients approach advanced CKD (Stage 4), options for renal replacement therapy, such as dialysis and/or transplantation should be discussed. Patients should be referred for access placement, to create arteriovenous fistulas or grafts to allow treatment with hemodialysis or abdominal catheter placement for those patients who elect treatment with peritoneal dialysis. Current policies allow patients to be listed on the cadaveric transplant list once the GFR is less than 20 mL/min. Some observational studies have shown that optimal management of complications in patients in stages before ESRD supervenes results in lower mortality. Perception of quality of life (QOL) may be impacted by factors related to chronic illness. Attention to these issues as well as symptoms of depression, pain, and sleep disturbances might enhance well-being and compliance in advanced stages of CKD.

FIGURE 37-3 Model for Stages in Initiation and Progression of Chronic Kidney Disease and Therapeutic Interventions.

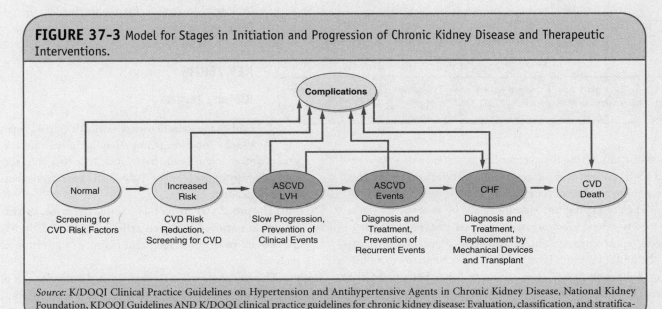

Source: K/DOQI Clinical Practice Guidelines on Hypertension and Antihypertensive Agents in Chronic Kidney Disease, National Kidney Foundation, KDOQI Guidelines AND K/DOQI clinical practice guidelines for chronic kidney disease: Evaluation, classification, and stratification. Kidney Disease Outcome Quality Initiative. *Am J Kidney Dis* 2002;39(Suppl 2):S1–S266.

The average age of an ESRD patient beginning therapy is approximately 60 years. About 84,000 ESRD patients died in 2004, with an annual mortality rate close to 25 percent! Cardiovascular disease is the most common cause of death in ESRD patients (Figure 37-4). The average life expectancy of a 60-year-old ESRD patient is 3.9 years, compared to 21.5 years among age-matched patients in the healthy general population. In addition, quality of life may be diminished in ESRD patients treated with dialysis compared with patients without chronic illness. Some of the symptoms commonly reported by ESRD patients include sexual dysfunction, insomnia, restless legs, and fatigue. Depression and diminished quality of life (QOL) have been shown to be associated with higher mortality in ESRD patients.[9,10] Time spent on dialysis, financial burden, medication burden, and change in relationships with the spouse or significant others are some of the psychosocial problems faced by ESRD patients.

Renal transplantation has been shown to be associated with better survival than age-, race-, and gender-matched patients treated with dialysis.[11] In 2004 there were more than 60,000 patients on the deceased donor transplant waiting list, but only 10,228 kidney transplants were performed. Over the years, the average wait time for a deceased donor renal transplant has increased. Current wait time for a cadaveric donor kidney transplant is three to five years or higher, depending on the region of the United States, in addition to various other

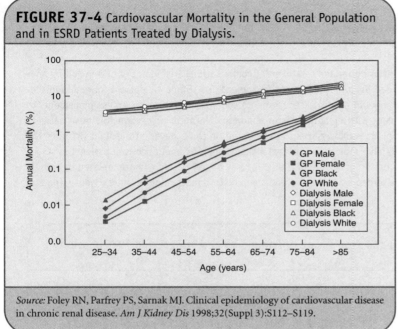

FIGURE 37-4 Cardiovascular Mortality in the General Population and in ESRD Patients Treated by Dialysis.

Source: Foley RN, Parfrey PS, Sarnak MJ. Clinical epidemiology of cardiovascular disease in chronic renal disease. *Am J Kidney Dis* 1998;32(Suppl 3):S112–S119.

ment adds a high burden of cost to the nation. Transplantation is associated with improved morbidity, mortality, and QOL as well as lower costs, for patients who are suited for this therapeutic option. CKD is one of the focus areas of Healthy People 2010. To achieve the goals of Healthy People 2010, a comprehensive plan of action focusing on early detection, optimizing management of risk factors of CKD, especially in high risk populations, and increasing patient and health care personnel awareness of the morbidity and mortality of CKD is needed. Programs should be devised at the national, regional, and local level to reduce the disease burden, for patients and society.

KEY TERMS

Biology Terms

End-Stage Renal Disease (ESRD): Occurs when kidney function is not adequate to sustain life, on an irreversible chronic basis, such that renal replacement therapy in the form of dialysis or a renal transplantation is needed.

Dialysis: The process where blood is cleared of toxins, and excess fluid removed using an artificial kidney, as in hemodialysis, or through the peritoneum, as in peritoneal dialysis.

Uremia: The syndrome in CKD Stage 5, which includes lack of appetite, nausea, vomiting, pericarditis, peripheral neuropathy, and mental status changes (ranging from loss of concentration and lethargy to seizures and coma).

Public Health Terms

Incidence: A measure of the risk of developing some new condition within a specified period of time, usually a year.

Prevalence: The total number of cases of the disease in the population at a given time, or the total number of cases in the population, divided by the number of individuals in the population.

Primary Prevention: Measures provided to individuals to prevent the onset of a targeted condition. Primary prevention measures include activities that help avoid a given healthcare problem.

Secondary Prevention: Measures that identify and result in treatment of asymptomatic persons who have already developed risk factors or preclinical disease but in whom

factors. Considering the average life expectancy of a 60-year-old ESRD patient is about four years, it is clear many patients die waiting for a renal transplant.

The ESRD program was established by an act of Congress in 1972 to extend Medicare coverage to patients requiring dialysis or renal transplantation to sustain life. Since then, the costs of the ESRD program have increased exponentially to 19 billion dollars in 2004. This accounts for 6 percent of the Medicare budget, which is allocated to less than 1 percent of the Medicare population.[2] Although there are no absolute contraindications, patients with terminal cancer, or terminal liver, lung, and heart disease are usually not offered dialysis or transplantation. Entry into a transplantation program necessitates evaluation to demonstrate that a patient can tolerate the stresses of the operation and treatment with immunosuppressive drugs, as well as an assessment of the ability of the patient to adhere to a complicated medical regimen. The morbidity, mortality, economic burden, and epidemic of chronic kidney disease are therefore enormous.

CONCLUSION

In conclusion, chronic kidney disease is a major public health problem in the United States. CKD, especially in its late stages, imposes a dramatic challenge to patients' quantity and quality of life. Although the United States maintains an entitlement program that provides care to patients with ESRD, its treat-the condition is not clinically apparent. These activities are focused on early case finding of asymptomatic disease that occurs commonly and has significant risk for negative outcome without treatment.

Tertiary Prevention: Activities involve the care of established disease, with attempts made to restore to highest func-tion, minimize the negative effects of disease, and prevent disease-related complications. Because the disease is now established, primary prevention activities may have been unsuccessful. Early detection through secondary preven-tion may have minimized the impact of the disease.

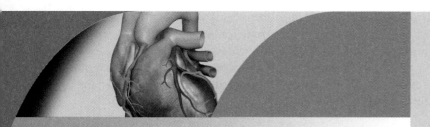

Questions for Further Research, Study, Reflection, and Discussion

For the Individual Student

In order to answer these questions, it may be necessary to research the primary literature.

- What are three major functions of the kidney? List the screening tests used to detect kidney disease.
- What is the most common cause of chronic kidney disease in the United States?
- What are the reasons for the increasing incidence of chronic kidney disease?
- Briefly describe the physiological process by which each the four major causes of ESRD produce kidney damage.
- Tables 37-2 and 37-3 are the Life Tables in the general population and in ESRD patients treated with dialysis. What is the life expectancy of a 65-year-old ESRD patient on dialysis compared to a 65-year-old healthy person? What are your conclusions?

TABLE 37-2 Life Table for the General Population

Age	All Races			White			Black		
	All	M	F	All	M	F	All	M	F
0	77.8	75.2	80.4	78.3	75.7	80.8	73.1	69.5	76.3
1	77.4	74.7	79.9	77.7	75.2	80.2	73.1	69.6	76.3
5	73.5	70.8	76.0	73.8	71.3	76.3	69.2	65.7	72.4
10	68.5	65.9	71.0	68.9	66.3	71.3	64.3	60.8	67.5
15	63.6	61.0	66.1	63.9	61.4	66.4	59.4	55.9	62.5
20	58.8	56.2	61.2	59.1	56.6	61.5	54.6	51.2	57.7
25	54.0	51.6	56.3	54.4	52.0	56.6	50.0	46.7	52.8
30	49.3	46.9	51.5	49.6	47.3	51.8	45.4	42.3	48.1
35	44.5	42.2	46.6	44.8	42.6	46.9	40.8	37.8	43.4
40	39.9	37.6	41.9	40.1	37.9	42.1	36.3	33.4	38.8
45	35.3	33.1	37.2	35.5	33.4	37.4	31.9	29.1	34.3
50	30.9	28.8	32.7	31.1	29.1	32.9	27.8	25.1	30.1
55	26.6	24.7	28.3	26.7	24.9	28.4	24.0	21.5	26.0
60	22.5	20.8	24.0	22.6	20.9	24.1	20.4	18.2	22.2
65	18.7	17.1	20.0	18.7	17.2	20.0	17.1	15.2	18.6
70	15.1	13.7	16.2	15.1	13.7	16.2	14.1	12.4	15.3
75	11.9	10.7	12.8	11.9	10.7	12.8	11.4	9.9	12.2
80	9.1	8.2	9.8	9.1	8.1	9.7	9.1	8.0	9.6
85	6.8	6.1	7.2	6.7	6.0	7.1	7.1	6.3	7.5
90	5.0	4.4	5.2	4.9	4.3	5.1	5.5	4.9	5.7
95	3.6	3.2	3.7	3.5	3.1	3.6	4.2	3.8	4.3
100	2.6	2.3	2.6	2.5	2.2	2.5	3.2	2.9	3.2

Source: United States Life Tables, 2004. NVSR Volume 56, Number 9.

TABLE 37-3 Life Table for Patients with End-Stage Renal Disease

Unadjusted	1980	1981	1982	1983	1984	1985	1986	1987	1988	1989	1990	1991	1992	1993	1994	1995
0–4	72.4	68.0	69.0	62.6	60.6	37.0	72.4	62.0	42.9	70.5	44.8	58.6	57.4	57.2	62.4	71.9
5–9	88.9	71.2	52.1	80.3	85.7	59.4	78.1	78.3	91.4	66.9	65.0	28.7	70.3	35.9	74.5	59.4
10–14	61.4	57.8	65.5	83.0	66.0	81.6	61.3	86.6	54.5	60.9	58.1	72.2	65.7	71.7	57.1	70.1
15–19	78.3	63.6	64.6	73.5	64.3	58.5	58.8	58.6	68.5	68.1	64.2	67.3	63.8	65.2	72.5	66.2
20–29	54.1	47.2	47.6	46.1	44.5	43.3	45.5	44.9	46.4	44.0	46.0	44.7	48.1	52.3	52.2	53.1
30–39	38.5	36.2	31.8	33.8	33.0	30.7	29.3	29.2	30.8	33.3	32.2	32.2	33.1	34.1	32.8	35.0
40–49	26.6	23.7	23.4	22.7	24.8	22.3	21.1	22.2	24.0	20.2	21.6	20.0	22.2	22.0	23.1	23.0
50–59	13.7	14.1	14.3	11.9	11.7	12.5	11.8	12.0	11.3	11.2	10.9	11.8	11.5	11.3	12.7	12.7
60–64	8.3	8.1	6.5	7.6	7.1	7.7	7.3	6.6	7.2	6.3	6.3	6.6	6.7	7.3	7.7	7.3
65–69	4.7	5.6	4.3	4.7	5.2	5.8	4.7	4.3	4.6	4.2	4.6	3.9	4.3	4.8	4.5	4.6
70–79	2.8	2.4	2.9	2.4	2.9	2.8	2.3	2.6	2.5	2.2	2.0	1.9	2.1	2.3	2.1	2.3
80+	1.9	1.0	1.6	0.2	1.3	0.8	0.8	0.7	0.6	0.8	0.4	0.6	0.6	0.7	0.7	0.8

Source: USRDS 2007 Annual Data Report available at www.usrds.org

For Small Group Discussion

- In the case study presented in the chapter, what are the factors that lead to the development of chronic kidney disease in Ms. Smith?
- How could these factors have been addressed so the progression of CKD could be slowed?

For Entire Class Discussion

- How would you design a campaign to increase awareness of chronic kidney disease at the state level, targeting the high-risk groups in particular?
- Should there be age limits for entry into ESRD program?
- Is the U.S. Medicare dollar well spent on this small entitlement group?
- How would the continued rise of chronic kidney disease impact Medicare resources, the health of the present and future populations, national resources, and provision of services?

EXERCISES/ACTIVITIES

- Obtain an automated blood pressure (BP) monitor and learn how to use it. What blood pressure reading would make you recommend a person to see a doctor?
- Obtain a urine dipstick and learn how to look for protein in the urine.
- One of limiting factors for kidney transplantation is the number of organs available. Find out how many in your class have signed up for organ donation.
- Think of two or three ideas on how you would encourage people to become organ donors.

Healthy People 2010

Indicator: Physical Activity

Focus Area: Nutrition and Overweight

Goal: Promote health and reduce chronic disease associated with diet and weight

Objectives:

19-10. Increase the proportion of persons aged 2 years and older who consume 2,400 mg or less of sodium daily

REFERENCES

1. The National Kidney Foundation. New York: NKF; 2008. Available at http://www.kidney.org. Accessed May 6, 2008.

2. United States Renal Data Service (USRDS), National Institutes for Diabetes and Digestive Kidney Diseases. USRDS 2006 Annual Data Report. Available at http://www.usrds.org. Accessed May 6, 2008.

3. Schoolwerth AC, Engelgau MM, Hostetter TH, Rufo KH, Chianchiano D, McClellan WM, et al. Chronic kidney disease: a public health problem that needs a public health action plan. *Prev Chronic Dis* 2006;3:A57.

4. Coresh J, Byrd-Holt D, Astor BC, Briggs JP, Eggers PW, Lacher DA, Hostetter TH. Chronic kidney disease awareness, prevalence, and trends among U.S. adults, 1999 to 2000. *J Am Soc Nephrol* 2005;16:180–188.

5. Coresh J, Astor BC, Greene T, Eknoyan G, Levey AS. Prevalence of chronic kidney disease and decreased kidney function in the adult US population: Third National Health and Nutrition Examination Survey. *Am J Kidney Dis* 2003;41:1–12.

6. Tarver-Carr ME, Powe NR, Eberhardt MS, LaVeist TA, Kington RS, Coresh J, Brancati FL. Excess risk of chronic kidney disease among African-American versus white subjects in the United States: a population-based study of potential explanatory factors. *J Am Soc Nephrol* 2002;13:2363–2670.

7. Merkin SS, Coresh J, Roux AV, Taylor HA, Powe NR. Area socioeconomic status and progressive CKD: the Atherosclerosis Risk in Communities (ARIC) Study. *Am J Kidney Dis* 2005;46:203–213

8. de Zeeuw D, Parving HE, Henning RH. Microalbuminuria as an early marker for cardiovascular disease. *J Am Soc Nephrol* 2006;17:2100–2105.

9. Mapes DL, Bragg-Gresham JL, et al. Health-related quality of life in the Dialysis Outcomes and Practice Patterns Study (DOPPS). *Am J Kidney Dis* 2004;44(Suppl 2):54–60.

10. Kimmel PL. Psychosocial factors in adult end-stage renal disease patients treated with hemodialysis: correlates and outcomes. *Am J Kidney Dis* 2000;35(Suppl 1):S132–S140.

11. Wolfe RA, Ashby VB, Milford VL, et al. Comparison of mortality in all patients on dialysis, patients on dialysis awaiting transplantation, and recipients of first cadaveric transplant. *N Engl J Med* 1999;341:1725–1730.

CROSS REFERENCES

Atherosclerosis

Diabetes

Hypertension

Inflammation

The Nutrition Transition

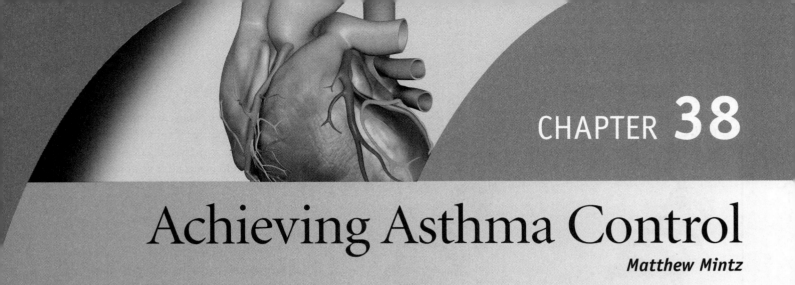

CHAPTER 38

Achieving Asthma Control

Matthew Mintz

> Approximately 11 people die from asthma each day. (Centers for Disease Control and Prevention)

LEARNING OBJECTIVES

By the end of this chapter, students will be able to:

- Describe the process of inflammation and how it causes symptoms in asthmatics.
- Classify asthma severity based on recently updated guidelines.
- List the factors that define asthma control.
- Discuss environmental and societal factors contributing to the burden of asthma as well as ways to overcome these factors.

HISTORY

Asthma along with chronic obstructive pulmonary disease (COPD) are among the 10 leading chronic conditions causing restricted activity. Asthma is only second to chronic sinusitis as the most common cause of chronic illness in children. Asthma, which is characterized by acute episodes of wheezing and shortness of breath, has been recognized for centuries. For many years asthma was thought to be a psychosomatic illness, likely due to the fact that emotional stress can indeed trigger asthma attacks. We now know much more about the biologic basis, primarily inflammation of the small airways in the lungs, that causes asthma. Similarly, many remedies for asthma, including asthma cigarettes, have been used throughout modern history. Fortunately, research has led to effective pharmaco-logical treatments, specifically inhaled corticosteroids, which are considered the mainstay of chronic asthma therapy and have been shown to improve morbidity and mortality. Public health also continues to play an important role in both ensuring proper delivery of care and reducing environmental factors that may lead to asthma.

BASIC SCIENCE FACTS/KEY CONCEPTS REVIEW

What Is Asthma?

Asthma is an obstructive airway disease characterized by episodic airway narrowing that resolves either spontaneously or with treatment. Two major factors that contribute to such narrowing are 1) airway hyperresponsiveness to stimuli that otherwise elicit minimal or no bronchoconstriction in non-asthmatics and 2) chronic inflammation.

The lungs are divided into branches, like an upside-down tree. The smaller airways are called bronchioles and are usually open, allowing air exchange (Figure 38-1). In an asthmatic, smooth muscles in the airway contract and close the airway in response to stimuli that are normally harmless. When the airways close, air cannot get out. This process is known as *bronchoconstriction*. Stimuli vary from individual to individual and may include various allergens, respiratory viruses, exercise, cold air, stress, and/or occupational exposures. In addition, inflammation is a key and critical component.

The inflammation triggered in asthmatics is a complex process that leads to marked airway swelling, mucus plug formation, and an increase in hyperresponsiveness, all of which contribute to airflow limitation. In addition, chronic inflammation over long periods of time can cause scarring and thickening of the airway walls, leading to further obstruction. This

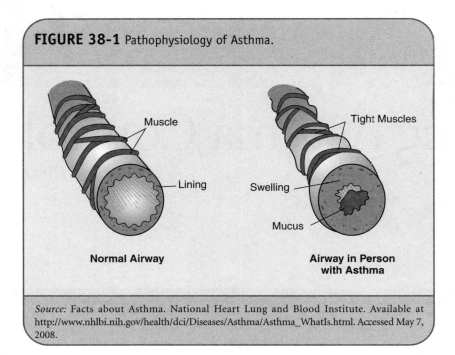

FIGURE 38-1 Pathophysiology of Asthma.

Muscle

Lining

Tight Muscles

Swelling

Mucus

Normal Airway

Airway in Person with Asthma

Source: Facts about Asthma. National Heart Lung and Blood Institute. Available at http://www.nhlbi.nih.gov/health/dci/Diseases/Asthma/Asthma_WhatIs.html. Accessed May 7, 2008.

utes to hours. Symptoms are often worse at night and in the early morning. In rare cases, acute episodes can persist for days or weeks either with mild obstructive symptoms with or without superimposed exacerbations or, in status asthmaticus, which is continuous severe obstructive symptoms. During acute exacerbations, asthma can be potentially fatal.

Patients with asthma have an increased IgE response to normal stimuli. IgE is one of the immunoglobulins or proteins in the body's immune system that normally protects the body from foreign invaders such as parasites. Asthma develops more often in childhood than in adulthood. *Atopy*, a genetic predisposition to an IgE-mediated response to environmental stimuli, is a major risk factor for the development of asthma in childhood. The relationship between atopy and asthma is complex. Allergic rhinosinusitis and eczema are also atopic diseases. Family members may have some or all of these illnesses.

process, known as *airway wall remodeling*, may cause permanent damage and over time lead to worsening asthma that no longer responds to treatment.

Acute airway obstruction results in paroxysms of wheezing, dyspnea, chest tightness, and cough, usually lasting minutes

Many cells and substances (mediators) produced by these cells play a major role in the onset and persistence of asthma. Cells include mast cells, eosinophils, macrophages, T lymphocytes, and epithelial cells (Figure 38-2). Once IgE combines

CASE STUDY

Scenario

JB is a seven-year-old African-American male living in the Southeast area of Washington, D.C. He currently attends public school and lives at home with his three-year-old sister and mother, who is separated from the children's father. His mother smokes cigarettes, but tries to do so only while she is at work, and goes outside to smoke when at home. JB was diagnosed with asthma by his pediatrician when he was age five. He is currently on montelukast, a **leukotriene modifier**, once daily. He uses an albuterol metered-dose inhaler for rescue medication, approximately three to four times a week. Both JB and his mother feel that JB's asthma is well controlled. JB does admit that he is not able to play soccer as well as his peers at school and blames this partially on his asthma. He is also reluctant to use his albuterol at school because he is afraid that he will be teased. JB has been to the emergency department twice in the past year for his asthma. His lung function has been tested by **spirometry** and found to be normal.

Defining the Issues and Patient's Understanding

The patient in this case is a seven-year-old child. As with all diseases with children, their developmental level is critical to their understanding of their disease and their role in treatment. As a seven-year-old, JB understands that asthma is a medical condition that causes his symptoms and prevents him from performing as well as his peers in recreational activities. This can be particularly troubling as peer relations and norms are just beginning to take more emotional importance. He is embarrassed about

FIGURE 38-2 Cellular Mechanisms Involved in Airway Inflammation and the Interaction of Multiple Cell Types and Mediators in Airway Inflammation. Abbreviations: IL, interleukin; Ig, immunoglobulin; LTB, leukotriene B.

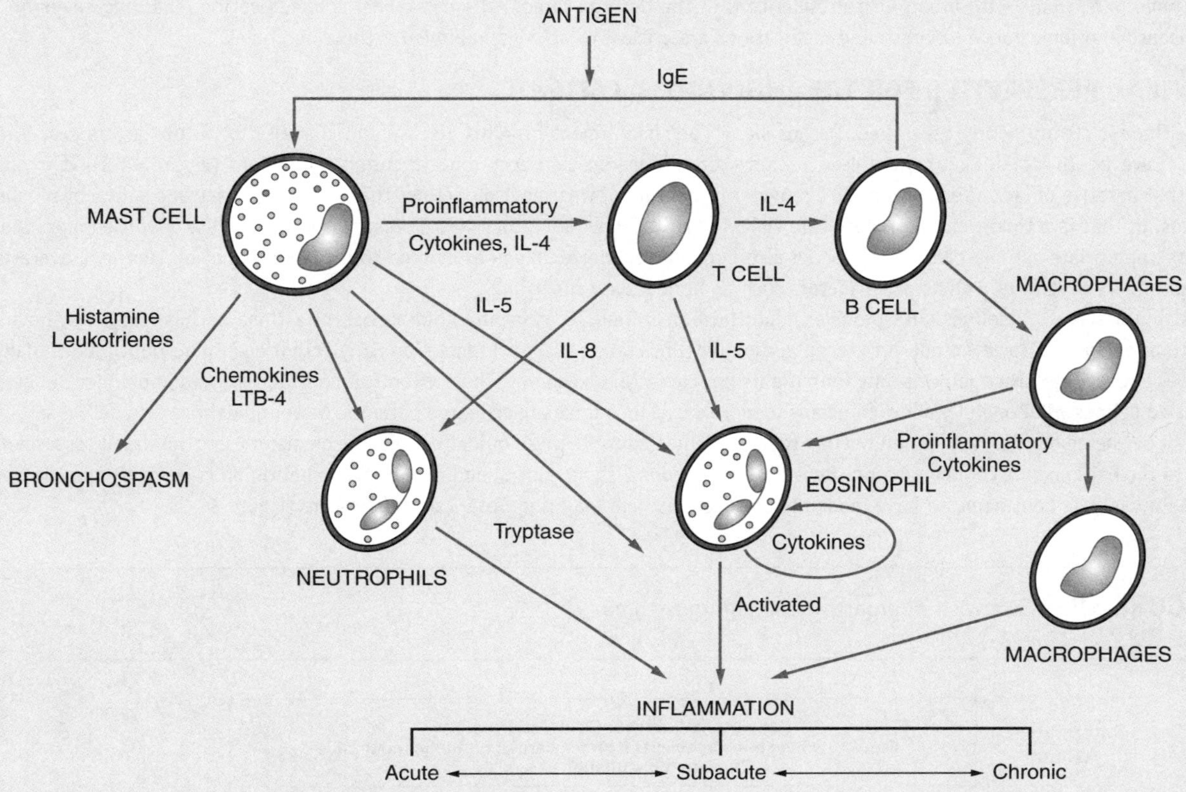

Source: Expert Panel Report-2, National Asthma Education and Prevention Program, NHLBI, 1997.

his disease, especially regarding the use of his rescue medication before or after soccer practice. However, he is aware that this medication does make him feel better.

The parent plays a crucial role in the management of childhood chronic disease. JB's mom is aware that her son has asthma, but she may not be aware of the seriousness of the disease, as evidenced by her continuing to smoke. It is common for parents and patients to normalize serious asthma and overestimate the degree of asthma control. One study showed that nearly two thirds of asthmatics classified as having moderate persistent asthma believed that their asthma was well controlled, and more than one third of asthmatics classified as having severe asthma also believed their asthma was well controlled. The fact the JB has been to the emergency room shows that he is at extreme risk for another severe attack. JB's mom needs to understand that asthma can be fatal, especially if not well controlled.

The fact that the patient is on a leukotriene modifier and not the preferred treatment of an **inhaled corticosteroid** in part may be due to JB's mother's reluctance to allow her son to take these medications. Patient misconceptions of inhaled steroids (confusing them with anabolic steroids), older data suggesting the medications may cause growth delay, and marketing by the manufacturers of these drugs touting once-daily pills that control asthma all lead to an overuse of these medications and an under-use of inhaled steroids, the preferred treatment for asthma.

Finally, JB and his mom's socioeconomic (single mom in a poor D.C. neighborhood) and potential cultural differences with her treating clinician also may impede optimal asthma care. There is a vast amount of data demonstrating healthcare disparities in asthma, particularly with urban African Americans in the United States. Patient-provider communication regarding **severity** of the disease and importance of controlled medications are critical to achieve improved asthma outcomes.

CLINICAL PERSPECTIVE FOR THE INDIVIDUAL PATIENT

JB's asthma is clearly poorly controlled. He has significant impairment from his disease and is at risk for future severe exacerbations. However, JB remains on montelukast, a non-preferred medication according to current guidelines (Figure 38-3). It is possible that because of lack of education, JB's provider is unaware of treatment guidelines that include efficacy and safety of inhaled steroids, or that in a time-limited primary care visit, the clinician would rather give a prescription for a pill to a worried mom than discuss appropriate asthma care. JB's provider also may not recognize JB's poor asthma control because of his mother's overestimation of JB's control as well as other factors such as normal lung function.

Using previous guidelines, JB's provider might have classified JB as having mild persistent asthma because he is not having symptoms every day. However, not until recently did guidelines take functional impact on daily activities into account. Additionally, previous severity classification was only for patients not currently on therapy. The concepts of control, risk, and impairment in more recent guidelines will hopefully allow clinicians to more easily recognize undertreated patients. Newer guidelines also define asthma severity by the amount of medication needed to gain asthma control. These guidelines also recommend using validated assessment tools to further enhance communication. Because JB has poor asthma control and risk for exacerbation on current asthma therapy, he would likely be considered to have moderate to severe asthma requiring Step 3 or greater care (Figure 38-3).

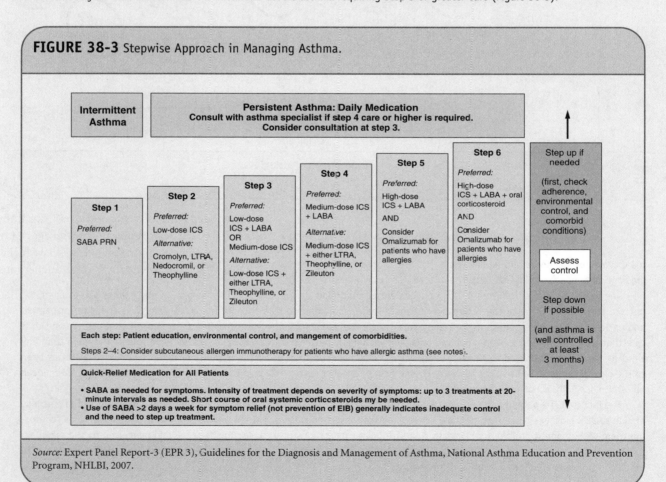

FIGURE 38-3 Stepwise Approach in Managing Asthma.

Source: Expert Panel Report-3 (EPR 3), Guidelines for the Diagnosis and Management of Asthma, National Asthma Education and Prevention Program, NHLBI, 2007.

JB's provider should switch him to an inhaled steroid **controller** inhaler alone or in combination with a **long-acting bronchodilator**. JB should be brought back to the clinician's office within a month to assess asthma control and either step-up or step-down therapy. The clinician may want to consider a **written action plan** with a **peak flow meter** to help JB and his mother identify an attack before it occurs and empower them to take a more active role in the management of JB's disease. Finally, the provider, patient, and mother must work on better communication to ensure that goals are recognized and met. The clinician should educate JB's mother on the seriousness of the disease as well as the importance of her continued smoking on her son's health.

Potential Level of Intervention Earlier

Earlier intervention could have happened both in selecting a more appropriate agent, starting treatment earlier, and making sure JB's parents understood his diagnosis and its potential consequences. As mentioned, inhaled corticosteroids are the agents of choice, even for very young children and infants. JB's mom may have been reluctant to take inhaled steroids, and the treating clinician could have reassured her of their safety. In addition, often the diagnosis of asthma itself is delayed. This happens in part because many infants wheeze, but not all infants will develop asthma. Providers that treat children are often overcautious about labeling a young child with a chronic disease. However, the potential risk is worsening asthma over time. Infants who have risk factors for developing asthma (parent history, allergic rhinitis, eczema) and have more than two wheezing episodes in a year, lasting more than one day should be treated with inhaled steroids. Finally, the clinician needs to educate the parent about how to manage this chronic illness, the purposes of the medication, and the risks if the disease is not well controlled.

with a trigger (*allergen*), this starts a cascade of activity by these inflammatory cells, which make several mediators to recruit additional cells. The inflammatory cells and their mediators all cause changes in the airway that eventually lead to symptoms. For example, histamine is a mediator released by macrophages that causes bronchoconstriction. Other changes triggered by inflammatory mediators include nerve stimulation, mucus secretion, and small blood vessel leakage.

The component of bronchial hyperresponsiveness is present apart from as well as potentiated by the inflammatory process. Bronchoconstriction contributes significantly to the symptoms of wheezing and difficulty breathing (dyspnea) and the degree of constriction correlates closely with clinical severity. Acute bronchoconstriction following allergen exposure results from IgE-dependent mast cell release of mediators such as histamine, tryptase, leukotrienes, and prostaglandins. The mechanism of airflow obstruction is less well understood for other stimuli such as exercise, cold air, irritants, and stress.

Measuring Lung Function

Other basic science concepts important in asthma involve measuring lung function, which is usually done with a device called a *spirometer*. When studying lung function on a spirometer, clinicians are generally concerned with how much one can breathe out and how fast. Therefore, three main parameters are looked at in most respiratory diseases: FEV1, FVC, and the ration between the two. The *forced vital capacity* (*FVC*) measures how much air you can breathe out of your lungs after a deep inspiration. *Total lung capacity* (*TLC*) is the FVC plus the amount of air left in your lungs after you breathe it all

out. The *forced expiratory volume* (*FEV1*) is the amount of air you can forcibly exhale in one second. In obstructive lung disease like asthma and COPD, patients are not able to exhale as fast (decreased FEV1) and as much (FEV1/FVC) as normal subjects.

PUBLIC HEALTH PERSPECTIVE FOR THE HEALTH OF THE GENERAL POPULATION AND OF HIGH RISK GROUPS

Asthma continues to be a growing burden in the United States despite the advent of multiple medications and an increased understanding of asthma pathophysiology. There are nearly 2 million emergency department visits and over 10 million physician office visits each year. Females, children ages 14 or less, and African Americans as compared to whites have higher rates of office visits. African Americans also have higher rates of asthma-related emergency department visits, hospitalizations, and deaths.

The lifetime prevalence of asthma in the United States is estimated at nearly 26.7 million people, with a 12-month attack prevalence (persons with one or more attacks) at nearly 11.1 million. Despite increased treatment options, the morbidity and mortality associated with asthma remains high. Asthma accounts for nearly 500,000 hospitalizations. Fortunately, asthma deaths that peaked in the mid 1990s have actually started to decline in the last decade. However, they are still high at over 4,000 deaths each year.

Reasons for the continued burden of asthma are multifactorial, but may be related to lack of implementation of guidelines, **disparities in care**, and **environmental factors**. Though guidelines have existed since the early nineties, efforts to implement them have been poor, especially in primary care settings. Studies continue to demonstrate a disproportionate rate of death, hospitalization, emergency room use, and disability from asthma occurs in specific age, gender, racial, and ethnic groups. Socioeconomic status seems to play a very important role. Though whites and non-whites have similar rates of asthma, non-whites have twice the rate of death, hospitalization, and emergency department visits. Finally, environmental factors may contribute to asthma morbidity and mortality, as indoor (tobacco smoke) and outdoor (ozone, sulfur dioxide, nitrogen dioxide, acid aerosols) pollutants may have both a causative and aggravating role.

Healthy People 2010 has clear goals and objectives to reduce the burden of disease from asthma. Public health workers should focus efforts on guideline implementation, reducing disparities, and working with regulatory agencies regarding environmental triggers. Educational efforts must be culturally sensitive and recognize barriers to care for disadvantaged minorities. Professional organizations, lay volunteer groups, federal agencies, and the private sector must work together with asthma experts to implement multiple programs at national, state, and community levels.

At the national level, multiple organizations engage in asthma surveillance and education programs. In 2006, the Centers for Disease Control and Prevention (CDC) awarded 32 million dollars worth of grants to states, cities, and other organizations to improve their surveillance systems and program activities. The National Heart, Lung, and Blood Institute, one of the CDC's chief implementation partners, makes multiple recommendations on how to improve public health programs addressing asthma. According to the NHLBI's guidelines, **community based** efforts should include the school systems, which has already been proven to be successful in several existing programs. Other NHLBI recommendations target access and environmental issues. Because healthcare access may be an issue, particularly for those groups who have a higher morbidity, outreach programs in the community such as mobile clinics or involving community pharmacists are examples of potential interventions. Finally, public health organizations need to initiate surveillance efforts and monitor both occupational and environmental exposures and their impact on illness and disability related to asthma.

KEY TERMS

Clinical Terms

Alternative Asthma Medications: The cornerstone of asthma therapy is inhaled corticoid sterones (ICSs). ICS dose can be increased or long-acting beta-2 agonists (LABAs) can be added for more severe asthma. In certain situations, leukotriene receptor antagonists (LTRAs) are also recommended. There are older medications that do not work as well and/or have side effects, and these include cromolyn and nedocromil (which stabilize mast cells) as well as theophylline (a bronchodilator). Omalizumab is a new, genetically engineered weekly injection reserved for only for the very severe patient.

Asthma: An obstructive airway disease characterized by episodic airway narrowing that resolves either spontaneously or with treatment, caused by hyperresponsiveness to otherwise normal stimuli and chronic inflammation.

Asthma Control: A more recent concept and focus of care that recognizes some of the limitations of severity classification (Figure 38-4). The parameters of impairment are similar to asthma severity, except that now patients are divided into well controlled, not well controlled, and very poorly controlled. The concept is that with appropriate therapy, most patients regardless of classification should be able to achieve control. Though treatment is initiated based on severity level, treatment is adjusted based on control (Figure 38-5). Providers can initiate higher doses and/or second medications if asthma is not controlled (step up), or decrease treatment if asthma is well controlled (step down).

Asthma Severity: A type of classification system used for patients with asthma since the early 1990s based on daytime and nighttime symptoms, pulmonary function as measured by spirometry, use of rescue medication, and most recently by impact of asthma on one's daily activities such as interference with work, school, and play (Figure 38-5). There are two components of severity, impairment (symptoms, lung function) and risk, specifically for exacerbations. Treatment for asthma should be initiated based on the current severity classification. A limitation of this classification system is that asthma is a variable disease, and even patients with mild persistent asthma can have poor asthma control.

Controller and Reliever Therapy: Patients with persistent asthma (asthma that is symptomatic more than twice a week) require two kinds of medications: controller and reliever. Controller medications, preferably inhaled corticosteroids, are taken every day, regardless of symptoms, to prevent exacerbations. Reliever medications are usually short-acting bronchodilators (albuterol) to be used only when patients are symptomatic. This concept is important to patient education, because it is common for patients to discontinue their preventative, controller medications when they are feeling well. In addition, over-

FIGURE 38-4 Classifying Asthma Severity and Initiating Treatment.

Components of Severity		Classification of Asthma Severity (≥12 years of age)			
			Persistent		
		Intermittent	**Mild**	**Moderate**	**Severe**
Impairment **Normal FEV_1/FVC:** 8–19 yr 85% 20–39 yr 80% 40–59 yr 75% 60–80 yr 70%	Symptoms	≤2 days/week	>2 days/week but not daily	Daily	Throughout the day
	Nighttime awakenings	≤2x/month	3–4x/month	>1x/week but not nightly	Often 7x/week
	Short-acting $beta_2$-agonist use for symptom control (not prevention of EIB)	≤2 days/week	>2 days/week but not >1x/day	Daily	Several times per day
	Interference with normal activity	None	Minor limitation	Some limitation	Extremely limited
	Lung function	• Normal FEV_1 between exacerbations • FEV_1 >80% predicted • FEV_1/FVC normal	• FEV_1 >80% predicted • FEV_1/FVC normal	• FEV_1 >60% but <80% predicted • FEV_1/FVC reduced 5%	• FEV_1 >60% predicted • FEV_1/FVC reduced >5%
Risk	**Exacerbations (consider frequency and severity)**	**0–2 year**	**>2/year →**		
		← Frequency and severity may fluctuate over time for patients in any severity category →			
		Relative annual risk of exacerbations may be related to FEV_1			
Recommended Step for Initiating Treatment		**Step 1**	**Step 2**	**Step 3** and consider short course of systemic oral corticosteroids	**Step 4 or 5** and consider short course of systemic oral corticosteroids
		In 2–6 weeks, evaluate level of asthma control that is achieved and adjust therapy accordingly.			

Source: Expert Panel Report-3 (EPR 3), Guidelines for the Diagnosis and Management of Asthma, National Asthma Education and Prevention Program, NHLBI, 2007.

use of reliever medications is a sign of poorly controlled asthma.

Inhaled Corticosteroids (ICSs): The cornerstone of asthma therapy and recommended for all patients with persistent asthma. Inhaled steroids have been shown to be superior than all other agents in the ability to improve lung function, reduce symptoms, prevent exacerbations, and even reduce death. One study showed that ICS given earlier in the course of the disease seemed to halt progression, but other studies have been unable to replicate these data.

Leukotriene Modifiers (also, **Leukotriene Receptor Antagonists [LTRA]**). A type of asthma medication that works by blocking leukotrienes, which is an important mediator in the inflammatory cascade. They have a low risk of side effects and can be taken in pill form; however, they are not as effective as ICS.

FIGURE 38-5 Assessing Asthma Control and Adjusting Therapy.

Components of Control		Classification of Asthma Control (≥12 years of age)		
		Well Controlled	Not Well Controlled	Very Poorly Controlled
Impairment	Symptoms	≤2 days/week	>2 days/week	Throughout the day
	Nighttime awakenings	≤2/month	1–3/week	≥4/week
	Interference with normal activity	None	Some limitation	Extremely limited
	Short-acting beta$_2$-agonist use for symptom control (not prevention of EIB)	≤2 days/week	>2 days/week	Several times per day
	FEV$_1$ or peak flow	>80% predicted/ personal best	60–80% predicted/ personal best	>60% predicted/ personal best
	Validated questionnaires ATAQ ACQ ACT	0 ≤0.75 ≥20	1–2 ≥1.5 16–19	3–4 N/A ≤15
Risk	**Exacerbations**	**0–1 per year**	**2–3 per year**	**>3 per year**
	Progressive loss of lung function	Evaluation requires long-term follow-up care		
	Treatment-related adverse effects	Medication side effects can vary in intensity from none to very troublesome and worrisome. The level of intensity does not correlate to specific levels of control but should be considered in the overall assessment of risk.		
Recommended Action for Treatment		• Maintain current step. • Consider step down if well controlled for at least 3 months.	• Step up 1 step and • Reevaluate in 2–6 weeks. • For side effects, consider alternative treatment options.	• Consider short course of systemic oral corticosteroids, • Step up 1–2 steps, and • Reevaluate in 2 weeks. • For side effects, consider alternative treatment options.

Source: Expert Panel Report-3 (EPR 3), Guidelines for the Diagnosis and Management of Asthma, National Asthma Education and Prevention Program, NHLBI, 2007.

Long-Acting Bronchodilators (LABA). In contrast to short acting bronchodilators (SABA) that are used for rescue/reliever medication, LABAs are used for asthma control. When combined with an ICS, they have been shown to improve both objective lung function measurements as well as patient factors such as improvement in peak flow readings and days without asthma symptoms. They should not be used without ICSs, as one study showed an increase in rates of asthma death when used alone.

Peak Flow Meters: Handheld devices used by asthmatic patients to track their daily airflow. Because patients' airflow is generally reduced prior to an asthma attack and they may not perceive this decrease, home measurement of peak flow may prevent serious exacerbations by allowing treatment before an asthma attack happens. Providers will help patients determine their "personal best" peak flow number and have them track this over time. Peak flow reading can be used in conjunction with asthma action plans. They are recommended for patients with moderate to severe asthma.

Spirometry: Pulmonary function testing (PFT) is done using a machine called a spirometer, a device that measures how much air one can breathe in or out (lung volumes) as well as how fast one is able to breathe air out (lung flow).

Asthma is an pulmonary obstructive disease, with relatively normal volumes, but reduced flow. To properly diagnose asthma and rule out any underlying condition, it is recommended that patients have spirometric assessment; it is also recommended to objectively measure response to treatment as well as recommended every one to two years to assess progressive decline in lung function. Spirometry can be performed in the primary care setting, but many primary care physicians do not have these devices. Specialists such as allergist and pulmonologists used spirometry as standard of care practice.

Written Action Plans: Directions from a healthcare provider to asthmatic patient or caregiver that instruct exactly what to do when patients are feeling well, when they are symptomatic, and when they are having asthma attacks. The instructions usually involve which medications to take and when, and also can be used in conjunction with peak flow meters. Other instructions may include trigger avoidance and contact information. Despite lack of evidence that written action plans improve asthma outcomes, they serve as an excellent communication tool between patients and providers and continue to be recommended by national guidelines.

Public Health Terms

Community Based Asthma Programs: Though individual patient and provider interactions can be improved, it is clear that in order to reduce the asthma burden, community programs are needed. Both school and pharmacy-based programs have shown some initial success. Mobile asthma vans also have shown promise, especially in minority and impoverished areas.

Environmental Triggers: Factors in the environment that contribute to asthma. Outdoor triggers include ozone, sulfur dioxide, nitrogen dioxide, and acid aerosols. Extremes in temperature or humidity may play a role. Indoor pollutants such as tobacco smoke also worsen asthma.

Healthcare Disparities: Difference in health outcomes between majority and minority populations that cannot be accounted for by socioeconomic factors alone. Asthma prevalence and morbidity is particular worse in African Americans. Though some genetic factors have been hypothesized and socioeconomic factors do play a role, other factors such as discrimination and culture insensitivity may an important part in asthma treatment disparities.

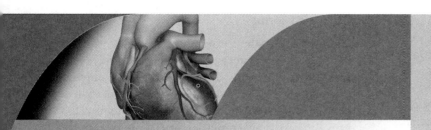

Questions for Further Research, Study, Reflection, and Discussion

For Individual Student

In order to answer these questions, it may be necessary to research the primary literature.

- Describe how inflammation and bronchoconstriction lead to asthma symptoms.
- How do currently marketed asthma products (to patients or healthcare professionals) treat asthma? How do these products fit with current evidence-based recommendations (guidelines)?

For Small Group Discussion

- Locate resources and educational material for JB and his mother. Are there any educational materials or programs specifically geared toward a seven-year-old with asthma?
- What is the impact of the family situation on JB's asthma?
- How would you counsel JB and his mother to keep his asthma under optimal control?
- Because the prevalence of asthma is common, and many public health students choose this career path due to their own personal illness, ask for volunteers in the class who have asthma to describe their experience. (Students can also discuss observed experience with asthma in a family member or close friend.)

For Entire Class Discussion

- What are the local statistical data for asthma in your community? Are there geographic areas or certain populations where the prevalence of asthma is higher? What might be some reasons for any variations?
- Plan an asthma initiative for the local community surrounding the school. What types of interventions might you use? Who would they be aimed at and why? Where might you go for resources (assuming a limited budget)?

EXERCISES/ACTIVITIES

- Obtain demonstrator devices from practitioner's office or pharmaceutical rep and learn how to use and teach inhalers to a patient and his/her family.
- Purchase or obtain a sample of a peak flow meter; learn how to use as well as teach to a patient.
- Go to a local elementary school and speak with school nurse. Is there an asthma program in school? If so, then describe it. How many students use inhalers in this school? Is quick relief inhaler use communicated with parent? Physician? How many asthma attacks does the school nurse see each year?

Healthy People 2010

Focus Area: Respiratory Diseases

Goal: Promote respiratory health through better prevention, detection, treatment, and education efforts.

Objectives:

24-1. Reduce asthma deaths.

24-2. Reduce hospitalizations for asthma.

24-3. Reduce hospital emergency department visits for asthma.

24-4. Reduce activity limitations among persons with asthma.

24-5. Reduce the number of school or workdays missed by persons with asthma due to asthma.

24-6. Increase the proportion of persons with asthma who receive formal patient education, including information about community and self-help resources, as an essential part of the management of their condition.

24-7. Increase the proportion of persons with asthma who receive appropriate asthma care according to the NAEPP Guidelines.

24-8. Establish in at least 25 states a surveillance system for tracking asthma death, illness, disability, impact of occupational and environmental factors on asthma, access to medical care, and asthma management.

RESOURCES

Mintz M, ed. *Disorders of the Respiratory Tract: Common Challenges for the Primary Care Practitioner.* Totowa, NJ: The Humana Press Inc.; 2006.

Mintz ML. Update in the diagnosis and treatment of asthma in adults and children—Part 1: diagnosis, monitoring and prevention of disease progression. *Am Fam Physician* 2004;70:893–898.

Mintz ML. Update in the diagnosis and treatment of asthma in adults and children—Part 2: medical management. *Am Fam Physician* 2004;70:1061–1066.

National Asthma Education and Prevention Program. *Expert panel report: guidelines for the diagnosis and management of asthma: update on selected topics—2002.* Bethesda: U.S. Department of Health and Human Services, Public Health Service, National Institutes of Health, National Heart, Lung, and Blood Institute, 2002; NIH publication no. 02-5074.

National Asthma Education and Prevention Program. *Expert Panel Report 3 (EPR 3): Guidelines for the Diagnosis and Management of Asthma.* Bethesda: U.S. Department of Health and Human Services, Public Health Service, National Institutes of Health, National Heart, Lung, and Blood Institute, 2007; NIH publication no. 08-4051 (prepublication copy). Available at http://www.nhlbi.nih.gov/guidelines/asthma/asthgdln.htm. Accessed May 7, 2008.

Healthy People 2010: Objectives for Improving Health. Chapter 24: Respiratory Diseases. Available at http://www.healthypeople.gov/Document/pdf/Volume2/24Respiratory.pdf. Accessed May 7, 2008.

Centers for Disease Control, National Center for Health Statistics. *Asthma prevalence, health care use and mortality: United States, 2003–05.* Available at http://www.cdc.gov/nchs/FASTATS/asthma.htm. Accessed May 7, 2008.

CROSS REFERENCES

Inflammation

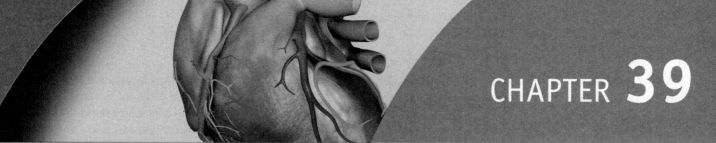

Arthritis: The Nation's Most Common Cause of Disability

Patience White

Arthritis is the most common cause of disability in the United States.[1]

LEARNING OBJECTIVES

By the end of this chapter, students will be able to:

- Describe arthritis and list the three most common types of arthritis.
- Discuss the risk factors for the most common form of arthritis, osteoarthritis.
- Discuss the nonpharmacological and pharmacological interventions for osteoarthritis.
- List the public health messages for arthritis.

HISTORY

Doctor-diagnosed **arthritis** affects one in five Americans and its prevalence will increase from 46 million U.S. adults today to 67 million (25 percent of the projected total adult population) by 2030. Arthritis prevalence increases with age and is higher among women than men in every age group. Arthritis is not an old person's disease; nearly two thirds of people with arthritis are younger than 65 years of age. A recent Centers for Disease Control and Prevention (CDC) study estimated that 294,000 U.S. children under age 18 (or 1 in 250 children) have been diagnosed with arthritis or another rheumatologic condition. Arthritis affects all race and ethnic groups: 37.2 million white adults, 4.6 million black adults, 3.1 million Hispanic

adults, and 1.6 million adults of other races have arthritis. Today 41 percent (19 million) of the 46 million U.S. adults report limitations in their usual activities due to their arthritis and this will grow to 25 million in 2030. Blacks with arthritis have more activity limitation than whites. In addition to activity limitations, 31 percent (8.2 million) of working age adults with doctor-diagnosed arthritis report being limited in work activities due to arthritis. Work limitations attributable to arthritis affect 5 percent of the general population and 30 percent of people with arthritis. Blacks and Hispanics with arthritis have more work limitation and severe joint pain from arthritis than whites.

By the year 2030, the number of people with doctor-diagnosed arthritis will increase an average of 34 percent in all 50 states. More alarming, 10 states are projected to have increases ranging from 50 percent to 99 percent, and three states (Arizona, Florida, and Nevada) are projected to see their numbers more than double. These estimates may be conservative as they do not account for the current trends in obesity, which may contribute to future cases of osteoarthritis, the most common cause of arthritis.

In 2003, the total cost attributed to arthritis and other rheumatic conditions in the United States was 128 billion dollars, up from 86.2 billion dollars in 1997 ($80.8 billion in medical care expenditures and $47 billion in earnings losses). Each year arthritis results in 750,000 hospitalizations and 36 million outpatient visits.

Arthritis is a major player in other chronic diseases, often making it difficult for people to exercise to improve their comorbid conditions. A total of 52.4 percent of people with diabetes, 57.8 percent people with heart disease, and 47.6 percent of people with hypertension have doctor diagnosed arthritis.

BASIC SCIENCE FACTS/KEY CONCEPTS REVIEW

The word *arthritis* literally means joint inflammation. The term *arthritis* is used to describe more than 100 rheumatic diseases and conditions that affect joints, the tissues that surround the joint and other connective tissue. The pattern, severity, and location of symptoms can vary depending on the specific form of the disease. Typically, rheumatic conditions are characterized by pain and stiffness in and around one or more joints. The symptoms can develop gradually or suddenly. Certain rheumatic conditions also can involve the immune system and various internal organs of the body. The three most common forms of arthritis are:

1. **Osteoarthritis (OA):** Osteoarthritis affects 27 million adults in the United States and is a disease characterized by degeneration of cartilage and its underlying bone within a joint as well as bony overgrowth. Osteoarthritis results in the failure of cartilage cells (*chondrocytes*) to maintain the balance between degradation and synthesis of supporting matrix. The symptoms of OA are pain, short-lasting stiffness, joint cracking, joint swelling, fatigue, and functional limitation. The joints most commonly affected are the apophyseal joints of the spine, knees, hips, and those in the hands. The specific causes of osteoarthritis are unknown. The risks for OA are age, mechanical (obesity and trauma), family history, female sex, and molecular events in the affected joint. Disease onset is gradual and usually begins after the age of 40. There is currently no cure for OA. Treatment for OA focuses on relieving symptoms and improving function, and can include a combination of patient education, physical therapy, weight control, and use of medications.

2. **Gout:** Gout affects 3.0 million Americans and is a rheumatic disease resulting from deposition of uric acid crystals (monosodium urate) in tissues and fluids within the body. This process is caused by an overproduction or underexcretion of uric acid. Certain common medications, alcohol, and dietary foods are known to be contributory factors. Acute gout will typically manifest itself as an acutely red, hot, and swollen joint with excruciating pain. These acute gouty flare-ups respond well to treatment with oral anti-inflammatory medicines and may be prevented with medication and diet changes. Recurrent bouts of acute gout can lead to a degenerative form of arthritis called gouty arthritis.

3. **Rheumatoid Arthritis (RA):** Rheumatoid arthritis affects 2.1 million Americans and is a systemic inflammatory disease that manifests itself in multiple joints of the body. The inflammatory process primarily affects the lining of the joints (synovial membrane), but can also affect other organs. The inflamed synovium leads to erosions of the cartilage and bone and sometimes joint deformity. Pain, swelling, and redness are common joint manifestations. Although the definitive causes are unknown, RA is believed to be the result of a faulty immune response. RA can begin at any age and is associated with fatigue and prolonged stiffness after rest. There is no cure for RA, but new drugs such as biological medications are increasingly available to treat the disease. In addition to medications and surgery, good self-management that includes exercise is known to reduce pain and disability.

Certain factors have been shown to be associated with a greater risk of arthritis. Some of these risk factors are modifiable while others are not.

Non-Modifiable Risk Factors

- **Age:** The risk of developing most types of arthritis increases with age.
- **Gender:** Most types of arthritis are more common in women; 60 percent of all people with arthritis are women. Gout is more common in men.
- **Genetic:** Specific genes are associated with a higher risk of certain types of arthritis, such as rheumatoid arthritis (RA), systemic lupus erythematosus (SLE), and ankylosing spondylitis.

Modifiable Risk Factors

- **Overweight and obesity:** Excess weight can contribute to both the onset and progression of knee osteoarthritis.
- **Joint injuries:** Damage to a joint can contribute to the development of osteoarthritis in that joint.
- **Infection:** Many microbial agents can infect joints or cause a reactive arthritis, both of which potentially cause the development of various forms of arthritis.
- **Occupation:** Certain occupations involving repetitive knee bending and squatting are associated with osteoarthritis of the knee.
- **Malignment of the joint** as well as joint laxity and developmental deformities can predispose the joint to be damaged and to have an earlier onset of osteoarthritis.

Obesity is a known risk factor for the development and progression of knee osteoarthritis and possibly osteoarthritis of other joints. For example, obese adults are up to four times more likely to develop knee osteoarthritis than normal weight adults.[1] Excess body weight is also associated with about 35 percent of adults with doctor-diagnosed arthritis who are obese compared to only 21 percent of those without arthritis. Figure 39-1 shows that reducing body weight results in significant improvements in the health-related quality of life of people with arthritis.

Despite the fact that physical activity and exercise have been shown to benefit people with arthritis by improving pain, function, and mental health, many people with arthritis report no leisure time physical activity. Almost 44 percent of adults with doctor-diagnosed arthritis report no leisure time physical activity, a considerably higher proportion compared with adults without arthritis (36 percent). Figure 39-2 shows that low levels of physical activity place individuals with arthritis at further risk of inactivity-associated conditions such as cardiovascular disease, diabetes, obesity, and functional limitations.

Treatments of Arthritis

The focus of treatment for arthritis is to control pain, minimize joint damage, and improve or maintain function and quality of life. According to the American College of Rheumatology, the treatment of arthritis might involve the following:

- Medication
- Nonpharmacological therapies
  - Physical or occupational therapy
  - Splints or joint assistive aids
  - Patient education and support
  - Weight loss
- Surgery

In conjunction with medical treatment, self-management of arthritis symptoms is very important as well. The Arthritis Foundation Self Help Program and the Chronic Disease Self-Management Program, both developed by Dr. Kate Lorig of Stanford University, are effective self-management education programs. The program helps people develop the skills needed to manage their arthritis on a day-to-day basis and gain the confidence to carry it out.

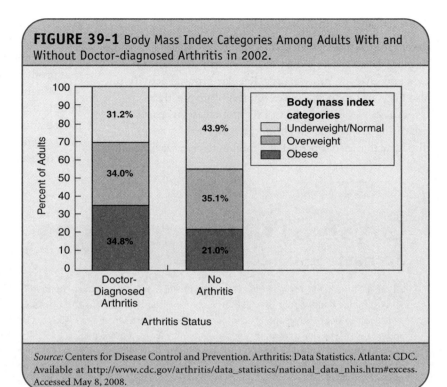

FIGURE 39-1 Body Mass Index Categories Among Adults With and Without Doctor-diagnosed Arthritis in 2002.

Source: Centers for Disease Control and Prevention. Arthritis: Data Statistics. Atlanta: CDC. Available at http://www.cdc.gov/arthritis/data_statistics/national_data_nhis.htm#excess. Accessed May 8, 2008.

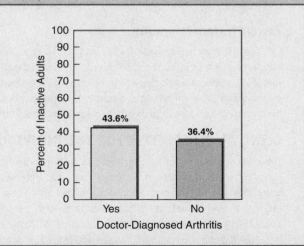

FIGURE 39-2 Proportion with Physical Inactivity Among Adults With and Without Doctor-diagnosed Arthritis, 2002.

Source: Data are from Shih M, Hootman JM, Kruger J, Helmick CG. Physical activity in men and women with arthritis, National Health Interview Survey, 2002. *Am J Prev Med* 2006;30:385–393. Centers for Disease Control and Prevention. *Arthritis: Data Statistics.* Atlanta: CDC; 2002. Available at: http://www.cdc.gov/arthritis/data_statistics/national_data_nhis.htm#excess. Accessed May 8, 2008.

Exercise and Weight Reduction

Recent studies have shown that moderate physical activity three or more days a week can help to relieve arthritis pain and stiffness and give you more energy. Regular physical activity can also lift your mood and make you feel more positive.

An activity that produces a slight increase in heart rate or breathing is considered moderate physical activity. Low-impact activities performed at a moderate pace work best for people with arthritis. These include walking, swimming, and riding a bicycle. Everyday activities such as dancing, gardening, and washing the car can be good if done at a moderate pace that produces slight breathing and heart rate changes.

Weight control is essential; research suggests that maintaining a healthy weight reduces the risk of developing osteoarthritis and may decrease disease progression. A loss of just 11 pounds can decrease the occurrence (incidence) of new knee osteoarthritis.

CASE STUDY

Scenario

C.S. is a 58-year-old African-American woman who came to her local community clinic with complaints of right knee pain. She is asking if she should apply to social security for disability because she thinks she has the arthritis her mother had that made her bedridden in her elder years. She notes the pain is worse when she walks or climbs stairs, which is a key activity for her job as a housekeeper. She does not participate in any non-work–related physical activity as she is always caring for the two grandchildren ages 10 and 8 and is tired once she comes home. She has steadily gained weight over the past 10 years as she finds that she eats to gain energy and deal with her stressful life. Her average weight is 180 lbs and she is 5'5". C.S. understands she needs to lose weight but she finds it hard to do any activity due to her knee pain. She is the major breadwinner for her two grandchildren who are living with her. Her daughter is in rehab for drug dependence. She had noted that her right leg is not straight and makes a lot of noise when she goes up stairs. She always wears sneakers at work. She completed an eighth-grade education.

Defining the Issues

This is a woman who does not have a regular healthcare provider and has not taken care of her routine health issues. She is living in a stressful situation with few supports. She is developing work-related limited activity due to her painful right knee. She needs to continue to bring in an income. Social security disability payments often result in recipients living in poverty.

Patient's Understanding

C.S. has little understanding of what arthritis is, that there are many kinds, and that there are treatments for arthritis that can improve her limitations. She is surprised that she has arthritis as she thinks "only old people have arthritis," because her mother had joint problems when she was in her 70s. She also assumes there is nothing she can do for her arthritis as it is a natural part of aging and there is nothing she can do to prevent arthritis. She thinks that Social Security disability will be a viable option for her income. She has not spoken to her employer about this situation.

CLINICAL PERSPECTIVE FOR THE INDIVIDUAL PATIENT

The clinical picture is of an obese woman with activity-related knee pain, no morning stiffness, and no immediate prior joint injury. This is most consistent with osteoarthritis. Her exam shows she does not have any joint warmth or redness but does have bony enlargement, and had genu valgus of her right knee. She has bilateral full knee extension but could flex her right knee only 60 degrees and her left to 100 degrees. One needs 90 degrees of knee flexion to walk up and down stairs easily. Measuring her quadriceps muscles revealed that she had greater than 2 cm difference between them with her right quadriceps smaller than her left even though she was right handed and legged, which indicates muscle atrophy of the right quadriceps. A standing radiograph of both knees demonstrates joint space loss, bony overgrowth (*osteophytes*), and changes in the subchondral bone on the right, which is diagnostic for OA.

The American College of Rheumatology has recommendations for the management of knee osteoarthritis that include non-pharmacological and pharmacological interventions. First, C.S. should understand the type of arthritis she has and be offered appropriate patient education materials that are available through the Arthritis Foundation, National Institutes of Health, American College of Rheumatology, WebMD, or the CDC arthritis Web sites. Focusing on self-management approaches is key as she is feeling overwhelmed to the point of discussing disability at a young age. Depression is a common comorbidity in people with arthritis. To manage her pain and learn self-management techniques, she could consider the Arthritis Self Help Course that is offered throughout the country through local Arthritis Foundation Chapters. At the same time, the healthcare provider should ascertain where she is in the stages of change with regards to weight loss and physical activity behavior modifications. Understanding the relationship between her weight, lack of physical activity, and her knee pain would be essential. Her body mass index (BMI) is 30 and some practical discussion of weight reduction strategies should be undertaken. She should understand her BMI (BMI Categories: Underweight ≤ 18.5, Normal weight = 18.5–24.9, Overweight = 25–29.9, Obesity ≥ 30 BMI) and develop a realistic goal for a weight reduction program. She should understand that only 15 pounds of weight loss can decrease her knee pain by up to 50 percent as well as decrease the progression of her osteoarthritis in her right knee and perhaps prevent the occurrence in her left knee. She should also improve the muscle strength and range of motion in her right knee. A consultation with a physical therapist would assist her in muscle strengthening and range of motion exercises.

An important part of her joint health and weight management program is participating in regular physical activity. Most weight loss occurs because of decreased caloric intake. Sustained physical activity is most helpful in the prevention of osteoarthritis and weight regain. In addition, exercise has a benefit of reducing risks of cardiovascular disease and diabetes, beyond that produced by weight reduction alone. She should be counseled to start exercising slowly, and gradually increase the intensity. Trying too hard at first can lead to injury and worsening pain. She could be given a referral to the local Arthritis Foundation if she would be interested in a group exercise program on land or in a pool or be referred to other group exercise programs. It is important for her to know that her exercise does not have to be done all at one time to improve her arthritis. Initial activities may be walking or swimming at a slow pace. She can start out by walking 30 minutes for three days a week with her grandchildren and can build to 45 minutes of more intense walking, at least five days a week. With this regimen, her sense of helplessness may improve and she can burn 100 to 200 calories more per day. All adults should set a long-term goal to accumulate at least 30 minutes or more of moderate-intensity physical activity on most—and preferably all—days of the week. This regimen can be adapted to other forms of physical activity, but walking is particularly attractive because of its safety and accessibility. Plan with her when and where she could do this walking activity in her community. Also, try to increase "every day" activity such as taking the stairs instead of the elevator or parking a distance from the grocery store. Reducing sedentary time is a good strategy to increase activity by undertaking frequent, less strenuous activities.

Consider assistive devices for ambulation such as a cane, knee brace, and/or foot inserts to improve the mechanics of the knee. Orthotists can be very helpful in finding the brace and insert that will fit the problem and be tolerated by the person with arthritis. Consider unloading the knee with prescribing a cane to be used on the opposite side and be sure she is using appropriate footwear.

Last but not least, consider such pain medications, interartciular steroid or hyaluronan injections or topical pain relief creams. Oral drugs like acetaminophen, other nonsteroidal anti-inflammatory drugs (NSAIDs) such as naprosyn or ibuprophen, or other analgesics such as tramadol or opiates are helpful. As NSAIDs increase blood pressure or can result in other gastrointestinal or cardiovascular side effects, discussing the risk/benefit profile of the drugs is essential. These medications can assist her to embark on her physical activity as well as strengthening and range of motion exercises that are the cornerstone to her improved function and decrease in disability. If she has refractory pain and disability despite the above approach, the next step would be a consultation from an orthopedic surgeon to learn if a procedure such as a total joint replacement is beneficial.

To keep her employment, she should discuss her situation with her employer and ask for a few simple accommodations until she has improved. She can keep her current income and not risk falling into poverty on social security disability income.

PUBLIC HEALTH PERSPECTIVE FOR THE HEALTH OF THE GENERAL POPULATION AND OF HIGH RISK GROUPS

Arthritis remains a major public health issue that will increase in the future. Since 1998, the Arthritis Foundation's public health activities have centered around the National Arthritis Act, the National Arthritis Action Plan, the arthritis section of Healthy People 2010, and National Committee on Quality Assurance (NCQA) to develop an arthritis-related Health Plan Employer Data and Information Set (HEDIS) measure. These are outlined below.

National Arthritis Act

In 1975, the Arthritis Foundation led a coalition to push the Congress to pass the National Arthritis Act, which initiated an expanded response to arthritis through research, training, public education and treatment. The Act called for a long-term strategy to address arthritis in the United States.

National Arthritis Action Plan

Over 40 partners and the Arthritis Foundation in 1999 created one of the first national road maps for a chronic illness in the United States: the National Arthritis Action Plan (NAAP). The NAAP is a blueprint for population-oriented efforts to combat arthritis and emphasizes four public health values: prevention; use and expand the science base; seek social equity; and build partnerships (see the text box for the aims and activities of NAAP). In 2000, the Federal Government funded the infrastructure for the Arthritis Program at the CDC that funds its infrastructure along with grants for implementation of the arthritis public health plan through the establishment of arthritis programs in state health departments (see http://www.cdc.gov/arthritis for a listing of states with arthritis action plans), a limited investigator-initiated grant program, and a CDC-funded peer reviewed grant to the Arthritis Foundation. With this funding, the Arthritis Foundation created effective public education and awareness activities in both English and Spanish ("Physical Activity: the Arthritis Pain Reliever" campaign) and has developed evidence-based programs for people with arthritis (see the Life Improvement Series descriptions at http://www.arthritis.org, which include an arthritis-specific self-help course and exercise and water exercise programs developed in conjunction with the YMCA). They are offered throughout the United States through Arthritis Foundation Chapters.

NATIONAL ARTHRITIS ACTION PLAN

The overarching aims of the NAAP are:

- Increase public awareness of arthritis as the leading cause of disability and an important public health problem.
- Prevent arthritis whenever possible.
- Promote early diagnosis and appropriate management for people with arthritis to ensure them the maximum number of years of healthy life.
- Minimize preventable pain and disability due to arthritis.
- Support people with arthritis in developing and accessing the resources they need to cope with their disease.
- Ensure that people with arthritis receive the family, peer, and community support they need.

The aims of the NAAP will be achieved through three major types of activities:

- Surveillance, epidemiology, and prevention research
- Communication and education
- Programs, policies, and systems

The Arthritis group at the Centers for Disease Control developed and collected arthritis data through the **Behavioral** **Risk Factor Surveillance System (BRFSS)**, the **National Health Interview Survey (NHIS)**, and the **National Health and Nutrition Examination Survey (NHANES)**, and it has published an annual arthritis data report during Arthritis Month in May (see http://www.cdc.gov/arthritis for the latest facts and statistics about arthritis in the United States).

Quality of Care Measures for People with Arthritis

As a part of the Arthritis Foundation Quality Indicators Project (AFQUIP), the Arthritis Foundation (AF) created indicators for treatment of rheumatoid arthritis and osteoarthritis and for analgesics and pain use. These were forwarded to and used by the American College of Rheumatology Quality Measures Committee. All three indicators were submitted to the National Quality Measures Clearing House and will be posted at the end of 2006.

The AF served as the patient constituency group on the NCQA Musculoskeletal Workgroup, the outcome of which was a HEDIS measure for disease-modifying antirheumatic drugs that took effect in the reporting year 2006 (http://www.ncqa.org/tabid/59/Default.aspx; accessed May 8, 2008).

The OA indicators have been used for the American Medical Association's Physician Consortium for Performance Improvement.

Key Public Health Arthritis Messages

The Arthritis Foundation and the Centers for Disease Control recommend the following key public health messages to reduce the impact of arthritis. Early diagnosis and appropriate management of arthritis, including self-management activities, can help people with arthritis by decreasing pain, improving function and productivity, and lowering healthcare costs. Key self-management activities include the following:

Develop Your Skills. Learning techniques to reduce pain and limitations can be beneficial to people with arthritis. Self-management education, such as the Arthritis Foundation Self Help Program (AFSHP), or the Chronic Disease Self Management Program (CDSMP) help you develop the skills and confidence to manage your arthritis on a day-to-day basis. For example, AFSHP has been shown to reduce pain even four years after participating in the program.

Be Active. Research has shown that physical activity decreases pain, improves function, helps build and maintain healthy bones, muscles and joints and delays disability. Walking just as little as 30 minutes—even 10 minutes three times a day—can ease joint pain, improve mobility, and reduce fatigue. The Arthritis Foundation offers joint-safe physical activity programs proven to decrease pain and increase flexibility and range of motion. (See http://www.arthritis.org for an Arthritis Foundation Chapter near you and register for the Arthritis Foundation Life Improvement Series: AF Self Help, AF Exercise, and AF Aquatic Programs).

Watch Your Weight. The prevalence of arthritis increases with increasing weight. Research suggests that maintaining a healthy weight reduces the risk of developing arthritis and may decrease disease progression. A loss of just 11 pounds can decrease the occurrence (incidence) of new knee osteoarthritis. For those living with symptoms, losing 15 pounds can cut knee pain in half.

See Your Doctor. Understand if you have arthritis and what type. Early diagnosis and appropriate management are important, especially for inflammatory types of arthritis. For example, early use of disease-modifying drugs can affect the course of rheumatoid arthritis. If you have symptoms of arthritis, see your doctor and begin appropriate management of your condition.

Protect Your Joints. Joint injury can lead to osteoarthritis. People who experience sports or occupational injuries or have jobs with repetitive motions (like repeated knee bending) have more osteoarthritis. Avoid joint injury to reduce your risk of developing osteoarthritis. Speak with a health care professional about ways to reduce strain on your joints.

The Arthritis Foundation, many other volunteer health associations, government agencies, and professional associations are working together to improve policies so that healthy food at reasonable prices and better places for physical activity are available in communities across the country.

KEY TERMS

Biology/Clinical Terms

Arthritis: Term used to describe more than 100 rheumatic diseases and conditions that affect the joints and tissues, causing inflammation around the joints.

Gout: Rheumatic disease resulting from an accumulation of uric acid crystals in tissues and fluids within the body.

Osteoarthritis: Degeneration of the cartilage and underlying bone within a joint, characterized by bony overgrowth.

Osteophytes: Bony overgrowth of joints caused by rheumatic diseases.

Rheumatoid Arthritis (RA): Systemic inflammatory disease manifesting in multiple joints in the body, primarily affecting the lining of the joints and sometimes other organs.

Public Health Terms

Behavioral Risk Factor Surveillance System (BRFSS): A routine, systematic epidemiological method of collecting information on certain health behaviors to analyze.

National Health Interview Survey (NHIS): A source of information collected on the overall health of the civilian population of the United States that consists of questionnaires on health, demographics, and socioeconomic status.

National Health and Nutrition Examination Survey (NHANES): A national health survey conducted to obtain information on the overall health and nutritional status of the general population of the United States.

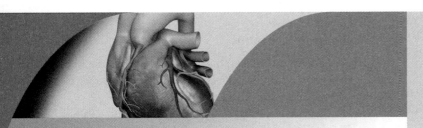

Questions for Further Research, Study, Reflection, and Discussion

For the Individual Student

In order to answer these questions, it may be necessary to research the primary literature.

- Describe the pathophysiology of osteoarthritis and link your findings to the current approaches to the therapy.
- Understand the major differences between osteoarthritis, gout, and rheumatoid arthritis, and formulate the public health messages for each. Compare and contrast your findings.
- Review the stages of change and decide where C.S. (see Case Study) is on the continuum.

For Small Group Discussion

- Locate resources for people with arthritis. Where are the best Web sites and culturally competent patient education materials?
- From the information provided in the Case Study, how would you counsel C.S. to begin her weight reduction and physical activity regimen, given her social situation?

- Research the Americans with Disabilities Act. What job accommodations would you recommend for C.S.?
- As arthritis is common, ask for volunteers in the class who have arthritis or have family members who have arthritis to describe the type and the impact that arthritis has had on the individual and the family.

For Entire Class Discussion

- Research other forms of arthritis and discuss how different forms of arthritis affect different racial and ethnic groups.
- Visit an orthotist to try on knee braces, learn who needs shoe inserts, and how to use a cane.
- Review the evidence for improved outcomes on the available weight reduction and physical activity programs for people with arthritis. Which have the best outcomes?

EXERCISES/ACTIVITIES

- Visit an Arthritis Foundation self-help, exercise, or aquatic program, and ask the participants how the class has helped them.
- Complete a community assessment of the places to get physical activity and healthy food, and plan how to improve the environment to increase the public's ability to be more physically active and eat a healthy diet.

Healthy People 2010

The nation's public health plan, Healthy People 2010 was created with consultation with the nation's health constituencies by the Department of Health and Human Services. It has several goals for arthritis.

Arthritis Components in Healthy People 2010

2-1. (Developmental) Increase the mean number of days without severe pain among adults who have chronic joint symptoms.

2-2. Reduce the proportion of adults with chronic joint symptoms who experience a limitation in activity due to arthritis.

2-3. Reduce the proportion of all adults with chronic joint symptoms who have difficulty in performing two or more personal care activities, thereby preserving independence.

2-4. (Developmental) Increase the proportion of adults aged 18 years and older with arthritis who seek help in coping if they experience personal and emotional problems.

2-5. Increase the employment rate among adults with arthritis in the working-aged population.

2-6. (Developmental) Eliminate racial disparities in the rate of total knee replacements.

2-7. (Developmental) Increase the proportion of adults who have seen a healthcare provider for their chronic joint symptoms.

2-8. (Developmental) Increase the proportion of persons with arthritis who have had effective, evidence-based arthritis education as an integral part of the management of their condition.

7-11. Increase the proportion of local health departments that have established culturally appropriate and linguistically competent community health promotion and disease prevention programs.

19-1. Increase the proportion of adults who are at a healthy weight.

19-2. Reduce the proportion of adults who are obese.

22-1. Reduce the proportion of adults who engage in no leisure-time physical activity.

22-2. Increase the proportion of adults who engage regularly, preferably daily, in moderate physical activity for at least 30 minutes per day.

22-4. Increase the proportion of adults who perform physical activities that enhance and maintain muscular strength and endurance.

22-5. Increase the proportion of adults who perform physical activities that enhance and maintain flexibility.

REFERENCE

1. Centers for Disease Control and Prevention (CDC). Atlanta: CDC. *Targeting Arthritis Reducing Disability for Nearly 19 Million Americans.* Available at: http://www.cdc.gov/nccdphp/publications/aag/arthritis.htm. Accessed May 8, 2008.

RESOURCES

Klippel JH, Stone JH, Crofford L, White PH, eds. *Primer on Rheumatic Diseases*, 13th ed. New York: Springer; 2007.

Arthritis Foundation (AF). *Home page.* Atlanta: AF; 2008. Available at http://www.arthritis.org. Accessed May 8, 2008.

Centers for Disease Control and Prevention (CDC). Atlanta, CDC. *Arthritis.* Available at http://www.cdc.gov/arthritis. Accessed May 8, 2008.

Loy B. Job Accommodations Network (JAN). Morgantown, WV: JAN. *Accomodation and Compliance Series: Employees with Arthritis.* Available at http://www.jan.wvu.edu/media/Arthritis.html. Accessed May 8, 2008.

Centers for Disease Control and Prevention (CDC). Atlanta: CDC. National Arthritis Action Plan: Executive Summary. Available at http://www.cdc.gov/arthritis/state_coordinators/pdf/naap_executive_summary.pdf. Accessed May 8, 2008.

Helmick C, Felson D, Lawrence R, Gabriel S, Hirsch R, et al. Establishment of the prevalence of arthritis and other rheumatic diseases in the United States. Part I. *Arthritis Rheum* 2008;58:15–25.

Lawrence R, Felson D, Helmick C, Arnold LM, Choi H, et al. Establishment of the prevalence of arthritis and other rheumatic diseases in the United States. Part II. *Arthritis Rheum* 2008;58:26–35.

Hootman J, Bolen J, Helmick C, Langmaid G. Prevalence of doctor-diagnosed arthritis and arthritis-attributable activity limitation—United States, 2003–2005. *MMWR Morbid Mortal Wkly Rep* 2006;55:1089–1092.

Hootman JM, Helmick CG. Projections of U.S. prevalence of arthritis and associated activity limitations. *Arthritis Rheum* 2006;54:266–229.

Shih M, Hootman JM, Kruger J, Helmick CG. Physical activity in men and women with arthritis, National Health Interview Survey, 2002. *Am J Prev Med* 2006;30:385–393.

Felson DT, Zhang Y. An update on the epidemiology of knee and hip osteoarthritis with a view to prevention. *Arthritis Rheum* 1998;41:1343–1355.

Brady TJ, Kruger JMS, Helmick CG, Callahan LF, Boutaugh ML. Intervention programs for arthritis and other rheumatic diseases. *Health Educ Behav* 2003;30:44–63.

Hootman JM, Sniezek JE, Helmick CG. Women and arthritis —burden, impact and prevention programs. *J Womens Health Gen Based Med* 2002;11:407–416.

Keefe FJ, Lefebvre JC, Kerns RD, Rosenberg R, Beaupre P, Prochaska J. Understanding the adoption of arthritis self management: stages of change profiles among arthritis patients. *Pain* 2000;87:303–313.

Kruger JMS, Helmick CG, Callahan LF, Haddix AC. Cost-effectiveness of the Arthritis Self-Help Course. *Arch Intern Med* 1998;158:1245–1249.

CROSS REFERENCES

Exercise
Inflammation
The Nutrition Transition

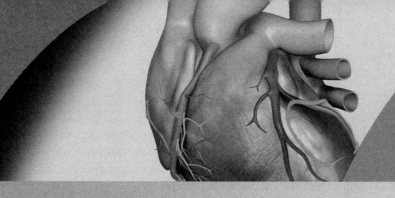

CHAPTER **40**

Osteoporosis: A Significant Cause of Disability and Mortality

Karen Kemmis
Dale Avers

A woman's risk of hip fracture is the same as the combined risk of breast, uterine and ovarian cancer.
National Osteoporosis Foundation. Fast Facts. Available at: http://www.nof.org/osteoporosis/diseasefacts.htm

LEARNING OBJECTIVES

By the end of this chapter, students will be able to:

- Describe the dynamic process of bone remodeling.
- Establish risk factors for osteoporosis.
- Identify areas for prevention of osteoporosis.
- Discuss the relationship of falls and osteoporosis.

HISTORY

Osteoporosis is defined as a skeletal disorder characterized by compromised bone strength predisposing a person to an increased risk of fracture, especially at the spine, hip, and wrist. Bone strength primarily reflects the integration of bone quality and bone density. Figure 40-1 shows photomicrographs comparing normal, healthy bone and osteoporotic bone.[1]

Osteoporosis is included as a focus area in Healthy People 2010. The 2004 *Surgeon General's Report on Bone Health and Osteoporosis*[2] demonstrates the importance of osteoporosis in public health. This report placed osteoporosis in the forefront of public health concerns, along with smoking, second-hand smoke exposure, mental health, youth violence, and physical activity.

Osteoporosis no longer be should considered a necessary result of aging but rather as a disease that can be prevented, diagnosed, and effectively treated. Former Surgeon General, Richard Carmona, MD, MPH, FACS, stated that, "with appropriate nutrition and physical activity throughout life, individuals can significantly reduce the risk of bone disease and fractures."[p.v] Some of this responsibility falls on health professionals who can assess, diagnose, and treat at-risk patients. However, the Surgeon General's primary message was that, "a coordinated public health approach that brings together a variety of public and private sector stakeholders in a collaborative effort is the most promising strategy for improving the bone health of Americans."[2p.v–vi] Much research has been performed to provide information about bone health and bone disease. As a result of this research, risk factors have been identified, the diagnosis of osteoporosis has become more noninvasive and accessible to many, and treatment options have increased and become more effective.

Prevention of osteoporosis starts at an early age by promoting adequate physical activity, and calcium and vitamin D intake in children and adolescents. Risk factors for osteoporosis and fracture can be identified throughout life, allowing modification where possible, and further evaluation and treat-

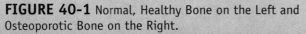

FIGURE 40-1 Normal, Healthy Bone on the Left and Osteoporotic Bone on the Right.

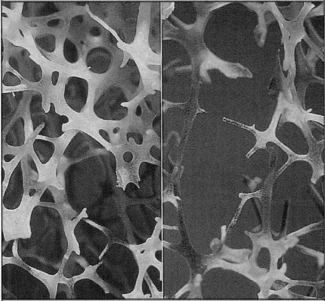

Source: International Osteoporosis Foundation. Image of normal and osteoporotic bone. Available at http://www.iofbonehealth.org/newsroom/resources/image-normal-osteoporotic-bone.html. Accessed May 12, 2008.

ment for non-modifiable risk factors. Many new treatments are available including drugs that can significantly reduce the risk of fracture. Many secondary causes of osteoporosis have been identified, such as use of glucocorticoids and certain diseases that harm bone health including those which cause malabsorption. These can be identified and interventions provided to limit the harmful effects to bone. Falls are a leading cause of fractures in the aging adult. Many risk factors for falls can be identified and interventions can be carried out to improve balance and decrease the incidence of injurious falls and fracture. Osteoporosis has changed from a "silent disease" that was diagnosed only after a fracture occurred, to a disease that can be prevented, diagnosed, and effectively treated.

BASIC SCIENCE FACTS/KEY CONCEPTS REVIEW

Function of the Skeleton

The bony skeleton serves many functions that include providing mobility, support, and protection for the body and storage of essential minerals required for other body functions. **Calcium** and **phosphorus** are two key minerals stored in the bones that are responsible for proper functioning of muscles and nerves. Bone is in a constant state of remodeling, where old bone is broken down by cells known as **osteoclasts** and new

bone is formed by cells that build bone known as **osteoblasts**. **Vitamin D** is necessary for absorption of calcium in the small intestine and to help maintain blood calcium levels within the normal ranges. It is required for proper muscle function and may have a direct effect on bone.

Magnitude of the Problem

Osteoporosis affects 44 million Americans, with 10 million diagnosed with the disease and 34 million with low bone mass, putting these Americans at risk for developing osteoporosis. Of the 10 million individuals believed to have osteoporosis, 8 million are women and 2 million are men. Osteoporosis occurs more frequently in people who are of Caucasian and Asian descent; however, osteoporosis is considered a significant risk in people of all ethnic backgrounds.

One in two women and one in four men over age 50 will have an osteoporosis-related fracture in her/his remaining lifetime. The risk of sustaining an osteoporotic fracture in women is greater than the combined risk of sustaining a heart attack, stroke, or breast cancer. Approximately 1.5 million fractures occur annually as a result of osteoporosis. This includes over 300,000 hip fractures, approximately 700,000 vertebral fractures, 250,000 wrist fractures, and 300,000 at other sites (that is, ribs and pelvis). The national direct care expenditure, including hospitalization, nursing homes, and outpatient services for osteoporotic fractures, is estimated at $18 billion per year in 2002 dollars.[3] As the population ages and inflation occurs, these costs will steadily increase in the future.

Risk Factors for Osteoporosis and Fractures

Many risk factors have been identified for osteoporosis and fractures. Some of the risk factors are considered modifiable and others are considered non-modifiable. Table 40-1[4] lists the risk factors that have been identified for osteoporosis and fractures.

Factors That Optimize Bone Health and Decrease Risk of Fractures[4]

Building strong bones during childhood and adolescence and maintaining strong bones during adulthood is critical in preventing osteoporosis and fracture later in life. The National Osteoporosis Foundation has identified five factors to optimize bone health and decrease the risk of fracture.[4] These 5 factors are:

1. A balanced diet rich in calcium and vitamin D
2. **Weight-bearing** and **resistance-training** exercises
3. A healthy lifestyle with no smoking or excessive alcohol intake

TABLE 40-1 Risk Factors for Osteoporosis and Fractures[4]

- Personal history of fracture after age 50
- Current low bone mass
- Female sex
- Small body size
- Advanced age
- Family history of osteoporosis or history of fracture in a first degree relative
- Estrogen deficiency as a result of **menopause**, especially early or surgically induced
- Abnormal absence of menstrual periods (amenorrhea)
- Anorexia nervosa
- Low lifetime calcium intake
- Vitamin D deficiency
- Use of certain medications (corticosteroids, chemotherapy, anticonvulsants, excessive thyroid replacement, and others)
- Certain chronic medical conditions such as those that cause poor intestinal absorption (Crohn disease, celiac disease, liver disease) and those associated with immobility or bed rest (stroke, Parkinson disease, multiple sclerosis)
- Low hormonal levels in men
- Sedentary lifestyle
- Current cigarette smoking
- Excessive use of alcohol
- Caucasian or Southeast Asian descent

Source: Data from National Osteoporosis Foundation. Fast facts. http://www.nof.org/osteoporosis/diseasefacts.htm. Accessed July 15, 2007.

4. Talking to one's healthcare professional about bone health
5. Bone density testing and medication when appropriate

Detection of Osteoporosis

In the past, osteoporosis was able to be detected only after a fracture was sustained or when a fracture was visualized by x-ray. Unfortunately, x-ray could not demonstrate the bone loss associated with osteoporosis until 40 percent to 50 percent of the bone loss had occurred. Now, new, noninvasive testing of bone density is available through various techniques. **Dual energy x-ray absorptiometry (DXA)** is a painless, noninvasive test that uses low-dose special x-ray beams. DXA of the hip and spine is the "gold standard" for detection of low bone mass at these sites, which are common sites of osteoporotic fractures. DXA testing is covered by most insurance plans including Medicare if it is considered medically necessary with a

physician's order. Medicare now provides coverage for bone mass measurements every two years in the person who:

- Is postmenopausal and at risk of osteoporosis
- Has primary hyperparathyroidism
- Has certain spinal abnormalities that might indicate a fracture
- Is on long-term corticosteroid therapy, such as prednisone
- Is being monitored to assess the response to FDA-approved osteoporosis medications[5]

Repeated bone density tests should be performed at the same location and on the same device when possible to allow for accurate and consistent results because of the differences in the technology.

Prevention and Treatment

Nutrition

Calcium and vitamin D are critical for bone health. Table 40-2 lists the goals for daily calcium intake by age.[6]

Calcium is available in dairy products and many other foods including those fortified with calcium. Food and supplement labels give calcium amounts in a percentage based on a requirement of 1,000 milligrams (mg) per day. Because people require varying amounts of calcium based on age and other factors, it is important to understand how to calculate the amount of calcium in milligrams.[7] Table 40-3 describes the calculation of calcium in mg from a food label. To determine if calcium supplements are needed, determine the daily calcium intake goal from Table 40-2 and subtract dietary calcium

TABLE 40-2 Goals for Daily Calcium Intake

Age	Calcium*
4–8	800 mg
9–18	1,300 mg
19–50	1,000 mg
51–65	1,200 mg
Over 65	1,200 mg

mg = milligrams.

*It may be unhealthy to take more than 2,500 milligrams per day of calcium, including food and supplements.

Source: Data from Standing Committee on the Scientific Evaluation of Dietary Reference Intakes. DRI Dietary Reference Intakes for Calcium, Phosphorus, Magnesium, Vitamin D, and Fluoride. Washington, DC: National Academy Press; 1997.

TABLE 40-3 Calculation of Milligrams (mg) Calcium from a Food Label

1. Find the percent calcium per serving
2. Drop the percent symbol (%)
3. Add a zero

For example, 30 percent calcium per serving is equal to 300 milligrams of calcium.

Source: Data from U.S. Food and Drug Administration. Calcium Education Program Leader's Guide. Accessed October 20, 2007. Available at: http://www.cfsan.fda.gove/~dms/ca-2.html and U.S. Food and Drug Administration. How to Understand and Use the Nutrition Facts Label. July 7, 2006; http://www.cfsanfda.gov/~dms/foodlab.html#ca. Accessed July 15, 2007.

intake from food and beverages. It is best to increase calcium through dietary means (calcium-rich or calcium-fortified foods) and then add supplements if necessary.

Vitamin D is available naturally from the sun. However, many individuals do not get adequate sun exposure (for example, those living in Northern latitudes and those who are not outdoors in the sunshine, or institutionalized) or limit sun exposure due to concern about skin cancer. Dietary sources of vitamin D are not readily available so foods fortified with vitamin D and supplements are often beneficial to maintain vitamin D levels in the body.[8]

Vitamin D Needs of Special Groups

Adequate vitamin D status, which depends on dietary intake and cutaneous synthesis, is important for optimal calcium absorption, and it can reduce the risk for bone loss. Two functionally relevant measures indicate that optimal vitamin D (serum 25-hydroxyvitamin D) may be as high as 80 nmol/L. Older adults and individuals with dark skin (because the ability to synthesize vitamin D from exposure to sunlight varies with degree of skin pigmentation) are at a greater risk of low serum 25-hydroxyvitamin D concentrations. Also at risk are those exposed to insufficient ultraviolet ra-diation (that is, sunlight) for the cutaneous production of vitamin D (for example, housebound individuals).[8]

For individuals within the high-risk groups, substantially higher daily intakes of vitamin D_3 (that is, 25 micrograms [μg] or 1,000 International Units [IU] of vitamin D_3 per day) have been recommended to reach and maintain serum 25-hydroxyvitamin D values of 80 nmol/L. Three cups of vitamin D-fortified milk (total equals 7.5 μg or 300 IU), 1 cup of vitamin D-fortified orange juice (2.5 μg or 100 IU), and 15 μg (600 IU) of supplemental vitamin D_3 would provide 25 μg (1,000 IU) of vitamin D_3 daily.[8]

Physical Activity and Exercise

Physical activity and exercise have the potential to increase bone density in youth and young adulthood, maintain and possibly modestly increase bone density in adulthood, increase muscle mass, decrease postural problems from osteoporosis through postural stability, improve balance and agility, and reduce the risk of fall-related fractures.[9,10] Physical activity, particularly high-impact activities, has been shown to have beneficial effects on **bone mineral density (BMD)** in children and female adolescents for many years afterwards, although BMD decreases upon cessation of the physical activity.[11] The two types of physical activity and exercise that have a direct benefit on bone health across all ages are weight-bearing and resistive strengthening exercises. Weight-bearing physical activity and exercises that put stress or impact through the bone include walking, hiking, dancing, and stair climbing (Table 40-4)[2] as opposed to activities such as cycling and swimming. Resistive strengthening exercise builds bone through muscle contraction.[12] This muscle contraction pulls on the bone, causing the

TABLE 40-4 Summary of Physical Activity Guidelines for Bone Health Across the Lifespan

	Children and Adolescents	Young to Middle Aged Adults	Older Adults
Duration and frequency of moderate-intensity physical activity	60 minutes on most, preferably all, days per week	30 minutes on most, preferably all, days per week	30 minutes on most, preferably all, days per week
Duration and frequency of high-intensity physical activity	20 minutes on 3 or more days per week	10 minutes of moderate to high impact as tolerated	No recommendations

Source: Data from U.S. Department of Health and Human Services. *Bone Health and Osteoporosis: A Report of the Surgeon General 2004.* Rockville, MD: U.S. Department of Health and Human Services Public Health Service Office of the Surgeon General; 2004.

bone to remodel. Resistance to any exercise can be achieved through the use of body weight, dumbbells, wrist/ankle weights, exercise bands and tubing, and exercise machines (Table 40-5)[13] and needs to be progressive.[10]

Exercise is the single most effective intervention to reduce falls.[14] Exercise can reduce falls through progressive, moderately intense strengthening exercise and balance training.[15] Because altered balance is the largest contributor to falls in older adults,[16] improving balance should be an objective in fall prevention programs, especially in the presence of osteoporosis.[15] Programs aimed at improving balance include Tai Chi,[17,18] strengthening exercises,[19] and dynamic balance skill development.[20]

TABLE 40-5 Guidelines for Strength Training Across the Lifespan

	Children and Adolescents	Young to Middle Aged Adults	Older Adults
Number of exercises		8–10 to train all major muscle groups	
Repetitions per set		8–12 repetitions	
Sets of exercise		1–2 sets	
Rate of perceived exertion (RPE)	Avoid maximal exertion	12 to 13 (somewhat hard)	12 to 13 (somewhat hard)
Frequency	2–3 times per week	At least 2 times per week	At least 2 times per week
Rest between sessions		At least 48 hours	
Emphasis	Proper form/training technique	Maintain bone mass and increase muscle strength and mass	Functional activities (sit to stand, stair climb, mini-squats)

Source: Data from American College of Sports Medicine. ACSM's Guidelines for Exercise Testing and Prescription. Seventh ed. Baltimore, MD: Lippincott Williams & Wilkins; 2005.

CASE STUDIES
Osteoporosis Along the Lifespan

Bone health can be best achieved by promoting optimal bone formation during childhood and adolescence. The following case study demonstrates the consequences of poor bone health in adolescence and thus a failure of primary prevention.

Scenario 1
A 16-Year-Old Caucasian Female

Megan is a 16-year-old Caucasian female who runs on her high school cross-country team. She is the second best runner on the team and hopes for a college scholarship for cross-country. She is 67 inches tall and weighs 108 pounds [body mass index (BMI) equals 17 kg/m^2, which is considered underweight]. She has a history of two stress fractures, one in each foot. She begins to experience shin pain during running. She continues to run until the pain prevents her from maintaining a normal stride. Megan's coach speaks to her parents, requesting she make an appointment with her physician. The physician examines Megan and requests an x-ray, which shows several stress fractures of the tibia.

Scenario 2
A 63-Year-Old Asian Female

Case 2 describes an opportunity for secondary prevention of osteoporosis in an individual who demonstrates several risk factors of osteoporosis.

Nora is a 63-year-old Asian female who is employed as a college professor. She has a petite build at 60 inches tall and weighs 98 pounds (BMI equals 19.1 kg/m^2, which is considered normal weight). She has chronic neck and low back pain due to arthritis and reports a 2 inch loss in height. Nora had smoked many years ago and has a history of oral steroid use for pain many years ago. She has an active lifestyle, walking four miles per day and doing all of her house- and yard work. She has postural faults with a forward head and rounded shoulders. She reports no history of falls or fractures. She has recently had a DXA test with T-scores in the −2.2 to −2.4 range for her hip and spine.

Scenario 3

An 81-Year-Old Caucasian Female

Case 3 describes an opportunity for tertiary prevention of osteoporosis. The individual described has developed osteoporosis; thus, the focus is on managing the disease and prevention of osteoporosis-related complications such as fractures and disability.

Evelyn is an 81-year-old widowed, Caucasian female who lives alone in a three-level house. She stands 65 inches tall but states that her maximum height was 67.5 inches. She weighs 132 pounds making her BMI 22 kg/m^2, which is considered normal weight. She has chronic low back pain with a history of lumbar stenosis, lumbar fusion, and multiple compression fractures with a subsequent scoliosis. She is taking narcotic medications for the pain. She also takes medications for hypertension, hypercholesterolemia, acid reflux, and congestive heart failure. Occasionally she uses a sedative to help her sleep.

Evelyn has a history of falls that have increased in frequency over the past two months without a known cause. She has not had any obvious fractures from the falls. Surgical history includes a right total hip arthroplasty for arthritis 15 years ago. She fractured her left radius skiing about 18 years ago. She reports noticing an increase in urinary incontinence, has acid reflux, and dyspnea on exertion (shortness of breath climbing stairs and walking at what she considers a moderate pace). She was taking a bisphosphonate medication for osteoporosis but had to stop due to gastric distress. She continues to work 10 hours per week as a financial planner, does light housework and all of her own personal care. She walked one hour per day until two years ago when she had to stop due to balance problems. Her back pain currently increases with walking and standing.

CLINICAL PERSPECTIVE FOR THE INDIVIDUAL PATIENT

Results of Fractures

Fractures can be a devastating and life-altering event, especially in older women with osteoporosis who have a greater likelihood of sustaining another fracture. In the year following a hip fracture, 24 percent of women who sustained the hip fracture will die. While the rate of hip fracture in men is about one third to one half the rate of women, mortality following a hip fracture in men is nearly twice that of women (approximately 40 percent). Only 10 percent of those sustaining a fracture will return to full activity. In addition to the personal consequences of hip fractures, there are enormous public health consequences. Twenty percent of Americans who were ambulatory prior to their hip fracture will require long-term care afterward. Only 15 percent of those who sustain an osteoporosis-related hip fracture can walk across a room unaided six months after the fracture implying an increased need for supportive services.

Fractures of the spine (vertebral fractures) also increase morbidity and mortality. Vertebral fractures are associated with an increased risk for spine and other non-spine fractures, decreased quality of life,[21] pain, deterioration of physical function,[22] loss of height,[23] an increased kyphosis, difficulty breathing, stomach pains and digestive discomfort, decreased mobility and energy,[24] and increased long-term morbidity and mortality.[25] Clearly, fractures have a significant relationship to morbidity and mortality.

PUBLIC HEALTH PERSPECTIVE FOR THE HEALTH OF THE GENERAL POPULATION AND OF HIGH RISK GROUPS

Public health interventions can target primary, secondary, or tertiary levels of osteoporosis.

Primary Prevention

Primary prevention of osteoporosis addresses the elimination of a disease before it starts by reducing or eliminating risk factors. This type of prevention can be achieved through education/counseling. Primary prevention begins at birth and continues as a lifelong challenge. Lifestyle factors are responsible for 10 percent to 50 percent of bone mass and structure. The promotion of bone health includes: following a bone-healthy diet including a well-balanced diet and sufficient calcium and vitamin D; engaging in regular physical activity; avoiding harmful behaviors including smoking and excessive alcohol consumption; and assessing for and treating secondary causes of osteoporosis. Children need age-appropriate teaching tools that encourage healthy bone-building habits (calcium, vitamin D, and exercise). Adolescents can positively affect bone health by supporting rapid growth with adequate calcium and vitamin D, one hour of daily exercise and through avoidance of behaviors that harm bone health, including eating disorders (anorexia nervosa and bulimia), over-exercising, smoking, alcohol, and anabolic steroids. The female athletic triad of disordered eating/over-training, amenorrhea, and osteoporosis can negatively affect peak bone mass in females. Case 1 describes an opportunity for primary prevention of osteoporosis.

Secondary Prevention

Secondary prevention of osteoporosis involves identifying a disease in the early stages, often before symptoms are present, thereby minimizing adverse outcomes and preventing harmful consequences. This is achieved through early detection of those at risk and initiation of appropriate treatments to prevent fractures. Bone density testing should be performed on those at risk of osteoporosis. Table 40-6 provides a list of those who should get a bone density test according to the New York State Osteoporosis Education and Prevention Program.

The diagnosis of osteoporosis is based on T-scores and defined by the World Health Organization (WHO). The T-score compares an individual's bone density to the average bone density of young healthy adults of the same gender. Figure 40-2[26] presents the status of bone health based on T-scores.

Low bone mass is a risk factor for osteoporosis and is diagnosed when the T-score is between −1 and −2.5. A person with low bone mass should take steps to prevent or slow the progression to osteoporosis. Osteoporosis is diagnosed when the T-score is at or below −2.5. The lower the bone mass, the greater the risk for fracture. Osteoporosis also can be diagnosed if a person has a history of fractures without trauma or with low trauma.[26]

If a person is diagnosed with osteoporosis or low bone mass, there are steps that should be taken to prevent progression and fracture. A healthy diet should be consumed, including adequate amounts of calcium and vitamin D. Maintenance of a healthy body weight should be promoted. Physical activity and exercise should be encouraged to maintain bone and muscle strength, flexibility, to improve or maintain best posture, and to challenge balance to decrease the risk of falls and subse-

---

TABLE 40-6 Guidelines of Those Who Should Get a Bone Mineral Density Test

In general, bone mineral density testing is recommended for the following individuals:

- All women aged 65 or older regardless of risk factors;
- Postmenopausal women under age 65 who have one or more risk factors (other than race, gender, and postmenopausal status);
- Postmenopausal women who have a current and/or previous fracture with minimal trauma;
- Adults (including postmenopausal women, premenopausal women, and men) on steroid medications for more than three months; and
- Men with a current/previous fracture or a major risk factor for osteoporosis such as low testosterone, alcoholism, or any other secondary cause of osteoporosis.

The decision to have a BMD test should be made in collaboration with a doctor or medical professional. If a bone density test is recommended, a prescription with a diagnosis is needed.

Source: New York State Osteoporosis Education and Prevention Program. *Who Should Have the Test?* New York: NYSOEPP; 2008. Available at http://www.nysopep.org/Diagnosis_WhoShouldHaveTest.shtm. Accessed May 8, 2008.

---

quent fractures. Yearly height checks on an accurate device should be performed to monitor changes in height as a height loss of greater than 2 inches from maximal height can be due to vertebral compression fractures, even in the absence of pain.[27,28] Smoking cessation and moderation of alcohol intake should be strongly encouraged.

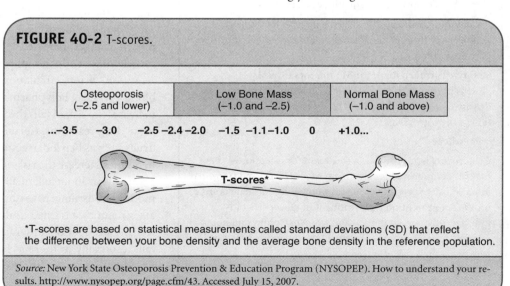

FIGURE 40-2 T-scores.

Osteoporosis (−2.5 and lower)	Low Bone Mass (−1.0 and −2.5)	Normal Bone Mass (−1.0 and above)

...−3.5   −3.0   −2.5 −2.4 −2.0   −1.5 −1.1 −1.0   0   +1.0...

T-scores*

*T-scores are based on statistical measurements called standard deviations (SD) that reflect the difference between your bone density and the average bone density in the reference population.

Source: New York State Osteoporosis Prevention & Education Program (NYSOPEP). How to understand your results. http://www.nysopep.org/page.cfm/43. Accessed July 15, 2007.

Several medications are FDA approved for the prevention and treatment of osteoporosis. Medication should be prescribed with a history of vertebral or hip fracture, the presence of vertebral deformities, or low BMD (T-score ≤ −2.5) by DXA testing. Consideration for treatment is indicated when the T-score is between −1.5 and −2.5 depending on other risk factors (prior adulthood fracture, older age, a family history of fracture, low body weight, high bone turnover, medications or diseases that are harmful to the bone, and those who smoke). Table 40-7[4] summarizes medications currently approved for osteoporosis.

Tertiary Prevention

Tertiary prevention of osteoporosis occurs when an existing, usually chronic disease is managed to prevent further func-

---

TABLE 40-7 Medications Approved for Osteoporosis

Bisphosphonates
This group of medications reduces bone resorption by inhibiting the activity of osteoclasts.
- Alendronate and alendronate plus vitamin D
- Ibandronate
- Risedronate and risedronate with calcium
- Calcitonin

Estrogen/Hormone Therapy
Estrogens increase bone density by counteracting the natural loss of estrogen in women during menopause.

- Estrogens
- Estrogens and progestins
- Parathyroid hormone: teriparatide [PTH (1-34)]

Parathyroid hormone (PTH), given intermittently, increases bone density through the formation of new bone in the osteoporotic skeleton.

Selective Estrogen Receptor Modulators (SERMs)
SERMs have an estrogen-like effect on bone, increasing bone density by reducing the resorption of bone through the inhibition of the osteoclasts.

- Raloxifene

Alendronate is approved as a treatment for osteoporosis in men and is approved for treatment of glucocorticoid (steroid)-induced osteoporosis in men and women. Risedronate is approved for prevention and treatment of glucocorticoid-induced osteoporosis in men and women. Parathyroid hormone is approved for the treatment of osteoporosis in men who are at high risk of fracture.

Source: Data from National Osteoporosis Foundation. Fast facts. http://www.nof.org/osteoporosis/diseasefacts.htm. Accessed July 15, 2007.

---

tional loss. Following an osteoporotic fracture, prevention should block or slow the progression of disability. Intervention should focus on improvement of posture, body mechanics, fall prevention, and exercises to maintain bone density. Rehabilitation following a fracture should maximize quality of life and prevent complications. Many people who have sustained a fracture do not get medically evaluated or treated for osteoporosis. If a person has undetected osteoporosis, the person is at an increased risk for sustaining another fracture, heightening the risk of disability and death.

Osteoporotic fractures increase morbidity and mortality. Many who sustain a fracture become isolated, depressed, have a fear of falls, and suffer chronic pain and disfigurement. Often a loss in independence occurs, especially with hip fractures where 20 percent of individuals have to reside in a nursing home. Mortality is three to four times greater in patients with a hip fracture in the first three to four months after fracture.

Aggressive intervention should be aimed at maximizing bone health, minimizing morbidity, and preventing future fractures. Calcium supplements reduce bone loss and fractures, Vitamin D supplements reduce fractures and falls, physical activity preserves bone mass, builds muscle mass, reduces falls, and delays the loss of independence, and medications reduce the risk of future fractures up to 50 percent.

A key component of intervention after a fracture should include fall prevention. One third of all people over the age 65 fall each year with half falling more than once.[29] One in 10 falls results in a serious injury[30] and 95 percent of hip fractures are the direct result of a fall.[31] Even if an injury does not occur, many people become more fearful of falling, consequently decreasing their activity level and becoming more deconditioned, thus increasing the likelihood of a subsequent fall.[32]

There are identifiable risk factors for falls. Certain age-related changes increase the risk of falls, including decreased muscle mass and strength; impaired balance, coordination, sensation, vision, circulation, and cognition; and changes in blood pressure. Polypharmacy of four or more medications increases the risk of falls through enhanced and combined adverse drug reactions. Certain drugs, especially psychoactive drugs such as benzodiazepine, antidepressants, and sedatives/hypnotics increase the risk of falls.[33–36] Environmental factors play a role in about half of all home-related falls.[37] While home modifications alone have not been shown to reduce falls, home assessment by a trained healthcare professional such as physical and occupational therapists may be effective in reducing falls, especially in those at high risk for falling.[14] Table 40-8 lists those home modification prevention strategies that may be effective.[14]

The Surgeon General's Report on Bone Health and Osteoporosis suggests that "Federal, State, and local govern-

TABLE 40-8 Home Modification Prevention Strategies

- Removing tripping hazards
- Using non-slip mats in the bathtub and on shower stall floors
- Installing grab bars next to the toilet and in the tub or shower
- Installing handrails on both sides of stairways
- Improving home lighting

ments (including State and local health departments) join forces with the private sector and community organizations in a coordinated, collaborative effort to promote bone health."[2] Current research provides knowledge about risk factors for osteoporosis, prevention strategies, methods of accurate diagnosis, and treatments for the prevention and treatment of osteoporosis. Applying knowledge about the risk factors and causes of osteoporosis into practice has the potential to decrease the monetary and personal costs of this devastating disease.

KEY TERMS

Biology Terms

Bone mineral density (BMD): A measure of the amount of calcium in the bones; used to diagnose osteoporosis.

Calcium: A key mineral stored in bones that is responsible for proper functioning of muscles and nerves.

Dual Energy X-Ray Absorptiometry (DXA): A type of test used to diagnose osteoporosis.

Estrogens: Female hormones produced by the ovaries. Estrogen deficiency can lead to osteoporosis.

Menopause: The time in a woman's life when menstrual periods permanently stop; also called the "change of life." Menopause is the opposite of the menarche.

Osteoblasts: Cells that build bone.

Osteoclasts: Cells that break down bone.

Osteoporosis: A skeletal disorder characterized by compromised bone strength predisposing a person to an increased risk of fracture, especially at the spine, hip, and wrist.

Phosphorus: An essential element in the diet and a major component of bone; also found in the blood, muscles, nerves, and teeth. It is a component of adenosine 5'-triphosphate (ATP), the primary energy source in the body.

Resistive Strength Exercise: A type of exercise that uses a force opposing the movement, such as a weight, to cause a strong muscle contraction. This type of exercise promotes low forces on bone that promote healthy bone formation.

Vitamin D: A vitamin that is necessary for absorption of calcium and phosphorus and to maintain blood calcium and phosphorus within normal levels. Under normal conditions of sunlight exposure, dietary supplementation may not be necessary.

Weight Bearing Activity: A type of physical activity that loads bones through their length such as when walking or running. This type of activity is essential for healthy bone formation.

Public Health Terms

Primary Prevention: Activities designed to help prevent the onset of a disease.

Secondary Prevention: Activities that address asymptomatic individuals who present with risk factors and/or signs of disease before the disease is present to delay or halt their progression.

Tertiary Prevention: Involves the management of individuals who have developed the disease in an attempt to restore them to their highest function, minimize the negative effects of disease, and prevent disease-related complications. Because the disease is now established, primary prevention activities may have been unsuccessful. Early detection through secondary prevention may have minimized the impact of the disease.

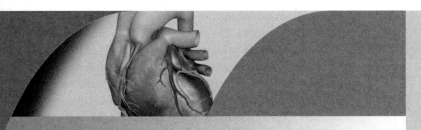

Questions for Further Research, Study, Reflection, and Discussion

For the Individual Student

In order to answer these questions, it may be necessary to research the primary literature.

- What osteoporosis risk factors do you currently have? How can you modify them?
- Thinking about your own family, who is at risk for osteoporosis? What can he/she do to minimize the risk?
- What are the consequences of osteoporosis?

For Small Group Discussion

Megan (Scenario 1, 16-Year-Old Caucasian Female)

- Does Megan have risk factors for osteoporosis? What are they?
- What further questions should be asked of Megan and her parents?
- What education should be presented to Megan and her parents as primary prevention to promote better bone health and decrease the risk of osteoporosis in the future?

Nora (Scenario 2, 63-Year-Old Asian Female)

- What risk factors does Nora have for osteoporosis?
- What is Nora currently doing that is healthy for her bones?

- What steps should she take to improve her bone health and decrease the risk of future fractures?
- What are her current calcium and vitamin D requirements?
- What would her optimal exercise program include?
- Should she consider medication for improving bone health?

Evelyn (81-Year-Old Caucasian Female)

- What are Evelyn's risk factors for osteoporosis?
- Was there a time in the past when she may have been alerted of her at-risk bone health?
- What steps should be taken to minimize the risk of future fractures?

For Entire Class Discussion

- Distinguish between consideration of osteoporosis as a health problem and osteoporosis as a public health problem.
- At what age group should public health efforts be targeted to prevent osteoporosis?
- Should public health strategies be different for different age groups? Defend your position.
- To effectively reduce the consequences of osteoporosis, what public health efforts should also be incorporated into a prevention strategy? What current efforts might also impact osteoporosis?

EXERCISES/ACTIVITIES

- Have each student complete an osteoporosis risk factor inventory that emphasizes diet, family history, and physical activity. Then have the student determine his/her risk. This could also be done for a parent or grandparent to emphasize the primary and secondary aspects of public health.
- As a class discussion, have students discuss ways to encourage children and adolescents to adopt bone-healthy habits.

Healthy People 2010

Focus Area: Osteoporosis

Goal: Prevent illness and disability related to arthritis and other rheumatic conditions, osteoporosis, and chronic back conditions.

Objectives:

2-9. Reduce the proportion of adults with osteoporosis.

2-10. Reduce the proportion of adults who are hospitalized for vertebral fractures associated with osteoporosis.

REFERENCES

1. International Osteoporosis Foundation. Image of normal and osteoporotic bone. http://www.iofbonehealth.org/newsroom/resources/image-normal-osteoporotic-bone.html. Accessed May 8, 2008.

2. U.S. Department of Health and Human Services. *Bone Health and Osteoporosis: A Report of the Surgeon General 2004*. Rockville, MD: U.S. Department of Health and Human Services Public Health Service, Office of the Surgeon General; 2004.

3. Gabriel S, Tosteson A, Leibson C, Crowson CS, Pond GR, et al. Direct medical costs attributable to osteoporotic fractures. *Osteoporosis International. Osteoporos Int* 2002;13:323–330.

4. National Osteoporosis Foundation. Fast facts. http://www.nof.org/osteoporosis/diseasefacts.htm. Accessed May 8, 2008.

5. Centers for Medicare and Medicaid Services. Bone Mass Measurement (BMM), revised 2007. Baltimore, MD. Available at http://www.cms.hhs.gov/BoneMassMeasurement/. Accessed May 8, 2008.

6. Standing Committee on the Scientific Evaluation of Dietary Reference Intakes. *DRI Dietary Reference Intakes for Calcium, Phosphorus, Magnesium, Vitamin D, and Fluoride*. Washington, DC: National Academy Press; 1997.

7. U.S. Food and Drug Administration. *How to Understand and Use the Nutrition Facts Label*. July 7, 2006. Available at http://www.cfsan.fda.gov/~dms/foodlab.html#ca. Accessed May 8, 2008.

8. U.S. Department of Health and Human Services and U.S. Department of Agriculture. Dietary Guidelines for Americans. Washington, DC: U.S. Government Printing Office; 2005.

9. Faulkner RA, Bailey DA. Osteoporosis: a pediatric concern? *Med Sport Sci* 2007;51:1–12.

10. Close JCT, Lord SL, Menz HB, Sherrington C. What is the role of falls? *Best Pract Res Clin Rheumatol* 2005;19:913–935.

11. Rautava E, Lehtonen-Veromaa M, Kautiainen H, Kjander S, Heinonen OJ, et al. The reduction of physical activity reflects on the bone mass among young females: a follow-up study of 142 adolescent girls. *Osteoporos Int* 2007;18:915–922.

12. Frost HM. From Wolff's law to the Utah paradigm: insights about bone physiology and its clinical applications. *Anat Rec* 2001;262:398–419.

13. American College of Sports Medicine. *ACSM's Guidelines for Exercise Testing and Prescription*, 7th ed. Baltimore: Lippincott Williams & Wilkins; 2005.

14. Stevens JA. Falls among older adults—risk factors and prevention strategies. *Falls Free: Promoting a National Falls Prevention Action Plan*. Washington, DC: National Council on Aging; 2005.

15. Madureira MM, Takayama L, Gallinaro AL, Caparbo VF, Costa RA, Pereira RM. Balance training program is highly effective in improving functional status and reducing the risk of falls in elderly women with osteoporosis: a randomized controlled trial. *Osteoporos Int* 2007;18:419–425.

16. Silsupadol P, Siu KC, Shumway-Cook A, Woollacott MH. Training of balance under single- and dual-task conditions in older adults with balance impairment. *Phys Ther* 2006;86:269–281.

17. Wolf SL, Barnhart HX, Kutner NG, McNeely E, Coogler C, Xu T. Reducing frailty and falls in older persons: an investigation of Tai Chi and computerized balance training. Atlanta FICSIT Group. Frailty and Injuries: Cooperative Studies of Intervention Techniques. *J Am Geriatr Soc* 1996;44:489–497.

18. Li F, Fisher KJ, Harmer P, McAuley E. Falls self-efficacy as a mediator of fear of falling in an exercise intervention for older adults. *J Gerontol B Psychol Sci Soc Sci* 2005;60:P34–P40.

19. Lord SR, Ward JA, Williams P, Strudwick M. The effect of a 12-month exercise trial on balance, strength, and falls in older women: a randomized controlled trial. *J Am Geriatr Soc* 1995;43:1198–1206.

20. Wolf B, Feys H, De W, van der Meer J, Noom M, Aufdemkampe G. Effect of a physical therapeutic intervention for balance problems in the elderly: a single-blind, randomized, controlled multicentre trial. *Clin Rehabil* 2001;15:624–636.

21. Fechtenbaum J, Cropet C, Kolta S, Horlait S, Orcel P, Roux C. The severity of vertebral fractures and health-related quality of life in osteoporotic postmenopausal women. *Osteoporos Int* 2005;16:2175–2179.

22. Oleksik AM, Ewing S, Shen W, van Schoor NM, Lips P. Impact of incident vertebral fractures on health related quality of life (HRQOL) in postmenopausal women with prevalent vertebral fractures. *Osteoporos Int* 2005;16:861–870.

23. Siminoski K, Jiang G, Adachi JD, Hanley DA, Cline G, et al. Accuracy of height loss during prospective monitoring for detection of incident vertebral fractures. *Osteoporos Int* 2005;16:403–410.

24. Cortet B, Houvenagel E, Puisieux F, Roches E, Garnier P, Delcambre B. Spinal curvatures and quality of life in women with vertebral fractures secondary to osteoporosis. *Spine* 1999;24:1921–1925.

25. Hasserius R, Karlsson MK, Jonsson B, Redlund-Johnell I, Johnell O. Long-term morbidity and mortality after a clinically diagnosed vertebral fracture in the elderly—a 12- and 22-year follow-up of 257 patients. *Calcif Tissue Int* 2005;76:235–242.

26. New York State Osteoporosis Prevention & Education Program (NYSOPEP). *How to Understand Your Results*. Available at http://www.nysopep.org/page.cfm/43. Accessed May 8, 2008.

27. Kantor SM, Ossa KS, Hoshaw-Woodard SL, Lemeshow S. Height loss and osteoporosis of the hip. *J Clin Densitom* 2004;7:65–70.

28. Tobias JH, Hutchinson AP, Hunt LP, McCloskey EV, Stone MD, et al. Use of clinical risk factors to identify postmenopausal women with vertebral fractures. *Osteoporosis Int* 2007;18:35–43.

29. Hornbrook MC, Stevens VJ, Wingfield DJ, Hollis JF, Greenlick MR, Ory MG. Preventing falls among community-dwelling older persons: results from a randomized trial. *Gerontologist* 1994;34:16–23.

30. Centers for Disease Control and Prevention, National Center for Injury Prevention and Control. Web-based injury statistics query and reporting system (WISQARS) [online]: CDC; 2006.

31. Grisso JA, Kelsey JL, Strom BL, et al. Risk factors for falls as a cause of hip fracture in women. The Northeast Hip Fracture Study Group. *N Engl J Med* 1991;324:1326–1331.

32. Murphy SL, Dubin JA, Gill TM. The development of fear of falling among community-living older women: predisposing factors and subsequent fall events. *J Gerontol A Biol Sci Med Sci* 2003;58:M943–M947.

33. Ray WA, Griffin MR, Malcolm E. Cyclic antidepressants and the risk of hip fracture. *Arch Intern Med* 1991;151:754–756.

34. Cumming RG. Epidemiology of medication-related falls and fractures in the elderly. *Drugs Aging* 1998;12:43–53.

35. Leipzig RM, Cumming RG, Tinetti ME. Drugs and falls in older people: a systematic review and meta-analysis: I. Psychotropic drugs. *J Am Geriatr Soc* 1999;47:30–39.

36. Ensrud KE, Blackwell T, Mangione CM, Bowman PJ, Bauer DC, et al. Central nervous system active medications and risk for fractures in older women. *Arch Intern Med* 2003;163:949–957.

37. Nevitt MC, Cummings SR, Kidd S, Black D. Risk factors for recurrent nonsyncopal falls: a prospective study. *JAMA* 1989;261:2663–2668.

CROSS REFERENCES

Exercise

The History of Nutrition

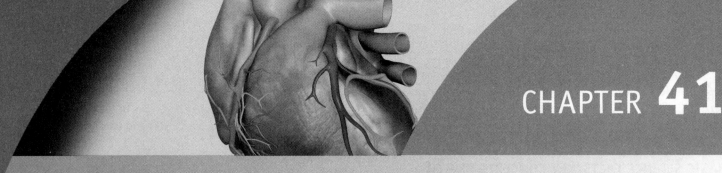

CHAPTER 41

Alzheimer's Disease: A Slow Death

Christopher J. Battle
Raluca Popovici

According to the Alzheimer's Association, in 2007 there were an estimated 5.1 million Americans with the disease, and by 2050 as many as 11 million to 16 million people may be affected.[1]

LEARNING OBJECTIVES

By the end of this chapter, students will be able to:

- Describe the primary causes of Alzheimer's disease.
- Analyze Alzheimer's disease's costs to society.
- Explain why Alzheimer's disease is a primary concern for public health officials.
- Evaluate methods to alleviate the burden of Alzheimer's disease on patients, their families, and caregivers.
- Design a plan for caregivers to care for an Alzheimer's patient and maintain their own health.

HISTORY

Alzheimer's disease (AD) is a progressive, neurodegenerative brain disorder characterized by cognitive decline, behavioral changes, and neuropsychiatric symptoms caused by the degeneration and eventual death of **neurons** (nerve cells) in several areas of the brain. In 1901, Dr. Alois Alzheimer examined a 51-year-old female patient named Mrs. Auguste D., who was complaining of memory loss. Dr. Alzheimer initially diagnosed her with "amnestic writing disorder" when she was unable to recall several objects he had presented to her just minutes before. When Mrs. Auguste D. died in April of 1906, Dr. Alzheimer examined her brain and found the **amyloid plaques** and **neurofibrillary tangles** that he later described and that

have become the defining physical features of the disease. Dr. Alzheimer's mentor, Dr. Emil Kraepelin, later described cases like Mrs. Auguste D.'s and others under "Alzheimer's disease" in his *Textbook for Students and Doctors.*[2]

From Dr. Alzheimer's time until the 1970s, the diagnosis of this disease was reserved generally for patients younger than 65 years old who exhibited memory loss and the neuropathologic findings described above. *Senile dementia* was considered an unfortunate companion of the normal aging process. More recently, the diagnosis of AD has been applied to all patients who exhibit the medical history, cognitive decline, neuropsychiatric symptoms, and neuropathologic signs of Alzheimer's disease. According to the National Mental Health Association, "The disease usually begins after age 65 and risk of AD goes up with age. While younger people may have AD, it is much less common. About 3% of men and women ages 65–74 have AD and nearly half of those over age 85 could have the disease."[3]

OVERVIEW

What Is Alzheimer's Disease?

AD is not a part of normal aging. Symptoms experienced by patients with AD include difficulty following conversations, repeating questions several times, difficulty performing everyday tasks such as cooking food, writing notes, and adding numbers. The patients can have problems using the toilet and forgetting to bathe and/or comb their hair. Some patients become very frustrated with their inability to perform tasks and remember as well as they used to. They can become agitated, restless, and may repeat movements over and over. Other patients wander, become paranoid, and have delusions and hallucinations. These symptoms are the result of the gradual loss of neurons due to AD. As the brain loses more neurons, it becomes atrophied, and the symptoms of AD worsen. In addition, connections between nerve cells become disrupted and this interferes with normal cognitive processes.

BASIC SCIENCE FACTS/KEY CONCEPTS REVIEW

The neuropathology of AD is characterized by amyloid plaques and neurofibrillary tangles (Figure 41-1). Amyloid plaques consist of abnormal congregations of the **beta amyloid** protein outside of the neurons. In a healthy brain, amyloid precursor protein is broken down and eliminated. In a brain affected by Alzheimer's disease, an enzyme called beta secretase trims the amyloid precursor protein and beta amyloid is one of the by-products.[4] Beta amyloid then accumulates to form the amyloid plaques. These plaques are eventually lethal to the neurons and lead to the memory loss and behavioral changes seen in Alzheimer's patients.

Neurofibrillary tangles consist mostly of the abnormally phosphorylated tau-protein.[5] Normal phosphorylation is the addition of a phosphate (PO_4) group to a protein. In AD, the **tau protein** is hyperphosphorylated, meaning extra phosphate groups are attached to the tau protein. These abnormal proteins aggregate within the cell and are insoluble. Tangles form inside cells. Most people have some plaques and tangles but those with Alzheimer's develop far more. The plaques and tangles first form in areas important in learning and memory and then spread to other areas of the brain. It is still uncertain if these two neuropathologic findings are primary causes of Alzheimer's disease or merely physical findings, particularly in the case of neurofibrillary tangles.

AD patients have deficits in several of the brain's chemical messengers, called **neurotransmitters**. The neurotransmitter primarily responsible, acetylcholine, aids in the process of forming memories and is scarce in the neurons of brain regions that are devastated by AD. Currently approved pharmaceutical therapies target the declining levels in acetylcholine levels to help restore acetylcholine levels. We will examine this later in the chapter. Serotonin, somatostatin, and noradrenaline are other neurotransmitters that can decline in Alzheimer's patients and may contribute to their memory and behavioral disturbances in these patients. Serotonin, for example, is implicated as a factor in depression, normal sleep cycle maintenance, and appropriate appetite,[6] which are all problems that affect many patients with Alzheimer's disease.

Complex multifactorial genetic factors play some role in developing AD. There are two recognized types of Alzheimer's disease: familial Alzheimer's disease (FAD) and late-onset or sporadic Alzheimer's disease. According to The National Institute on Aging, FAD affects less than 10 percent of AD patients. FAD develops in patients before the age of 65. Mutated genes on three different chromosomes can play a part in causing AD. If one of the mutated genes is inherited, the patient will almost always develop FAD.

Late-onset or sporadic AD generally occurs after the age of 65 and its inheritability is less clear. Lifetime risk of developing AD is approximately 11 percent to 16 percent. People who have a first degree relative with AD have a lifetime risk of 26 percent to 45 percent. Women are more likely to develop AD, but this seems due to the fact that women live longer than men, and that the incidence of late-onset AD is tied to age. The most studied gene for late-onset AD is apolipoprotein-E (APOE). There are three **alleles** (or types) of APOE and one of these types is tied to an increased chance of developing AD, but people with one or even two copies of this gene only have an increased chance and not a certainty of developing AD. While certain individuals are genetically predisposed to AD, they won't necessarily have AD as they age, suggesting that environmental factors play a large role in AD. These factors are not well-established though.[7]

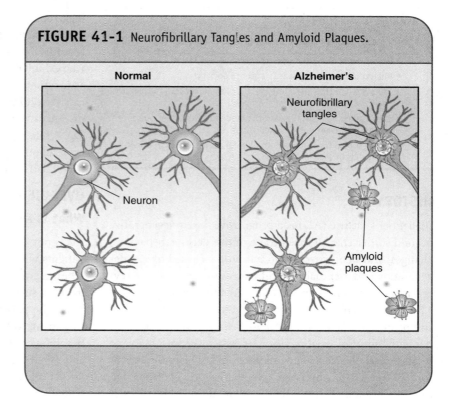

FIGURE 41-1 Neurofibrillary Tangles and Amyloid Plaques.

CASE STUDY

Scenario

A 63-year-old female, Mrs. B, presents to her primary care physician (PCP) complaining of forgetfulness. She reports that she walks across her home, into a room, and forgets why she went there. She also has trouble remembering names of people she sees every week at church. Her PCP asks her if either of her parents had AD and she says that her father went "senile" before he died. The doctor performs a **Mini-Mental Status Examination (MMSE)** and the patient scores a 30 out of 30. The doctor tells her that she does not have AD but that he will continue to monitor her reported memory loss.

Four years later, the now 67-year-old patient returns to her PCP accompanied by her 45-year-old daughter and granddaughter. The patient no longer drives and has increased episodes of forgetfulness. Six months ago, she got lost while driving and couldn't find her way home from the supermarket. Finally, a police officer assisted her in getting home six hours after she was scheduled to meet her daughter at home. In addition, the daughter has come to the patient's home to find the stove burners turned on despite no meal preparation. The daughter also found unopened envelopes containing unpaid bills after her mother's telephone service was suspended.

The PCP performs another MMSE. This time, the patient scores 22 out of 30. The PCP refers the patient to a neurologist. The daughter, who is now visiting her mother daily, brings the patient to the neurologist three months later. The neurologist repeats the MMSE (score 23) and orders an MRI of the brain and basic blood work as well as tests for thyroid activity and B_{12} levels. The neurologist asks the patient and the daughter, who is now the *de facto* caregiver, to come back in two weeks.

The neurologist informs them that all of the tests, except for the MMSE, are essentially normal for the patient's age. Having ruled out the most common causes of **dementia** other than AD, the neurologist diagnoses her with AD. The patient immediately becomes agitated and says, "I'm not going crazy. I don't have any Alzheimer's disease." She then tells her daughter she wants to go home. The neurologist prescribes donepezil HCl and asks the caregiver to schedule another appointment in six months.

Over the course of the next few years, Mrs. B continues to decline. One year after the initial AD diagnosis, the patient is forced to move in with her daughter's family because they cannot afford $6,000 per month for the assisted living facility. The patient makes several attempts to take the car on errands and finally the caregiver has to remove the car battery. One day, a neighbor found the patient wandering in the street one half mile from home. The caregiver ultimately has to cut back to part-time at her job in order to care for her mother. Money becomes even more of an issue. The patient becomes increasingly agitated and combative and will not taker her medication. After subsequent visits to the PCP and neurologist, she is prescribed antidepressants and anxiolytics. The caregiver has difficulty getting the patient to take the medication.

At the age of 74, eleven years after complaining of memory loss and seven years after the AD diagnosis, the patient passes away during the night of heart failure.

Defining the Issues

1. Patient is worried she is losing her mind and wondering what will happen to her. Will she recognize her family? Will she remember to pay bills? Will she injure herself or someone else?
2. The caregiver is concerned about her mother's well-being. She also wonders how she will handle the myriad duties of a caregiver. Will she be able to afford caring for her mother and simultaneously supporting her own family? How will her own health fare given the increased physical stresses of caring for her mother? Will she be able to spend enough time with her own children? Finally, will she develop AD someday?

Patient's Understanding of the Issues

The patient knows that something is wrong with her ability to process routine information and remember mundane tasks and events. She doesn't understand why everyone is so impatient and frustrated with her. If anyone should be frustrated, it should be she. The patient feels she is losing control of her life and that her daughter and the physician are forcing her to take medications, stop driving, and visit the doctor's office unnecessarily.

Caregiver's Understanding of the Issues (Figure 41-2)

The caregiver understands that she and her mother have essentially reversed roles; the caregiver must now remind her mother to brush her teeth when her mother once pestered her to do this same task. She knows her mother won't get better and that her caregiving role will only expand with time. She understands that she must remain patient with her mother but she does get frustrated with the constant demands.

CLINICAL PERSPECTIVE FOR THE INDIVIDUAL PATIENT AND FOR THE HEALTHCARE PROVIDER

Diagnosis of AD

All AD is dementia, but not all dementia is AD. Dementia is not a disease itself, but rather a collection of symptoms characterized by decline in cognitive and intellectual function and inability to perform the routine activities of daily living, as was the case of Mrs. B. Approximately 50 percent to 60 percent of all dementias are caused by AD.[8] The remaining cases of dementia are caused by cerebrovascular disease (particularly stroke), alcohol-related dementia, psychiatric disorders (depression), delirium, head injury, infection (encephalitis, syphilis, AIDS), hypothyroidism, vitamin B_{12} deficiency, Lyme disease, variant-Creutzfeldt-Jakob disease (human form of mad cow disease).

Typically, an elderly patient reports memory loss to the physician, or a family member or friend reports that the patient is having difficulty remembering, is getting lost, or might not be cleaning the house or handling bill payments properly. After establishing the nature of the problem, the physician begins ruling out causes for dementia other than Alzheimer's. AD cannot be diagnosed for sure without examining brain tissue and noting the amyloid plaques and neurofibrillary tangles discussed earlier; ethically this is not possible in live patients. In order to diagnose AD clinically, the physician must rule out other dementing illnesses.

The Mini-Mental State Examination (MMSE) is the most commonly used assessment tool. MMSE tests orientation to place and time, memory, attention and calculation, naming, reading, writing, copying, and the ability to follow a three step command.[9] The test can be performed in a clinic in about ten minutes and is scored on a scale of 0 to 30.[10] Test scores are not adjusted for level of education. Well-educated individuals score higher and this masks cognitive deficits. Lower scores are seen with declining cognitive function, arithmetic and visuospatial abilities, poor word-retrieval, and impaired judgment and problem solving.

Other medical conditions can mimic the symptoms of dementia. Hypothyroidism and anemia include in their symptoms the temporary loss of mental ability and must be ruled out as causes of dementia. Routine blood tests can reveal whether the thyroid gland is functioning normally and whether the person may be vitamin B_{12} deficient. Both of these conditions are treatable with synthetic thyroid medications or supplemental vitamin B_{12}, respectively. Blood tests also can reveal infections such as syphilis or Lyme disease, and even other signs of disorder that might be causing the dementia so the patient can be treated appropriately.

Symptoms such as fatigue, memory problems, difficulty learning and retaining material, and sleep disorders could be a sign of several diseases. When performing the differential diagnosis, the physician has to rule out other illnesses before establishing that the individual is affected by AD. For example, if a patient presents with the symptoms described above, the patient may be suffering from depression. If the physician suspects the patient suffers from depression, there are several treatments available including professional counseling, support groups, and antidepressant medications.

Brain imaging on computed tomography (CT) or magnetic resonance imaging (MRI) is a valuable tool in diagnosing AD. Imaging techniques give the clinician a view of the brain to determine whether or not the patient has a tumor, or more likely

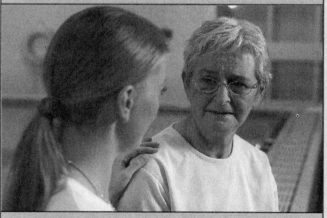

FIGURE 41-2 Elderly Woman with her Caregiver.

Source: © AbleStock.

for a dementing illness, such as a stroke. In stroke, a portion of the brain is deprived of blood flow and thus oxygen, which can lead to death of the neurons in the area affected by the stroke. Depending on where the stroke occurs, the damage can affect memory, movement, and or behavior. These two methods (CT and MRI) reveal differences in density. For example, when a group of neurons is missing because a stroke affected the area, the cerebrospinal fluid (CSF) that fills the missing space in is less dense than the brain tissue surrounding it. The imaging method exploits this difference and shows where there is more dense brain tissue and where there is less dense CSF. Cognitive function loss due to stroke is called cerebrovascular dementia. Imaging of brains with pure AD usually shows atrophy and few other abnormalities as well as characteristic wasting away of areas important to memory and cognitive functioning. This atrophy is due to loss of neurons caused by the toxic effects of amyloid plaque and neurofibrillary tangle aggregation. AD neuron loss is diffuse and stroke neuron loss is localized to the area where the stroke or lack of blood flow occurred. Multi-infarct dementia, where a patient has multiple mini-strokes over a period of time, can mimic Alzheimer's disease as well. The series of mini-strokes can cause cognitive decline gradually and must be differentiated from AD using the techniques described and evaluating cerebrovascular risk factors like advanced age, male gender, smoking, obesity, and cardiac disease. In the absence of signs of stroke, cerebrovascular risk factors indicating that cerebrovascular damage may be responsible for memory loss, or other findings inconsistent with AD, the physician can make a more educated assessment that AD is responsible for symptoms the patient exhibits.

Another useful diagnosing tool is the positron emission tomography (PET). PET scans show deficits in brain activity rather than providing structural detail of the brain. Before the scan is initiated, the patient is injected with glucose combined with a radiotracer, a radioactive substance. Areas of the brain, or another organ of interest, which are the most metabolically active appear brighter on the scan. In the case of Alzheimer's patients, the PET scan will show that the brain uses less glucose than the normal brain, and, more importantly, it will show this before any symptoms appear.[11]

Once the physician has ruled out other causes of dementia such as stroke, infection, depression, or any of the other conditions already addressed, the most likely diagnosis remaining is AD. AD is thus a diagnosis of exclusion.

Course or Stages of Alzheimer's Disease

Early AD

Typically, early stage Alzheimer's disease patients exhibit word-finding difficulty, episodes of spatial disorientation, problems with simple arithmetic or spelling, and poor judgment. AD patients might leave the stove burners on or they may have problems paying their bills and handling their checkbook. These patients have difficulties but usually retain enough faculties to live on their own.

Moderate AD

Moderate Alzheimer's patients experience worsening of cognitive functions. Language problems accelerate, memory deteriorates, and orientation to time and place decline. Newer memories are lost. The ability to form any new memories is lost. Moderate stage patients are typically less aware that they have problems with cognition and these problems begin to significantly affect daily routines. The patients are at increased risk of falls. Psychiatric symptoms and behavioral disturbances cause difficulties for the patient and caregiver. Moderate patients usually can't live by themselves or at least need frequent outside intervention to maintain their safety and daily activities. These patients lose track of conversations and may not know to whom they are speaking. Conversation becomes more general; moderate AD patients will leave out details of a recent vacation or they will fabricate details in an attempt to appear socially normal. Asking more specific questions can be frustrating for both the patient and the questioner.

Severe AD

Severe AD patients show more physical symptoms than earlier stage patients. Many are in wheelchairs or bedridden. They lose bladder and bowel control. As neurodegeneration affects more basic parts of the brain, breathing and digestion are affected. Patients stop seeking food and water. Many are significantly dehydrated unless caregivers make a concerted effort to ensure hydration. Severe patients might stop talking altogether and may be unresponsive to any stimulus.

Current Therapies

Understanding how neurotransmitters work is crucial to understanding current therapies. Neurons do not physically touch each other; they are separated by a very small space called the *synapse*. They must rely chemical messengers that they release to span this synapse in order to communicate to the next neuron whether or not to "fire" or produce an electrical impulse that travels the length of the neuron and eventually terminates at the end of the neuron. If this electrical impulse is strong enough, the neuron will release neurotransmitters, like acetylcholine, into the next synapse. If enough acetylcholine is released, the strength of this "chemical message" is strong enough to pass the signal along.

As addressed earlier, acetylcholine levels decline in the AD brain. Acetylcholine is an important chemical messenger that facilitates in forming memories. Because the AD brain's acetylcholine levels are deficient, the brain cannot properly form memories. Acetylcholinesterase is an enzyme (a protein that catalyzes chemical reactions) that breaks down acetylcholine present in the synapse. This natural process helps to recycle the acetylcholine for the neurons to reabsorb and use later.

It is important to note that before 1993, there were no therapies approved by the Food and Drug Administration (FDA) specifically for treating AD. Tacrine was approved that year and it is now part of a class of drugs called acetylcholinesterase inhibitors (AChEI's), although it is now rarely used because newer and better medications are available. AChEI's inhibit acetylcholinesterase. That is, they inhibit the enzyme that causes breakdown of acetylcholine in the synapse, resulting in more acetylcholine available to the neurons. The AD brain needs help in maintaining acetylcholine levels in order to preserve function and help maintain memory. In addition, other pharmaceutical therapies involve treating the symptoms associated with AD, including psychosis, anxiety, and depression. It is common to find an AD patient taking AD medications as well as antidepressants, anxiolytics (anti-anxiety medications), and antipsychotics.

The most commonly prescribed drugs for AD are AChEI's donepezil HCl, rivastigmine, and galantamine, and the NMDA-receptor agonist memantine. Memantine is a different type of drug that works by regulating calcium intake of neurons. Calcium also serves as a chemical messenger in many of the body's cells. In the AD brain, some neurons continually allow calcium into the cell. The continuous calcium intake creates "noise" for the cell and makes it difficult for the cell to differentiate when an actual signal is being sent. Memantine serves as a neuronal "crossing guard," where calcium is no longer continually signaling the neurons, but appropriate calcium signals get through. Memantine also protects the cell because continual influx of calcium is toxic to the neuron, so if too much calcium is allowed into the cell, the cell will die.

None of these drugs is a cure. The aim of these medications is to slow the progression of the disease and to treat the symptoms of AD. AChEIs inhibit the breakdown of acetylcholine in the AD brain, but they do not reverse the brain's loss of neurons and the cognitive abilities of patients on these drugs continue to decline. New therapies are under development. Examples of such therapies are vaccines that work by combating the formation of plaques, cholesterol-lowering drugs, and blood pressure medications. People who take these medications have a reduced risk of vascular dementia, and because vascular dementia and AD appear to be linked, controlling high blood pressure may also help prevent AD.

Stem cell research is not likely to assist in the near future because it is not well understood and because of the nature of AD. Stem cells have shown promise in diseases such as diabetes and Parkinson's because they are localized to specific types of cells in one part of the body. As AD causes diffuse neuron loss across several parts of the brain, it is a much more difficult disease to target with stem cells. In addition to discovering how stem cells might be able to help replace dying neurons and retain the brain's memories, scientists will have to find a way to place these stem cells in the exact spot that a dying neuron occupies. Neuronal loss is not centralized in AD; there are thousands of areas that would have to be targeted by stem cells in order for stem cell therapy to be effective.

PUBLIC HEALTH PERSPECTIVE FOR THE HEALTH OF THE GENERAL POPULATION AND OF HIGH RISK GROUPS

Even though the molecular mechanisms of AD are better understood now than they were a century ago, AD's etiological agent remains unknown. Not knowing what causes AD combined with the fact that the disease onset is impossible to detect makes primary and secondary prevention challenging. Tertiary prevention, which aims at treating symptoms and slowing progression of disease, remains important despite its minimal impact on the incidence and prevalence of AD. Prevention programs affecting the onset of disease will have the greatest public health impact.

If no major therapeutic advances occur and if the prevalence rate remains constant, it is expected that in 2050 approximately 10.2 million persons will have AD.[12] Of these, 3.8 million will have a mild form and 6.5 million will experience moderate or severe AD.[12] Most of the persons in the moderate and severe group will require nursing care due to the debilitating nature of AD. In 2000, the total estimated Medicare spending for persons with AD was 62 billion dollars and the average per capita spending for someone aged 65 and older was $13,207.[13]

Age is considered to be a risk factor for many illnesses including the family of cognitive diseases, which includes AD. As the U.S. population continues to live longer, the risk of developing AD increases. Developing AD is not a *sine-qua-non* consequence of getting old, and research has shown that in a healthy aging brain synapses do continue to form. Furthermore, advancing in years, unfortunately, is one risk factor no one can alter. It is thus important to find out what other addressable factors contribute to a decline in cognitive ability.

In the fall of 2005, the Centers for Disease Control and Prevention (CDC) and the Alzheimer's Association formed a partnership that aims to bring a public health perspective to cognitive health. The Healthy Brain Initiative and its byproduct the National Public Health Road Map to Maintaining Cognitive Health were thus created. This map encompasses 44 action items, with 10 of those considered to be of highest priority for immediate action[14]:

1. Determine how diverse audiences think about cognitive health and its associations with lifestyle factors.
2. Disseminate the latest science to increase public understanding of cognitive health and to dispel common misconceptions.
3. Help people understand the connection between risk and protective factors and cognitive health.
4. Conduct systematic literature reviews on proposed risk factors (vascular risk and physical inactivity) and related interventions for relationships with cognitive health, harms, gaps, and effectiveness.
5. Conduct controlled clinical trials to determine the effect of reducing vascular risk factors on lowering the risk of cognitive decline and improving cognitive function.
6. Conduct controlled clinical trials to determine the effect of physical activity on reducing the risk of cognitive decline and improving cognitive function.
7. Conduct research on other areas potentially affecting cognitive health such as nutrition, mental activity, and social engagement.
8. Develop a population-based surveillance system with longitudinal follow-up that is dedicated to measuring the public health burden of cognitive impairment in the United States.
9. Initiate policy changes at the federal, state, and local levels to promote cognitive health by engaging public officials.
10. Include cognitive health in *Healthy People 2020,* a set of health objectives for the nation that will serve as the foundation for state and community public health plans.

The Alzheimer's Association developed the Maintain Your Brain® initiative that contains 10 steps to care for one's brain.[15] These strategies present ways in which one may reduce the odds of developing AD.

1. *Head first.* The brain is a vital organ that needs care as much as other parts of the body.
2. *Take brain health to heart.* The heart pumps the oxygenated blood needed in day-to-day brain function. Damage to the heart in the form of heart disease will affect circulation and thus the blood flow to the brain.
3. *Your numbers count.* Body weight, blood pressure, and cholesterol and sugar level are important for the overall health of the individual, brain health included.
4. *Feed your brain.* A healthy diet rich in fruits, vegetables, and Omega 3 fatty acids will be beneficial to the brain.
5. *Work your body.* Physical exercise, even as little as 30 minutes a day, increases oxygenation of the brain.
6. *Jog your mind.* Any form of stimulating mental activity increases the vitality of the brain.
7. *Connect with others.* Interacting with other persons in activities that combine physical and mental elements may help keep the brain healthy.
8. *Heads up! Protect your brain.* Using protective gear when needed helps protect the brain from unnecessary injury.
9. *Use your head.* Avoiding unhealthy habits such as smoking, excessive drinking, and recreational drugs may reduce the risk of developing a cognitive condition.
10. *Think ahead—start today!* Prevention is generally better than disease management.

Even though great advances have been made in what it is known about AD, key elements remain unknown. Research has shown that a healthy older brain continues to form synapses, implying that AD is not an automatic consequence of aging; lifestyle is possibly as important as the genetic makeup in affecting the odds of developing AD. Maintaining a healthy way of life is beneficial for well-being in general and mental health in particular. With the US population living longer, if no preventive measures against AD are taken at the individual level, the strain on the public health system will be even greater than it is today.

Current and Future Impact of Alzheimer's Disease

The costs of AD are myriad. When considering AD's impact on society, we must include not only the costs of doctor visits, blood and imaging tests, medications, adult daycare, and nursing homes, but also the costs and stress associated with family and paid caregivers. According to the Alzheimer's Association, most Americans over the age of 65 participate in Medicare. In 2000, Medicare spent nearly three times as much on average per dementia patient as they do for beneficiaries without dementia ($13,207 versus $4,207). Demented beneficiaries made 3.4 times the number of hospital visits and those visits cost 3.2 times as much as the average for non-demented beneficiaries ($7,704 versus $2,204).[16] The financial costs of AD are tremendous and will continue to grow as AD becomes more prevalent with the aging of the American population.

Alzheimer's patients gradually lose the ability to take care of themselves. At first, they may need help with ordinary household chores, handling bills, or being driven. Later, they may need help getting out of bed or getting dressed and bathed properly. Some even need assistance maintaining a proper diet and being fed. The Alzheimer's Association and National Institute on Aging estimate "the current direct and indirect costs of caring for the 4.5 million Americans living with Alzheimer's disease to be 100 billion dollars *annually*. . . . By 2030, when the entire baby boomer population is over 65 years of age, the number of Americans with Alzheimer's disease will soar to levels that may exceed our ability to absorb the added cost."[17] By 2050 as many at 16 million Americans may have AD.[18]

In addition to the costs directly associated with AD patients, there are significant costs for caregivers. Caregivers need to take time off from work to take the patient to numerous doctors and some caregivers quit jobs to be the primary caregiver. Caregivers can suffer from the increased physical and psychological stress of their task. "Alzheimer's caregivers are known as the hidden or second victims of the disease. They commonly suffer from fatigue, stomach problems, headaches, difficulty sleeping, anger, sadness, and especially depression. The cause is clear. Because more than 70 percent of sufferers live at home, they are cared for by relatives and friends day and night for as many as 20 years. An average Alzheimer's caregiver spends on average, 69 hours a week caring for a relative stricken with the disease—and has done so for at least four years. Fifty percent of Alzheimer's caregivers live with their loved one."[18]

KEY TERMS

Clinical Terms

Allele: A version of a gene at a given location on a chromosome. One allele is inherited from each parent.

Amyloid Plaques: Abnormal protein aggregates found outside of the neurons of Alzheimer's patients.

Beta Amyloid: The main constituent of amyloid plaques in the brains of patients with Alzheimer's disease formed when beta secretase cleaves with amyloid protein.

Dementia: The loss of cognitive abilities, including memory, judgment, and intellectual ability, that interferes with activities of daily living.

Mini-Mental Status Examination (MMSE): The MMSE is a brief quantitative measure of cognitive status in adults; it can be used to screen for cognitive impairment, to estimate the severity of cognitive impairment at a given point in time, to follow the course of cognitive changes in an individual over time, and to document an individual's response to treatment (definition from http://www.minimental.com).

Neurofibrillary Tangles: Abnormal protein aggregates found inside the neurons of patients with Alzheimer's disease.

Neurons: Basic nerve cell of the brain and nervous system. Neurons receive and send electrical messages to and from the brain to the body.

Neurotransmitter: A chemical messenger that bridges the gap between neurons to convey signals.

Tau Protein: Major component of neurofibrillary tangles in Alzheimer's disease.

Public Health Terms

Sensitivity: The percent of people correctly identified by a test as having the disease out of the total number of people with the disease. It is expressed as TP/TP + FN, where TP is true positive, and FN is false negative. Sensitivity shows how good the test is in correctly identifying those people who truly have the disease.

Specificity: The percent of people correctly identified by the test as being disease-free among those without the disease. It is expressed TN/TN + FP, where TN is true negative and FP is false positive. Specificity shows how good the test is in correctly identifying those who are disease free.

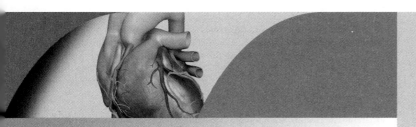

Questions for Further Research, Study, Reflection, and Discussion

For the Individual Student

In order to answer these questions, it may be necessary to research the primary literature.

- What are the risk factors associated with AD?
- Who is at the greatest risk of developing AD?
- How are amyloid plaques formed?
- Describe the relationship between dementia and AD.
- What steps are necessary to diagnose AD?

For Small Group Discussion

- What treatment options are available to patients with AD like Mrs. B?
- What should caregivers consider when caring for their AD patient? What should they consider with regard to their own health?
- What can be done to reduce the costs of AD?

For Entire Class Discussion

- Even though the etiological agent is unknown, there are brain imaging techniques such as CT, MRI, and PET scans that may detect the disease in its early stages. At this time, treatment cannot cure but will slow the disease progression. The **sensitivity** and **specificity** of these techniques are not very well researched, possibly with the exception of PET scans. Would you recommend that Medicare/Medicaid cover the cost of the scan in everybody over the age of 65? Defend your position.

EXERCISE/ACTIVITY

- Students should arrange to observe the administration of the MMSE to a patient, or should administer the exam to a fellow student and discuss what the MMSE assesses.
- Visit the Alzheimer's Unit in a nursing home to observe and discuss the challenges of caregiving for these patients, and report back to the class.

REFERENCES

1. Alzheimer's Association. *Alzheimer's Disease Facts and Figures, 2007.* Chicago: Alzheimer's Association. Available at http://www.alz.org/national/documents/report_alzfactsfigures2007.pdf. Accessed May 12, 2008.

2. Maurer K, Maurer U. *Alzheimer The Life of a Physician and Career of a Disease.* New York: Columbia University Press; 2003.

3. Mental Health America. *Alzheimer's Disease.* Alexandria, VQ: Mental Health America. Available at http://www.nmha.org/index.cfm?objectId=C7DF8E58-1372-4D20-C8536BAD8B0D0360. Accessed May 12, 2008.

4. Vassar R, Bennet BD, Baku-Khan S, Kahn S, Mendiaz EA, et al. Beta-secretase cleavage of Alzheimer's amyloid precursor protein by the transmembrane aspartic protease BACE. *Science* 1999;286:735–740.

5. Jicha GA, Lane E, Vincent I, Otvos L Jr, Hoffmann R, Davies P. A conformation and phosphorylation dependent antibody recognizing the paired helical filaments of Alzheimer's disease. *J Neurochem* 1997;69:2087–2095.

6. National Advisory Mental Health Council. Healthcare reform for Americans with severe mental illnesses. *Am J Psychiatry* 1993;150:1447–1465.

7. Reynolds CA, Wetherell JL, Gatz M. Heritability of Alzheimer's Disease, vol 2. In: Vellas B, eds. *Research and Practice in Alzheimer's Disease.* New York: Springer Publishing Co.; 1999:175–191.

8. Adelman AM, Daly MP. Initial evaluation of the patient with suspected dementia. *Am Fam Physician* 2005;71:1745–1750.

9. Crum RM, Anthony JC, Bassett SS, Folstein MF. Population-based norms for the Mini-Mental State Examination by age and educational level. *JAMA* 1993;269:2386–2391.

10. Folstein MF, Folstein SE, McHugh PR. "MINI-MENTAL STATE." A practical method for grading the cognitive state of patients for the clinician. *J Psychiatr Res J Psychiatr Res* 1975;12:189–198.

11. Mayo Clinic. Positron emission tomography (PET) scan: detecting conditions early. Available at: http://www.mayoclinic.com/health/pet-scan/CA00052. Accessed May 12, 2008.

12. Sloane PD, Zimmerman S, Suchindran C, Reed P, Wang L, Boustani M, Sdha S. The public health impact of Alzheimer's disease, 2000–2050: potential implication of treatment advances. *Ann Rev Public Health* 2002;23:213–231.

13. The Lewin Group. 2003. *Saving Lives, Saving Money: Dividends for Americans Investing in Alzheimer's Research.* Chicago: Alzheimer's Association. Available at: http://alz.org/national/documents/report_savinglivessavingmoney.pdf. Accessed May 12, 2008.

14. Centers for Disease Control and Prevention and the Alzheimer's Association. The Healthy Brain Initiative: a national public health road map to maintaining cognitive health. Atlanta: CDC; 2007. Available at http://www.cdc.gov/aging/pdf/TheHealthyBrainInitiative.pdf. Accessed May 12, 2008.

15. Alzheimer's Association. *Maintain Your Brain.* Chicago: Alzheimer's Association; 2006. Available at http://alz.org/national/documents/brochure_maintainyourbrain.pdf. Accessed May 12, 2008.

16. Alzheimer's Association. *Alzheimer's Disease and Chronic Health Conditions: The Real Challenge for 21st Century Medicare.* Washington, DC: Alzheimer's Association; 2003.

17. Alzheimer's Association and the National Alliance for Caregiving, Ernst RL, Hay JW. The U.S. economic and social costs of Alzheimer's disease revisited. *Am J Public Health* 1994;84:1261–1264.

18. National Institutes of Health. Press release to 1994 figures. *Cited in 2001–2002 Alzheimer's Disease Progress Report.* Bethesda: NIH publication number 03-5333; July 2003:2.

CROSS REFERENCES

Epidemiology of Aging

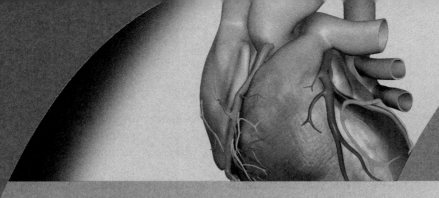

CHAPTER 42

Perinatal Depression: A Worldwide Problem in Women's Health

Julia Frank

One out of every ten women experiences a serious depression within three months of giving birth.

According to the World Health Organization, depression is the second worldwide cause of **DALYs (disability adjusted life years)** in both sexes between the ages of 15 and 44 and the primary source of DALYs for women.[1]

LEARNING OBJECTIVES

By the end of this chapter, students will be able to:

- Identify the burden of depressive illness on women and their societies around the world.
- Define descriptive psychiatric diagnosis.
- Describe contemporary theories of the biological and psychosocial aspects of major depression.
- Recognize the importance of epidemiology, **screening**, and preventive intervention as useful public health approaches to improving care for **perinatal** depression.
- Discuss discriminatory health insurance coverage and other barriers to receiving care for psychiatric disorders.

HISTORY

The illness of depression stands at the intersection of women's reproductive biology and social stressors in relation to women's health and mental health around the world.

Since 1977, most mental health professionals have identified and studied psychiatric disorders based on the pattern of their signs (observable manifestations) and symptoms (experiences reported by patients). Psychiatric disorders are classified by their signs and symptoms, as laid out in the *Diagnostic and Statistical Manual* (*DSM-IV-TR*) published by the American Psychiatric Association.[2] Such descriptive diagnosis has many advantages for public health: it allows different people with different types of training to arrive at the same diagnosis simply by recording answers to the appropriate questions (high reliability). Such standardization, in turn, has facilitated population-based research that supports a public health agenda to identify **risk factors**, vulnerable populations, and opportunities for prevention.

DSM IV CRITERIA FOR MAJOR DEPRESSIVE DISORDER

Criterion	Description
A	Symptoms must be present for at least a two week period and represent a change from prior functioning. Criterion symptoms are either sad mood or a pervasive loss of interest or pleasure in most activities for most of the day, every day *AND* four of seven other symptoms.
	1. Gain or loss of weight

2. Difficulty falling or staying asleep (insomnia) or sleeping more than usual (hypersomnia)

3. Being visibly agitated or slowed down

4. Fatigue or diminished energy

5. Thoughts of worthlessness or extreme guilt

6. Difficulty thinking, concentrating, or making decisions

7. Frequent thoughts of death or suicide or a suicide attempt

B   Symptoms do not meet criteria for a Mixed Episode.

C   Symptoms cause clinically significant distress or impairment in social, occupational, or other important areas of functioning.

D   Symptoms are not caused by a substance (such as medication or substance abuse) or a general medical condition (such as hyperthyroidism).

E   Symptoms are not accounted for by the bereavement of a loved one.

Source: Adapted from the American PsychiatricAssociation. *Diagnostic and Statistical Manual (DSM IV TR)*. Washington, DC: APA Press; 2006.

Depression as a psychiatric diagnosis has a meaning beyond that of the word as commonly used. Psychiatry speaks, in particular, of *Major Depressive Disorder*, defined as an episodic condition that manifests itself in mood, "vegetative signs" (dysregulated sleep, appetite, energy), and thought. To be diagnosed with major depression, a person must reach a threshold of criteria ("caseness"), which include core criteria and a defined level of associated findings.

The diagnosis of a major depressive episode includes several qualifiers. It must represent a significant change from a person's normal state. The symptoms must be present most of the time during the period of the illness (minimum of two weeks) and must impair the person's social or occupational functioning. If the syndrome is related to a known physical cause—for example, substance abuse or an underlying medical condition—then it would receive the label of "depression secondary to general medical condition" or "substance induced mood disorder–depressive type." Recent bereavement, though it may have similar symptoms, is also excluded. However, depression in reaction to other events—losses, disappointments, maltreatment, or trauma—is diagnosed as major depression without reference to its cause, which may or may not be known.

Descriptive psychiatric diagnosis is far from ideal. The *DSM* defines disorders without reference to their ultimate or proximal causes (*etiology* or *pathophysiology*). Widely different processes, possibly requiring quite different treatment, may all receive the same label. Conversely, the same pathological process may produce syndromes (patterns of signs and symptoms) that receive different labels. This disjunction between diagnosis and underlying causes impedes the development of specific treatments. Thus, most psychiatric disorders, as currently diagnosed and defined, may respond (or not respond) to a wide variety of interventions, from drugs to psychotherapy or environmental change.

BASIC SCIENCE FACTS/KEY CONCEPTS REVIEW

The symptoms of major depression, thus defined, reflect a variety of brain processes as well as patterned responses to a variety of social conditions. Human beings are biological organisms with unique psychological qualities who are constantly adapting to changing physical and psychosocial environments. Successful adaptation involves biological, psychological, and behavioral adjustments, and depression is best understood as patterned maladaptation, encompassing problems in all three domains. Current research has illuminated both the biological and the psychological dysfunctions seen in major depression.

Neurobiology of Depression

Disruptions of nervous system activity in major depression reflect a dysregulation of many normally coordinated processes. In the normal brain, activity in nerve cells (**neurons**) in various areas produces such responses as subjective pleasure following eating, having sex, or a rewarding social interaction. A sensation of curiosity leading to exploratory behavior is another neuropsychological process, as is the coordinated set of responses to threat known as the fight–flight reaction. These processes all require communication between neurons in identifiable brain areas, communication that occurs when one neuron releases a chemical messenger (**neurotransmitter**) that binds to a receptor on another neuron and stimulates or inhibits its activity. There are literally billions of messages fizzing constantly among neurons in the living brain. Research tracing the activity of different neurotransmitters has localized the neurotransmitter activity associated with pleasure, fear, and rage to specific brain areas or networks.

Neurobiological models of depression characterize both the neurochemical changes associated with dysregulation of these processes and the brain areas where these dysregulations occur.[3]

Neuroanatomy in Relation to Mood

Figure 42-1[4] shows the inner surface of a side (medial) view of the brain, highlighting the anatomical regions that seem to be most involved in the illness of depression. Taken together, these brain areas are called the **limbic system**. Limbic structures that seem to function abnormally in depression include the hippocampus, which is necessary for short-term memory, the amygdala, which is involved in motivation, rage and fear responses, the nucleus accumbens (not shown), which subserves the sensation of reward, and the hypothalamus (not shown), a center of transmitters (releasing factors) that regulate the release of hormones from the pituitary gland (stimulating factors) that in turn regulate the release of hormones from glands throughout the body (thyroid, sex glands, and adrenal glands). The cascade of events regulating hormonal release is referred to as the **hypothalamic-pituitary-adrenal axis** (**HPA axis**; Figure 42-2).[5]

Table 42-1 lists each brain structure, one or two of its functions relative to depression, and some of the area's associated neurotransmitters or hormones.

The areas of the limbic system all regulate and are influenced by other brain regions also involved in depression. The reception of sensory messages, language production, the initiation of behavior and any voluntary function requires an intact cerebral cortex (the surface of the brain), which interacts reciprocally with limbic structures (Figure 42-3).[6]

Thus, depressive ideation (thoughts of worthlessness, hopelessness, guilt) reflects disrupted cortical function. The part of the brain closest to the forehead—the frontal or prefrontal cortex—is involved in so-called executive functions, including the ability to initiate or inhibit behavior, filter or prioritize stimuli, and pay sustained attention. Signs of impaired executive function in depression include problems making decisions, impaired concentration, and lack of motivation. The physical agitation or slowing of motor activity that occurs in depression implicates dysfunction in areas of the brain that regulate the activity of voluntary muscle, especially a cluster of cells regulated by both the cortex and the limbic system, designated the basal ganglia (not shown).

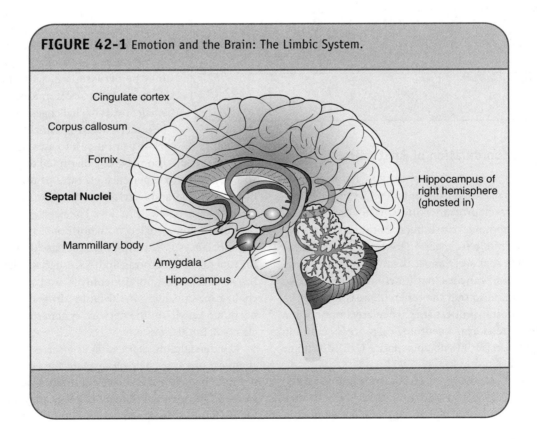

FIGURE 42-1 Emotion and the Brain: The Limbic System.

Cingulate cortex

Corpus callosum

Fornix

Septal Nuclei

Mammillary body

Amygdala

Hippocampus

Hippocampus of right hemisphere (ghosted in)

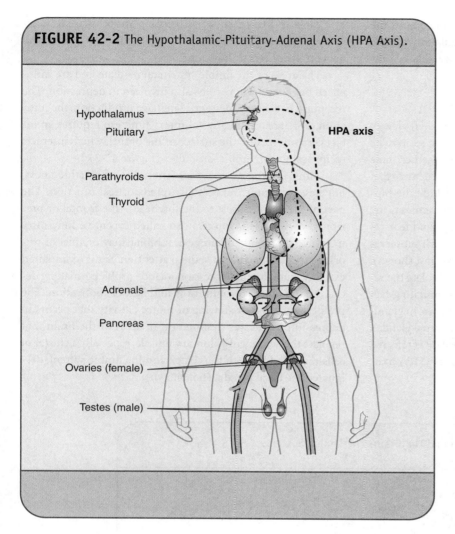

FIGURE 42-2 The Hypothalamic-Pituitary-Adrenal Axis (HPA Axis).

Hypothalamus
Pituitary

HPA axis

Parathyroids

Thyroid

Adrenals

Pancreas

Ovaries (female)

Testes (male)

Neurochemical Coordination of Anatomical Structures

Remember that depression is a disruption of patterns of activities coordinated by neurotransmitters. While hundreds of molecules and compounds may influence brain activity, a relatively small number of cell clusters in the brain synthesize the neurotransmitters that seem most involved in depression. These cells send out branches that touch on cells dispersed throughout the brain, so that the different areas function in concert. Four neurotransmitters are particularly important in understanding depression as a neurological process: serotonin (5 hydroxytryptophan [5HT]), norepinephrine (NE), dopamine (DA), and acetylcholine (ACH).

Figure 42-4[7] shows the brain areas (caudal raphe nuclei) where cells make serotonin and how these cells branch throughout the brain. Acetylcholine, dopamine, and norepi-

nephrine are distributed in a similar pattern. Cell bodies in the brainstem synthesize these transmitters, which are released in widely dispersed higher brain areas. Table 42-2 links each transmitter to the name of the cell cluster (nucleus) where it is made.

To complicate matters, serotonin is a metaregulator that modulates the actions of dopamine and norepinephrine. In addition, many other substances, including hormones like estrogen/progesterone/testosterone, thyroid hormone, and cortisol, regulate nerve cells and coordinate brain activity.[3]

Depression: A Disorder of Neuroregulation

Understanding this anatomical and neurochemical circuitry is necessary to conceptualizing depression as a disorder of neuroregulation. Research has identified many aspects of this dysregulation. For example, depression involves decreased brain serotonin regulation of norepinephrine (either from decreased levels of serotonin or abnormal functioning of serotonin or norepinephrine receptors). This dysfunction results in inappropriate levels of general arousal. A depressed person may be overaroused, with the inability to sleep or to turn off anxious responses to small threats or challenges, or the person may be underaroused and unable to respond with curiosity or interest to aspects of the environment. He or she also may have disrupted dopamine function and be unable to experience pleasure or reward. Hormones, norepinephrine, and acetylcholine function together to regulate cycles of sleep and wakefulness. The sleeplessness or sleepiness of depression may reflect both hormonal and neurotransmitter imbalances. Most drug therapies are designed to change the function of neurotransmitters, especially drugs that stabilize serotonin and norepinephrine, and secondarily acetylcholine and dopamine. In the future, drugs designed to regulate hormone activity in the nervous system may develop as new classes of antidepressants.

Understanding depression as a series of interconnected chemical processes helps to explain the association between reproductive events, especially childbirth, and depression in women. The physical changes of pregnancy may account for the finding that the **postpartum** period is associated with el-

TABLE 42-1 Brain Structures and Functions

Structure	Function	Transmitter(s)	Depressive Symptom
hippocampus	short-term memory	acetylcholine	cognitive inefficiency
amygdala	fear, rage, selective attention	serotonin, norepinephrine	anxiety, irritability, vigilance hypersensitivity to negative environmental cues (threat or deficiencies)
nucleus accumbens	reward	dopamine	lack of pleasure, decreased motivation
HPA axis	sleep, appetite, sexual behavior, metabolic rate, adaptation to acute and chronic environmental or social stress	releasing and inhibitory factors, stimulating hormones	vegetative changes (insomnia, anhedonia, lack of libido, weight changes)

evated risk of depression in nearly all societies. Recall that sex hormones like estrogen and progesterone are regulators and coordinators of brain activity. Both work directly in the brain and indirectly by affecting the activity of other neurotransmitters, especially serotonin. Estrogen and progesterone rise to their highest possible levels during pregnancy, and fall precipitously at delivery. In fact, it is normal for women to experience sudden, brief bouts of tearfulness in the first two weeks after delivery, often called the "Baby Blues." Between 60 percent and 80 percent of women describe this phenomenon, which is probably the direct manifestation of the sudden fall of sex steroid activity in the normal female brain. In women vulnerable to depression, these hormonal changes may lead to changes in neurotransmitter function that do not spontaneously go back to normal, leading to persistent depressive symptoms.

Psychological/Behavioral Aspects of Depression: Individual and Cultural Variation

Neurobiological models of depression do not tell the whole story. In humans, depression is more than a manifestation of disrupted brain function. Most neurobiological research is done on people who are severely depressed, with prominent neurovegetative symptoms. In other depressed patients, the disruptions of brain regulation are subtle and may not differ markedly from the brain processes of people who are not depressed. The explanation of this paradox is that humans have a uniquely broad repertoire of psychological and behavioral responses to their environments, patterns organized by language, social activity, and even by cultural traditions as well as by brain activity. In human populations, characteristic patterns of depression do not correspond directly to underlying brain activity. Someone may experience a major depressive episode, diagnosed by the person's thought patterns and behavior, but still have grossly normal brain function. Indeed, most cases of depression do not involve identifiable brain dysfunction, at least as measured by currently available tools. The factors that have been identified; for example, low brain serotonin levels in people who commit suicide represent group rather than individual differences.

The neurobiological dysfunctions of depression, when present, are universal; that is, they appear across human populations, and analogous dysfunctions occur in other mammals under various conditions. By contrast, the psychological and

FIGURE 42-3 Surface of the Brain.

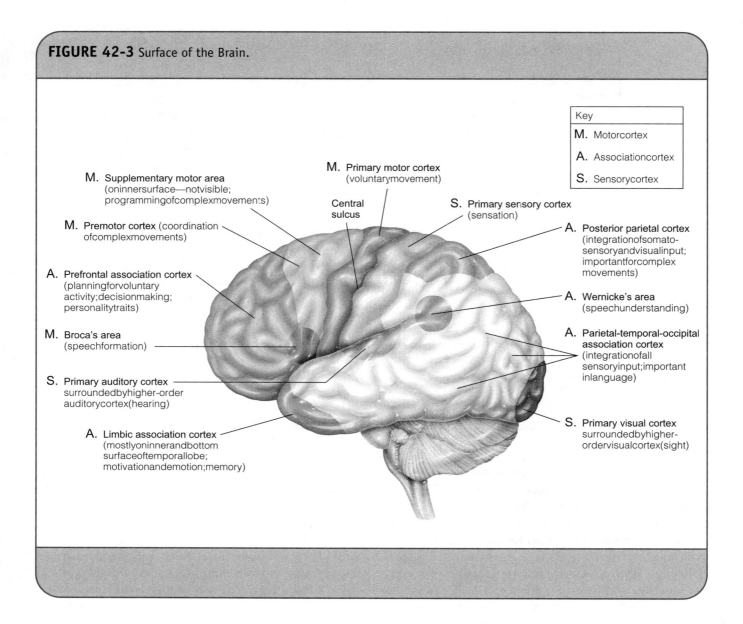

Key
M. Motorcortex
A. Associationcortex
S. Sensorycortex

M. Supplementary motor area (oninnersurface—notvisible; programmingofcomplexmovements)

M. Premotor cortex (coordination ofcomplexmovements)

A. Prefrontal association cortex (planningforvoluntary activity;decisionmaking; personalitytraits)

M. Broca's area (speechformation)

S. Primary auditory cortex surroundedbyhigher-order auditorycortex(hearing)

A. Limbic association cortex (mostlyoninnerandbottom surfaceoftemporallobe; motivationandemotion;memory)

M. Primary motor cortex (voluntarymovement)

Central sulcus

S. Primary sensory cortex (sensation)

A. Posterior parietal cortex (integrationofsomato-sensoryandvisualinput; importantforcomplex movements)

A. Wernicke's area (speechunderstanding)

A. Parietal-temporal-occipital association cortex (integrationofall sensoryinput;important inlanguage)

S. Primary visual cortex surroundedbyhigher-ordervisualcortex(sight)

behavioral manifestations of human depression vary around the globe. Personal history and culture shape how we respond to the world around us and influence what people in different societies recognize as core symptoms of depression. In Western cultures, for example, people typically express depression in terms of sadness, low self-esteem, and feelings of despair (hopelessness) or powerlessness (helplessness). These are the recognized cognitive patterns of depression in countries with Western European values. Around the world, people in similarly unrewarding, frustrating, or threatening circumstances may have similar thoughts but recognize other dimensions of

depressive illness as core features. Rather than tell a healer of feeling sad or helpless, they may seek help for pain, unexplained physical symptoms, or behavioral outbursts.

In addition to the different "idioms of distress"[8] offered by different cultures, past personal history shapes our responses to the world. Early loss of a parent, being maltreated in childhood, or always being made to feel at fault all may contribute to the development of depression in an adult, but the nature of the person's depressive experience may be different in each context. For one depressed person, guilt may be the most prominent symptom, while another person may feel prima-

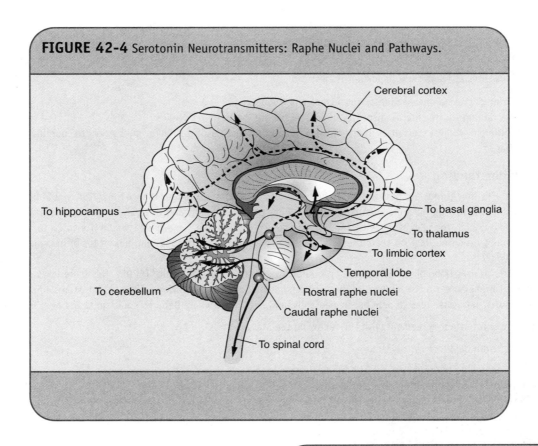

FIGURE 42-4 Serotonin Neurotransmitters: Raphe Nuclei and Pathways.

rily inadequate or helpless. Patterns of thought also influence behavior, so that the person who feels hopeless and helpless may be withdrawn and lacking in initiative, while a person who feels threatened may be agitated or aggressive. The heterogeneity of depressive illness reflects the complexity of human experience and of the conditions in which humans live.

In summary, depression is a biospsychosocial condition. To fully understand a depressed patient requires understanding basic biology, personal history, and present conditions.

TABLE 42-2 Nuclei and Chemical Transmitters in the Brain

Transmitter Factory	Transmitter
Locus ceruleus	Norepinephrine (NE)
Raphe nuclei	Serotonin (5HT)
Nucleus basalis	Acetylcholine (ACH)
Basal ganglia	Dopamine (DA)

CASE STUDY
Scenario

Deborah S., a 25-year-old woman whose husband is stationed in Iraq, brings her eight-week-old child to the pediatrician for a well baby check. Although clean and well nourished, the child is not smiling spontaneously, and the woman seems distracted and tired.

Defining the Issues

This vignette illustrates at least three important issues:

- Recognizing depression as an illness, not a transient mood
- Role of screening for psychiatric disorders in general medical settings
- Role of different medical specialties in diagnosing and treating psychiatric disorders, and barriers to coordinating care across specialties

Patient's Understanding

The pediatrician asks how things are going, and Deborah says, "This is so much harder than I thought it would be. I never seem to get enough sleep. It was OK until my mom left, but now I can't think straight, and when the baby cries, sometimes I feel like breaking down and crying, too! I'm at my wit's end. To tell you the truth, I feel sometimes I would like to go to sleep and never wake up." Deborah's eyes well up with tears then she forces a smile and says, "I guess you hear a lot of new mothers say stuff like this, don't you?"

The pediatrician asks Deborah to fill out the Edinburgh Postnatal Depression Scale[9] (EPDS). Her score is 14, which prompts the pediatrician to take an extra ten minutes to discuss with her that she may be suffering from major depression. Her doctor explains the diagnosis, suggests steps to help her immediately, and negotiates where Deborah could go to get help for the problem.

> EPDS: Mothers rate their agreement with the following ten statements.
>
> In the past seven days:
>
> 1. I have been able to laugh and see the funny side of things.
> 2. I have looked forward with enjoyment to things.
> 3. I have blamed myself unnecessarily when things went wrong.
> 4. I have been anxious or worried for no reason.
> 5. I have felt scared or panicky for no very good reason.
> 6. Things have been getting on top of me.
> 7. I have been so unhappy that I had difficulty sleeping.
> 8. I have felt sad or miserable.
> 9. I have been so unhappy that I have been crying.
> 10. The thought of harming myself had occurred to me.

CLINICAL PERSPECTIVE FOR THE INDIVIDUAL PATIENT

In this Case Study, Deborah is a young mother seeking advice from a doctor as to whether her experience is normal, given her situation, or something that requires treatment. Because mothers and those around them expect the arrival of a baby to be a joyous event, to feel sad and be unable to experience pleasure are particularly disturbing in this context. What makes Deborah's experience a disorder, however, is not that it confounds expectation, but that it follows a recognized pattern of dysfunction and is disrupting her functioning, albeit in subtle ways. Specifically, this new mother feels overwhelmed and helpless and describes exhaustion and sleep problems. Her behavior may be causing developmental delays in her infant (lack of social smiling by 8 weeks). In other words, her condition may have serious consequences, and not just for herself. Her desire to sleep and never wake up suggests possible suicidal thoughts as well.

The idea of mental illness generally is fearful to patients, because of the association with bizarre experiences and irrationality. However, this mother knows she is not her normal self, and having her experience validated by a professional is a helpful step, necessary to her recovery.

The clinician in this situation needs to avoid arbitrary judgments about where to draw a boundary between normal and disordered. Because the normal perinatal symptoms of poor sleep and fatigue may also be signs of depression, clinicians need tools to separate normal and abnormal postpartum states. The Edinburgh Postnatal Depression Scale is a *screening* questionnaire that has been given to thousands of new mothers (and pregnant women) to identify and quantify symptoms. Research has then correlated responses with data from extensive clinical interviews in which trained mental health professionals probe to uncover the entire range of depressive symptoms and signs, and the significant impairment needed to make the diagnosis according to *DSM IV* criteria. A score above 10, or the endorsement of suicidal ideation, or both, suggests the woman is suffering from diagnosable major depression. Such a woman may benefit from treatment, but the woman in the vignette is not the pediatrician's patient, so she requires referral to adult medicine or mental health. Use of a screening tool allows people without specialty training to identify needs quickly and to open up a discussion of problems that were not the purpose of a given appointment.

Health Policy and Barriers to Mental Health Care

The need for specialized, coordinated health and mental health services for the treatment of perinatal depression is obvious but unmet. Pregnant and postpartum women see obstetricians and pediatricians frequently during the period of risk. Unfortunately, access to general health providers does not guarantee access to mental health care. Discrimination against payment for mental healthcare is widespread. It is currently legal for an insurer to "carve out" mental health from general health care in order to apply special limits to what the insurer will pay for the mental health care. Psychiatric services are often not available in the types of clinics where an uninsured woman gets her care.

Government-sponsored health programs like Medicaid and Medicare both facilitate and put up many barriers to patients getting mental health care. Medicare, for example, covers psychiatric care but requires that patients pay 50 percent of the cost of a mental health visit out of pocket, compared to a 20 percent copay for a medical visit. Medicaid benefits vary by state. In many states, Medicaid coverage for pregnant women expires after the first month postpartum, which is earlier than most women recognize they may have depression. Correcting these inequities will require reforms in governmental regulation of health insurance, but campaigns for "mental health parity" have not, so far, succeeded at either the federal level (for Medicare/Medicaid) or the state level (for Medicaid and private insurance).

Other Barriers to Mental Health Care

Even if a woman has financial resources to pay for care, being pregnant or tied down with an infant may make her unable to keep appointments for herself. Pediatricians typically do not regard mothers as their patients and believe that screening for depression should be someone else's responsibility. Although obstetricians are supposed to screen their patients, many in practice focus on the physical pregnancy and are reluctant to deal with other conditions. The stigma attached to a mental health diagnosis makes some women reluctant to describe their symptoms, and the doctors who see them are also often reluctant to probe, for fear of shaming or embarrassing their patients. As a result, population surveys have shown repeatedly that perinatal depression often goes unrecognized. Even when recognized, the condition may go untreated, at great cost to mother and child.

The many barriers to accessing psychiatric treatment are unfortunate, because perinatal depression is quite responsive to treatment.[10] Medications (many of which are reasonably safe to take while pregnant or nursing) work as well in this situation as in depression occurring in other circumstances. Psychotherapy is also an effective treatment for perinatal depression. It helps women find social support, manage their anxiety, understand the meaning of the life changes that come with having a new baby, and rethink old sorrows and conflicts that may come up during this period of adjustment. Untreated depression may last several years and may adversely affect both the mother's health and the infant's development.

PUBLIC HEALTH PERSPECTIVE ON PERINATAL DEPRESSION: EPIDEMIOLOGY, SCREENING, PREVENTION, AND SERVICE DELIVERY

The values of pubic health, including population-based research, screening, prevention, and the development of efficient, effective services, are crucial to addressing the challenge that perinatal depression poses to medicine and to society.

Epidemiology

Epidemiological research based on the *DSM* criteria has proven conclusively that women suffer depression at roughly double the rate of men. This finding is true around the world, across social classes, and under many different conditions.[11] The percentage of women in a given society who suffer from depression may reflect social factors such as poverty, lack of rights, or protections from exploitation, but the rate of depression relative to men is invariably two to one or greater. More detailed examination of these data suggests that female reproductive biology contributes to this increase of relative risk. Rates of new onset major depression are twice as high in women relative to men during the years between menarche and menopause. Rates before and after, as well as rates of recurrence of depression once established, are roughly equal in both sexes.[12]

Research also has shown that pregnancy and the year following childbirth are periods of particular increased risk of depression, either new onset or recurrence, for women. Roughly 10 percent of women will meet criteria for depression during pregnancy, although rates of hospitalization and treatment for depression decrease in this period. After giving birth, about half these women recover, but another group of women become symptomatic, so that the rate of depression postpartum is still 10 percent to 12 percent. In countries with good population-based health statistics and universal health care, the six months following childbirth are those in which women have the highest lifetime likelihood of being hospitalized for depression. Childbirth, as a biopsychosocial event, is a conclusively proven risk factor for major depressive disorder in women.

DSM IV acknowledges the relationship between childbirth and depression by providing a specifier to the diagnostic label. A woman who is depressed in pregnancy does not get a special diagnosis, but the manual contains the category of "major depression with postpartum onset." There is no diagnosis of "depression secondary to pregnancy" or "depression secondary to childbirth." As normal states, pregnancy and parturition cannot be considered sole or adequate causes of an illness. Ninety percent of pregnant and postpartum women are not depressed. Pregnancy increases the likelihood a woman will become depressed, but one must search for other factors to explain why this occurs.

Again, public health research methods, specifically, statistical models for identifying risk factors, have been crucial in explaining this finding.[13] Past personal history of depression or a family history of depression turn out to be major risk factors for women to develop perinatal depression. Current stressors such as inadequate social support or accumulated recent life changes are also risk factors. Being pregnant as a teenager, which is associated with other types of social adversities, is another major risk factor. Taken together, these findings suggest that the biopsychosocial changes of pregnancy and childbirth bring on depression in women who are already vulnerable based on genes, past personal history, or social adversity.

In addition to risk factors present before and during pregnancy and at birth, the extended postpartum period presents many psychological challenges, accompanied by both rapid and slow biological adjustments. Hormones present during pregnancy disappear within days of delivery, and mothers recover ordinary hormonal cycles at widely varying rates. Psychologically, a baby can make its mother feel helpless, trapped, and unable to work on the life goals she had before pregnancy. Babies also may disrupt women's relationships with their partners or with other people close to them. Anxiety for the baby's well-being can generalize to a state of constant vigilance and reactivity. When a woman is physically, psychologically, or behaviorally unable to adapt to these circumstances, she may fall ill with depression.

Screening

Medical care, strictly speaking, is reactive. Patients are supposed to experience or recognize some health problem and seek out expert help to understand and manage it. Public health has broadened the concept of health care to include screening, that is, developing ways to identify illness or risk of illness in the absence of overt symptoms or active care-seeking by the patient. Screening may be either population based or a part of clinical care. In the case of perinatal depression, sophisticated screening tools are available to use in identifying the psychiatric problem in the course of providing pediatric, obstetrical, or general medical care.

As illustrated in the Case Study in this chapter,[10] the Edinburgh Perinatal Depression Scale (EPDS) is a well-validated screening tool. It is a self-administered test in simple language that takes a minute to score. It quickly identifies women who need further evaluation for depression, based either on the number and level of their symptoms or on the presence of suicidal ideation. Studies have demonstrated its validity in many different cultures, social classes, language groups, and clinical settings.

Prevention

Treating maternal depression is preventive care for the infant, who is otherwise at risk for delays in social, physical, and cognitive development.[14] Preventing depression in mothers is harder; women who are at very high risk for postpartum depression (for example, because of a previous postpartum episode) sometimes will start treatment late in pregnancy or immediately after delivery, a form of secondary prevention that may be effective. Research into primary prevention has been less fruitful, though some evidence suggests that improving social support during pregnancy or providing brief home visits from trained workers weekly for six weeks after delivery may lower the rate of postpartum depression.[15] This low cost practice is common in England.

Education of both potential patients and healthcare providers is another essential method for improving detection and treatment of this condition. Testimony from heroic survivors of the illness such as the actress Brooke Shields[16] has been particularly effective in reducing the stigma associated with postpartum depression, especially the misconception that depression may make mothers into monsters who may harm their children.

Public health also suggests other ways to improve society's approach to perinatal depression. For example, the development of a personal medical record that includes information about risk factors such as personal or family history of depression might improve coordination of services for women who seek pregnancy care from obstetricians but mental health care from primary care physicians or mental health providers.

CONCLUSION

Major depression is a common, often untreated, complication of pregnancy and childbirth worldwide. Neurobiological models of depression account for the shared features of the condition across societies and individuals. Personal and cultural factors account for the marked heterogeneity in how the illness appears in individuals. Epidemiological research has done a great deal to improve our understanding of the scope of this problem and to identify risk factors and the range of treatment outcomes. Such research depends on the availability of sound screening tools for identifying and following the course of the disorder. The Edinburgh Postnatal Depression Scale is one such instrument that has facilitated such research in many contexts. More information will not, by itself, guarantee that women will receive appropriate care for perinatal depression. The removal of institutional barriers to receiving mental health care, in particular, legislating parity for mental and physical health care in the structure of insurance benefits, would improve women's access to care in the United States. Both clinical medicine and public health have much to contribute to the ultimate goal of developing better methods of prevention and treatment and implementing more broadly the pharmacological and psychosocial treatment modalities already known to be effective for this common, disabling disorder.

KEY TERMS
Biology Terms

HPA Axis: A neurochemical network that coordinates the functions of the hypothalamus, pituitary and adrenal glands.

Limbic System: A network of brain areas essential for memory, motivated behavior, the ability to experience pleasure, and response to environmental threat (specifically includes hippocampus, amygdala, and hypothalamus).

Neuron: Single nerve cell, a building block of the central nervous system.

Neurotransmitters: Molecule released by one nerve cell that activates or suppresses another nerve cell. Examples: dopamine, acetylcholine, norepinephrine, and serotonin.

Perinatal (also **Peripartum**): Associated with pregnancy and childbirth.

Postpartum: After childbirth.

Public Health Terms

DALY (Disability Adjusted Life Years): A summary measure that combines the impact of illness, disability, and mortality on population health (WHO definition).

Risk Factor: Something that increases a person's chance of developing a disorder.

Screening: Efforts to detect illness in individuals before they are obviously sick or disordered, or when they have not sought care for a specific problem.

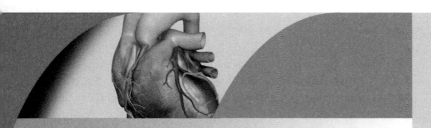

Questions for Further Research, Study, Reflection, and Discussion

For the Individual Student

In order to answer these questions, it may be necessary to research the primary literature.

- What is a Disability Adjusted Life Year, and how does this measure apply to depression?
- What other psychiatric disorders besides depression involve dysregulation in the serotonergic neurotransmitter system? (*Hint:* what other disorders respond to serotonergic medications?)
- If fluctuations in estrogen and progesterone are implicated in the pathophysiology of major depression in women during their reproductive years, how does one account for the presence of major depression in men?
- What are the advantages and disadvantages of a descriptive diagnostic system, such as the *DSM IV* for psychiatric disorders? What are the alternatives?

For Small Group Discussion

- How accurate is the EPDS in identifying depression in pregnant or postpartum women? What are some of the reasons that practitioners should use it, and what are some of the reasons that many still don't?
- Military service often separates men from their wives during the perinatal period (pregnancy and after delivery). Based on the role of social support in preventing or improving the course of depression in new mothers, what types of programs might the military develop to anticipate and address the likelihood of perinatal depression in military families?
- Every student in your group should have some form of health insurance. Different policies have different limits and procedures for covering psychiatric care. Each group member should find out what his/her policy covers, and how this differs from or resembles the policy's general medical benefit. Does this policy require referral by a non-mental health provider (gatekeeping)? Does the policy require the subscriber to choose a provider from a particular network or group? How do you find a covered provider and how long does it typically take to get an appointment? Does the policy have any coverage for an out-of-network provider?

For Entire Class Discussion

- Why is the cost of depression in DALYs so high?

EXERCISE/ACTIVITY

- Any group of women of childbearing age is likely to have members who can provide personal testimony about the physical and emotional challenges of the perinatal period (from conception through the first year of a child's life). Ask parents in your group (or invite a panel of parents) to reflect on the perinatal period: what did he/she expect beforehand and how was the experience different from this expectation? What were some of the challenges (biological, psychological, or social) to general adaptation he/she experienced in relation to this pregnancy, and what helped or hindered the response to these challenges?

Healthy People 2010

Indicator: Mental Health

Focus Area: Maternal, Infant, and Child Health

Goal: Improve the health and well-being of women, infants, children, and families.

Objectives:

16-5. Reduce maternal illness and complications due to pregnancy.

REFERENCES

1. World Health Organization. Mental Health. Depression. Available at http://www.who.int/mental_health/management/depression/definition/en/. Accessed May 13, 2008.

2. American Psychiatric Association. *Diagnostic and Statistical Manual IV TR.* Washington, DC: APA Press; 2006.

3. Plizska SR. *Neuroscience for the Mental Health Clinician.* New York: Guilford Press; 2003.

4. http://web.lemoyne.edu/~hevern/psy340/graphics/limbic.system.jpg.

5. Simon Fraser University, Burnaby, B.C., Canada. *HPA Axis.* Available at http://www.sfu.ca/~vkyrylov/Research/Physiology/major-endo2.gif. Accessed May 13, 2008.

6. A Review of the Universe: Structures, Evolutions, Observations, and Theories. Profile of the brain. Available at http://universe-review.ca/I10-80-prefrontal.jpg. Accessed May 13, 2008.

7. The Lundbenk Institute, Skodsborg, Denmark. CNSforum. Neurological pathways. Available at http://www.cnsforum.com/content/pictures/imagebank/hirespng/Neuro_path_SN_PHB.png. Accessed May 13, 2008.

8. Nichter R. Idioms of distress: alternatives in the expression of psychosocial distress: a case study from South India. *Cult Med Psychiatry* 1981;5:379–408.

9. Cox JL, Holden JM, Sagovsky R. Detection of postnatal depression: development of the 10-item Edinburgh Postnatal Depression Scale. *Brit J Psychiatry* 1987;150:782–786.

10. Wisner KL, Parry BL, Piontek CM. Postpartum depression. *N Engl J Med* 2002;347:194–1998.

11. Weissman MM, Bland R, Joyce PR, Newman S, Wells JE, Wittchen Hu. Sex differences in rates of depression: cross-national perspectives. *J Affect Disord* 1993;29:77–84.

12. Cyranowski JM, Frank E, Young E, Shear MK, Cyranowski JM, et al. Adolescent onset of the gender difference in lifetime rates of major depression, a theoretical model. *Arch Gen Psychiatry* 2000;57:21–27.

13. Robertson E, Grace S, Wallington T, Stewart DE. Antinatal risk factors for postpartum depression: a synthesis of recent literature. *Gen Hosp Psychiatry* 2004;26:289–295.

14. Weinberg MK, Tronick EZ. The impact of maternal psychiatric illness on infant development. *J Clin Psychiatry* 1998;59(Suppl 2):53–61.

15. Dennis CL, Creedy D. Psychosocial and psychological interventions for preventing postpartum depression. *Cochrane Database Syst Rev* 2007:2.

16. Shields B. *Down Came the Rain: My Journey through Postpartum Depression.* New York: Hyperion Books; 2005.

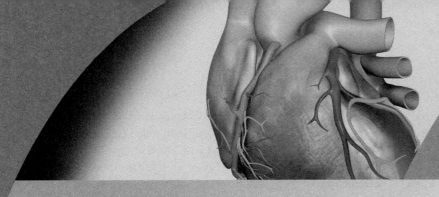

CHAPTER 43

The Science of Sleep

Michele Wagner
Daniel Webb

Drowsy driving kills more than 1,550 people a year in the United States and causes 71,000 injuries, according to the National Highway Traffic Safety Administration, which estimates there are 100,000 sleep-related crashes a year.[1]

LEARNING OBJECTIVES

By the end of this chapter, students will be able to:

- Describe the physiological processes that control sleepiness and wakefulness.
- Connect how disruptions in those processes place an individual at risk for injury or other disease.
- List the most common sleep disorders.
- Discuss how sleep disorders impact the public's health.

INTRODUCTION

No doubt, the consequences of **sleep** loss are significant. Historic tragedies have been linked to fatigue-related human error, among them the Exxon *Valdez* oil spill[1] and the NASA *Challenger* shuttle explosion.[2] The grave outcomes of events like these are just some of the reasons why improved understanding of the biology of sleep and wake can lead to improved quality of life and safety.

Emerging science and advances in technology now are allowing us to examine sleep at a level of detail never before possible. In addition to documenting the more obvious consequences of poor sleep, scientists are increasingly exploring what happens during sleep at the neurological and physiolog-

ical levels. What they are discovering is that sleep provides more benefits than previously thought and is absolutely crucial to promoting health and maintaining physiological processes.

So why is sleep so important? Although we naturally think of sleep as a time of rest and recovery from the stresses of everyday life, research is revealing that sleep is a dynamic activity, during which many processes vital to health and well-being take place. New evidence shows that sleep is essential to helping maintain mood, memory, and cognitive performance. It also plays a pivotal role in the normal function of the endocrine and immune systems. In fact, studies show a growing link between sleep duration and a variety of serious health problems, including obesity, diabetes, hypertension, and depression.

It is no exaggeration to say that some of the most pressing problems we face as a society may be linked to poor sleep. Drowsiness in sleep-deprived drivers is likely the cause of more than 100,000 crashes, 71,000 injuries, and more than 1,550 deaths each year.[3] In addition, sleep disorders are estimated to cost Americans over $100 billion annually in lost productivity, medical expenses, sick leave, and property and environmental damage.[4] On a personal level, we all know how miserable we feel after a night of poor sleep.

Despite the fact that at least 40 million Americans report having sleep problems, more than 60 percent of adults have never been asked about the quality of their sleep by a physician, and fewer than 20 percent ever initiated a discussion about it.[5] Clearly, sleep's impact on health and well-being is underrecognized. But the growing body of knowledge about the complex structure, function, and mechanisms of sleep as well as the consequences when sleep is lost or disturbed, should serve as a wake-up call for making sleep a public health priority.

BASIC SCIENCE FACTS/KEY CONCEPTS REVIEW

To understand the importance of sleep, it is helpful to know something about the basic mechanisms of the **sleep-wake cycle**. This cycle, which consists of roughly 8 hours of nocturnal sleep and 16 hours of daytime wakefulness in humans, is controlled by a combination of two internal influences: sleep **homeostasis** and **circadian rhythms**.

Homeostasis is the process by which the body maintains a "steady state" of internal conditions such as blood pressure, body temperature, and acid-base balance. The amount of sleep each night is also under homeostatic control. From the time that we wake up, the homeostatic drive for sleep accumulates, reaching its maximum in the late evening when most individuals fall asleep. Although the neurotransmitters of this sleep homeostatic process are not fully understood, there is evidence to indicate that one may be the sleep-inducing chemical, adenosine. As long as we are awake, blood levels of adenosine rise continuously, resulting in a growing need for sleep that becomes more and more difficult to resist. Conversely, during sleep, levels of adenosine decrease, thereby reducing the need for sleep. Certain drugs, like caffeine, work by blocking the adenosine **receptor**, disrupting this process.

Sleep loss results in the accumulation of a sleep debt that must eventually be repaid. When we stay up all night, for example, our bodies will demand that we make up each hour of lost sleep—by napping or sleeping longer in later cycles—or suffer the consequences. Even the loss of one hour of sleep time that accumulates for several days can have a powerful negative effect on daytime performance, thinking, and mood.

Circadian rhythms refer to the cyclical changes—like fluctuations in body temperature, hormone levels, and sleep—that occur over a 24-hour period, driven by the brain's biological "clock." In humans, the biological clock consists of a group of neurons in the **hypothalamus** of the brain called the **suprachiasmatic nucleus** (SCN) (Figure 43-1). These internal 24-hour rhythms in physiology and behavior are synchronized to the external physical environment and social/work schedules. In humans, light is the strongest synchronizing agent. Light and darkness are external signals that "set" the biological clock and help determine when we feel the need to wake up or go to sleep. In addition to providing synchronization in time between various rhythms, the circadian clock also helps promote wakefulness.

Thus, the homeostatic system tends to make us sleepier as time goes on throughout the waking period, regardless of whether it's night or day, while the circadian system tends to keep us awake as long as there is daylight, prompting us to sleep as soon as it becomes dark. Because of the complexity of this interaction, it is generally agreed that sleep quality and restfulness are best when the sleep schedule is regularly synchronized to the internal circadian rhythms and that of the external light-dark cycle: when we try to go to bed and wake up at around the same time each day, even on days off and

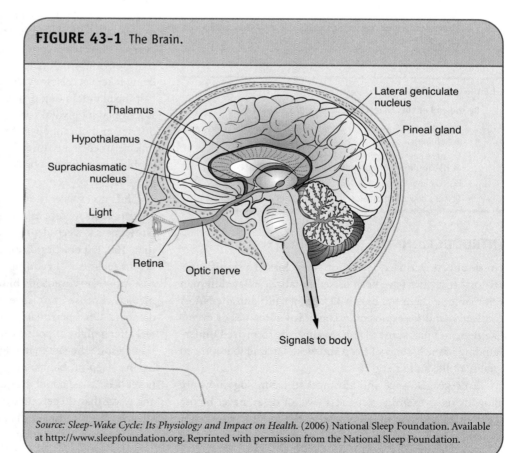

FIGURE 43-1 The Brain.

Thalamus

Hypothalamus

Suprachiasmatic nucleus

Light

Retina

Optic nerve

Lateral geniculate nucleus

Pineal gland

Signals to body

Source: Sleep-Wake Cycle: Its Physiology and Impact on Health. (2006) National Sleep Foundation. Available at http://www.sleepfoundation.org. Reprinted with permission from the National Sleep Foundation.

weekends. Moreover, the circadian system is particularly intolerant of major alterations in sleep and wake schedules, as anyone who has traveled cross-country by plane or worked the graveyard shift can attest.

Disruptions of the Circadian System

What happens when circadian rhythms are disrupted? Not surprisingly, when we attempt to stay awake against the schedule dictated by our circadian clock, our mental and physical performance is greatly diminished. Conditions associated with a disruption of circadian rhythms include shift work, jet lag, and other circadian rhythm sleep disorders. In jet lag, times for sleep and wakefulness dictated by the internal circadian clock do not correspond with external cues in the new time zone. The result is excessive sleepiness, poor sleep, loss of concentration, poor motor control, slowed reflexes, nausea, and irritability. Those who perform shift work, particularly on night shifts, also may experience the effects of a disrupted circadian sleep-wake cycle; research shows that 10 percent to 20 percent of shift workers report falling asleep on the job. They also may suffer from diminished performance and alertness, and may be more prone to accidents. Strategies to re-align circadian rhythm, such as using light and **melatonin** can help. There is also evidence that taking a nap in the middle of a night shift may help. Naps—even as short as 20 minutes—can maintain or improve alertness, performance, and mood.

The Stages of Sleep

Although it is common to think of sleep as a time of "shutting down," sleep is actually an active physiological process. While metabolism generally slows down during sleep, all major organs and regulatory systems continue to function. In fact, sleep can be categorized into distinct stages. There are two types of sleep: *rapid eye movement (REM) sleep* and *non-REM (NREM) sleep*. Changes in brain activity that take place are measured using an electroencephalogram (EEG).

NREM Sleep

NREM sleep is characterized by a reduction in physiological activity. As sleep gets deeper, the brain waves as measured by an electroencephalogram (EEG) get slower and have greater amplitude, breathing and heart rate slow down, and blood pressure drops. The NREM phase consists of four stages[6] (Figure 43-2):

- Stage 1 is a time of drowsiness or transition from being awake to falling asleep. Brain waves and muscle activity begin to slow down during this stage. People in stage 1 sleep may experience sudden muscle jerks, preceded by a falling sensation.

- Stage 2 is a period of light sleep during which eye movements stop. Brain waves become slower, with occasional bursts of rapid waves called sleep spindles, coupled with spontaneous periods of muscle tone mixed with periods of muscle relaxation. The heart rate slows and body temperature decreases.

- Stages 3 and 4 (which together are called slow wave sleep) are characterized by the presence of slow brain waves called delta waves interspersed with smaller, faster waves. Blood pressure falls, breathing slows, and body temperature drops even lower, with the body becoming immobile. Sleep is deeper, with no eye movement and decreased muscle activity, though muscles retain their ability to function. It is most difficult to be awakened during slow wave sleep. People who are awakened during these stages of sleep may feel groggy or disoriented for several minutes after they wake up. It also is during this stage that some children experience bedwetting, night terrors, or sleepwalking.

REM Sleep

REM sleep is an active period of sleep marked by intense brain activity. Brain waves are fast and desynchronized, similar to those in the waking state. Breathing becomes more rapid, irregular, and shallow; eyes move rapidly in various directions and limb muscles become temporarily paralyzed. Heart rate increases and blood pressure rises. This also is the sleep stage in which most dreams occur. Although the role each of these states plays in overall health is uncertain, having the right balance between them is believed to be important for obtaining restful, restorative sleep and for promoting processes such as learning, memory, mood, and ability to concentrate.

Sleep Architecture: The Right Mix of Sleep

Sleep research shows that adults of every age need, on average, a range of seven to nine hours of sleep each night; teenagers need about 9.5 hours, and infants generally require around 16 hours per day.[7] But just as important as the quantity of sleep is getting the right mix of REM and NREM sleep as well as shallow and deep sleep. In normal sleep, REM and NREM sleep alternate throughout the night according to a predictable pattern referred to as the "sleep architecture."[8] A complete sleep cycle consists of NREM and REM cycles that alternate every 90 to 110 minutes and is repeated four to six times per night.[9] Adults, on average, spend more than half of their total daily sleep time in stage 2 sleep, about 20 percent in REM sleep, and the remaining time in the other stages, but the amount of time spent in any given stage is not constant over the course of a night.[10] The first sleep cycles each night contain

FIGURE 43-2 Progression of Sleep Stages During a Single Night in a Normal Young Adult.

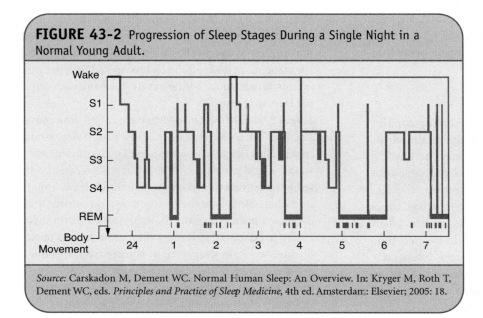

Source: Carskadon M, Dement WC. Normal Human Sleep: An Overview. In: Kryger M, Roth T, Dement WC, eds. *Principles and Practice of Sleep Medicine*, 4th ed. Amsterdam: Elsevier; 2005: 18.

fairly short periods of REM sleep and longer periods of slow wave sleep. As the night wears on, REM periods increase in length while the amount of slow wave sleep decreases. By morning, nearly all sleep is in stages 1, 2, and REM.[6] In addition to these nightly changes, the sleep architecture also varies over the course of a lifetime. Normal adults spend 20 percent to 25 percent of sleep time in REM, which is constant throughout adulthood, but newborn babies spend about half their time in REM sleep. Young children also have substantial amounts of deep NREM sleep, but as people age, the amounts of stages 3 and 4 NREM sleep decrease, with lighter sleep predominating. Although sleep may become more fragile in older people, the need for sleep does not decrease with age (Figure 43-3).[9]

Why Sleep Matters: The Impact of Sleep and Sleep Loss

Although scientists still are trying to find out why people need sleep, research on the sleep of animals shows that sleep is necessary for survival. Some experts believe sleep allows the body to repair itself; during sleep many cells show increased production of proteins, the essential building blocks needed for cell growth and repair of damage from stress and ultraviolet rays. The fact that many biochemical and physiological processes take place during sleep has led to a consensus among researchers that adequate sleep is essential to health and wellness. A look at the impact of sleep loss on physiological and cognitive functions also can help shed light on the purpose of sleep. Some of these functions include memory and attention,

complex thought, motor response, and emotional control. But sleep loss does far more than make us grumpy and groggy. In the past few years, investigators have found that sleep loss may have harmful consequences for our immune and endocrine systems as well as contribute to serious illnesses such as obesity, diabetes, and hypertension.

Sleep, Cognitive Performance, and Mood

The evidence that sleep deprivation adversely affects cognition and motor performance is striking. One study showed that people who were awake for up to 19 hours scored substantially worse on performance and alertness than those who were legally intoxicated.[10] Other studies have found:

- After one night of total sleep deprivation, subjects scored significantly lower on tests of judgment, simple reaction time, explicit recall, and inverse word reading.[7]
- Daytime alertness and memory are impaired by the loss of eight hours of sleep, especially when sleep loss is sustained over a few nights.[7]

Getting three, five, or less than seven hours of sleep a night for seven consecutive nights can significantly impair alertness and motor performance.[7] In addition, researchers at Stanford University found that people with mild to moderate **sleep apnea**, a health condition in which breathing stops periodically during sleep and disrupts sleep, did as badly or worse on reaction-time tests as those who would be considered to be inebriated in most states.[7] It is well documented that sleep loss can adversely affect mood. We all know how irritable we become after a night spent tossing and turning. A growing body of medical evidence links inadequate sleep with anger, anxiety, sadness, and dangerous risk-taking behavior. University of Pennsylvania researchers found that when study subjects were only allowed to sleep 4.5 hours a night for one week, they reported feeling more stressed, angry, sad, and mentally exhausted, with overall scores for mood and vigor declining steadily during the test period. When the subjects were allowed to get enough sleep, their mood scores improved dramatically.[11]

Hormones and Metabolism

Sleep is the time when the body secretes many important hormones that affect growth, regulate energy, and control metabolic and endocrine functions. For example, blood levels of the stress hormone, ***cortisol***, which can promote wakefulness, increase near the end of a complete sleep cycle. Growth hormone, which contributes to childhood growth and helps regulate muscle mass in adults, also is secreted during sleep. Follicle-stimulating hormone and luteinizing hormone, both involved in reproduction, also are released during sleep; the sleep-dependent release of luteinizing hormone is thought to initiate puberty. Further, the sleep cycle affects secretion of hormones influencing appetite and weight. Sleep loss has powerful potential implications for obesity and diabetes, both of which have grown to epidemic proportions in recent years.

Obesity and Diabetes

According to the Centers for Disease Control and Prevention, about 65 percent of Americans now are overweight or obese. Why is the nation getting fatter? Most experts attribute it to our sedentary lifestyle combined with our caloric intake. But we're also getting less sleep than we used to, a factor whose role in obesity is just coming to light. Researchers have measured the impact of sleep deprivation on certain hormones that affect the tendency toward obesity. For example, decreased slow wave sleep in young men is associated with decreased production in growth hormone.[12] Because growth hormone plays an important role during adulthood in controlling the body's proportions of fat and muscle, having less of it as men age increases the tendency toward becoming overweight and having a paunch in middle age. Other short-term studies have found a correlation between inadequate sleep and insufficient levels of the hormone leptin, a hunger suppressing hormone that regulates carbohydrate metabolism. Low levels of leptin cause the body to crave carbohydrates regardless of the amount of calories consumed. Further, short sleep increases production of the hormone ghrelin, a hunger-stimulating hormone. The growing problem of obesity also is linked to diabetes. A 1999 study at the University of Chicago found that a sleep debt accumulated over a matter of days can impair sugar metabolism and disrupt hormone levels. After 11 healthy young adults were allowed only a restricted amount of sleep (four hours) for several nights, their ability to process blood glucose had declined, in some cases to a pre-diabetic state, prompting their bodies to produce more insulin.[13]

Immune System

We often automatically retreat to bed when we have a cold or sore throat, instinctively perceiving that sleep helps us heal. Growing evidence suggests this is not mere wishful thinking but scientific fact. The best evidence for sleep's impact on the immune system comes from a recent study showing that the effectiveness of flu vaccinations is severely delayed in individuals who are sleep deprived. Flu shots were administered to men who had been restricted to just four hours of sleep per night for four straight nights and to those who had slept normally. Ten days after vaccination, those in the sleep-deprived group had a substantially lower immune response compared with those who got adequate sleep, producing less than half as many flu-fighting antibodies.[14] Cytokines, chemicals our immune systems use to help fight an infection, also are powerful sleep inducers. This suggests that sleep may help the body conserve energy and other resources it needs to mount an immune response and fight disease.

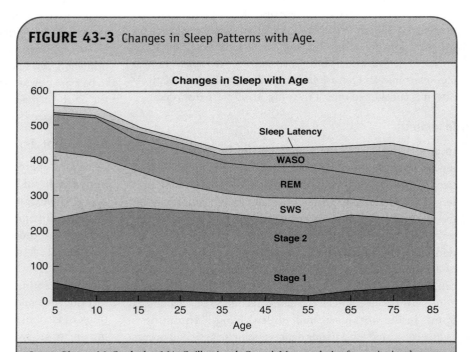

FIGURE 43-3 Changes in Sleep Patterns with Age.

Source: Ohayon M, Carskadon MA, Guilleminault C, et al. Meta-analysis of quantitative sleep parameters from childhood to old age in healthy individuals: Developing normative sleep values across the human lifespan. *Sleep* 2004;27:1255–1273. Used with permission from Associated Professional Sleep Societies, LLC; Carskadon M, Dement WC. Normal Human Sleep: An Overview. In: Kryger M, Roth T, Dement WC, eds. *Principles and Practice of Sleep Medicine*, 4th ed. Amsterdam: Elsevier; 2005:19.

Cardiovascular Disease

A growing amount of evidence shows a relationship between long- and short-term sleep loss and cardiovascular disease, including increased blood pressure and increased risk of stroke in addition to other long-term health consequences. Sleep deprivation has been associated with a rise in blood pressure during the night that lasts through the following day.[15] Evidence suggests an association between too much or too little sleep and an increased risk of coronary heart disease in women.[16] There is a high prevalence of sleep apnea (a breathing disorder during sleep) among people with cardiovascular problems. People with this common sleep disorder are at increased risk of hypertension as well as sudden death from cardiac causes during the night and early morning hours.[17]

Sleep Disorders

Anything that disrupts normal sleep affects the sleep-wake cycle, potentially leading to an imbalance in sleep homeostasis and circadian factors that regulate sleep. For some people, poor sleep constitutes a medical problem. Each year, at least 40 million people in the United States suffer from chronic sleep disorders, and another 30 million are troubled by transient or occasional sleep problems.[6] These disorders account for an estimated $16 billion in medical costs alone, wreaking havoc on people's work lives, driving, and social activities.[6] The most prevalent sleep disorders include **insomnia**, *sleep apnea*, **restless legs syndrome**, and **parasomnias**. While **narcolepsy** is relatively rare, it is considered one of the only "true" sleep disorders.

Insomnia

Insomnia is the complaint of difficulty initiating or maintaining sleep, waking too early and not being able to get back to sleep, or waking feeling unrefreshed and lethargic. Data presented at a National Institutes of Health (NIH) conference on management of chronic insomnia suggest that about 30 percent of the general population has complaints of sleep disruption, while approximately 10 percent have associated symptoms of daytime functional impairment.[18] The effects of insomnia can include daytime fatigue, impaired mood and judgment, poor performance, and an increased likelihood of accidents at home, in the workplace, and while driving.[19] Insomnia is highly comorbid with major depression or anxiety and occurs more often among women, the elderly, individuals of low socioeconomic status, and those who are widowed, divorced, or separated than in other individuals.[19] It may be *primary*, or not directly associated with any other health condition or problem, or *secondary* to some underlying health condition, such as depression, heartburn, cancer, asthma, or arthritis, or as a result of medications or drugs, including alcohol and caffeine. In some people insomnia is *transient*, can last up to one month, and may be caused by many things, among them jet lag, stress, a major life change such as a new job or loss of a relationship, environmental factors like noise, or even consuming too much caffeine.[19]

Chronic insomnia occurs when a person has insomnia a minimum of three nights a week for a month or longer. Chronic insomnia is present in either the primary or secondary forms mentioned above. In the secondary forms it usually is caused by a psychiatric or medical condition, medication taken for other disorders, or by alcohol consumption.[19]

Patients with chronic insomnia should be evaluated to ensure the sleep problem is not due to an underlying medical or psychiatric condition that may require treatment.

Depression and anxiety are the most common causes of insomnia, but insomnia can also lead to depression and anxiety. They are often comorbid, obfuscating efforts to discern which disorder is the primary cause of the other. In addition, certain behaviors can contribute to insomnia, such as excessive caffeine intake, drinking alcohol or smoking cigarettes before bedtime, excessive daytime napping, and irregular or continually disrupted sleep-wake cycles. As yet, little is known about the neurobiology of insomnia; however, hyperactivity of the systems in the brain that cause arousal is believed to be involved.

As evidence mounts on the importance of sleep, the development of safe and effective treatment for insomnia continues to be a priority for sleep researchers. The approach to treatment for poor sleep generally falls into two categories: behavioral and pharmacologic.

Behavioral Approach to Insomnia Treatment

Behavioral approaches and **sleep hygiene** are the cornerstones of treatment for insomnia.

Lifestyle changes, such as decreasing caffeine and alcohol intake, adjusting exercise, regulating not only diet but the amount and time we eat (contrary to conventional wisdom, heavy meals actually keep us awake), and stopping smoking all can contribute to more regular sleep patterns. Caffeine and nicotine are stimulants that can make it difficult to sleep, and nicotine also may cause nightmares. Although many people think of alcohol as a sedative, it actually disrupts sleep, causing nighttime awakenings.

Good sleep hygiene is equally important to achieving quality restorative sleep. These practices include maintaining the same sleep and wake patterns every day, avoiding stimulants late in the day, ensuring adequate exposure to natural daylight, and maintaining an environment conducive to sleep: one that is dark, cool, and noise-free.

In the 1970s and 1980s, *behavioral therapy* techniques for sleep were developed and became popular.[20]

Stimulus-control therapy conditions the patient to associate the bed and bedroom with sleep only, instructing the individual to get out of bed if unable to sleep and to avoid eating, reading, or watching television in bed. **Relaxation therapy** includes muscle relaxation, biofeedback, meditation, and breathing techniques, all aimed at helping the patient fall asleep faster and stay asleep longer. **Sleep-restriction therapy**, as its name suggests, restricts the individual's time in bed, resulting in sleep deprivation that allows the individual to fall asleep.

At the physiological level, *behavioral treatments* work in the same way as medications—by decreasing the activity of the arousal systems in the brain producing wakefulness—and 14 have been shown in some instances to be as or more effective than most medications in treating insomnia. However, if this treatment is not satisfactory, a pharmacological approach may be recommended, especially when more immediate relief is needed, or to break a cycle of sleeplessness before it becomes a chronic problem.

Pharmacological Approach to Insomnia Treatment

Over-the-Counter Products A variety of over-the-counter products are promoted as sleep aids, but these drugs often have many side effects and may not provide effective and sustained relief. They include *antihistamines* such as diphenhydramine and doxylamine, which induce sleep, but also may lead to daytime drowsiness, blurred vision, and dry mouth. Researchers continue to investigate whether other nonprescription therapies, such as herbal remedies or nutritional supplements, may effectively treat insomnia. Because of its role in the circadian system of promoting sleep, the nutritional supplement *melatonin* has been widely touted as a sleep aid. However, clinical studies on the safety, efficacy, and dosing of melatonin have yielded inconsistent results. Because much is still unknown about its potential effects, it is recommended that people talk to their doctors before taking melatonin.

Prescription Sleep Medications Until the 1960s, barbiturates, such as phenobarbital, were widely used as sedatives, despite their association with such dangerous side effects as addiction, tolerance, and abuse. In 1964, *benzodiazepines* (also known as *benzodiazepine receptor agonists*) were introduced and soon became the mainstay of pharmacological treatment. Some benzodiazepines in use today include flurazepam, triazolam, and temazepam.

Benzodiazepines are central nervous system depressants that work by enhancing the actions of the inhibitory neurotransmitter **gamma-aminobutyric acid (GABA)** at its receptor. GABA is believed to be one of the factors that help promote sleep and also is involved in cognitive, memory, and psychomotor functions. Because benzodiazepines bind nonspecifically to GABA receptors, they actually may be more active in reducing anxiety, inducing muscle relaxation, and inhibiting convulsions than in promoting sleep. Their side effects, such as memory loss, rebound insomnia, and drug dependence, may make them inappropriate for some people.[21]

In the early 1990s, a new generation of *nonbenzodiazepines* (or *nonbenzodiazepine receptor agonists*) was introduced that target only certain receptor subtypes of the GABA complex. These drugs, which include zolpidem and zaleplon, have the advantage of being much shorter acting compounds with less likelihood for daytime sleepiness or impairment of memory. However, they still may have some side effects, including rebound insomnia, dependence, drowsiness, dizziness, lightheadedness, and difficulty with coordination.[22]

Two medications for the treatment of insomnia—eszopiclone and ramelteon—recently received approval from the U.S. Food and Drug Administration (FDA). Based on published clinical reports, eszopiclone has demonstrated safety and efficacy of long-term nightly use, and helps people fall asleep and stay asleep throughout the night.

Unlike other prescription sleep aids, ramelteon is thought to work by selectively affecting melatonin receptors (neurons) in the suprachiasmatic nucleus (SCN), a part of the brain that functions to regulate times for sleep and times for optimal alertness or wakefulness. This contrasts with other hypnotic medications that work by binding to GABA receptors, which reduce central nervous system (CNS) activity.[23] Ramelteon has been found to be effective in helping those who have difficulty falling asleep. Because there has been no evidence that ramelteon has a potential for abuse or dependence, it can be prescribed for long-term use in adults and those with a history of drug dependence and abuse.

Evidence supports the efficacy of cognitive behavioral therapy and benzodiazepine receptor agonists in the treatment of chronic insomnia.[18] Very little evidence supports the efficacy of other treatments, despite their widespread use.

Obstructive Sleep Apnea

An estimated 18 million Americans have sleep apnea, a serious, potentially life-threatening disorder characterized by episodes of interrupted breathing during sleep.

Obstructive sleep apnea, affecting about 5 percent of the population, occurs when anatomical obstruction prevents air from flowing into or out of the person's airway despite efforts to breathe. It usually is associated with fat buildup, loss of muscle tone with aging, a narrow windpipe, or enlarged tonsils or adenoids that block the windpipe during breathing. *Central sleep* apnea, which is relatively rare, occurs when the system that controls breathing is abnormal and there are decreased efforts to breathe during sleep. In sleep apnea, the brain has to awaken the sufferer in order for breathing to start again. Frequent arousals from apneic events during the night prevent the person from getting enough deep, restorative sleep. Because of the constant interruption of their normal sleep patterns, people with sleep apnea often feel very sleepy, causing problems with daytime concentration and performance. Studies have shown that sleep apnea contributes to high blood pressure.[24] Risks for heart attack, irregular heartbeat, and stroke also are increased in those with sleep apnea in part due to the oxygen desaturation in the blood when breathing is disrupted. Other consequences of sleep apnea include depression, irritability, sexual dysfunction, learning and memory difficulties, and falling asleep while at work, on the phone, or driving. Sleep apnea's association with obesity can create a vicious cycle for some patients, who may find it harder to exercise because of their sleepiness. Successful treatment, usually with nasal *continuous positive airway pressure* (CPAP) or an oral appliance to advance the jaw, alleviates disruptions in breathing and can reduce sleepiness, motivating patients to effectively lose weight. People with sleep apnea should not take sedatives or sleeping pills, because they may prevent them from awakening to breathe.

Restless Legs Syndrome (RLS)

Recent research suggests that anywhere from 5 percent to 15 percent of Americans suffer from restless legs syndrome, a condition characterized by uncomfortable sensations in the legs, including creeping, tingling, cramping, burning, and pain that tend to worsen upon lying down or at rest (could be just sitting). These unpleasant sensations usually occur in the afternoon and early evening as they follow a circadian rhythm. People with RLS may find it difficult to relax and fall asleep because of their strong urge to walk or move to relieve the sensations in their legs. Although the cause is unknown, factors associated with RLS include:

- Family history
- Pregnancy
- Low iron or folate levels or anemia
- Chronic diseases, including kidney failure, diabetes, rheumatoid arthritis, and peripheral neuropathy
- Caffeine intake

Treatment options for people with RLS include both behavioral and pharmacological approaches. Making lifestyle changes (such as eating a balanced diet, avoiding caffeinated products, and avoiding drinking alcohol in the evening) and practicing good sleep hygiene have been shown to help lessen the severity and impact of RLS symptoms. If an iron deficiency is identified as the cause of symptoms, iron supplements, vitamin B_{12}, or folate (as indicated) may provide relief.[25]

Recent studies demonstrate that RLS may be caused by dopamine deficiency, a key chemical messenger in the brain responsible for smooth, coordinated movement and other motor and cognitive functions.[6] Some RLS patients have been found to respond positively to treatment with precursors of dopamine. Most recently, drugs classified as dopaminergic agonists such as ropinerole and pramipexole have become the treatment of choice for this debilitating sleep disorder.[26]

Parasomnias

When the transition from one sleep state to another doesn't progress in an orderly fashion or a person is aroused from sleep, bizarre and often complex behaviors known as parasomnias may occur. Parasomnias include sleepwalking, night terrors, and bedwetting, which are *NREM disorders* that occur early in the night. Night terrors are characterized by agitation, large pupils, sweating, and increased blood pressure. Many of the parasomnias are more common in children, who usually outgrow them and don't require treatment. Superficially resembling night terrors but more common in adults is *REM sleep behavior disorder*, which is characterized by vigorous or violent behaviors that occur later in the night. In this disorder, the temporary muscle paralysis that normally characterizes REM sleep is absent, allowing individuals to act out vivid dreams during sleep and potentially injure themselves or their bed partners. This disorder usually affects middle aged or elderly individuals who frequently also have a neurological disorder. Fortunately, most of these parasomnias can be treated effectively. A relative of the NREM parasomnias is *sleep-related eating disorder*, in which a person eats food during the night while he or she appears to be asleep. Two thirds of patients with this disorder are women. It may be induced by taking certain medications, such as amitriptyline (a sedating antidepressant) or zolpidem (a hypnotic), but it also may be triggered by other sleep disorders, such as obstructive sleep apnea or restless legs syndrome. Although many medicines have been tried to treat the disorder, their success has been limited.[27]

Narcolepsy

About one in 2,000 people suffers from narcolepsy, a chronic neurological disorder that causes the sufferer to fall asleep at times when he or she wants to be awake. In addition to an overwhelming and recurring need to sleep at inappropriate times, features of narcolepsy include cataplexy, sleep paralysis, hypnagogic hallucinations, and autonomic behavior; not all narcoleptics experience all of these symptoms.

- *Cataplexy*: a sudden loss of muscle control ranging from slight weakness (head droop, facial sagging, jaw drop, slurred speech, buckling of knees) to total collapse. It is commonly triggered by intense emotion (laughter, anger, surprise, fear) or strenuous physical activity.
- *Sleep paralysis*: being unable to talk or move for a brief period when falling asleep or waking up.
- *Hypnagogic hallucinations*: vivid and often frightening dreams and sounds reported when falling asleep.
- *Autonomic behavior*: performing familiar tasks without full awareness or later memory of them.

Recent discoveries indicate that people with narcolepsy lack a neuropeptide in the brain called orexin (also known as hypocretin), which normally is released during wakefulness and stimulates arousal. The loss of orexin-producing neurons in people with narcolepsy is probably caused by an autoimmune or neurodegenerative process.[28]

It is estimated that 125,000 to 200,000 Americans suffer from narcolepsy; however, fewer than 50,000 are properly diagnosed, in part because physicians may not always consider narcolepsy when evaluating symptoms of sleepiness and problems with concentration, attention, memory, and performance. Once diagnosed, an important part of the treatment can be involvement in a patient support group such as those organized by the Narcolepsy Network (http://www.narcolepsynetwork.org). Regularly scheduled daytime naps, a regular nightly bedtime schedule, and avoidance of heavy meals and alcohol are among the recommended behavioral approaches to treating narcolepsy. Stimulants, antidepressants, and other medications such as modafinil or methylphenidate can help control the symptoms of narcolepsy. Sodium oxybate, fluoxetine, and venlafaxine (for adults and children) are used for treating cataplexy.[29] Because sodium oxybate improves nighttime sleep in these patients, it also may reduce their excessive daytime sleepiness.

Acknowledgment

The preceding material, prepared by the National Sleep Foundation in a pamphlet entitled Sleep-Wake Cycle: Its Physiology and Impact on Health (2006), *has been included with permission of the National Sleep Foundation. It is available online at http://www.sleepfoundation.org. Accessed May 14, 2008.*

CASE STUDY

Scenario

Carl, a 52-year-old white male, is being seen for back pain following his second automobile accident in a year. He says he just passed out and ran off the road. His wife, who has accompanied him, says he has had several other near accidents. She has come with him because he seems to have problems remembering things of late. Additional history discloses they no longer sleep in the same room because of his loud snoring. This has not solved her sleeping problem, however, because she stays awake to be sure he is still breathing.

A physical exam shows a drowsy overweight male with mild hypertension. He has swelling of the legs, occasional irregular heartbeat, and a large tongue and small throat that taken together create a reduced airspace.

Nocturnal pulse oximetry, a test to measure oxygen concentration in the blood, is ordered pending scheduling of *polysomnography*. Sleep study discloses breathing disruptions of 83 per hour consistent with severe sleep apnea of an obstructive nature.

Defining the Issues

- Recurring drowsiness and daytime sleepiness, including while driving
- Possible sleep apnea
- Hypertension
- Loud snoring at night disturbs the sleep of other members of the household

Patient's Understanding

Carl has a family history of hypertension. He recalls that as a boy, his parents also slept in separate bedrooms on account of his father's snoring. He is aware of the dangers of falling asleep behind the wheel, but with no access to alternative transportation, he has no other option for getting to and from work.

CLINICAL PERSPECTIVE

Level of Intervention Now

CPAP titration performed in lab during last two hours of sleep study showed that a level of 14 cm pressure and 2 liters of oxygen eliminated oxygen desaturations below 90 percent and returned nighttime breathing to normal levels. Carl will therefore use CPAP therapy each night as he sleeps to help his breathing, which should improve sleep and reduce daytime drowsiness.

Potential Level Earlier

Early intervention would require early recognition of signs of sleep apnea. In this case, loud snoring and frank apaneic spells recognized by the spouse should raise a red flag. Most often the patient's bed partner is aware of a potential sleep disorder long before the patient. With sleep apnea, 95 percent of cases are undiagnosed, and physicians are especially likely to overlook cases occurring in people who are not white, middle-aged males. Screening efforts need to be aware of cases occurring in people who are not the stereotypical patient.

PUBLIC HEALTH PERSPECTIVE FOR THE HEALTH OF THE GENERAL POPULATION AND OF HIGH RISK GROUPS

When it comes to public health, sleep disorders are important not only for the acute suffering and fatigue they cause, but also for the additional accidents and injuries that result from drowsiness and chronic lack of sleep. Perhaps more germane to the average student, studying sleep as a public health issue requires considering all sources of sleep deprivation, both from recurring sleep disorders and from conscious decisions to reduce sleep. Sleep loss for any reason, whether due to a chronic disorder or to a late night of studying or socializing, places an individual at increased risk of injury and disease.

It is estimated that 50 to 70 million Americans chronically suffer from a sleep disorder, and on any given day, many more people are likely to experience drowsiness from a poor night's sleep. As this chapter has discussed, although chronic sleep deficits have been associated with a wide range of negative health effects, including obesity, diabetes, acute infection, and cardiovascular disease, a detailed understanding of the exact pathways and processes linking sleep and health has yet to be discovered. Much more certain, however, are the short-term cognitive deficits associated with both chronic and acute sleep loss.

Drowsiness caused from inadequate sleep is a major contributor to motor vehicle accidents. According to a 2007 study by the National Sleep Foundation, 60 percent of American drivers reported operating a vehicle while feeling drowsy in the past year, and more than one third (37 percent) have actually fallen asleep.[29] The National Highway Traffic Safety Administration conservatively estimates that 100,000 police-reported crashes are the direct result of driver fatigue each year.[30] Independent of alcohol effects, driver sleepiness accounts for almost 20 percent of all serious car crash injuries. Overall, drowsy drivers cause an estimated 1,550 deaths, 71,000 injuries, and $12.5 billion in monetary losses. In fact, drowsy driving causes nearly the same number of injuries and fatalities each year as drunk driving even though it receives a considerably lesser amount of attention. These statistics may be the tip of the iceberg because currently it is difficult to attribute crashes to sleepiness.

Inadequate sleep and drowsiness are also significant contributors to workplace injuries and, according to some studies, to falls involving older people. Fewer studies have attempted to connect sleep to injuries and falls than to motor vehicle accidents, and future research should assess what interventions can help prevent injuries stemming from sleep disorders and drowsiness.

Despite its relevance to our daily health and functioning, sleep is commonly overlooked as a significant contributor to disease and to public health. Thanks to the efforts of several organizations, however, sleep is finally garnering more of the attention it deserves from researchers and clinicians. In 2006, at the behest of the National Sleep Foundation and several other partners, the Institute of Medicine released a report discussing health as a public health problem. In addition to researching the rates of sleep disorders and their health outcome, the report also identified several key steps that could strengthen the capacity to research sleep as a contributor or detractor from health. The steps they identify are:

- Establish the workforce required to meet the clinical and scientific demands of the field
- Increase awareness of the burden of sleep loss and sleep disorders among the general public
- Improve surveillance and monitoring of the public health burden of sleep loss and sleep disorders
- Expand awareness among healthcare professionals through education and training
- Develop and validate new and existing diagnostic and therapeutic technologies
- Expand accreditation criteria to emphasize treatment, long-term patient care, and chronic disease management strategies
- Strengthen the national research infrastructure to connect individual investigators, research programs, and research centers
- Increase the investment in interdisciplinary sleep programs in academic health centers that emphasize long-term clinical care, training, and research[31]

CONCLUSION

Unfortunately, sleep is sometimes given a low priority in modern life, taking a back seat to our busy schedules and lifestyles. Yet, as scientists in the field of sleep medicine continue to discover, sleep is a dynamic activity in its own right that is as essential to good health as diet and exercise, and as necessary for survival as food and water. Sleep research continues to expand and attract more notice from scientists and clinicians alike. More research and public education, however, are needed to make sleep a top health priority. As one of the most crucial, yet most overlooked, indicators of overall health, it is important that doctors and primary health care professionals begin an ongoing dialogue with their patients about sleep.

KEY TERMS

Circadian Rhythms: Cyclical changes—like fluctuations in body temperature, hormone levels, and sleep—that occur over a 24-hour period, driven by the body's biological "clock."

Cortisol: One of several stress hormones produced by the adrenal cortex that is secreted near the end of sleep to stimulate alertness.

Gamma-Aminobutyric Acid (GABA): An amino acid in the central nervous system associated with the transmission of nerve impulses.

Homeostasis: Process by which the body maintains a "steady state" of internal conditions such as blood pressure, body temperature, acid-base balance, and sleep.

Hypothalamus: Region of the forebrain below the thalamus, controlling body temperature, thirst, and hunger, and involved in sleep and emotional activity.

Insomnia: Sleep disorder characterized by an inability to initiate sleep or to remain asleep for a reasonable period or waking feeling unrefreshed.

Melatonin: Hormone secreted by the pineal gland especially in response to darkness that promotes sleep.

Narcolepsy: A sleep disorder characterized by sudden and uncontrollable episodes of deep sleep.

Non-Rapid Eye Movement (NREM) Sleep: Collectively describes the four stages of sleep preceding REM sleep that are characterized by a reduction in physiological activity and a slowing of brain waves.

Parasomnia: A category of sleep disorders in which abnormal physiological or behavioral events occur during sleep, including night terrors and sleepwalking.

Pineal Gland: A small cone-shaped organ of the brain that secretes the hormone melatonin into the bloodstream.

Polysomnography: A sleep study. A diagnostic test measuring several physiological variables including brain electrical activity, eye and jaw muscle movement, leg muscle movement, and airflow.

Receptor: A molecular structure within a cell or on the surface characterized by selective binding of a specific substance and a specific physiological effect that accompanies the binding.

Rapid Eye Movement (REM) Sleep: A recurring sleep state characterized by rapid eye movement and intense brain activity, during which dreaming occurs.

Relaxation Therapy: A form of sleep behavioral therapy including muscle relaxation, biofeedback, meditation, and breathing techniques aimed at helping the patient fall asleep faster and stay asleep longer.

Restless Legs Syndrome: A sleep disorder primarily characterized by leg discomfort during sleep, which is only relieved by frequent movements of the legs.

Sleep: A natural and periodic state during which consciousness of the environment is suspended.

Sleep Apnea: A serious, potentially life-threatening sleep disorder characterized by episodes of interrupted breathing during sleep.

Sleep Architecture: The predictable pattern of alternating REM and NREM sleep that occurs throughout the night, consisting of four NREM phases and one REM phase.

Sleep Hygiene: Practices conducive to good sleep including maintaining the same sleep and wake patterns every day, avoiding stimulants late in the day, ensuring adequate exposure to natural daylight, and maintaining a cool, dark, and quiet sleep environment.

Sleep-Restriction Therapy: A form of sleep behavioral therapy that restricts the individual's time in bed, resulting in sleep deprivation that allows the individual to fall asleep.

Sleep-Wake Cycle: The biological pattern of alternating sleep and wakefulness, in humans roughly 8 hours of nocturnal sleep and 16 hours of daytime activity.

Stimulus-Control Therapy: A form of sleep behavioral therapy that conditions the patient to associate the bed and bedroom with sleep.

Suprachiasmatic Nucleus (SCN): A region in the hypothalamus that regulates circadian rhythms, acting as the body's sleep-wake center or "biological clock."

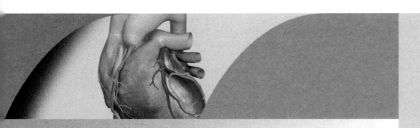

Questions for Further Research, Study, Reflection, and Discussion

For the Individual Student

In order to answer these questions, it may be necessary to research the primary literature.

- What are some of the major chronic diseases associated with inadequate sleep and/or sleep disorders?
- What are some of the major hormones, neurotransmitters, and dietary and environmental factors that interfere with the circadian rhythm and homeostatic process? Provide an overview of the physiological mechanisms each hormone/chemical interrupts.
- Describe physiological differences between REM and non-REM sleep.
- Identify several of the major physiological processes that occur both in the brain and in the body while we sleep. How does lack of sleep interfere with these processes, and what health outcomes may result from their disruption?
- List three sleep disorders and discuss possible treatments and outcomes.

For Small Group Discussion

- How might Carl's sleep apnea have been detected sooner (see Case Study)?

- Apart from sleep disorders, what other diseases might impair someone's ability to achieve restful sleep?

For Entire Class Discussion

- Given the large health and economic burden associated with inadequate sleep and sleep disorders, what role would each of the following groups play in addressing the problem: health care providers, employers, school systems, law enforcement agencies, individuals.

EXERCISE/ACTIVITY

- Over the course of several weeks, keep a journal of your own sleep patterns, noting the time you went to bed, the time you got out of bed, how many hours you slept each night, how many times you woke up, the quantity and content of your dreams, and how refreshed you felt each morning. In the same journal, keep track of any times during the day when you become tired or drowsy. Also keep track of how many and what types of stimulants you consume each day, including what time you consumed them (example: 1 cup of coffee at 3 pm). At the end of your journaling period, go back and look for trends in your sleep habits. What might you do to improve your sleep habits? Overall, how would you reduce or increase your sleep hygiene? After reading this chapter and learning about the impact of sleep deprivation, how do you think your sleep schedule is affecting your performance at school and/or work?

REFERENCES

1. National Transportation Safety Board. *Grounding of the U.S. Tankship EXXON VALDEZ on Bligh Reef, Prince William Sound near Valdez, AK March 24, 1989.* Washington, DC: National Transportation Safety Board; 1990; NTIS Report Number PB90-916405.

2. *Report of the Presidential Commission on the Space Shuttle Challenger Accident,* vol 2. Appendix G. *Human Factors Analysis.* Washington, DC: U.S. Government Printing Office; 1986.

3. Knipling R, Wang J. Revised estimates of the U.S. drowsy driver crash problem size based on general estimates system case reviews. In: *Thirty-Ninth Annual Proceedings of the Association for the Advancement of Automotive Medicine.* Des Plaines, IL: Association for the Advancement of Automotive Medicine; 1995:415–466.

4. Stoller MK. Economic effects of insomnia. *Clin Ther* 1994;16:873–897.

5. National Sleep Foundation. Survey: *Sleep in America.* Washington, DC: National Sleep Foundation; 2000.

6. National Institute of Neurological Disorders and Stroke (NINDS). *Brain Basics: Understanding Sleep.* Available at http://www.ninds.nih.gov/disorders/brain_basics/understanding_sleep.htm. Accessed May 14, 2008.

7. National Sleep Foundation. *How Much Sleep Is Enough.* Available at: http://www.sleepfoundation.org/site/c.huIXKjM0IxF/b.2419131/k.6C23/How_Much_Sleep_is_Enough.htm. Accessed on May 29, 2008.

8. National Sleep Foundation. *Survey: Sleep in America.* Washington, DC: National Sleep Foundation; 2000.

9. National Heart, Lung, and Blood Institute (NHLBI). Information about sleep. In: *Sleep, Sleep Disorders, and Biological Rhythms* (Teacher's Guide). Colorado Springs, CO: BSCS; 2003:19–38. Available at: http://science.education.nih.gov/supplements/nih3/sleep/guide/nih_sleep_curr-supp.pdf. Accessed May 14, 2008.

10. Kuo AA. Does sleep deprivation impair cognitive and motor performance as much as alcohol intoxication? *West J Med* 2001;174:180.

11. Dement WC, Vaughan CC. *The Promise of Sleep.* New York: Delacorte Press; 1999: 274.

12. Van Cauter E, Leproult R, Plat L. Age-related changes in slow wave sleep and REM sleep and relationship with growth hormone and cortisol levels in healthy men. *JAMA* 2000;284:861–868.

13. Spiegel K, Leproult R, Van Cauter E. Impact of sleep debt on metabolic and endocrine function. *Lancet* 1999;354:1425–1429.

14. Spiegel K, Sheridan JF, Van Cauter E. Effect of sleep deprivation on response to immunization, *JAMA* 2002;288:1471–1472.

15. Rosansky SJ; Menachery SJ, Whittman D, Rosenberg JC. The relationship between sleep deprivation and the nocturnal decline of blood pressure. *Am J Hypertens* 1996;9:1136–1138.

16. Ayas NT, White DP, Manson JE, Stampfer MJ, Speizer FE, et al. A prospective study of sleep duration and coronary heart disease in women. *Arch Intern Med* 2003;163:205–209.

17. Gami AS, Howard DE, Olson EJ, Somers VK. Day-night pattern of sudden death in obstructive sleep apnea. *N Engl J Med* 2005;352:1206–1214.

18. National Institutes of Health (NIH) Consensus Development Program. *State-of-the-Science Conference Statement on Manifestations and Management of Chronic Insomnia in Adults.* Final Statement, August 18, 2005. Available at http://consensus.nih.gov/2005/2005InsomniaSOS026PDF.pdf. Accessed May 14, 2008.

19. Edinger JD, Means MK. Overview of insomnia: definitions, epidemiology, differential diagnosis, and assessment. In: Kryger MH, Roth T, Dement WC, eds. *Principles and Practice of Sleep Medicine,* 4th ed. Philadelphia: Elsevier/Saunders; 2005.

20. Morin CM. Psychological and behavioral treatments for primary insomnia. In: Kryger MH, Roth T, Dement WC, eds. *Principles and Practice of Sleep Medicine,* 4th ed. Philadelphia: Elsevier/Saunders; 2005:726–737.

21. Woods JH, Katz JL, Winger G. Abuse and therapeutic use of benzodiazepines and benzodiazepine-like drugs. In: Bloom FE, Kupfer DJ, eds. *Psychopharmacology, The Fourth Generation of Progress.* New York: Raven Press; 1995. Available at: http://www.acnp.org/G4/GN401000172/CH168.html. Accessed May 14, 2008.

22. Wagner J, Wagner M. Nonbenzodiazepines for the treatment of insomnia. *Sleep Med Rev* 2000;4:551–581.

23. National Sleep Foundation. NSF Alert, July 26, 2005. *Is Rozerem a new kind of sleeping pill?* Available at http://www.sleepfoundation.org/nsfalert/index.php?secid=&id=32. Accessed January 18, 2006.

24. Peppard PE, Young T, Palta M, Skatrud J. Prospective study on the association between sleep disordered breathing and hypertension. *N Engl J Med* 2000;342:1378–1384.

25. Restless Legs Syndrome Foundation. *Restless Legs Syndrome: Causes, Diagnosis and Treatment.* Available at http://www.rls.org/NetCommunity/Document.Doc?&id=3. Accessed May 14, 2008..

26. Montplaisir J, Allen R, Walters A, et al. Restless legs syndrome and periodic limb movements in sleep. In: Kryger MH, Roth T, Dement WC, eds. *Principles and Practice of Sleep Medicine,* 4th ed. Philadelphia: Elsevier/Saunders; 2005:839–852.

27. National Sleep Foundation. *Sleepmatters. Sleep-Related Eating Disorder.* Available at: http://www.sleepfoundation.org/site/c.huIXKjM0IxF/b.2421125/k.6662/Most_Common_Sleep_Problems_in_Women.htm. Accessed January 18, 2006.

28. Scammell TE. The regulation of sleep and circadian rhythms. *Sleep Medicine Alert.* National Sleep Foundation. 2004;8(1).

29. National Sleep Foundation. *State of the States Report on Drowsy Driving.* November 2007. Available at http://www.drowsydriving.org. Accessed May 14, 2008.

30. National Center on Sleep Disorders Research (NCSDR) and the National Highway and Traffic Safety Administration(NHTSA) Expert Panel on Driver Fatigue and Sleepiness. *Drowsy Driving and Automobile Crashes.* Available at http://www.nhtsa.dot.gov/people/injury/drowsy_driving1/drowsy.html#NCSDR/NHTSA. Accessed May 14, 2008.

31. Institute of Medicine of the National Academies. *Sleep Disorders and Sleep Deprivation: An Unmet Public Health Problem.* April 2006. Available at http://www.iom.edu/CMS/3740/23160/33668.aspx. Accessed May 14, 2008.

RESOURCES

National Sleep Foundation: http://www.sleepfoundation.org
Sleep Research Society: http://www.sleepresearchsociety.org

CROSS REFERENCES

Behavioral Determinants of Health

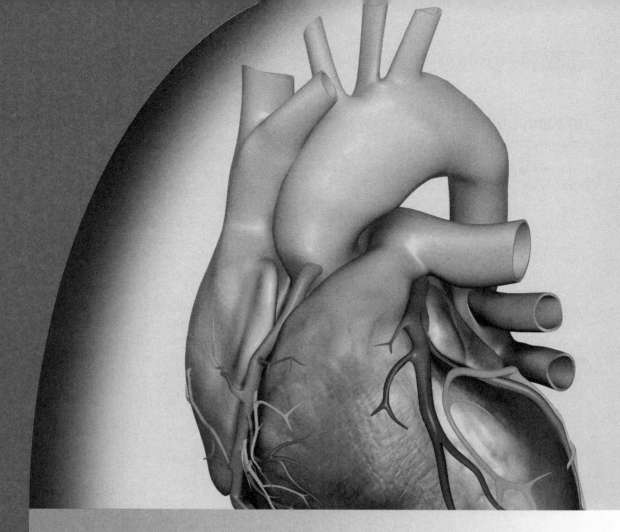

PART **VI**

Skills and Tools of Public Health

INTRODUCTION

Constance Battle

It is a very sad thing that nowadays there is so little useless information.

—Oscar Wilde
Irish dramatist, novelist, poet (1854–1900)

Analysis of the national public health workforce is difficult to achieve. It is clear, however, that critical healthcare shortages exist in some areas and that there is increasing national demand for education in public health. Although the resulting shortage crises are more pronounced in developing countries, the developed world is also unable to produce enough workers to keep up with escalating demand. To build a sustainable, capable public health system, public health workers must learn to adapt to the changing landscape. For all levels of health pro-fessionals, including healthcare providers and public health workers, learning new information search skills and health communication strategies and integrating information technology into existing workflow will be critical. The following two chapters will help students develop the basic professional skills needed to become productive contributors to the evolving world of health care. The first chapter addresses information search approaches, a skill that is ever harder to master given the unfettered growth of new health-related information, some of it poor. This chapter will help you learn how to search, sort, and understand the mass of health-related information currently available as you try to become health literate. The second chapter on communication will help you to learn how to interact with and to educate consumers as they too struggle to become health literate, a difficult task given the overwhelming amount of information.

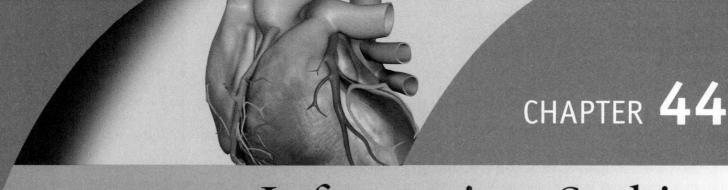

CHAPTER 44

Information-Seeking Strategies in Public Health

Cynthia Kahn
Elaine Sullo

> Of all the sciences, public health has the most diversity: diversity in its subject matter, its audience, and its workforce, and therefore, its information needs.[1,2]

LEARNING OBJECTIVES

By the end of this chapter, the student will be able to:

- Recognize the value of information in public health.
- Identify challenges in using information professionally: information overload, information literacy, bias in the literature, and the multidisciplinary nature of public health.
- Distinguish between the levels of information sources—primary, secondary, and tertiary—and the resources available to obtain appropriate information.
- Locate and critically appraise the literature, especially non-scholarly sources.
- Construct Internet and databases searches.

INTRODUCTION

This chapter illustrates the importance of information-seeking strategies for the public health student and practitioner. Information is everywhere; we are constantly inundated from newspapers, magazines, and books to advertisements on radio and television, and even gossip. Consequently, the professional public health practitioner needs to cultivate the appropriate skills for finding and assessing information, as it is an attribute of efficient, high-quality practice.

This chapter presents both theoretical and practical information. Context aids in understanding and, therefore, systems of information organization will be explained along with an overview of how information is created. The challenges that the current systems present are explained as are tips and ideas for getting around these issues. Once an overview of the information environment is presented, an in-depth look at using them is offered. How do you choose the correct database to find information that addresses your question? Will one database provide the information or will you have to use several? Practical advice on database selection is one component; examples on effectively searching databases and using **search engines** will also be provided. To begin, a list of definitions is provided.

WHAT DO WE MEAN BY "PROFESSIONAL USE OF INFORMATION"?

The opening statement is about the importance of finding information. Are you thinking about Google (http://www.google.com) or Wikipedia (http://en.wikipedia.org) right now? Well, you are not alone. Recent statistics reveal that users conduct more than 91 million searches *per day* in Google. Furthermore, when the top seven search engines are added together, there are 231 million searches conducted in the United States each day. Wikipedia is similarly popular. The number of Wikipedia articles has grown from 19,700 in 2002 to 1,560,000 in 2007. So, yes, there is information on the **Internet**, and yes, lots of people know how to access that information. Unfortunately, for academic and professional work, a search engine may not be the right option.

Search engines, such as Google, search the "free" **World Wide Web**. For the most part, this refers to Web pages published by companies, organizations, and individuals. Scholarly information is published in peer-reviewed journals. Because most journal publishers charge subscription fees to access their materials, you will not find their articles freely available on the Web. In fact, it has been estimated that only about 7 percent of what you might find on the free Web is suitable for academic or professional work.

Metamend, a company that bills itself as search engine marketing experts, infer from the number of Web hosts that there are 171 billion pages of content on the Web. This is one example of the challenge Eppler and Mengis call "information overload." They define *information overload* as a term "often used to convey the simple notion of receiving too much information."[3] How else do we feel inundated by information? Here are some general examples:

1. an increase in the number of television and cable channels (over 600 channels)
2. an explosion of Web pages
3. search engine results which number in the millions
4. exposure to commercials and advertising. American corporations spend over $15 billion yearly on marketing to children; the average American child sees about 40,000 television commercials every year.[4]
5. piles of newspapers, magazines, and journals waiting to be read
6. daily intrusion of telecommunications such as e-mail, cell phones, personal digital assistants (PDAs), instant messages

There are negative consequences to information overload, namely, a possible decrease in a person's ability to make good decisions (Figure 44-1). This is manifested by a person's diffi-

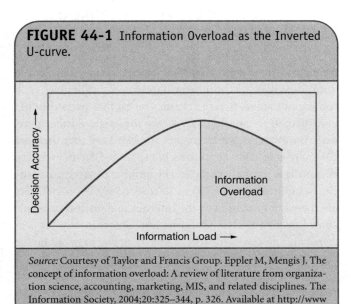

FIGURE 44-1 Information Overload as the Inverted U-curve.

Source: Courtesy of Taylor and Francis Group. Eppler M, Mengis J. The concept of information overload: A review of literature from organization science, accounting, marketing, MIS, and related disciplines. The Information Society, 2004;20:325–344, p. 326. Available at http://www.informaworld.com. Accessed May 16, 2008.

culty "in identifying the relevant information, becoming highly selective and ignoring a large amount of information, having difficulties in identifying the relationship between details and the overall perspective, needing more time to reach a decision, and finally not reaching a decision of adequate accuracy."[5]

In the professional literature for medicine and public health, information overload is a similar problem. Here are examples for medicine and public health:

1. Medical knowledge doubles every six to eight years with new medical procedures emerging every day.[6]
2. Public health is both interdisciplinary and multidisciplinary, making information volume and access a challenge.
3. A Google search on *public health* brings up 448,000,000 results.
4. A search on *public health* as a subject heading in MEDLINE results in 3,513,435 citations.
   a. *The National Library of Medicine currently reports that MEDLINE contains bibliographic citations and author abstracts from more than 5,000 biomedical journals published in the United States and 80 other countries.* The database contains over 15 million citations dating back to the mid-1950s.[7] *These numbers compound when other health databases such as CINAHL (Cumulative Index of Nursing and Allied Health Literature) or PsycINFO are included, even when overlap is considered.*

INFORMATION LITERACY

In an era when today's truths become tomorrow's outdated concepts, individuals who are unable to gather pertinent information are equally as illiterate as those who are unable to read or write.

E. Gordon Gee and Patricia Senn Breivik
Libraries and Learning, 1987[8]

The traditional measures of literacy are reading and writing. In addition to these, **computer** and **digital literacy** is required for today's graduates. The practical skills showcased at the end of the chapter—selecting the right database(s) to search, utilizing the steps for a successful search, and conducting effective Internet research—are an aspect of computer and digital literacy. Putting these concepts together provides the broad understanding of what information literacy is, namely, a person's ability to effectively find and evaluate answers to questions using a variety of information resources. These skills are important; they not only enable the public health student or practitioner to deal with information overload, but done right, they are the cornerstone of successful evidence-based practice.

Example: When asked to write a grant proposal to the Bill and Melinda Gates Foundation, the information illiterate goes to Google, finds the Bill and Melinda Gates Foundation Web site and takes at face value what the Foundation says about itself. In contrast, the information literate accesses the library online and searches a variety of databases. The path of the information literate will go from business and management information (such as *Hoover's Company Records*), to read an unbiased company record, to news sources in broad databases such as ProQuest Research Library, Lexis-Nexis or Scopus, and finally, to the research databases, including Global Health and MEDLINE, to assess the types of projects funded by the Foundation and the science generated from the research.

Have you heard the term **evidence-based medicine**? It is a widely used term that most people do not understand. Essentially, evidence-based medicine is decision-making based on scientific reasoning and systematic uses of data and information systems. While evidence-based medicine refers specifically to the clinical environment, the practice has expanded to other fields: **evidence-based public health**, evidence-based nursing, evidence-based librarianship, evidence-based management, etc. Done right, the evidence-based model is not ANY use of the literature; it is the use of evaluated, reproducible evidence. O'Neal and Brownson note that the "increasing technical sophistication of public health problems and approaches emphasizes the importance for an evidence-based approach to developing policy and interventions."[9]

In fact, the problems and approaches that public health practitioners deal with were categorized into essential public health services by a steering committee that included representatives from U.S. Public Health Service agencies and other major public health organizations. There are three broad categories of services: assessment, policy development, and assurance. Every one of these categories and subsequent interventions are all dependent on appropriate use of information. The public health workforce has an especially critical need for information seeking skills (Figure 44-2).

The Essential Public Health Services

1. Monitor health status to identify and solve community health problems.
2. Diagnose and investigate health problems and health hazards in the community.
3. Inform, educate, and empower people about health issues.

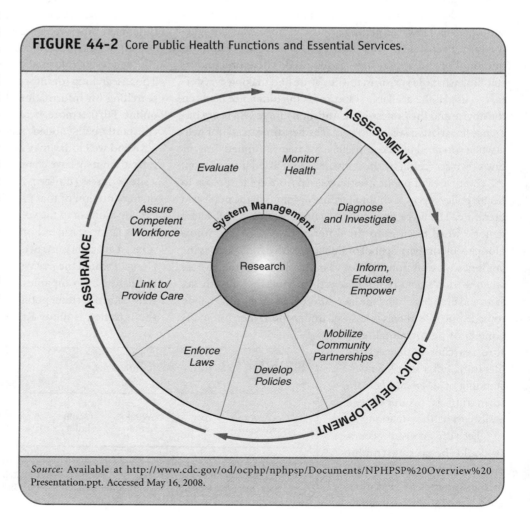

FIGURE 44-2 Core Public Health Functions and Essential Services.

Source: Available at http://www.cdc.gov/od/ocphp/nphpsp/Documents/NPHPSP%20Overview%20Presentation.ppt. Accessed May 16, 2008.

4. Mobilize community partnerships and action to identify and solve health problems.

5. Develop policies and plans that support individual and community health efforts.

6. Enforce laws and regulations that protect health and ensure safety.

7. Link people to needed personal health services and assure the provision of healthcare when otherwise unavailable.

8. Assure competent public and personal healthcare workforce.

9. Evaluate effectiveness, accessibility, and quality of personal and population-based health services.

10. Research for new insights and innovative solutions to health problems.

Are you curious, persistent, analytical, and thoughtful? These traits are required for public health work and are also traits needed in information seeking. An inquisitive mind and an active desire to learn and to know are the attributes of a curious person. However, getting answers is not always straightforward. Persistence—not taking answers at face-value but questioning and appraising—is required. Therefore, understanding what **bias** exists in the literature and making every effort to use all the available resources is the difference between the novice and the professional. And, don't forget, there are reference librarians available to help. The best time to ask for help is when you need to be comprehensive, there is limited time, or one's own searching has not revealed the needed information.

Every area of public health research from epidemiology to health policy report their findings and opinions in the published literature. The literature, though, is not one-size-fits-all, and a generic word to sum up the differences is *bias*. The Johns Hopkins Bloomberg School of Public Health defines bias as the amount we are off from the true value. It asks: how wrong we are when we don't get it right?[10] From the perspective of study design, and even of reading the literature, bias is a well-understood topic.[11] The role of bias is less well understood when put in the context of performing literature searches and accessing literature, but a simple understanding of *when and how* information is produced can easily correct the situation.

Let's say an event occurs. It could be a catastrophic event, such as September 11th or the tsunamis of December 2004, although it does not have to be traumatic. Information about the event is created and disseminated, and the passage of time—or when information is produced in relation to the event—as well as the medium, can tell you a lot about the quality of the information (Figure 44-3 and Table 44-1). What can you expect to find the closer you are to an event?

When closer to the event itself, the information provided is simple: who, what, when. Typical **sources** are social networks (**blogs** or **Wikis**) or news sources (cable news websites); both are available through the World Wide Web (Web).

As more time passes, the type of author changes from those with little or no expertise to professionals, experts, and scholars. Further, bias is limited through the use of **peer review**, footnotes, and bibliographies. So, what you find at the other end of the spectrum—years after the event has occurred—is true research being produced and disseminated.

WORLD WIDE WEB

One of the advantages of using the Web is its scope; the fact that such a wealth of information is available anywhere at any time makes the Web an attractive resource. There is no one person or organization that controls the Web or its content and, as a result, information is unorganized and unstructured. Those searching for information on the Web can spend hours searching for information that may or may not be available online. Furthermore, because the Web is organic—content is constantly being added, removed, or changed—a site that is alive and well today may not be in existence tomorrow, or information may have changed or been deleted. Careful note of a site's address (uniform resource locator [URL]) can provide documentation of that page for reference.

In addition to the volatile nature of the Web, quality control is lacking. Anyone, anywhere, with any qualifications or none at all, can construct a Web page. Search engines (such as Google) search the *free* Web, which includes mostly Web pages published by companies, organizations, and individuals. A well-known cartoon published in the *New Yorker* quipped, "On the Internet, Nobody Knows You're a Dog."[12] The cartoon

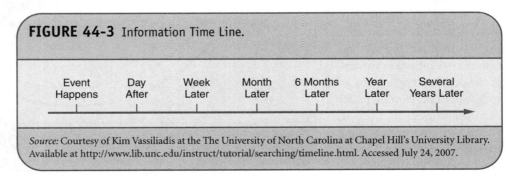

FIGURE 44-3 Information Time Line.

Event Happens	Day After	Week Later	Month Later	6 Months Later	Year Later	Several Years Later

Source: Courtesy of Kim Vassiliadis at the The University of North Carolina at Chapel Hill's University Library. Available at http://www.lib.unc.edu/instruct/tutorial/searching/timeline.html. Accessed July 24, 2007.

TABLE 44-1 Information Time Line

Time	Source(s)	Type of Information/Audience	Author(s)
Event Happens	News sources, like newspapers, news Web sites, and radio and television broadcasts	General: who, what, where	Journalists or writers who may or may not have any expertise in the article's topic
Week Later	Popular magazines and other sources of news	General	Journalists or writers who may or may not have any expertise in the article's topic
One Month Later	Professional magazines and more in-depth news reports and analyses	Professional; scholarly	Practitioners or professionals who have at least some background in or experience with the topics.
Six Months Later	Professional journals and conference proceedings	Researchers or experts (are peer-reviewed, contain citations, bibliographies)	Practitioners or professionals
One Year Later	Books, government reports, and articles in scholarly journals	Researchers or experts	Researchers, scholars, or practitioners who are considered experts in their field
Several Years Later	Scholarly books and journal articles, and even reference works	Researchers or experts	Researchers, scholars, or practitioners who are considered experts in their field

refers to the anonymous nature of the Web. As a Web user, care must be taken to verify an author's background, qualifications, authority in a certain subject area, expertise, etc.

Many online resources are more current than their print counterparts. When you consider the amount of time consumed in writing a textbook, editing, revising, and then printing, publishing on the Web is advantageous because items can be updated instantaneously and continuously. Although the Web is useful for finding current information, please do not assume that documents and Web pages have been updated or revised in some time. It is important to note the date that a site or document was created, along with a date the page was revised. Any page lacking such information should be used with extreme caution.

With the amount of material available—even freely available—and the fact that it is quick and easy to use, it is tempting to simply turn to the Web for research needs. Because you are now aware that information on the Web can be extremely biased, you will be more *discerning* and *critical* of what you find and how it is used.

GREY LITERATURE

A format that is often overlooked is **grey literature**. This format is noteworthy for public health—an interdisciplinary pro-

fession—because significant public health information is generated through academic, governmental, and nonprofit organizations. Grey literature is defined as literature that is *not* produced or distributed by commercial publishers. It can be in the form of program reports, newsletters, conference proceedings, meeting notes and abstracts, interviews, data sets, policy briefs, and other formats.

This type of information is not usually indexed by databases as it is not published by scholarly journals, and often the Web is the only place grey literature is available. Due to its volume, diversity, and nontraditional formats, the greatest challenge involved with grey literature is identification. There is limited indexing and acquisition by libraries, so only the persistent public health student or worker will be aware that grey literature exists and make every effort to find relevant sources.

Noteworthy collections or gateways of grey literature exist, such as The New York Academy of Medicine (NYAM) Library, which catalogs grey literature from more than 175 organizations and publishes them in the online *Grey Literature Report* on a quarterly basis (available at http://www.nyam.org/library/pages/grey_literature_report. Accessed May 15, 2008).

Not only is the NYAM Library collecting these items and making them available for their clients, but they are paving the way for other libraries to collect and catalog in this area as well.[13] Despite the difficulties in identifying and accessing grey literature, pubic health students and practitioners must keep in mind the importance of these resources as it enables them to learn and build on the activities and research of other professionals in the field, provides examples of successful assessments or interventions to their stakeholders or constituents, and provides support for policy and decision making.[14]

THE MEDLINE DATABASE

MEDLINE, maintained by the National Library of Medicine (NLM), is the most widely used database for searching the biomedical literature; this database contains over 15 million references to journal articles in biomedicine and health, but also has broad coverage of public health, health policy development, behavior sciences, and others. Most publications indexed for MEDLINE are scholarly journals, with coverage going back to the 1950s.[15] MEDLINE is available through several commercial vendors, such as OVID, or is free to the public via PubMed. Public health students typically have access to MEDLINE through their university library's subscription or they can access PubMed on the Web at http://www.pubmed.gov.

CASE STUDIES

As noted earlier, each essential public health services category—assessment, assurance, and policy development—is an information-intensive activity. The following case studies, representing each of these categories, give examples of the use of information by public health professionals. The first case study illustrates an assessment activity. It profiles the U.S. Public Health Service in the 1950s when it began looking for a link between tobacco and health. Assurance is the focus of the second case study. A more recent topic, this case study is from the late 1990s when researchers sought to ameliorate the correlation of low educational attainment and infant mortality by using appropriate interventions. The final case study illustrates the use of information in health policy using the development of a smallpox vaccination policy as its topic.

CASE #1. ASSESSMENT: TOBACCO AND HEALTH

Dr. Leroy E. Burney was Surgeon General of the U.S. Public Health Service from 1956 to 1961. During his tenure, he was aware of a growing body of research examining the effect of tobacco smoke on human health. The research consistently showed an association between cigarette smoking and lung cancer and other forms of morbidity. Under the auspices of the United States Surgeon General, a scientific study group, sponsored by the National Cancer Institute, the National Heart Institute, the American Cancer Society, and the American Heart Association, was organized in June 1956. The purpose of the group was to review the problem and to recommend further avenues of research.

The seven members of the study group, led by biochemist Dr. Frank M. Strong, Professor of Biochemistry, University of Wisconsin, held six two-day conferences to review what was known about the effects of tobacco smoking on human health. To achieve this objective, the group was comprehensive in its investigation. They examined the published literature, unpublished literature, and consulted with experts. The bibliography to the study group's report—"Joint Report on Smoking and Health"—included 76 references. Not only did it contain a large number of references, but there was also a significant amount of depth to what was included. For example, the references spanned 31 years (1926–1957, when the report was published), and included English and non-English language publications, unpublished data as well as human and animal studies. After reviewing the available evidence for the reader, the study group concluded: "the sum total of scientific evidence establishes beyond a reasonable doubt that cigarette smoking is a causative factor in the rapidly increasing incidence of human epidermoid carcinoma of the lung."

The "Joint Report" was published on June 7, 1957, in the journal *Science*. Not long after, Dr. Burney issued a statement titled "Smoking and Lung Cancer." In his statement, Dr. Burney said, "the Public Health Service is deeply concerned with the increasing death rate from lung cancer in the United States and in other parts of the world." The numbers were striking. The death rate from lung cancer for white males had risen from 3.8 per 100,000 population in 1930 to 31.0 in 1956, a 715 percent increase in the incidence of lung cancer in 26 years. Dr. Burney concluded his statement by saying, "it is a statutory responsibility of the Public Health Service to inform members of the medical profession and the public on all matters relating to important public health issues. The relationship between smoking and lung cancer constitutes such an issue and falls with the responsibility of the Public Health Service."

The goals of assessment services in public health are to monitor health status to identify and solve community health problems; diagnose and investigate health problems and health hazards in the community; and inform, educate, and empower people about health issues. Certainly, the work done by Dr. Burney as the U.S. Surgeon General and the identification and quantification of the problem by the U.S. Public Health Service and the Study Group are evidence of these activities. The importance of information-seeking skills and access to the literature is clear in this case.

CASE #2. ASSURANCE: PARENTAL LOW LITERACY AND INFANT MORTALITY

Syracuse Healthy Start (SHS) is a federally funded initiative run by the Onondaga County Health Department. The goal of SHS is to prevent infant mortality and reduce racial and ethnic disparity in birth outcomes. In 1997, the group received a Healthy Start grant from the Health Resources and Services Administration (HRSA). With this grant, SHS sought to implement a set of evidence-based interventions to address parental low literacy as a risk factor for infant mortality.

Creation of evidence-based interventions required local data analysis, published study review, material assessment, programmatic intervention initiation, and outcome evaluation. Efforts to analyze local data included a review of epidemiological data on adult literacy, maternal education, and infant mortality from the New York State Vital Records and the Literacy Coalition of Onondaga County. In considering all births in Syracuse from 1996 to 1997, mothers with only a high school education or less was the leading risk factor for infant death. Review of published studies on the topic, conducted over a two-year period, was done by searching MEDLINE, and the review revealed that information distributed by healthcare providers must be easy to read, of a literacy level that is common to most consumers, and culturally relevant to the population at hand. The SHS staff members were also in contact with researchers and consultants who had experience in this area; for example, Sue Stableford, the Director of the University of New England's AHEC Health Literacy Center, was a consultant to SHS and a resource for this project. Current health education materials that are given to pregnant women were analyzed and evaluated according to three predetermined criteria. Of these documents, 78.5 percent were above the seventh-grade reading level, while 100 percent were above the sixth-grade reading level.

Interventions by the SHS to ameliorate the correlation of low educational attainment and infant mortality consisted of five strategies/programs including: 1) provision of written health materials; 2) health education; 3) initiatives to ensure that adolescents complete school; 4) screening and referral of parents to adult literacy programs; and 5) increased paternal involvement. SHS conducted an evaluation of these interventions for all births in Syracuse from 2000 to 2001 and found that participation in these programs resulted in lower post-neonatal deaths for infants whose mothers had with fewer than twelve years of education. Overall, these findings suggest that the evidence-based initiatives in place are effective in reducing infant mortality for this group.[16]

CASE #3. POLICY DEVELOPMENT: A MODEL FOR A SMALLPOX VACCINATION POLICY

Due to recent global and national events, bioterrorism is a frightening, yet real threat and as such, discussion has been ensuing regarding the reintroduction of the smallpox vaccine. To inform the debate regarding a smallpox-vaccination policy for the United States, seven researchers came together in 2002 and developed six possible scenarios of smallpox attacks, while considering potential threats, and produced a mathematical model that describes policy effects based on estimated parameters. The researchers then identified and analyzed the probability of attack and assessed the trade-offs between vaccination-related harms and benefits.

Researchers wanted to develop detailed, realistic scenarios for smallpox bioterrorist attacks and therefore needed to identify literature on the smallpox vaccine, the natural history of smallpox, and the spread of smallpox after World War II in Europe and North America, as the social structure, health status, and population immunity during this time period may have been similar to that of the current United States population. Researchers used several databases for their search, including the National Library of Medicine's LOCATORplus, MEDLINE, EMBASE, BIOSIS, the Cochrane Collaboration, and the Defense Technical Information Center. Based on the literature, researchers identified 25 smaller and 20 larger outbreaks of smallpox after World War II, explored relationships between reproductive rate and outbreak, identified three patterns of the spread of smallpox, and developed significant assumptions about the natural history of smallpox.

Based on this literature review, researchers built a "multipart policy model" that took into account potential threats, predicted the number of deaths with the use of various measures to control the spread of smallpox, and highlighted the consequences of various policies. The researchers noted that based on their models, a smallpox-vaccination policy must be based on judgments about the probability of an attack and on the recognition that the probability may be increased by military engagements abroad or decreased by preparedness at home.

Researchers represented the RAND Center for Domestic and International Health Security, Santa Monica, California, and Arlington, Virginia; the Center for Research in Patient-Oriented Care, Veterans Affairs San Diego Healthcare System and the University of California, San Diego; and Erasmus University, Rotterdam, the Netherlands.

SEARCHING THE LITERATURE

Hopefully, you are now feeling empowered to conduct expert searches to meet your educational and professional obligations. You now know the theory behind the creation and dissemination of information as well as how to determine its bias and value. This section takes a turn from discussing what it is to presenting practical skills for finding and using public health information. Answers to public health questions are found across a multiplicity of disciplines, such as education, psychology, and medicine, and in a range of source material: primary, secondary, and tertiary. By learning the fundamentals of searching you will know where to search, have a better idea of what you need, and, most importantly, be able to apply this skill in a multidisciplinary setting.

STEPS IN BIBLIOGRAPHIC DATABASE SEARCHING

There are seven steps used to conduct an effective database search. The steps are listed, and an example, using each of the steps, follows:

1. Define the topic.
2. Select database or databases to search (Table 44-2).
3. Choose search topics: keywords and controlled vocabulary.
4. Perform individual searches and combine terms.
5. Apply limits to retrieved results.
6. Review results (read and evaluate).
7. Select the results that will best answer the question.

An Example
Cardiovascular Disease Prevention in Women

1. Define the topic.
   I am interested in researching cardiovascular disease prevention in women. I would like to find primary and secondary sources of a scholarly value.
2. Select databases to search.
   Primary sources: Census, Centers for Disease Control and Prevention (CDC), NYAM Grey Literature.
   Secondary sources: MEDLINE, CINAHL, Library Catalog.
3. Choose search topics: key words and controlled vocabulary.
   Concept 1: Cardiovascular Diseases
   Concept 2: Women or Women's Health
   Concept 3: Prevention or Public Health or Community
4. Perform individual searches and combine terms. In this example, the search was conducted in the MEDLINE database (Figure 44-4).

TABLE 44-2 Database Suggestions by Format

Source	Database
News Sources	Ethnic News Watch
	Factiva
	Lexis-Nexis Academic Universe
	National Journal Policy Central
Popular Magazines	EBSCOHost Academic Search Premier
	EBSCOHost Business Source Premier
	Lexis-Nexis Academic Universe
	ProQuest ABI/Inform
	ProQuest Research Library
Scientific, Technical, or Medical Professional, and Scholarly Articles	MEDLINE
	Global Health
	OSH-ROM (Occupational Safety and Health)
	PsycINFO
	Scopus
Books and Reference Materials	Library Catalog
	OCLC Worldcat

5. Apply limits to retrieved results. This example limits the search results to English language, humans, and the years "2000–2007."
6. Review the results. There are 36 results matching the search terms and limits applied. For most articles, the bibliographic information (author, title, source) and the abstract are available. For some, the full text is linked as well.
7. Select the results that will best answer the question. Here are results to consider:
   • Jilcott SB, Keyserling TC, Samuel-Hodge CD, Rosamond W, Garcia B, Will JC, Farris RP, Ammerman AS. Linking clinical care to community resources for cardiovascular disease prevention: the North Carolina Enhanced WISEWOMAN project. *J Women Health* 2006;15:569–583.
   • Rosenfeld AG. State of the heart: building science to improve women's cardiovascular health. [Review] *Commun Nurs Res* 2006;39:33–50.

FIGURE 44-4 Medline Database.

#	Search History	Results	Display
1	Cardiovascular Diseases/	52792	DISPLAY
2	Women/	10281	DISPLAY
3	Women's Health/	11532	DISPLAY
4	Primary Prevention/	8798	DISPLAY
5	Public Health/	40122	DISPLAY
6	Community Health Planning/	3142	DISPLAY
7	1 and (2 or 3) and (4 or 5 or 6)	44	DISPLAY

Combine Searches   Delete Searches   Save Search/Alert

8	Limit 7 to (english language and humans and yr = "2000 – 2007")	36	DISPLAY

Source: © Ovid Technologies. New York: WoltersKluwer Health. Reprinted with permission of Ovid Technologies.

- Roberts BH, Thompson PD. Is there evidence for the evidence-based guidelines for cardiovascular disease prevention in women? [Review] *Gender Med* 2006;3:5–12.
- Albright C, Thompson DL. The effectiveness of walking in preventing cardiovascular disease in women: a review of the current literature. [Review] *J Womens Health* 2006;15:271–280.
- Yngve A, Hambraeus L, Lissner L, Serra Majem L, Vaz de Almeida MD, Berg C, Hughes R, Cannon G, Thorsdottir I, Kearney J. Gustafsson JA, Rafter J, Elmadfa I, Kennedy N. The Women's Health Initiative. What is on trial: nutrition and chronic disease? Or misinterpreted science, media havoc and the sound of silence from peers? *Public Health Nutr* 2006;9:269–272.

From a search of CDC National Center for Health Statistics (NCHS), two reports were identified that provide excellent primary data for researching this question.[17]

- United States Centers for Disease Control and Prevention. Health, United States, 2006 contains information about the population, on women's health (even specific to women's health and cardiovascular risk factors such as cholesterol, cigarette smoking, and hypertension).
- Barnes, Patricia. Physical activity among adults: United States, 2000 and 2005.

From a search of the library catalog, two books were identified that would be helpful in answering this research question.

- Goldman MB, Hatch MC. *Women and Health*. San Diego: Academic Press; 2000.
- Douglas PS. *Cardiovascular Health and Disease in Women*, 2nd ed. Philadelphia: W.B. Saunders; 2002.

STEPS TO SUCCESSFUL INTERNET RESEARCH

In addition to database searching, many students and practitioners now turn to information on the Web. There are steps to an effective Internet search just as we saw there are steps to an effective database search. Before you begin searching, you will want to ask yourself an important question: *Is the Web the right tool for your research topic?* Remember, only a small amount of professional, scholarly, or scientific information is available through the free Web. Depending on what type of information you are searching for, would a textbook or journal article be better suited to your needs?

1. *Use the appropriate search tool.* Consider that the use of search engines, meta-search engines, and directories may result in different results. Learning the differences between each type of search tool will allow you to search more efficiently. You may also decide to search more than one search engine and compare the results.

2. *Use appropriate search techniques.* This step is the most important in differentiating between a novice search and an experienced searcher. As with a searching a database, it is important to be familiar with the search engine's interface and rules of use. For example, is the search engine case sensitive? Can you limit your search to a certain domain, such as *.edu*? Can you use quotation marks to search for a phrase?

3. *Use the correct Boolean operators.* Search engines are built and maintained by vastly different companies that are often competitors. Therefore, they do not all look or work the same. Becoming an effective Internet searcher requires some familiarity with how the search engine works, so that you know what operators are allowed and recognized. For example, Google automatically inserts AND in between search terms. So if you include AND in your search, Google will tell you, "The 'AND' operator is unnecessary—we include all search terms by default." Most search engines have a "help" or "about" section that will explain how to construct effective searches.

4. *Evaluate search results.* Thinking critically about any information you use in a professional or academic environment is a necessity, and even more so when finding information on the Web. Be sure to consider the authority, bias, currency, design, and evaluate the sites you review.[18]

EVALUATING INTERNET RESOURCES

A—Authority

Who wrote the information? What are their credentials?
Are the information sources cited? Are these reliable sources?
Check domain (.gov, .org, or .edu versus .com)

B—Bias

Who sponsors the site? Do they have a financial interest? Is there a conflict of interest?
Are there ads present? Can you identify them as ads?

C—Currency

When was the information published? Updated?
More important in some areas (legislation, drug information) than in others (developmental milestones, anatomy)

D—Design

Is it easy to navigate the Web site?
Is the information well organized?
Are all the links working and current?

E—Evaluate

Is the information clear and easy to understand?
In English (or another language you read)?
Is the information fact or opinion?
Compare with another reliable source.
Cite your sources.

CONCLUSION

This chapter illustrates the importance of information to the public health field from theoretical and practical perspectives. The chapter presented terminology and concepts such as Boolean operators that are essential for developing effective strategies to search for information. In addition, a discussion of information overload and the challenges of finding quality information in an Internet environment were presented. The essential public health services and examples of information use in each categories—assurance, assessment, and policy development—were described. Once the theory of information use encompassing information overload, bias, the Internet, and the multi-disciplinary nature of public health were understood, practice skill-building examples and exercises were presented. The development of information-seeking skill is crucial to one's ability to work in public health. It is a foundation upon which competency is based. It is an art and a science and requires curiosity, questioning, flexibility in thinking as well as persistence and analysis in practice.

KEY TERMS

Bias: A systematic error that occurs in a study and leads to a distorted result. Examples of bias are selection bias, information bias, or confounding factors.[19]

Bibliographic Database: An electronic version of a catalog or index; allows the user to identify publications by author, subject, title, or other search terms. It generally provides at least a full citation to the item, and often other information such as abstracts, assigned subject headings, and sometimes the full text. Examples of bibliographic databases include MEDLINE, CINAHL, Academic Search Premier, and Scopus.

Blogs: Short for Web log, a Web page that serves as a publicly accessible personal journal for an individual; are frequently updated and often reflect the personality of the author. A typical blog combines text, images, and links to other blogs, Web pages, and other media related to its topic.

Boolean Operators: Named after the British mathematician, George Frederick Boole (1815–1864), who developed a system of logic to show the relationship among terms or concepts. There are three primary Boolean operators (AND, OR, and NOT) and they can be used to group search terms when conducting a literature search (Figure 44-5).

Computer Literacy: A familiarity with computing concepts and the ability to use common applications.

Digital Literacy: The productive use of the Internet to present, access, and use information.

Evidence-Based Medicine: The conscientious, explicit, and judicious use of current best evidence in making decisions about the care of individual patients. "The practice of evidence-based medicine means integrating individual clinical expertise with the best available external clinical evidence from systematic research."[20]

Evidence-Based Public Health: Effectively finding and evaluating answers to questions about populations and disease or health.

Grey Literature: Material disseminated outside of the traditional peer-reviewed journal or scholarly book. Examples include conference papers, newsletters, research reports, and position papers. As some researchers do not submit their work to scholarly journals, grey literature may be the only source in which their research can be located.[21]

Information Literacy: A set of abilities requiring individuals to recognize when information is needed and have the ability to locate, evaluate, and use effectively the needed information.

Internet: A vast infrastructure connecting computers and networks around the world.

Peer Review: Refers to a journal's policy of having experts in a given field examine a submitted article before accepting it for publication. This process assures that only high quality articles based on sound research that offer a significant contribution to the field are included for publication in the journal.[22]

Search Engine: Used to find Web pages and information from the free Web on the Internet about a particular subject. "Free Web" pages are published by companies, organizations, and individuals. Unlike a database, it is an unstructured environment.

Sources: Works (source book, data, document, material, study) that supply information or evidence.

Primary Sources are the "raw data" of public health research. Data are collected on the population at all levels (local, state, and national) in order to assess, assure, and plan for the health of the nation.

Secondary Sources are research reports. A review article, for example, is a secondary source.

Tertiary Sources are based on secondary sources. They synthesize and explain research.

Wikis: A Web site that allows visitors to easily add, remove, and otherwise edit available content. Any user can edit the site content, including other users' contributions, using a regular Web browser.

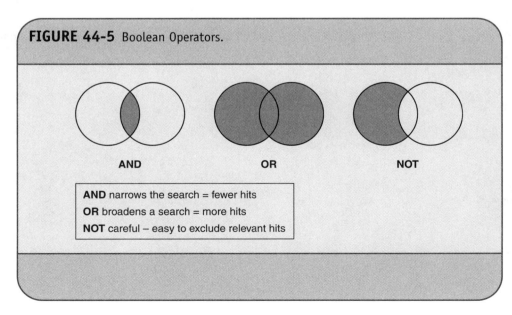

FIGURE 44-5 Boolean Operators.

AND   OR   NOT

AND narrows the search = fewer hits
OR broadens a search = more hits
NOT careful – easy to exclude relevant hits

World Wide Web (Web or WWW): One of the avenues information is disseminated over the Internet; a way of accessing information via the hypertext transfer protocol (http), utilizing browsers to access Web pages through hyperlinks. When users turn to the Web for information, they do so for many reasons. However, the simple act of "googling" a term to an inexperienced searcher could result in thousands or even millions of results to sift through. A discussion of this medium is the key to using this resource to its most effective advantage.

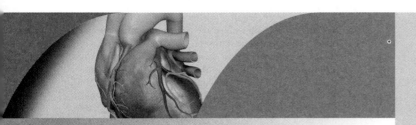

Questions for Further Research, Study, Reflection, and Discussion

For the Individual Student

In order to answer these questions, it may be necessary to research the primary literature.

- Define *information overload*. Give a general example and an example specific to public health.
- Explain the difference between what you find when using a search engine versus a database.
- Describe the steps required to conduct a successful Internet research.

For Small Group Discussion

- Pick a public health topic of your choice, perhaps one of the leading health indicators defined in the Healthy People 2010 project of the CDC. Using a Web search engine, find several Web sites on the topic. Discuss your evaluation of these sites for use in academic or professional work.
- Talk about sources of information—Web, news sources, magazines, journals, books—and the level of bias (from little or no review to peer review) that can be expected. How does this impact the range of resources you would consult to conduct professional or academic work?

For Entire Class Discussion

- Using the search engine of your choice, find Web sites related to pandemic flu and discuss your evaluation of these sites for use in academic or professional work.
- Pick a public health service area (assurance, assessment, policy development) and discuss the primary, secondary, and tertiary sources you would expect to use for that type of work.
- Public health relies on a variety of information resources. Think about data sources and grey literature. How do these fit into creating answers to questions in public health?

EXERCISES/ACTIVITIES

- Define the terms *bias* and *evidence-based medicine*.
- Go to the library Web site and find at least two databases that are unfamiliar to you. What time period and topics can you expect to find? Do you plan to use these resources in the future?
- Create a research strategy to investigate whether high-fructose corn syrup is responsible for the obesity epidemic. Think about what material will be useful (news stories, grey literature, journal articles, books), where you will search (Web search engine, library catalog, database[s]), how you will formulate questions, and how you will evaluate the information you would find.

Healthy People 2010

Focus Area: Health Communication

Goal: Use communication strategically to improve health.

Objectives:

11-2. Improve the health literacy of persons with inadequate or marginal literacy skills.

11-3. Increase the proportion of health communication activities that include research and evaluation.

11-4. Increase the proportion of health-related World Wide Web sites that disclose information that can be used to assess the quality of the site.

REFERENCES

1. O'Carroll PW, Cahn MA, Auston I, Selden CR. Information needs in public health and health policy: results of recent studies. [Review]. *J Urban Health* 1998;75:785–793. [No abstract available. PMID: 9854240, PubMed–indexed for MEDLINE from p. 791.]

2. LaPelle NR, Luckmann R, Simpson EH, Martin ER. Identifying strategies to improve access to credible and relevant information for public health professionals: a qualitative study. *BMC Public Health* 2006;6:89. Available at http://www.biomedcentral.com/content/pdf/1471-2458-6-89.pdf. Accessed May 15, 2008. [PMID: 16597331 PubMed—indexed for MEDLINE.]

3. Eppler M, Mengis J. The concept of information overload: a review of literature from organization science, accounting, marketing, MIS, and related disciplines. [Electronic version.] *Inf Soc* 2004;20:325–344. [Retrieved 7/5/2007, from Academic Search Premier database; p. 326]

4. Linn S. *Consuming Kids: Protecting Our Children From the Onslaught of Marketing and Advertising.* New York: Anchor Books; 2005.

5. Eppler M, Mengis J. The concept of information overload: a review of literature from organization science, accounting, marketing, MIS, and related disciplines. [Electronic version.] *Information Society* 2004;20:325–344. [Retrieved 7/5/2007, from Academic Search Premier database; pp. 331, 333.]

6. Mantovani F, Castelnuovo G, Gaggioli A, Riva G. Virtual reality training for health-care professionals. [Electronic version.] *CyberPsychol Behav* 2003;6:389. [Retrieved 7/5/2007, from Academic Search Premier database.]

7. National Institutes of Health. *PubMed Overview.* (updated 2007) Available at http://www.ncbi.nlm.nih.gov/entrez/query/static/overview.html#Database%20Coverage. Accessed May 15, 2008.

8. Gee EG, Breivik PS. *Libraries and Learning.* Proceedings of the Arden House symposium, New York. (1987, March 15). [ERIC Document Reproduction Service No. ED 284 593; As quoted in Verhey, M. P. (1999). Information literacy in an undergraduate nursing curriculum: Development, implementation, and evaluation. *The Journal of Nursing Education, 38*(6), 252–259.]

9. O'Neall MA, Brownson RC. Teaching evidence-based public health to public health practitioners. [Electronic version.] *Ann Epidemiol* 2005; 15:540–544.

10. John's Hopkins Bloomberg School of Public Health. (2008) *Epidemiology—Glossary.* Available at http://www.jhsph.edu/publichealthexperts/Glossary.htm. Accessed May 15, 2008.

11. Richard Riegelman, M.D. has written *Studying a Study and Testing a Test: How to Read the Medical Evidence* (Baltimore: Lippincott Williams and Wilkins; 2000) to help those in the medical field understand the professional literature. Similar texts exist in public health. For example, Brownson RC. *Evidence Based Public Health.* Oxford, New York: Oxford University Press; 2003.

12. Steiner P. "On the Internet nobody knows you are a dog (cartoon)." *The New Yorker,* July 5, 1993;69:61.

13. The New York Academy of Medicine. Library (2004). *Grey Literature Report.* Available at http://www.nyam.org/library/pages/grey_literature_report. Accessed May 16, 2008.

14. Turner AM, Liddy ED, Bradley J, Wheatley JA. Modeling public health interventions for improved access to the grey literature. *J Med Libr Assoc* 2005;93:487–494. Available at http://www.pubmedcentral.nih.gov/tocrender.fcgi?iid=122940. Accessed May 16, 2008.

15. National Library of Medicine. *Fact sheet MEDLINE.* (Updated April 2008.) Available at http://www.nlm.nih.gov/pubs/factsheets/medline.html. Accessed May 16, 2008.

16. Levandowski BA, Sharma P, Lane SD, Webster N, Nestor AM, Cibula DA, et al. Parental literacy and infant health: an evidence-based healthy start intervention. *Health Promot Pract* 2006;7:95–102.

17. Centers for Disease Control and Prevention. *National Center for Health Statistics.* Available at http://www.cdc.gov/nchs/. Accessed May 16, 2008.

18. Cassell KA, Hiremath U. *Reference and Information Services in the 21st Century: An Introduction.* New York: Neal-Schuman Publishers; 2006.

19. Greenberg, R. S. (2005). *Medical epidemiology* (4th ed.). New York: Lange Medical Books/McGraw-Hill.

20. Sackett DL, Rosenberg WM, Gray JA, Haynes RB, Richardson WS. Evidence based medicine: What it is and what it isn't (see comment). *BMJ* 1996;312:71–72.

21. Arnold SJ, Bender VF, Brown SA. A review and comparison of psychology-related electronic resources. *Journal of Electronic Resources in Medical Libraries* 2006;3:61–80.

22. Flatley RK, Weber MA. Professional development opportunities for new academic librarians. *Journal of Academic Librarianship* 2004;30:488–492.

CROSS REFERENCE

Communicating Health Information

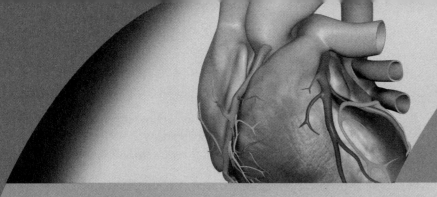

CHAPTER 45

Communicating Public Health Information

Pamela Poe

In 2003, the National Assessment of Adult Literacy (NAAL)[1] included questions to measure health literacy as part of a large national survey. Astonishingly, very few tested "proficient" at understanding and using health information.

LEARNING OBJECTIVES

By the end of this chapter, the student will be able to:

- List the four areas of communication study.
- Define the terms *health communication* and *health literacy*, and be familiar with related terms and definitions pertaining to the health communication field.
- Discuss the differences between prevention, risk, and crisis communication situations.
- Outline a basic approach to planning strategies for health communication campaigns.
- Discuss the role of health literacy and health communication in *Healthy People 2010*'s Focus Area 11 Health Communication objectives.

OVERVIEW: HEALTH LITERACY WITHIN HEALTH COMMUNICATION

The federal Department of Health and Human Services included six **health communication** objectives for the first time in its *Healthy People 2010* agenda for health objectives for the United States.[2] These six objectives covered disparate areas sharing a primary focus on some aspect of health communication and reflected concerns about Internet access and quality of health information, the quality of health communication research, healthcare provider communication skills, and efforts to improve health literacy.

The initial section of *Healthy People 2010*'s Focus Area 11 (Health Communication) defines health communication as follows:

> "Health communication encompasses the study and use of communication strategies to inform and influence individual and community decisions that enhance health. It links the domains of communication and health and is increasingly recognized as a necessary element of efforts to improve personal and public health. Health communication can contribute to all aspects of disease prevention and health promotion and is relevant in a number of contexts..."[2]

Even more simply, researcher, communication theorist, and teacher E. Rogers defined health communication as follows:

> "Health communication is any type of human communication whose content is concerned with health.... Communication is a vital ingredient in almost every form of medicine and health."[3]

Health literacy provides a way to assess how well health communication messages are understood by audiences. The targeting of messages to appropriate levels is an essential ingredient to constructing successful health communication campaigns. Improving health literacy is the goal of *Healthy People 2010*'s second objective within the health communication objectives of Focus Area 11. Health literacy may be defined as:

> The degree to which individuals have the capacity to obtain, process, and understand basic

health information and services needed to make appropriate health decisions.[2]

An understanding of health literacy principles is vital to reach diverse audiences with appropriate health communication messages and health campaign strategies. There are many quality sources of information on health literacy, and host of approaches to study, define, and address ways to improve this aspect of health communication.

The first national assessment of health literacy was developed by several federal agencies and included in a national literacy test in 2003. This test examined three types of health literacy skills and included these aspects of health literacy in the Health Literacy Component (HLC) of the 2003 National Assessment of Adult Literacy (NAAL):[1]

1. **Clinical type:** Questions addressed aspects of the process of interaction between doctors and patients, diagnosis and treatments, and clinical protocols such as medication and following health regimens.

2. **Prevention type:** Questions related to the actions people can take to maintain health such as exercise, nutrition, knowing when to seek medical care, and health screenings.

3. **Navigation of the healthcare system type:** Questions included how well test-takers could understand insurance procedures, healthcare system details, and patient rights or responsibilities under existing laws.[4]

Some questions arose during the analysis of these HLC questionaire results, which were published in detail on the Internet,[1] including how to consider those with limited or no fluency in English, and those with very limited reading ability. Ultimately, the test suggested that relatively few Americans possess the health literacy skills needed to make accurate assessments and arrive at the understandings that public health professionals may assume will result from health campaigns. If health literacy concerns are taken into account when health communication messages are constructed, this is likely to result in much more successful communication if tailored to the abilities of those intended as targets for the campaign.

Some critics of health literacy allege that testing the readability of materials by assessing grade levels (e.g., SMOG and Fry formulas)[5] may not be as useful as other means of coming to understand the power of audiences to comprehend specific health information. Simultaneously, others use these formulas to establish health literacy levels, viewing them as a vital tool. Other types of understandings or literacies that define health literacy are considered by Bernhardt and Cameron[6] to include *numeracy*, which is the ability to understand and work with numbers, *computer literacy*, that is, the ease with which con-

sumers can access health information online (also known as *e-health literacy*), and *media literacy*, the ability to be aware of and critically analyze media health messages including pictures, words, symbols and moving images.

In the *Healthy People 2010*[2] health communication objectives, Objective 11-2 specifically addresses the improvement of health literacy as a national health objective. Health literacy in this objective relates to any aspect of understanding and using health information and thereby reaching specific audiences at understandable levels.

HISTORY

Two Decades of Health Communication

In 1989, researcher Jon Nussbaum remarked in the first issue of the peer-reviewed journal *Health Communication* that, "health communication as a legitimate field of inquiry has finally arrived."[7] The addition of the *Journal of Health Communication* in 1996 further confirmed health communication as a distinct discipline. A published retrospective article in 2004 by Beck et al. suggests that the field of health communication began to emerge and be taken seriously as a discipline in the late 1980s.[8] This relatively recent field is of enormous potential benefit to the student of public health who desires to communicate effectively to patients and stakeholders.

The goals of this chapter are: 1) to define terms and aspects of health communication as it is currently being used in public health; 2) to examine a case study in which a social marketing campaign strategy was used for health communication; 3) to offer practical suggestions to use principles of health communication to construct public health campaigns and communicate messages about public health to diverse audiences; and 4) to consider the media context of current health communication efforts in an age of varied technologies, evolving digital media, and increasingly fragmented audiences.

BASIC SCIENCE FACTS/KEY CONCEPTS REVIEW

The study of communication includes:

- *interpersonal communication* between one or two individuals
- *organizational communication* within the organization or between the organization and external audiences
- *mass communication* industrialized products aimed at large public audiences
- *intrapersonal communication* messages occurring within the individual

The Field of Communication

In considering the general field of communication, it is important to begin by defining the various aspects of communication that scholars study, before addressing ways in which these areas of study relate to public health communication. We begin with the following areas of communication research:

- **Interpersonal communication** is the study of communication between a small group of two or three people, and includes attention to verbal, vocal, and nonverbal communication signals. This scholarly perspective is reflected in the study of patient and healthcare provider communication, communication between parents and children on health topics, or communication between caregivers and elderly relatives or children.
- **Organizational communication** is the study of communication practiced within organizations. Kreps and Thornton describe three types of message flow within organizations according to the organization's structure of managers and employees, including downward communication, upward communication, and horizontal communication.[9] A healthcare system such as a hospital would be concerned with the effectiveness of organizational communication to disparate external audiences or "publics" such as community partners, patients, advocacy organizations, the news media, or potential employees. Internal audiences would include clinical and administrative staff, stakeholders, and investors.
- **Mass communication** focuses on the study of communication that is mass-produced in an industrialized manner for large audiences through technological means.[10] Mass communication embraces a large area within health communication research and practice, including public health campaigns, the effects of advertising involving health products, and informational or news programming related to health. However, as the technological media landscape changes, this field is less likely to involve traditional one-way media messaging using such platforms as print, television, or radio. Interactive, Web-based and new media are increasingly included in the realm of mass communication. Researchers are facing the need to redefine terms as media usage becomes increasingly varied and interactive.
- **Mass media** (*plural of a single mass medium*) are the technological vehicles that allow mass communication messages to reach audiences. Radio, broadcast television, cable television, and Web-based or digital media are mass mediated platforms commonly used to reach audiences. The use of new media such as Webcasts, video streaming, or podcasts are increasingly included in the array of choices available for conveying these messages.
- **Intrapersonal communication** is the study of an individual's inner communication with the self. Examples of

this type of communication in relation to health would include a patient's self-talk while preparing to undergo surgery, an inner dialogue reflecting decisions about treatment options, or thought processes that precede health behaviors such as smoking cessation.

Within the general field of communication scholarship, a researcher often specializes in one of these areas. Health communication as a field of research may at times embrace multiple aspects of these communication areas.

Types of Health Communication

Public health purposes of health communication include:

- Prevention
- Risk communication
- Crisis communication

In the health communication arena, more than one communication area may be considered in light of the specific health-related research goals being studied.

Health communication can be used for a wide range of public health purposes, including prevention, risk communication, and crisis communication. **Prevention**, or disease prevention and health promotion, saves time and money by preventing disease instead of treating it later. Prevention information would most likely be targeted to audiences who may be unaware of the need for activities such as screenings, smoking cessation, or immunizations. According to Kreps and Thornton, the main goals of health promotion are to help people identify health risks, avoid them, and seek treatment if necessary.[9]

Risk communication involves the need to communicate to the public about specific health risks in a timely manner. In a communication guide for health practitioners, this definition of risk communication is used:

Risk communication is the interactive process of exchange of information and opinion among individuals, groups, and institutions. It involves providing messages about the nature of risk as well as other messages that express concerns, opinions, or reactions to risk messages.[11]

Kreps and Thornton include urgent public health crises such as West Nile virus and anthrax detection under the umbrella of risk communication, while others prefer to set aside a specific area of risk communication, with the designation of **crisis communication**. This provides a useful means of separating health communication tasks involving chronic risks to the public from those deemed urgent and in need of more rapid communication strategies.

Ultimately, it saves time to begin with a plan to strategize the nature of the risk, the needs of audiences for information, and the concerns of stakeholders. Consider these elements separately: staff plans, audience concerns, resources, target audiences, objectives, messages, strategies, time line, and evaluation.[11] Whether these or similar categories are used, the most important aspect of risk communication and in particular crisis communication is to begin with a structured plan based upon what is known, what is not yet known, and the specific information that needs to be communicated along with accurate audience targeting.

Health Communication in the New Media and the Digital Age

With the advent of interactive and new media, the rise of blogging, and other participatory media that narrowcast to specific audiences, public health professionals are facing a health communication landscape different from anything seen before. At the same time, some audiences may not be able to take full advantage of the technological opportunities available to others. The changing media landscape raises a number of questions:

- Which communication strategies that have worked before continue to work as media technology evolves?
- Will audiences be best reached via traditional media or will they require interactive involvement and nontraditional media channels?
- How can public health messages be made to stand out in an increasingly saturated media environment?
- What targeting strategies will yield the most effective results for reaching the intended audiences and stakeholders?

As communication technology continues to evolve at an astonishing rate, the emerging public health professional must keep in mind both proven health communication techniques and the need for innovative strategies. New ways to promote health messages will continue to evolve, as the consumer's use of advanced technologies changes in the social marketplace of ideas. At times, this evolution may create divisions between more and less savvy media consumers. If so, it is important to consider the best ways to define and reach each segment of the public.

KEY TERMS

Editor's Note:

Although integrating the **Key Terms** section into the text here departs from the standard chapter sequence, Dr. Poe has anchored the key concepts with critical relevant terms. Each definition serves as a window that provides a view to the field and, when taken together, they provide a useful overview of health communication.

Terms Related to Health Campaigns

Now we will examine terms relevant to the design of health communication strategies for public health awareness or behavior change. **Health campaign** (or *media campaign*) is a term often used to describe a systematic, purposeful strategy to achieve a health-related goal with an intended population. Targeted audiences, anticipated responses, and strategies used to appeal to the intended audiences are part of the planned approach of designing a health campaign.[12]

Two federal agency sources of information in the U.S. Department of Health and Human Services have provided valuable information about health campaigns and strategies: the Centers for Disease Control and Prevention (CDC)[13] and the National Cancer Institute (NCI) of the National Institutes of Health (NIH).[14]

Health Marketing or Social Marketing

Health marketing is a term developed for use by CDC[13] and is commonly referred to as **social marketing**[15] in studies on health campaign strategies. Health marketing includes "creating, communicating, and delivering health information and interventions"[13] and uses a customer-centered approach and scientific basis for developing and implementing these strategies to targeted audiences. This approach was founded on principles first used in the commercial sector and involves the use of marketing tactics that have traditionally been used to develop marketing and advertising campaigns. When applied to health-related strategic initiatives such as promoting health or preventing disease, the health marketing or social marketing approach has proved to be an effective strategy to understand audiences, develop and implement health campaigns.

The following definitions help to explain the stages of health campaign design, as summarized in the National Cancer Institute's publication, *Making Health Communication Programs Work*, which is also referred to as the "Pink Book."[14] This free publication offers detailed information of use to current and future health professionals related to designing, implementing, and evaluating health campaigns.

Formative evaluation, also known as **formative research**, is the research conducted before beginning a health campaign, in the initial stages of development. Pilot testing and pretesting are examples of using this type of research as an introductory method of beginning strategic message development.

Process evaluation or **formative research** is the research used to assess how well different aspects of the campaign are functioning during the implementation phase of a health campaign. Distribution of materials, the occurrence of program activities, and similar measures are examples of the activities used to assess the campaign during an active phase.

Outcome evaluation or **evaluative research** occurs after the completion of the campaign and is a vital research component to assess how close the campaign came to achieving its goals after completion.

Segmentation is the process of dividing the target population into subsets of individuals who are likely to share key characteristics. This strategy is used to heighten the effectiveness of social or health marketing and may reflect attention to **demographics**, which refer to characteristics of an audience segment or **psychographics** consisting of attitudes, beliefs, or opinions about an issue.

Communication strategy is a statement or document that expresses a planned process of assembling the components needed for an effective campaign. Elements of a communication strategy should include but are not limited to the following attributes: intended or target audiences, communication channels, key images, intended actions of audiences, benefits audiences will receive, and ways to convince audiences of these benefits.

Terms Related to Communication Theory and Health Behavioral Theory

The following definitions, while not specific to the design and implementation of health campaigns, are needed to understanding the underlying premises and key factors relating to the success of communication endeavors in the public health arena.

Communication theories[12] are ways to explain how communication works, that have been tested through research and added to the body of knowledge of the communication discipline. While communication theory is a vast area of research and study, one finds certain theories applicable to health communication. Each theory works with an underlying premise or series of assumptions collected and based upon prior research, which then furnish a scientific basis upon which to construct health communication campaigns. Many communication theories have relevance to the pursuit of health-related research agendas. An overview of the literature reveals a wide array of theories used as the basis for health communication studies, and while theory is not always used as the basis for this type of research, it provides a strong fundamental basis.[6]

Health behavior theories[16] are also tested by research and used as underlying bases for health communication strategies. However, these explanations of how and why people are motivated to consider and act upon intentions to change health behaviors differ from communication theories in their specific attention to predicting and understanding human behavior in response to interventions. As with communication theories, a vast number of health behavior theories have arisen over time based on research and tested in practice. These theories provide a scientific basis upon which to base effective strategic planning that builds upon the existing knowledge base of the discipline of health research.

CASE STUDY

The Canadian "Think Again" HIV/AIDS Prevention Campaign

One example of the use of social marketing strategies is the "Think Again" Canadian public health campaign.[17] This campaign was designed to promote HIV/AIDS prevention by encouraging gay men to examine assumptions about their partners and medical HIV status. The campaign was based on an original "Assumptions" social marketing campaign conducted in San Francisco, California, which consisted of phase one in 1999 and a second phase in 2001. The original campaign was designed by the marketing firm Cabra Diseno and sponsored by the San Francisco AIDS Foundation. This campaign was later sold to AIDS Vancouver for adaptation in Canada and was conducted as a national campaign called "Think Again" in June 2004 over a six-week period. AIDS Vancouver coordinated the project via partnerships with many other regional agencies and communities across Canada.[17]

Canadian public health officials were concerned about increasing rates of HIV infections among men who have sex with men. This target population had experienced an increasing number of positive HIV test results since 2001 and constituted the greatest number of HIV infections in the overall population, according to rates reported by the Public Health Agency of Canada. The original campaign in San Francisco had been based upon research indicating that many gay men engaged in unprotected sexual activities because of assumptions about the HIV status of their partners that might in fact be incorrect.

Based on these findings and the rising rates of infection, the campaign in Canada was developed with an overall message of "Think Again: How Do You Know What You Know?" targeted specifically to gay men who were risking unprotected sex with partners of unknown HIV status. The message suggested an aspect of intrapersonal communication reflecting the inner decision-making process a gay man might undergo while considering unprotected sexual activity with a partner.

The campaign used a variety of mass media to carry the message, including bilingual print ads, public transit and bathroom ads, a variety of give-away items, and national Web sites in both English and French. Only the city of Toronto permitted transit and billboard ads because the private media owners in other cities considered the ads unsuitable for public viewing. The Web sites contained statistical data on HIV/AIDS occurrence, a campaign description including background and visuals, health information related to the campaign, a forum for discussion, information on organizational partners sponsoring the campaign, and a bank of related articles.

For the evaluation report, 417 men were surveyed in a random sample selected from known spaces where gay men were likely to congregate. Average exposure to the national campaign was 79 percent. Three of the top messages received a range of from 47 percent to 35 percent and included "rethink risks," "protect self and partner," and "use condoms." Of those surveyed, 73 percent responded positively to the message, and 76 percent believed the message of the campaign had encouraged them to rethink an aspect of their sexual behavior. However, only 48 percent of those surveyed said that the campaign message actually caused them to change some aspect of their sexual behavior.

These results furnish an example of the important differences between awareness of public health messages, declared intention to change future behavior, and actual rates of behavior change as a result of public health communication efforts. High rates of awareness of public health messages do not mean that target audiences intend to change their behavior and, similarly, behavioral intention may not highly correlate with actual behavior. Outcome evaluations must address awareness, intention to change, and actual behavioral change separately to create a more realistic picture of the actual impact of communications.

PUBLIC HEALTH PERSPECTIVE FOR THE HEALTH OF THE GENERAL POPULATION AND OF HIGH RISK GROUPS

When applying concepts in public health communication, it is important to adapt a strategic approach even in the initial stages of a public health campaign. It can seem overwhelming to consider all of the variables, but the more systematic your approach, the better your chances for success and the more accurately you will be able to evaluate and measure results to see if you did in fact succeed in specific communication goals.

At the outset, practical strategies for constructing a campaign include setting up the parameters of timing, targets, and message delivery:

- *Time frame:* How soon does the public need to know this information? Is it an ongoing chronic situation or an acute need for information? This will help you determine if a prevention, risk communication, or crisis communication approach would work best.
- *Target audience(s):* Who do you need to reach the most with this information? The channels they use to gain information about health issues are likely to furnish key points of access. If you are not sure how to reach these audiences, it is advisable to examine what has been tried before.
- *Mass media points of contact:* What forms of mass media do your target audience(s) likely use? What would be reasonable ways to assess these media usage patterns?
- *Message testing:* What strategies would work best to test your message effectiveness? How often would you need to test and refine these messages during the campaign?
- *Alternate plans:* What if the status of your campaign issue suddenly changes or insufficient information is available? What strategies would you use in urgent crises or rapidly changing communication situations, and how would you communicate this aspect of the situation to the public?

One structured approach to constructing health campaigns is included in the planning guide *Making Health Communication Programs Work*, also known as the "Pink Book" published by the National Cancer Institute of the National Institutes of Health.[14] We will now review the elements contained in this guide, from the practical vantage point of assembling helpful tools to use in the specific health message design and testing for eventual health campaign strategies.

The National Cancer Institute's Pink Book Approach

The four stages in constructing a targeted campaign are:

Stage 1: Planning and Strategy Development
Stage 2: Developing and Pretesting Concepts, Messages, and Materials
Stage 3: Implementing the Program
Stage 4: Assessing Effectiveness and Making Refinements

This suggested health communication approach is based on the four stages and planning steps in NCI's Pink Book, also known as *Making Health Communication Programs Work*.[14] These stages operate in a cyclical fashion, and the final stage becomes the basis for the next round as refinements and adaptations are required. These stages are described in detail in this section to help initiate the process of using these tools as guides for constructing a targeted campaign.

Stage 1: Planning and Strategy Development

Good planning is essential for any health communication endeavor, as it is likely to save considerable costs in the long run. The more comprehensive the initial planning process, the less you will need to make potentially costly changes later.

The following six planning steps provide a framework upon which to launch the first phase of a health campaign: 1) assess a health situation or problem; 2) define your communication objectives; 3) define and explore target audiences; 4) consider the media channels you would need to reach your intended target audiences; 5) identify partners and consider the attributes of these partnerships; and 6) draft a communication plan for each of the target audiences tailored to their interests, media preferences, and cultural or language preferences. These steps are elements of the formative research needed to assess the initial landscape in which you will conduct your campaign. Ideally, the final step would include attention to the health literacy skills of audiences, and take into consideration their facility with prose, document-reading, and numerical tables or charts, as assessed in the NAAL data.[1]

Stage 2: Developing and Pretesting Concepts, Messages, and Materials

In the second stage of the process of planning a public health campaign, begin by considering what is already available before you design or test new materials. In this way, you are able to build on the knowledge gained in prior communication projects. The steps suggested by the NCI Pink Book for this stage are: 1) review existing materials, sometimes known as an **environmental scan**; 2) develop and test initial messages; 3) se-

lect the most viable messages to develop in greater depth; 4) design the second phase of message development; 5) pretest and refine the messages and materials for your campaign. It is likely that there will be cycling back and forth within these steps, as messages are tested and refined, and then retested with more focused materials as a result.

Stage 3: Implementing the Program

As this tends to be the most costly of the four phases, be sure to begin with a launch plan that specifies the activities, quantities of materials, and staff preparation needed to implement your program. Each event of the program implementation should have a valid rationale, as widely varying events will suit the audiences you intend to reach. For instance, a press conference might or might not be advisable unless you have a news "angle" that would be of sufficient interest to reporters.

A kick-off event is a good way to establish a time frame for a campaign, but these are most effective if tied to the community, partners, or newsworthy events in some way. Remember to: 1) promote good relationships with the news media, before, during, and after your campaign launch; 2) consider the best spokespersons available; 3) work with them to stay focused on the appropriate campaign messages; 4) monitor how the implementation phase is going through such tools as process evaluation, and solve problems as they arise; and 5) maintain good working partnerships with community leaders and other stakeholders. Active monitoring during this phase may reveal some misconceptions embedded in the initial planning stages, so be alert to aspects of your communication strategy that may now require adjustment in the face of realistic applied settings.

Stage 4: Assessing Effectiveness and Making Refinements

The importance of an outcome evaluation cannot be underestimated. It is the main means of assessing the degree to which you have accomplished your goals and objectives as set forth in the initial planning stage. An outcome evaluation justifies health communication strategies to organizational management and allows for greater understanding of the project for community partners or stakeholders. In particular, it provides a way to decide whether success has been achieved or more work is needed. The Pink Book advocates nine steps in order to conduct a meaningful outcome evaluation. These steps include a consideration of the information needed; the data, data collection methods, and testing instruments that would be appropriate to provide this information; the actual collecting, processing, and analysis of data; and the process of writing and distributing the final evaluation report.

As these four stages are a cyclical process, it is expected that the outcome evaluation report will yield recommendations for future health communication initiatives related to the particular public health issue that launched the study. As part of this report, it is important to consider how your planning began, how it has evolved, and the lessons learned during the course of your project. It is mainly through repeated application of these principles that public health communicators are able to establish a flowing relationship between the various stages, and an intuitive sense of when strategies are succeeding and when they are in need of adjustment or fine-tuning.

When applying the process described above to construct and evaluate public health campaigns, remember to return periodically if needed to the initial reason for the campaign. In this way, you will be able to ensure that the overall aim of your communication plan does not counteract or leave out important elements of the main idea behind your health communication effort.

CONCLUSION

Ultimately, effective health communication strategies must evolve to meet the needs of diverse and changing audiences and situations. Strategies that may have worked before may not be as effective in an ever-changing and increasingly interactive era characterized by new technologies and fragmented audiences. The communication culture of globally conducted business environments reveals shifting priorities, as new technologies are used and discarded or expanded based on audience adoption patterns in the context of economic, political, and social principles.

In this rapidly changing media environment, it is necessary to know when to plan, adapt, test, and revisit strategies. Become aware of media in your own experience, and the ubiquitous nature of media messages in your daily life. Media is likely to be a shifting landscape for many of the audiences you are trying to reach as a health professional. Consider the new media trends that have already taken place in a single lifetime. In this busy and confusing culture of competing messages, ask: what place does health communication occupy? What will help your message stand out? Getting public health messages across requires more than the use of the latest technologies. It begins and ends with strategic planning and carefully applied research and testing to use the best resources available.

The myth of the "general public" may no longer exist. To accommodate the sheer diversity of segmentation possible in the many "publics" to reach, the best preparation for commencing a health communication is an open-minded approach. Never assume that based on past experience, the rapidly evolving landscape of health communication will be the same. In the blink of an eye, technology can require significant adjustments. The degree to which you encompass and adapt to rapidly changing media environments is a good indication of the success you are likely to achieve in communicating health messages.

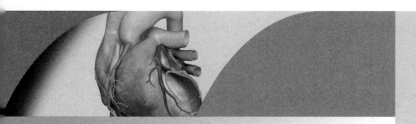

Questions for Further Research, Study, Reflection, and Discussion

For the Individual Student

In order to answer these questions, it may be necessary to research the primary literature.

- What are the differences between prevention, risk, and crisis communication?
- What are the three types of research discussed in this chapter, and what does each one entail?

For Small Group Discussion

- Reflect on public health issues in your community and select several to consider in light of health communication strategies. Find a health issue or devise a fictional scenario that would be appropriate for each of these categories: prevention, risk, and crisis communication. Consider your target audiences and specific media channels for the issue you have selected. Which types of mass media access would be most relevant to the audiences you are trying to reach? How could you use the three types of research (formative, process, outcome) to monitor the effectiveness of your campaign?
- Design a preliminary structured campaign strategy using the approach described in NCI's Pink Book. Analyze the key points needed to plan, launch, and evaluate a health communication campaign on a public health biological issue, using each of the four stages as a basis for planning.

- Select a potential risk or crisis communication scenario. Using the planning categories advocated by Tinker and Vaughan (2002),[11] begin a small group discussion with staff plans, audience concerns, objectives, and messages. What strategic resources might be available in your community to reach target audiences in a rapidly changing public health situation? Construct a fictional time line, including periods of evaluation.
- Consider the four types of communication: interpersonal, intrapersonal, organizational, and mass communication. Consider a public health issue in light of these four aspects. In a fictional scenario, how might these four different forms of communication relate to the dissemination of information, follow-up care, and compliance with care? What problems might you expect in each of these four areas, in relation to your scenario?

For Entire Class Discussion

- As a class, compile three visual lists on a white board, chalkboard or newsprint pad sheets: a. health issues, b. target audiences, and c. media strategies. During class discussion, note the ways in which characteristics of diverse potential audiences based on ethnic, cultural, racial, language, geographical location, age, or gender categories would affect the planning of effective health communication campaigns.

EXERCISE/ACTIVITY

- Identify a population with a specific health need in your community, and develop a communication campaign with a preventative, risk communication, or crisis communication message. Test your message by organizing a focus group comprised of members of that population. Prepare a poster or a brief write-up to present the findings of your focus group.

Healthy People 2010

Focus Area: Health Communication

Goal: Use communication strategically to improve health.

Objectives:

11-1. Increase the proportion of households with access to the Internet at home.

11-2. Improve the health literacy of persons with inadequate or marginal literacy skills.

11-3. Increase the proportion of health communication activities that include research and evaluation.

11-4. Increase the proportion of health-related World Wide Web sites that disclose information that can be used to assess the quality of the site.

11-5. Increase the number of centers for excellence that seek to advance the research and practice of health communication.

11-6. Increase the proportion of persons who report that their health care providers have satisfactory communication skills.

REFERENCES

1. Kutner M, Greenberg E, Jin Y, Paulsen C. (2006 September). *The Health Literacy of America's Adults: Results from the 2003 National Assessment of Adult Literacy.* Available at http://nces.ed.gov/pubsearch/pubsinfo.asp?pubid=2006483. Accessed May 26, 2008.

2. Office of Disease Prevention and Health Promotion. (n.d.). *Healthy People 2010 Health Communication Focus Area.* Washington, DC: U.S. Department of Health and Human Services. Available at http://www.healthy people.gov/document/HTML/Volume1/11HealthCom.htm. Accessed May 26, 2008.

3. Rogers EM. Up-to-Date Report. *J Health Commun* 1996;1:15–23.

4. U.S. Department of Health and Human Services. *Communicating Health: Priorities and Strategies for Progress.* Washington, DC: U.S. Department of Health and Human Services; 2003.

5. Doak CC, Doak LG, Root JH. *Teaching Patients with Low Literacy Skills.* Philadelphia: J.B. Lippincott; 1985.

6. Bernhardt JM, Cameron KA. Accessing, understanding, and applying health communication messages: the challenge of health literacy. In: Thompson TL, Dorsey AM, Miller KI, Parrott R, eds. *Handbook of Health Communication.* Mahwah, NJ: Lawrence Erlbaum; 2003:583–605.

7. Nussbaum J. Directions for research within health communication. *Health Commun* 1989;1:35–40.

8. Beck CS, Benitez JL, Edwards A, et al. Enacting "health communication": the field of health communication as constructed through publication in scholarly journals. *Health Commun* 2004;16:475–492.

9. Kreps GL, Thornton BC. *Health Communication: Theory and Practice,* 2nd ed. Prospect Heights, IL: Waveland Press; 1992.

10. Turow J. *Media Today: An Introduction to Mass Communication,* 2nd ed. New York: Houghton Mifflin; 2003.

11. Tinker T, Vaughan E. Risk communication. In: Nelson DE, Brownson RC, Remington PL, Parvanta C, eds. *Communicating Public Health Information Effectively: A Guide for Practitioners.* Washington, DC: American Public Health Association; 2002:185–203.

12. Salmon CT, Atkin C. Using media campaigns for health promotion. In: Thompson TL, Dorsey AM, Miller KI, Parrott R, eds. *Handbook of Health Communication.* Mahwah, NJ: Lawrence Erlbaum; 2003:449–472.

13. Centers for Disease Control and Prevention. Health Marketing: Creating, Communicating, Delivering. (2006). Atlanta, GA: National Center for Health Marketing. Available at http://www.cdc.gov/healthmarketing/. Accessed May 27, 2008.

14. National Cancer Institute. Pink Book – Making Health Communication Work. (2001). Bethesda: National Institutes of Health. Available at http://www.cancer.gov/pinkbook. Accessed May 27, 2008.

15. Maibach EW, Rothschild ML, Novelli WD. Social marketing. In: Glanz K, Rimer BK, Lewis FM, eds. *Health Behavior and Health Education: Theory, Research and Practice,* 3rd ed. San Francisco: Jossey-Bass; 2002:437–461.

16. Glanz K, Rimer BK, Lewis FM, eds. *Health Behavior and Health Education: Theory, Research and Practice,* 3rd ed. San Francisco: Jossey-Bass; 2002.

17. Lombardo AP, Léger YA. Thinking About "Think Again" in Canada: Assessing a Social Marketing HIV/AIDS Prevention Campaign. *J Health Commun* 2007;12:377–397.

CROSS REFERENCE

Information-Seeking Strategies in Public Health

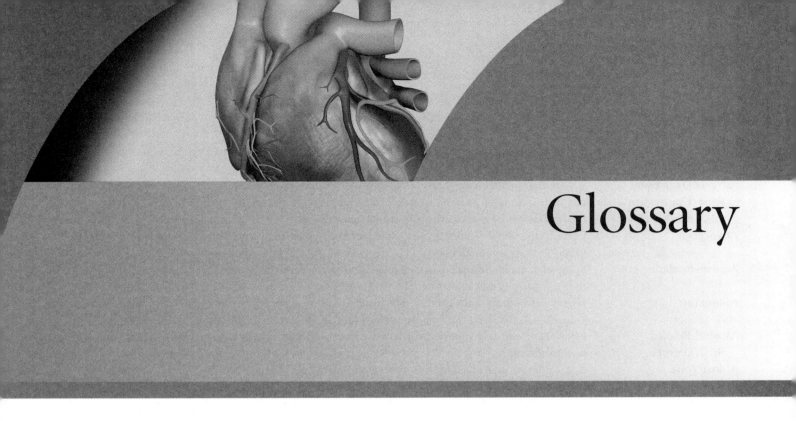

Glossary

Abscess:	A localized pocket of suppurative exudate (pus) and liquifactive necrosis that is entirely within, and surrounded by, tissue of an organ or body cavity.
Acetylcholine:	A particular chemical that functions as the chemical messenger of the parasympathetic nervous system.
Acquired Immuno-deficiency Syndrome (AIDS):	A condition of the immune system caused by the human immunodeficiency virus (HIV); characterized as having a CD4 cell count of less than 200 cells per cubic milliliter of blood (see *Human Immunodeficiency Syndrome*).
Active Immunity:	Adaptive immunity developed after exposure to an infection with a microorganism or following vaccination.
Active-Life Expectancy (also, *Disability-Free Life Expectancy*):	The average number of years an individual is expected to live free of disability if current patterns of mortality and disability continue to apply.
Active Tuberculosis:	State of people infected with *Mycobacterium tuberculosis* whose infection is not contained by the immune system and who are sick, frequently symptomatic, and very often contagious.
Activities of Daily Living (ADLs):	A scale to score physical ability/disability based on responses to questions about mobility and self-care; used to measure outcomes of interventions for various chronic disabling conditions such as arthritis.
Acute:	A sudden onset of a health effect (or exposure) that is often brief; sometimes loosely used to mean severe.
Adaptive Immunity:	An immune response developed following exposure to a foreign agent, which results in antigen recognition by T and B lymphocytes with development of specificity and memory.
Adaptive Skills:	Knowledge and ability to accomplish tasks of daily living including basic self-care, maintenance of personal hygiene, dressing, social judgment, and communication.
Addiction (also, *Dependence*):	Compulsive use of a drug, even in the face of significant adverse effects and consequences.
Adduct:	A new chemical species AB, each molecular entity of which is formed by direct combination of two separate molecular entities A and B in such a way that there is change in connectivity, but no loss, of atoms within the moieties A and B.
Adenocarcinoma:	Cancer that arises from glandular tissue.
Adjuvant:	A substance that enhances an immune response by prolonging exposure to the antigen within the body.

Adrenaline (also, *Epinephrine*):	The main hormone released from the adrenal medulla.
Adverse Drug Event (ADE):	Patient harm (including morbidity and mortality) linked to the use of a medication or substance.
Adverse Drug Event Reporting System (also, *MedWatch*):	A system implemented by the FDA to ensure the safety and efficacy of regulated, marketed medical products. The system allows reports of adverse events that are suspected to be related to a drug or medical device by healthcare professionals and patients.
Advocacy:	Communication directed at policy- and decision-makers to promote policies, regulations, and programs to bring about change.
Aerosol Spread:	Spray of virus in airborne particles less than five micrometers in size that can be carried in the air over long distances; can be filtered only by an N95 rated mask.
Aflatoxins:	Highly toxic compounds produced by mold fungus in agricultural crops, especially peanuts, and in animal feeds that have not been carefully stored; high-level exposure can cause liver cancer.
Alcohol-Related Birth Defects:	Fetal or infant body system disorders of structure or function associated with alcohol exposure during gestation.
Aldosterone:	A steroid hormone released from the adrenal cortex; acts in the distal tubule and collecting duct.
Alleles:	Alternate versions of the same gene. One allele is inherited from each parent. A gene might have multiple alleles, but each individual can have only two different alleles for any given gene.
Allostasis:	Where organisms maintain stability through change. By analogy, one can keep a home's temperature at different but constant levels by changing the thermostat setting.
Allostatic Load:	Prolonged activation of effectors involved in allostasis that contributes to wear and tear on the body; this idea provides a basis for studying the long-term health consequences of stress.
Alpha Cell:	A type of cell in the pancreas (in areas called the islets of Langerhans); these cells make and release a hormone called glucagon, which raises the level of glucose (sugar) in the blood.
Alternative Asthma Medications:	A class of drugs used to alleviate respiratory distress. The cornerstones of asthma therapy are ICS's, the dose of which can be increased or long-acting β2-agonists (LABAs) added for more severe asthma; in certain situations, leukotriene receptor antagonists (LTRAs) are also recommended. There are older medications that do not work as well and/or have side effects: chromolyn and nedocromil (which stabilize mast cells) as well as theophylline (a bronchodilator). Omalizumab is a new, genetically engineered weekly injection reserved for only for the very severe patient (see *Inhaled Corticosteroids*).
Amyloid Plaques:	Abnormal protein aggregates found outside the neurons of patients with Alzheimer's disease.
Angiogenesis:	Blood vessel formation. Tumor angiogenesis is the growth of blood vessels from surrounding tissue of a solid tumor, caused by the release of chemicals by the tumor.
Anomaly:	Abnormal development of a body system.
Anopheles:	The genus of mosquito capable of transmitting malaria to humans.
Anthelminthic Drugs:	A type of medication used to treat intestinal helminth infections. Albendazole or mebendazole are currently the standard anthelminthic treatments; although anthelminthic drugs treat the current infection, they do not prevent future reinfection.
Anthropogenic:	Ideas, actions, products, or effects that are caused or produced by humans.
Anthropozoonosis (pl., Anthropozoonoses):	Infectious diseases that can be transmitted from humans to animals.
Antibody:	A protein made in response to exposure to a foreign antigen that can bind to the antigen to facilitate elimination of the antigen.
Anticarcinogen:	Any chemical that reduces the occurrence or severity of cancers or acts against cancers that do occur, based on scientific evidence.
Antigen:	A foreign agent that can stimulate an immune response and bind to antibodies and T cells.
Antigenic Drift:	Minor genetic changes to circulating influenza viruses that occur seasonally and cause small, localized outbreaks of varying severity and extent.

Antigenic Shift: Major genetic re-assortment between two different influenza A viruses, resulting in a pandemic strain.

Antioxidants: Compounds that protect others from oxidation by being oxidized themselves. This prevents the breakdown of substances in food or the body, particularly lipids.

Aorta: The main arterial pipeline of the body. It originates at the top of the heart, curves up into the neck supplying the arteries to the head, face, and arms, and then dives down following the spinal column to finally divide at the level of the umbilicus into the main arteries to the lower extremities.

Apoptosis: Programmed cell death ("cell suicide"); a controlled sequence of events (or program) that leads to the elimination of cells without releasing harmful substances into the surrounding area.

Artemisinin-Based Combination Therapy (ACT): Treatment for malaria that combines an artemisinin-based compound with a drug or drugs from a different class. WHO recommends this drug combination as the first-line treatment for malaria in most regions in the world.

Artemisinins: A class of antimalarial drugs originally developed in China that is derived from the sweet wormwood plant (*Artemisia annua*).

Arthritis: An umbrella term to describe more than 100 rheumatic diseases and conditions that affect the joints and tissues, causing inflammation around the joints.

Asthma: An obstructive airway disease characterized by episodic airway narrowing that resolves either spontaneously or with treatment; it is caused by hyperresponsiveness to otherwise normal stimuli and chronic inflammation.

Asthma Control: A concept and focus of care to describe asthma severity, where patients are divided into well controlled, not well controlled, and very poorly controlled categories. With appropriate therapy, most patients regardless of classification should be able to achieve control. Though treatment is initiated based on severity level, treatment is adjusted based on control; providers can initiate higher doses and/or second medications if asthma is not controlled (step up) or decrease treatment if asthma is well controlled (step down).

Asthma Severity: Classification of patients with asthma since the early 1990s; based on daytime and nighttime symptoms, pulmonary function as measured by spirometry, use of rescue medication, and most recently by impact of asthma on one's daily activities (i.e., interference with work, school, and play). There are two components of severity—impairment (symptoms, lung function) and risk—specifically for exacerbations. Treatment for asthma should be initiated based on the current severity classification. A limitation of this classification system is that asthma is a variable disease, and even patients with mild persistent asthma can have poor asthma control.

Atherosclerosis (also, *Hardening of the Arteries*)**:** Artery walls become progressively thickened due to the accumulation of fatty deposits, smooth muscle cells, and fibrous connective tissue. Narrowing of the lumen of an artery occurs, restricting blood flow; too much cholesterol in the blood increases the risk that fatty deposits (plaque) will form in arteries.

Attenuation: A process in which a pathogen is altered so it is less virulent.

Attitudes: An individual's behavioral beliefs that performing certain actions will be associated with certain outcomes or attributes, and an individual's personal evaluation of the importance or value of those outcomes.

Autonomic Nervous System: The body's system comprising sympathetic and parasympathetic neurons, responsible for many automatic, usually unconscious processes to maintain the body's homeostasis (e.g., respiration, digestion and taste, heart rate, perspiration, micturation, and sexual arousal).

Autosomal Dominant Trait: A type of inherited disease or syndrome that is carried on an autosome (a non-sex chromosome) and requires only one copy of the associated allele for expression of the phenotype.

Autosomal Recessive Trait:	A type of inherited disease or syndrome that is carried on an autosome (a non-sex chromosome) and requires two copies of the associated allele for expression of the phenotype.
Avian Influenza:	A virulent strain of influenza A that infects birds; potentially could cause a pandemic in humans if the virus were to undergo antigenic shift and become easily transmissible from human-to-human.
Barrier Precautions:	Use of gloves, gowns, and hand washing to prevent contact spread of infections.
Bacille de Calmette et Guérin (BCG):	First vaccine developed to treat tuberculosis.
Behavioral Intention:	An individual's perception of his or her likelihood of modifying a certain behavior.
Behavioral Risk Factor Surveillance System (BRFSS):	A routine, systematic epidemiological method of collecting information on certain health behaviors to analyze.
Beta Amyloid:	The main constituent of amyloid plaques in the brains of Alzheimer's patients; formed when β-secretase cleaves amyloid protein.
Beta Cell:	A type of cell in the pancreas in areas called the islets of Langerhans; these cells make and release insulin, a hormone that controls the level of glucose (sugar) in the blood.
Bias:	A systematic error that occurs in a study and leads to a distorted result. Examples of bias are selection bias, information bias, or confounding factors.
Bibliographic Database:	An electronic version of a catalog or index that allows the user to identify publications by author, subject, title, or other search terms. It generally provides at least a full citation to the item, and often other information such as abstracts, assigned subject headings, and sometimes the complete text. Examples include MEDLINE, CINAHL, Academic Search Premier, and Scopus.
Bioavailability:	The quantity of vitamins provided by a food itself, and the amount of vitamins the body is able to absorb and use, which is often less than the total nutrients present in a food.
Biodiversity:	Number, variety, and range of different organisms (and their genes) located within an ecosystem.
Biofortification:	Genetically modifying agricultural products to improve their nutritional content.
Biological Plausibility (also, *Coherence*):	Epidemiological findings of association between the proposed causal agent and the biological disorder supported by existing knowledge of biological systems. If biological knowledge is absent, replication studies in other populations may be necessary to prove biological plausibility.
Biologically Active Substance (BAS):	Has the ability to alter a biological function of an organism.
Biomagnification:	The accumulation of an element or compound up the food chain.
Biopsy:	Removal of a small amount of tissue for examination under a microscope.
Blogs:	Short for Web log; a Web page on the Internet that serves as a publicly accessible personal journal for an individual. Blogs are frequently updated and often reflect the personality of the author; typically combines text, images, and links to other blogs, Web pages, and other media related to its topic.
Blood Glucose:	The main sugar found in the blood and the body's primary source of energy.
Blood Glucose Level:	The amount of glucose in a given amount of blood; noted in milligrams in a deciliter (mg/dL).
Blood Pressure (BP):	Force of blood exerted on the inside walls of blood vessels; expressed as a ratio (e.g., 120/80, read as "120 over 80") where the first number denotes the systolic pressure (defined as the pressure when the heart pushes blood out into the arteries) and the second number is the diastolic pressure (the pressure when the heart rests).
Body Mass Index (BMI):	A measure of underweight and overweight calculated as weight (kg) divided by height squared (m^2); a formula that uses weight and height to estimate body fat and health risks. In adults, a BMI between 19 and 24 is considered to be a healthy weight range for height. A BMI between 25 and 29 is considered overweight and a BMI of 30 or greater is considered obese. Anyone with a BMI of 30 or greater should talk to a health provider about losing weight for his or her health.
Body System:	Group of organs that function together (e.g., cardiovascular system, gastrointestinal system, neurological system, respiratory system, etc.).

Bone Mineral Density (BMD):	A measure of the amount of calcium in the bones used to diagnose osteoporosis.
Boolean Operators:	Named after the British mathematician George Frederick Boole (1815–1864), who developed a system of logic to show the relationship among terms or concepts. Three primary Boolean operators—AND, OR, and NOT—can be used to group search terms when conducting a literature search on the Internet or World Wide Web.
Brand Name (also, *Trade Name*)**:**	In medicine, a type of copyright or ownership of a drug or substance provided by a pharmaceutical company to link it to the reputation of the company; used in advertising and marketing to differentiate the company's drug from generic or similar drugs/substances marketed by other companies (e.g., Zantac® is the trade name for the generic drug, ranitidine).
Budding:	Having the ability to reproduce asexually through the pinching of genetic component of a parent cell.
Calcium:	Key mineral stored in bones that is responsible for proper functioning of muscles and nerves.
Cancer:	Abnormal cells that reproduce out of control, hijacking normal surrounding cells' genetic material (DNA), invading surrounding tissue and, if not halted, other organs as it replaces normal cells; metastasis occurs as the cancer cells invade the bloodstream or lymph vessels. DNA can be repaired in normal cells, but in cancerous cells the damage is not repaired. People can inherit damaged DNA, which accounts for inherited cancers, or their DNA is damaged by exposure to something in the environment (e.g., smoking tobacco).
Capsid:	A protein shell that covers the nucleic acid component of a virus.
Capsular Polysaccharide:	Water soluble, acidic, thick layer of carbohydrate produced by certain bacteria to prevent the host from being able to destroy it. They are linear and consist of regularly repeating subunits of one to six monosaccharides. Capsular polysaccharides displayed on the capsular surface allow for subtying or grouping of bacteria (e.g., *Neisseria meningitidis* has 13 serogroups based on antigens displayed on the surface of the capsule).
Carbohydrate:	One of the four main nutrients in food (others are lipids, proteins, nucleic acids) and is responsible for storing and transporting energy as well as help with process of development, immune system, blood clotting, pathogenesis, and fertilization. Foods that provide carbohydrates are starches, vegetables, fruits, dairy products, and sugars.
Carcinogen:	A substance with the potential to cause cancer (see *Cancer*).
Carcinogenesis:	Generation of cancer from normal cells; correctly, the formation of a carcinoma, but often used synonymously with transformation or tumorigenesis.
Cardiovascular Disease:	A range of heart and blood vessel (arteries, veins, and capillaries) conditions.
Case Fatality Rate:	Number of deaths/total number of injuries × 100; essentially, it is the percentage of people with that type of injury who die.
Cell-Mediated Immunity:	A protective mechanism mediated by antigen-specific T lymphocytes and other cells that combats challenges such as intracellular organisms, viruses, and tumor cells.
Cellular Exudate (also, *Inflammatory Edema*)**:**	An accumulation of protein-rich fluid in an extravascular space or tissue. When the exudate includes an influx of leukocytes, neutrophils, or other leukocytes, it is referred to as a cellular exudate.
Cerebrovascular Disease:	Damage to blood vessels in the brain where vessels can burst and bleed or become clogged with fatty deposits. When blood flow is interrupted, brain cells die or are damaged, resulting in a stroke.
Chemoprophylaxis:	Prevention of disease by the use of chemicals or drugs.
Chemotaxis and Chemoattractants:	In the inflammatory response, chemotaxis is the ameboid movement of cells (particularly neutrophils, monocytes, and macrophages) out of vessels and toward a site of

injury in response to a chemically attracting signal. Chemoattractant factors include some bacterial products and products released from necrotic cells, fibrinopeptides, C5a derived from activation of the complement cascade (C5a), and factors produced by stimulated macrophages and other cells, including leukotriene B4 and the chemokine interleukin-8 (IL-8).

Cholesterol: A soft, waxy substance found among fats circulating in the bloodstream and found in all other cells. The body manufactures some cholesterol and the rest comes from animal products ingested (i.e., meat, poultry, fish, eggs, butter, cheese, and whole and 2% milk). It is not found in foods from plants.

Chromosomes: Thread-like structures in the nucleus of a cell that are made of DNA and structural proteins. Human cells other than egg and sperm normally have 46 chromosomes (23 pairs). Egg and sperm cells have 23 chromosomes.

Chronic: A health-related state (or exposure) lasting a long time. The U.S. National Center for Health Statistics defines a chronic condition as one of three months' duration or longer.

Circadian Rhythms: Cyclical changes (e.g., fluctuations in body temperature, hormone levels, and sleep) that occur over a 24-hour period, driven by the body's biological "clock."

Close Contacts: In disease states, people in direct proximity with a patient. In the case of someone with meningococcal disease, this could include 1) household members; 2) child-care center contacts; and 3) persons directly exposed to the patient's oral secretions (e.g., by kissing, mouth-to-mouth resuscitation, endotracheal intubation, or endotracheal tube management).

Cofactors: Organic and inorganic molecules that influence the effect of other conditions.

Colectomy: Surgical removal of the colon performed in patients with high risk forms of colon or colorectal disease.

Colonoscopy: Visual examination of the inner surface of the colon using a flexible lighted scope passed into the body under sedation.

Colostomy: An opening in the abdominal wall to allow the passage of stool.

Comorbidity: Disease(s) that coexist(s) in a study participant in addition to the index condition that is the subject of study.

Community-Based Asthma Programs: Types of public awareness, therapeutic, and/or prevention strategies. Examples include school- and pharmacy based programs as well as mobile asthma vans in minority and impoverished areas.

Community-Based Outbreak: Occurrence of three or more confirmed or likely cases of a disease within three months among persons who are not in close contact, but reside in the same area, who do not share a common affiliation, and with a primary disease attack rate of ≥ 10 cases/100,000 persons.

Comorbid Factors: The coexistence of two or more disease processes, or indicates medical conditions already existing at the time of an injury.

Computer Literacy: A familiarity with computing concepts and the ability to use common applications to research questions on the Internet and the World Wide Web (see *Internet, World Wide Web*).

Conservation Medicine: A dynamic biological discipline that describes the relationship among human-induced environmental impact, public health, and the preservation and growth of endangered species or ecosystems.

Construct: An explicit idea derived for and applied to a specific theory.

Contact Spread: The infection of a virus, bacterium, or disease via touching a contaminated surface and self-inoculation of mucous membranes; can occur person to person (touch, cough, kiss, sexual intercourse, blood transfusion), animal to person (scratching, biting, handling feces), or mother to unborn child (e.g., AIDS virus, parasite).

Contagion (also, *Communicable Disease Transmission* [preferred]): The passing of disease or transmission of infection by direct contact, droplet spread, or contaminated matter.

Containment Strategy: Multifaceted plan to control a disease outbreak and prevent its further spread.

Controller and Reliever Therapy: Two types of medications for patients with persistent asthma (asthma symptomatic more than twice a week). Controller medications (preferably inhaled corticosteroids) are taken every day, regardless of symptoms, to prevent exacerbations. Reliever medications are usually short-acting bronchodilators (albuterol) to be used only when patients are symptomatic.

Cornea: The thin clear part of the eye that allows images to enter the eye and reach the retina so vision can occur.

Cortisol: One of several stress hormones produced by the adrenal cortex that is secreted near the end of sleep to stimulate alertness.

Cues to Action: External triggers that stimulate an individual to take action.

Culling: Depopulation of a group. To prevent avian influenza, infected birds from a localized area are killed to prevent its spread and lessen the chance of human disease involvement

Cutaneous: Relating to the skin (e.g., cutaneous anthrax is infection of the skin resulting from direct contact with the bacterium *Bacillus anthracis*).

Cytotoxic T Cells: Type of cells capable of destroying other immune and nonimmune cells.

DALY (see *Disability Adjusted Life Years*).

DASH Diet (see *Dietary Approaches to Stop Hypertension*).

Definitive Host: Location where parasites undergo sexual reproduction.

Delta Cell: A type of pancreatic cell located in the islets of Langerhans that makes somatostatin, a hormone that is believed to control how the beta cells make and release insulin and how the alpha cells make and release glucagon (see Alpha cells, Beta cells).

Dementia: An organic mental disorder that results in permanent or progressive loss of intellectual abilities (i.e., impairment in memory, judgment, and abstract thinking) and changes in personality.

Dental Caries: Destruction of the tooth by a formation of plaque in the oral cavity.

Dental Plaque: Oral flora that adhere to the surface of teeth and initiate breakdown of the tooth enamel.

Deoxyribonucleic Acid (DNA): The universal genetic material; the information molecule that carries hereditary information from one generation of cells to the next and from one generation of individuals to the next. Genes are made of DNA, which is the molecular basis of heredity.

Depression: A mental state or chronic mental disorder characterized by feelings of sadness, loneliness, despair, low self-esteem, and self-reproach; accompanying signs include psychomotor retardation (or less frequently, agitation), withdrawal from social contact, loss of appetite, and insomnia.

Detention: Those diagnosed with a communicable disease who fail to comply with public health orders and whose movements are legally restricted to a health facility or hospital (not a prison; see *Incarceration*).

Diabetes Mellitus: A condition characterized by hyperglycemia resulting from the body's inability to use blood glucose for energy. In type 1 diabetes, the pancreas no longer makes insulin and therefore blood glucose cannot enter the cells to be used for energy. In type 2 diabetes, either the pancreas does not make enough insulin or the body is unable to use insulin correctly.

Diabetic Ketoacidosis (DKA): Severe, out-of-control diabetes (high blood sugar) that needs emergency treatment; caused by a profound lack of circulating insulin. This may happen because of illness, taking too little insulin, or getting too little exercise. The body starts using stored fat for energy, and ketone bodies (acids) build up in the blood.

Dialysis: Process where blood is cleared of toxins and excess fluid is removed using an artificial kidney, as in hemodialysis, or through the peritoneum, as in peritoneal dialysis.

Diastolic Blood Pressure: In a blood pressure reading, the bottom number; represents the pressure in the arteries when the heart is at rest.

Diet Diversity: Describes the number of nutrients available to a population based on the foods they are able to access. Populations that are sustained on two or three major crops would have low diet diversity.

Dietary Approaches to Stop Hypertension (DASH diet): A type of diet developed by the U.S. Department of Health and Human Services and designed to reduce blood pressure due to generous amounts of potassium.

Dietary Fiber: Plant food components, including plant cell walls, pectins, gums, and brans, which cannot be digested; sources include fruits, nuts, grains, vegetables. Fiber is classified as soluble or insoluble; it increases fecal bulk, allowing its quick passage through the colon. Benefits of a high fiber diet include lower blood cholesterol levels, and prevention and treatment of constipation.

Dietary Guidelines for Americans: A report published by the U.S. Department of Agriculture and U.S. Department of Health and Human Services that explains how to eat to maintain health. The guidelines form the basis of national nutrition policy and are revised every five years.

Digital Literacy: The productive use of the Internet to present, access, and use information.

Directly Observed Therapy (DOT): The World Health Organizations' recommended strategy for delivering the basics of tuberculosis cure; combines a clinical approach (patients' drug intake is monitored daily by a nurse or a trained healthcare worker to ensure patient compliance) and a management strategy for public health systems that includes political commitment, maintenance of adequate drug supply, and viable recording and reporting systems.

Disability Adjusted Life Years (DALYs): A calculated estimate of the number of healthy, productive years of life lost due to morbidity or premature mortality from a disease, derived by applying disability "weights" to different conditions and multiplying that weight by the number of years that an infected person is affected by that condition.

Discretionary Calories: After fulfilling the daily recommended values of all food categories for his or her body type, each individual will still usually need between 100 and 300 additional calories to meet the recommended daily caloric intake; the individual can decide for him- or herself what to eat to consume the extra needed calories.

Distress: A form of stress that is consciously experienced in which the individual senses an inability to cope, attempts to avoid or escape the situation, elicits instinctively communicated signs, and has activation of the adrenal gland.

Diuretic: A drug that increases urine flow, usually by inhibiting sodium reabsorption.

DNA (see *Deoxyribonucleic Acid*).

Dopamine: One of the body's three catecholamines that is converted to norepinephrine, which then is converted to adrenaline.

Dose Response: As the exposure to the proposed causal agent increases, the response (risk) of the biological disorder increases.

Droplet Spread: Airborne particles of a virus, disease, or bacterium greater than five micrometers in size that travel only several feet (e.g., a sneeze from a person with influenza carries droplets of contagious virus).

Drug-Induced Disease: Unintended effect of a medication or substance resulting in morbidity or mortality; symptoms may cause a patient to seek medical care and/or require hospitalization.

Drug-Drug, Drug-Food, and Drug-Herbal Interactions: Chemical, physical, or physiological interactions between one drug product and another drug, food, or herbal substance that a patient might be receiving; interactions may result in an increase or decrease in the activity of the original drug and could therefore result in toxicity or lack of therapeutic efficacy.

Drug Susceptibility Testing (DST): Determination of the resistance profile of a specific tuberculosis (TB) strain, usually by culture on media (either solid or liquid) containing the different antibiotics and by monitoring subsequent growth. DST allows for the screening of MDR-TB and XDR-TB strains, and can be performed for first-line or second-line drugs.

Dual Energy X-Ray Absorptiometry (DXA): A diagnostic imaging test to measure bone density; used to diagnose osteoporosis.

Electrophile: An atom, molecule, or ion able to accept an electron pair.

ELSI: Acronym for "ethical, legal, and social implications" of human genome research. The ELSI program began as a central component of the Human Genome Project (q.v.), with the goal to support research and education about the applications of knowledge derived from research in genetics and genomics. The term ELSI now has come to signify any such category of issues, even if they are not directly related to the Human Genome Project.

Endemic: A disease that is constantly present to a greater or lesser degree in a particular group of people or in a particular location.

Endogenous: Developing or originating within the organisms or arising from causes within the organism.

Endoscopy: Visual examination of the inner surface of the esophagus, stomach, and/or small bowel performed using a lighted scope passed into the body under sedation.

End-Stage Renal Disease (ESRD): Occurs when kidney function is not adequate to sustain life, on an irreversible chronic basis, such that renal replacement therapy in the form of dialysis or a renal transplantation is needed.

Environment: Any factor that is physically external to an individual.

Environmental Tobacco Smoke (also, *Second Hand Smoke*)**:** Cigarette smoke blown into the environment by active smokers; proven to cause respiratory illnesses, cancer, and death in non-smokers.

Environmental Triggers: Factors outside of the individual that may contribute to asthma. Includes: ozone, sulfur dioxide, nitrogen dioxide, acid aerosols. Extremes in temperature or humidity may also play a role. Indoor pollutants such as tobacco smoke also worsen asthma.

Enzyme-Linked Immuno-sorbent Assay (ELISA) Test: One of the most common tests used to detect HIV antibodies; used in medicine as a diagnostic test and in industry for quality control.

Epidemic: Widespread outbreak of a disease, or a rapidly expanding cluster of cases of a disease in a single community or relatively small area.

Epidemiological Investigation: The process of discovery that determines the presence of an outbreak or biological attack, confirms the diagnosis, establishes the case definition, traces exposures and contacts, and characterizes the outbreak or attack (where, when, etc.).

Epidemiology: The study of the distribution and determinates of health-related states or events in specified populations, and the application of this study to control the health problems.

Epigastrium: Area of the abdomen located between the costal margins and the subcostal plane.

Epigenetic: Refers to the state of the DNA with respect to heritable changes in function without a change in the nucleotide sequence; can be caused by DNA modification (e.g., by methylation).

Epitope: A small portion of an antigen that can stimulate an immune response and serve as a binding site for antibody.

Erythrocytic Cycle: The part of the parasite life cycle in humans that occurs in blood cells.

Estrogens: Female hormones produced by the ovaries; deficiency can lead to osteoporosis.

Ethical, Legal, and Social Implications (see *ELSI*).

Evidence-Based Medicine: The conscientious, explicit, and judicious use of current best evidence in making decisions about the care of individual patients; integrates clinical experience with findings from strongly designed and executed study findings.

Evidence-Based Public Health: Effectively finding and evaluating answers to questions regarding the well-being of local, community, and national residents.

Evolution: The change in gene frequencies in populations of organisms over time, potentially leading to the production of new species; helps to determine the genetic structure of human populations, thereby helping to determine the nature and extent of disease in those populations.

Exo-Erythrocytic Cycle: The part of the parasite life cycle in humans that occurs in the liver, prior to release of parasites into the bloodstream.

Exogenous:	Produced outside of, originating from, or due to external causes.
Extra-Pulmonary Tuberculosis:	Active tuberculosis that is localized in an organ other than the lungs (not non-respiratory disease).
Extensively Drug-Resistant Tuberculosis (XDR-TB):	A strain of tuberculosis (TB) that is at least MDR-TB, and also includes resistance to fluoroquinolone (one class of second-line drugs) and at least one of the second-line injectable drugs (such as capreomycin or amikacin). XDR-TB strains are virtually untreatable (see *Tuberculosis*).
Fetal Alcohol Effects (FAE) (also, *Partial FAS* or *Possible Fetal Alcohol Effects*):	Includes individuals with intrauterine alcohol exposure who meet some of the facial features and at least one of the other criteria of fetal alcohol syndrome, including growth retardation, neurodevelopmental abnormalities, or behavioral or cognitive disorders.
Fetal Alcohol Syndrome (FAS):	Includes individuals with a history intrauterine alcohol exposure who have the identifiable facial features, growth retardation, and neurobehavioral dysfunction.
Fight or Flight:	A phrase coined by Walter Cannon that refers to the adrenaline-mediated response the body produces when confronted with an external stress that threatens homeostasis. Although Cannon believed the "fight" and "flight" responses to be physiologically identical, subsequent research has proven there are significant differences between them.
First-Degree Relatives:	Parents, siblings, children.
First-Line Drugs:	A group of five antibiotics (rifampicin, isoniazid, ethambutol, pyrazinamide, and streptomycin) used against tuberculosis that are the most effective and potent treatment options for TB patients.
Five C's (MRSA):	Factors that closely link an occurrence of methicillin-resistant *Staphylococcus aureus* (MRSA) in communities commonly known to have outbreaks. The 5 C's are: crowding, contact, compromised skin, contaminated items, and cleanliness.
Fluoroapatite:	Structural element of teeth composed of mineralized calcium, phosphate, and fluoride ions, causing tooth surface to become harder and less prone to decay.
Food Insecurity:	Limited or uncertain availability of nutritionally adequate and safe foods, or limited or uncertain ability to acquire acceptable foods in socially acceptable ways.
Fortification:	The addition of one or more nutrients to a food source, so as to correct a micronutrient deficiency.
Free Radical:	A highly chemically reactive atom, molecule, or molecular fragment with a free or unpaired electron; free radicals are produced in normal metabolic processes and UV radiation from the sun. Implicated in aging, cancer, cardiovascular disease, and other kinds of damage to the body.
Functional Foods:	A substance that provides nutritional benefits beyond its caloric or basic nutritional value when ingested (e.g., foods containing antioxidants).
Gamma-Aminobutyric Acid (GABA):	An amino acid in the central nervous system associated with the transmission of nerve impulses.
Gastritis:	Inflammation of the lining of the stomach.
Gene:	A segment of DNA that contains instructions for making a specific protein or proteins required by the body; are found in succession along the length of chromosomes. Human beings have about 20,000 genes.
Generic Name:	The chemical name of the drug (not the name used by the pharmaceutical company to market the agent; e.g., ranitidine is the generic name of the product Zantac®).
Genetics:	The branch of science concerned with the means and consequences of inherited biological variation.
Genetic Counseling:	"The process of helping people understand and adapt to the medical, psychological and familial implications of genetic contributions to disease. This process integrates interpretation of family and medical histories to assess the chance of disease occurrence or recurrence, education about inheritance, testing, management, prevention, resources and research, counseling to promote informed choices and adaptation to the risk or condition." (National Society of Genetic Counselors).
Genome:	All of the DNA of a given organism; e.g., the human genome or the mouse genome).
Genomics:	The study of whole genomes, usually focusing on extensive DNA sequences.
Genotype:	The genetic constitution of an organism or cell; the set of alleles inherited at a locus.
GFR	(see *Glomerular Filtration Rate*).

Gingivitis:	The first stage of gum disease characterized by inflammation and infection of the oral soft tissue (gums).
Glomerular Filtration Rate (GFR):	The volume of filtrate formed in both kidneys and passing into the proximal tubule. In adults it averages about 120 mL/min.
Glucagon:	A hormone secreted by alpha cells in the pancreas in response to low blood glucose concentration, which elicits release of glucose from liver glycogen stores.
Glucose:	A monosaccharide; sometimes known as blood sugar.
Gluteal Muscles:	Muscle group in the buttock that rotates and extends (straightens) the hip.
Glycogen:	A substance made up of sugars. Manufactured and stored in the liver and muscles as a storage form of glucose, it releases glucose (sugar) into the blood when needed by cells. Glycogen is the chief source of stored fuel in the body.
Good Source:	Label for a nutrient that provides 10 percent to 19 percent of the daily value of that nutrient per serving.
Gout:	Rheumatic disease resulting from an accumulation of uric acid crystals in tissues and fluids within the body.
Granulation Tissue:	The histological appearance of tissue during the early healing phase of acute inflammation when there is an influx of macrophages, and a proliferation of connective tissue cells and matrix disproportionate to the predominance of fibrosis and scar that is seen in the later stages of healing. The new connective tissue is loosely woven and includes many macrophages, proliferating endothelial cells, new blood vessels (angiogenesis), and an increasing number of myofibroblasts producing fine collagen strands.
Granuloma:	An aggregate of macrophages surrounded by a rim of lymphocytes. Although granulomas can be formed as a nonspecific response to indigestible matter, such as suture material, it also can form due to infectious and immune-mediated causes. Immune-stimulated macrophages take on a distinctive appearance referred to as "epithelioid" and may form giant cells with multiple nuclei ringing the periphery of the enlarged macrophage (Langhans giant cell). Tuberculosis is the most likely etiology of the granulomas, if caseous necrosis is seen within the granulomas.
Grey Literature:	Material disseminated outside of the traditional peer-reviewed journal or scholarly book. Examples include: conference papers, newsletters, research reports, and position papers. As some researchers do not submit their work to scholarly journals, this may be the only source in which their research can be located.
Habitat Modification:	The human addition or subtraction of plants, animals, or human-made products to an ecosystem.
Hamstrings:	Muscles in the back of the leg that extend or straighten the hip.
Health Communication:	The art and technique of informing, influencing, and motivating individual, institutional, and public audiences about important health issues. The scope of health communication includes disease prevention, health promotion, health care policy, and the business of health care as well as enhancement of the quality of life and health of individuals within the community.
Health Promotion:	Any planned combination of educational, political, regulatory, and organizational supports for actions and conditions of living conducive to the health of individuals, groups, or communities.
Healthcare Disparities:	A difference in health outcomes between majority and minority populations that cannot be accounted for by socioeconomic factors alone. For example, asthma prevalence and morbidity is particular worse in African Americans, the disparities possibly due to genetic and socioeconomic factors as well as racial discrimination and cultural insensitivity.
Healthy (Food):	Implies that a food is low in fat, saturated fat, sodium, and cholesterol and contains at least 10 percent of the daily value of one or more of the following nutrients: vitamin A, C, iron, calcium, fiber, or protein.

Healthy People 2010: Provides a framework for prevention of diseases in the United States; a statement of national health objectives designed to identify the most significant preventable threats to health and to establish national goals to reduce these threats.

Hemagglutinin: Surface protein on influenza A that attaches to respiratory tract cells to cause infection; the abbreviation of it and its numbered type is used as a component of the virus name (i.e., H5).

Hematemesis: The vomiting of blood.

Hematochezia: The passage of bloody stools.

Herd Immunity: The ability of a group of individuals to resist specific pathogens either through widespread natural exposure or by vaccination.

High-Density-Lipoprotein Cholesterol (HDL): A fat found in the blood that takes extra cholesterol from the blood to the liver for removal. It is sometimes referred to as "good" cholesterol.

Hip Fracture: A break near the top of the femur where it angles into the hip socket of the pelvis.

Homeostasis: State of equilibrium of the internal environment of the body that is maintained by dynamic processes of feedback and regulation. Homeostasis is a dynamic equilibrium.

HPA Axis: A neurochemical network that coordinates the functions of the hypothalamus, pituitary, and adrenal glands.

Human Genome Project: The effort, completed in 2003, to determine the sequence of all 3.2 billion base pairs of human DNA. The results of the project are in public databases that are accessible to all interested parties.

Human Immuno-deficiency Virus (HIV): A member of the retroviral family that causes AIDS by infecting and destroying T helper cells, which causes a gradual decline in the immune system.

Humoral immunity: A type of protection against disease that involves antibody-mediated responses.

Hunger: The internal, physiological drive to find and consume food; often experienced as a negative sensation and manifests as an uneasy or painful sensation. The recurrent and involuntary lack of access to food may produce malnutrition over time.

Hydroxyapatite: Structural element of teeth composed of mineralized calcium and phosphate ions.

Hyperglycemia: Too high a level of glucose (sugar) in the blood; a sign that diabetes is out of control. Many things can cause hyperglycemia. It occurs when the body does not have enough insulin or cannot use the insulin it does have to turn glucose into energy. Signs of hyperglycemia are a great thirst, a dry mouth, and a need to urinate often. For people with type 1 diabetes, hyperglycemia may lead to diabetic ketoacidosis.

Hyperlipidemia: Elevations of lipids (cholesterol, triglycerides) in the plasma.

Hypertension (also, *High Blood Pressure*): A condition present when blood flows through the blood vessels with a force greater than normal. Hypertension can strain the heart, damage blood vessels, and increase the risk of heart attack, stroke, kidney problems, and death. It is categorized as transitory or sustained elevation of systolic and diastolic blood pressure above 140/90 mm Hg.

Hypoglycemia: Too low a level of glucose (sugar) in the blood. This occurs when a person with diabetes has injected too much insulin, eaten too little food, or has exercised without extra food. A person with hypoglycemia may feel nervous, shaky, weak, or sweaty and have a headache, blurred vision, and hunger. Taking small amounts of sugar, sweet juice, or food with sugar will usually help the person feel better within 10 to 15 minutes.

Hypothalamus: Region of the forebrain, below the thalamus, that controls body temperature, thirst, and hunger and is involved in sleep and emotional activity.

Hypotholamic-Pituitary-Adrenocortical: A major stress effector system in which release of chemicals in the hypothalamus of the upper brainstem effect release of corticotrophin (ACTH) from the pituitary gland, and the ACTH stimulates release of steroid hormones from the adrenal cortex.

Iatrogenic: A disease or disorder attributed to medical therapy or intervention.

ICS (see *Inhaled Corticosteroids*).

Immune Evasion: The capability of invading microorganisms to avoid detection and/or destruction by the immune system.

Immunity:	A state of protection from disease created by innate and specific mechanisms.
Immunization:	Protection of individuals against disease by vaccination.
Impetigo:	A common skin infection characterized by vesicles or pustules that can rupture and have a characteristic "honey yellow" crust that can mimic a herpetic outbreak.
Incarceration:	Imprisonment of patients with tuberculosis who break the law of specific public health orders imposed on them.
Incidence:	The number of specified new events, during a specified period on a specified population.
Incontinence:	The lack of voluntary control of excretory functions.
Incubation Period:	Time lapse between exposure to a biological agent (infection) and the onset of clinical symptoms, usually several days to several weeks.
Independent Assortment:	The principle that different genes (and versions of genes, i.e., alleles) are distributed independently into egg and sperm; explains why it is possible to look like a certain family member, but not to have the same medical conditions or traits, and vice versa.
Indicated Prevention (also, *Tertiary Prevention*)**:**	Specific prevention strategies are applied to populations who demonstrate the disease (disorder or behavior) to prevent further morbidity or illness.
Indoor Residual Spraying (IRS):	When insecticide is sprayed on the interior walls of a house, leaving a residue on the walls that remains for three to six months depending on the housing construction and the type of insecticide used.
Inelastic Collision:	An impact in which some or all of the kinetic energy of the colliding bodies is absorbed by at least one of the partners.
Infectious Disease (also, *Communicable Disease*)**:**	An illness due to a specific infectious agent or its toxic products that arises through transmission of that agent or its products from an infected person, animal, or reservoir to a susceptible host, either directly or indirectly through an intermediate plant or animal host, vector, or the inanimate environment.
Inferior Vena Cava:	Large vein that collects the blood flow from the legs and abdominal organs and carries it back to the heart.
Inflammation:	A vascular and cellular host response that marshals leukocytes and essential proteins into tissues affected by infection or injury in order to kill or neutralize organisms, contain damage, and set in place those factors that can result in healing and repair.
Influenza:	Illness caused by any of several types (A, B, and C) of influenza virus, spread by airborne and tactile routes, and causing both upper and lower respiratory disease of varying degrees of severity.
Information Literacy:	A set of abilities requiring individuals to recognize when information is needed and have the ability to locate, evaluate, and use effectively the needed information.
Inhaled Corticosteroids (ICS):	The cornerstone medication for asthma and recommended for all patients with persistent asthma. Studies have shown them to be superior than all other agents in the ability to improve lung function, reduce symptoms, prevent exacerbations, and even reduce death.
Initiation:	Preneoplastic change in the genetic material of a cell.
Innate Immunity:	Nonspecific mechanisms involved in the early response to pathogens invading the body, which lack specificity and involve anatomical, physiological, phagocytic, and inflammatory mechanisms. Includes physical barriers such as mucosa or skin; leukocytes such as neutrophils and monocytes in circulation or macrophages in tissue, natural killer cells, eosinophils; and many proteins and cytokines such as complement, TNF, IL-1, and others.
Insecticide-Treated Bed Net (ITN):	A mosquito net of fiber that has been treated with insecticide. Bed nets can be treated by dipping in an insecticide mixture (traditional ITN) or the insecticide can be bound to the fabric, allowing it to remain on the netting for periods of three to five years (*long-lasting insecticide-treated net [LLIN]*).
Insomnia:	Sleep disorder characterized by an inability to initiate sleep or to remain asleep for a reasonable period or waking up feeling refreshed.

Instrumental Activities of Daily Living (IADLs): A scale of activities related to independent living that includes preparing meals, managing money, shopping for groceries or personal items, performing light or heavy housework, and using a telephone.

Insulin: A hormone that helps the body use glucose (sugar) for energy. The beta cells of the pancreas (in the islets of Langerhans) make the insulin. When the body cannot make enough insulin on its own, a person with diabetes must inject insulin made from other sources (i.e., beef, pork, or human insulin [recombinant DNA in origin or pork derived, semisynthetic]).

Insulin Resistance: The body's inability to respond to and use the insulin it produces. Insulin resistance may be linked to obesity, hypertension, and high levels of fat in the blood.

Integrase: An enzyme characteristic to retrovirals that allows viral genetic material to be integrated into the host DNA.

Intermittent Preventive Treatment (IPTi/p): Administration of treatment doses of an antimalarial drug or drug combination to persons who do not have the symptoms of malaria in order to prevent the onset of clinical malaria. The "i/p" denotes IPT given to infants or pregnant women.

Internet: A vast infrastructure connecting computers and networks around the world.

Intracellular: Existing within the cell.

Iron Deficiency Anemia: The intersection of two health conditions: iron deficiency, caused by inadequate iron absorption and/or iron loss, and anemia, which is caused by insufficient circulating red blood cells. Many individuals in the developing world infected with helminth infections suffer from both iron deficiency and anemia.

Islets of Langerhans (pronunciation: EYE-let). The clumps of cells within the pancreas that include those cells that make insulin and other hormones; includes several subvarieties, including: alpha cells, which make glucagon; beta cells, which make insulin; delta cells, which make somatostatin; and PP cells and D1 cells, about which little is known.

Isolation: Separation of patients with a communicable disease from non-infected individuals, preventing transmission of infection to others and allowing focused care.

Isozyme: Multiple forms of an enzyme that catalyze the same reaction but whose synthesis is controlled by more than one gene.

Jersey Barrier: Large, prism-shaped concrete blocks that separate lanes of traffic (often opposing lanes of traffic) with a goal of minimizing vehicle crossover in the case of accidents. The shape is designed to use the vehicle's momentum to send it back into the flow of traffic in the same direction rather than into oncoming traffic lanes or across lanes.

Larva: Immature stage of helminth prior to developing to adult worm.

Latent Tuberculosis Infection: State of people infected with *Mycobacterium tuberculosis* whose infection is contained by the immune system and who are not sick (and therefore not symptomatic) and not contagious.

Leukotriene Modifiers (also, *Leukotriene Receptor Antagonists [LTRA]*): A class of drugs used to treat asthma; they work by blocking leukotrienes, an important mediator in the inflammatory cascasde, and have a low risk of side effects but are not as effective as inhaled corticosteroids.

Life Expectancy (also, *Expectation of Life*): The average number of years an individual of a given age is expected to live if current mortality rates continue to apply.

Ligament: Fibrous tissue that connects one bone to another.

Limbic System: A network of brain areas essential for memory, motivated behavior, the ability to experience pleasure, and response to environmental threat (specifically includes hippocampus, amygdala, and hypothalamus).

Lipid: A type of fat in the body that can be broken down and used for energy.

Liver: Organ of the gastrointestinal system that resides in the right upper quadrant of the abdomen.

Long Acting Bronchodilators (LABA): Medication used for asthma control. When combined with an inhaled corticosteroid (ICS), they have been shown to improve both objective lung function measurements as well as patient factors such as improvement in peak flow readings and days without asthma symptoms. They should not be used without ICSs, as one study showed an increase in rates of asthma death when used alone.

Long-Term Care: Services, care, or items (e.g., assistive devices), including disease prevention and health promotion services, in-home services, and case management services, intended to assist individuals in coping with, and to the extent practicable, compensate for functional impairments in carrying out activities of daily living.

Low-Density Lipoprotein Cholesterol (LDL) (also, *"Bad" Cholesterol*): A type of fat found in the blood that distributes cholesterol around the body to where it is needed for cell repair and also deposits it on the inside of artery walls.

Lumbar Puncture (also, *Spinal Tap*): A diagnostic and sometimes therapeutic surgical procedure in which a needle is inserted into an area in the lower back and into the spinal canal to obtain spinal fluid, which is analyzed.

Lynch Syndrome: A hereditary form of colon cancer characterized by multiple polyps; accounts for 5 percent to 10 percent of all cases.

M2 Ion Channel Inhibitors: Class of antiviral medications including amantadine and rimantadine, to which greater than 90 percent of circulating seasonal influenza is resistant.

Macronutrients: Nutrients needed in large quantities, including carbohydrates, proteins, and fats.

Macrophage Activation: Antigen-presenting factors that secrete pro-inflammatory and antimicrobial mediators and synthesize products that have an important role in the inflammatory response (e.g., IL-1, TNF-α). Macrophages can be activated by the binding of microbial products, such as endotoxin or double-stranded viral RNA that bind to Toll-like receptors. which are constitutively expressed on the plasma membrane. Activation can also be triggered by the binding of opsonins (i.e., C3b and the Fc fragment of antibodies) and stimulated by action of cytokines, especially interferon-γ.

Malignant: Refers to cells or tumors growing in an uncontrolled fashion causing severe symptoms and progressively worsening disease that may result in death; such growths invade nearby normal tissue to take over its DNA so only cancerous cells reproduce, and eventually may reach more distant organs via the bloodstream (see *Cancer*).

Malnutrition: Failure to achieve nutrient requirements, which can impair physical and/or mental health; may result from consuming too little food or a shortage or imbalance of key nutrients.

Mass Drug Administration (MDA): The process of treating an entire community for a condition, as opposed to only treating infected individuals.

MDR-TB (see *Multidrug-Resistant Tuberculosis*).

Medicaid: A state-run health insurance program intended for low-income individuals.

Medical Nutrition Therapy: Use of specific nutrition counseling and interventions, based on an assessment of nutritional status, to manage a condition or treat an illness or injury.

Medication Reconciliation: A process that identifies, maintains, and updates the most accurate list of all medications (including non-prescription medications, herbals, and alternative medicines) that patients are taking, including dosage and route of administration.

Melatonin: Hormone secreted by the pineal gland, especially in response to darkness that promotes sleep.

Melena: Black "tarry" blood traces found in the stool; indicative of hemorrhage in the upper gastrointestinal tract (e.g., peptic ulcer).

Memory Cells: B and T cells, which "remember" a certain antigen after an initial exposure to the antigen.

Memory Impairment: A neuropathological state indicative of a disease process or toxic exposure affecting the brain such that memory loss has progressed to an extent that normal independent function is impossible.

Mendelian Inheritance: The principles of heredity first described by Gregor Mendel in 1865. Mendelian (single-gene) traits follow well-defined patterns of inheritance.

Meningitis:	An infection of the lining of the brain and or spinal cord; can be caused by bacteria or viruses.
Menopause (also, *the Change of Life*):	The time in a woman's life when menstrual periods permanently stop; the opposite of the menarche.
Mental Retardation:	Intellectual deficit measured by intelligence quotient (IQ) and adaptive tests. An individual must have both IQ and adaptive skills test scores less than two standard deviations below the mean (≤ 70) to meet diagnostic criteria for mental retardation. Mental retardation is divided into mild (70–55), moderate (54–40), severe (39–25), and profound (<25). Approximately 2.5 percent of the population has mental retardation; 85 percent of individuals with mental retardation are in the mild category.
Metabolic Syndrome:	The tendency of several conditions to occur together, including obesity, insulin resistance, diabetes or pre-diabetes, hypertension, and high lipids.
Methicillin-Resistant *Staphylococcus aureus* (MRSA):	Bacterial strains resistant to beta-lactam antibiotics. Benign MRSA infections typically colonize on the skin and mucous membranes but may cause severe infections.
Microarray:	A technology using a high-density array of nucleic acids, protein, or tissue for examining complex biological interactions simultaneously that are identified by specific location on a slide array.
Micronutrients:	Vitamins and minerals required in small amounts daily (e.g., vitamin A and iron).
Midbrain Reward Pathway:	A dopaminergic pathway in the brain that is activated by certain beneficial behaviors such as eating and sex, as well as by addictive drugs, to produce a sensation of pleasure.
Minerals:	Inorganic compounds needed for growth and for regulation of body processes.
Mini Mental State Examination (MMSE):	A brief, quantitative measure of cognitive status in adults that can be used to screen for cognitive impairment, estimate the severity of cognitive impairment at a given point in time, follow the course of cognitive changes in an individual over time, and document an individual's response to treatment.
Modifiable Risk Factor:	Condition present within an individual that increases the risk of disease occurrence but can be changed to alter subsequent risk of disease occurrence.
Morbidity:	Any departure, subjective or objective, from a state of physiological or psychological well-being.
Mortality:	The number of deaths in a given time or place.
MRSA	(see *Methicillin-Resistant* Staphylococcus aureus).
Mucosal-Associated-Lymphoid-Type (MALT) Lymphoma:	A rare form of lymphoid cancer associated with tissues distributed throughout mucosal linings of the digestive tract.
Multidrug-Resistant Tuberculosis (MDR-TB):	Strain of tuberculosis that is resistant to at least isoniazid and rifampicin, the two most potent first-line therapeutic drugs. MDR-TB strains are more difficult to treat and require the use of second line drugs.
Narcolepsy:	A sleep disorder characterized by sudden and uncontrollable episodes of deep sleep.
National Institutes of Health (NIH):	Federal agency responsible for overseeing government-sponsored biomedical research. It is divided into 27 institutes and research centers.
National Health Interview Survey (NHIS):	A source of information collected on the overall health of the civilian population of the United States that consists of questionnaires on health, demographics, and socioeconomic status of the general population.
National Health and Nutrition Examination Survey (NHANES):	A national health survey consisting of interviews and questionnaires conducted to obtain information on the overall health and nutritional status of the general population of the United States.
Negative Feedback:	A way in which homeostatic systems keep levels of monitored variables stable. If the sensed level is too high, the system directs changes in effectors that bring the level down; if the sensed level is too low, the system directs changes bringing the level up.
Neoplastic:	Characterized by the presence of new and uncontrolled cellular growth (see *Cancer*).
Nephron:	The functional unit of the kidney. Each human kidney has about one million of these tiny tubular structures.

Newton's First Law:	Objects in motion remain in motion until an external force is applied. The converse is also true: an object at rest tends to stay at rest until acted upon.
Newton's Second Law:	The acceleration of an object as produced by a net force is directly proportional to the magnitude of the net force, in the same direction as the net force, and inversely proportional to the mass of the object. More succinctly, Force = mass $\times$ acceleration (F = ma).
Neuraminidase:	Surface protein that releases new viruses from infected cells; the abbreviation of it and its numbered type is used as a component of the virus name (i.e., N1).
Neuraminidase Inhibitors:	Class of antiviral medications including oseltamivir and zanamivir.
Neurofibrillary Tangles:	Abnormal protein aggregates found inside the neurons of Alzheimer's patients.
Neurons:	The basic nerve cell of the brain and nervous system. Neurons receive and send electrical messages to and from the brain to the body.
Neurotransmitters:	Molecule released by one nerve cell that activates or suppresses another nerve cell. Examples: dopamine, acetylcholine, norepinephrine, and serotonin.
NHANES	(see *National Health and Nutrition Examination Survey*).
NIH	(see *National Institutes of Health*).
Non-Modifiable Risk Factor:	Condition present within an individual that increases the risk of disease occurrence but cannot be changed.
Non-Rapid Eye Movement (NREM) Sleep:	Collectively describes the four stages of sleep, preceding REM sleep, and is characterized by a reduction in physiological activity and a slowing of brain waves.
Non-Smoking as the Norm:	Movement that seeks to isolate smokers, discourage initiation, and eliminate the proven hazards of environmental smoke by emphasizing everyone's right to breathe air free of toxic tobacco smoke.
Noradrenaline (Norepinephrine):	The main chemical messenger of the sympathetic nervous system; responsible for much of regulation of the cardiovascular system by the brain.
Nutrient Density:	A quantitative measure of a food's nutrient value, measuring the amount of nutrients per kilocalorie.
Nutritional Monitoring:	A system of continuously measuring nutritional intake and status of a population; an important epidemiological tool for nutritional public health.
Obesity:	A condition in which a greater than normal amount of fat is in the body; more severe than overweight; having a body mass index of 30 or more.
Observational Learning:	Behavioral learning that occurs by watching the behaviors of others and the outcomes that result from others' actions.
Oncogenic:	Leading to the development of cancer.
Opsonin:	An opsonin is a protein that coats particulate matter in a way that enhances uptake in phagocytic leukocytes through binding of that protein to specific receptors (i.e., the C3b receptor in the case of complement factor C3b or the Fc receptor in the case of an antibody).
Oral Health:	Freedom from diseases and disorders that affect the craniofacial complex.
Organization-Based Outbreak:	The occurrence of three or more confirmed or likely cases of meningococcal disease of the same serogroup within three months among persons with a common affiliation but without close contact, resulting in primary disease attack rate of 10 cases/100,000 persons.
Osteoarthritis:	Degeneration of the cartilage and underlying bone within a joint, characterized by bony overgrowth.
Osteoblasts:	Type of cells that build bone.
Osteoclasts:	Type of cells that break down bone.
Osteophytes:	Bony overgrowth of joints caused by rheumatic diseases.
Osteoporosis:	A skeletal disorder characterized by compromised bone strength and predisposing a person to an increased risk of fracture, especially at the spine, hip, and wrist.

Outcome Expectancy: An individual's belief that a certain behavior or action will produce a certain outcome.

Overweight: An above-normal body weight; having a body mass index of 25 to 29.9.

Oxidative Stress: A condition of the cell in which there is an increase in the formation of reactive oxygen species that stresses the cell's ability to support its inherent protective mechanisms, resulting in injury to cellular membranes and a stimulation of gene expression that favors the synthesis of pro-inflammatory cytokines (i.e., interleukin-1 [IL-1], tumor necrosis factor-α [TNF-α]) and other mediators of the inflammatory response.

Pancreas: An organ that makes insulin and enzymes for digestion. The pancreas is located behind the lower part of the stomach and is about the size of a hand.

Pandemic Influenza: An influenza virus that has spread to cause epidemic disease on a continental or worldwide level, regardless of source (i.e., avian)

Papanicolaou Test (also, Pap Smear, Pap Test, Cervical Smear, Smear Test)**:** A type of screening for women used to identify abnormal cervical tissues that may be in neoplastic transformation as well as diseases (i.e., human papillomavirus [HPV] infection).

Parasomnia: A category of sleep disorders in which abnormal physiological or behavioral events occur during sleep, including night terrors and sleepwalking.

Parasympathetic Nervous System: One of the main components of the autonomic nervous system, responsible for many "vegetative" functions (i.e., gastrointestinal movements after a meal) (see *Autonomic Nervous System*).

Parkinson Disease: A progressive nervous system disease that produces slow movements, a form of limb rigidity called "cogwheel rigidity," and a "pill-roll" tremor that is present when the patient is at rest and decreases with intentional movement. Other features include a masklike facial expression, stooped posture, difficulty initiating or stopping movements, small handwriting, and improvement of the movement disorder by treatment with levodopa.

Passive Immunity: A type of disease prevention acquired by natural or acquired transfer of preformed antibodies.

Pathogen: An infectious biological agent that causes disease.

Peak Flow Meters: Handheld devices used by asthmatic patients to track their daily airflow. Because patients' airflow is generally reduced prior to an asthma attack and they may not perceive this decrease, home measurement of peak flow may prevent serious exacerbations by allowing treatment before an asthma attack happens. Providers will help patients determine their "personal best" peak flow number, and have each patient track their numbers over time. Peak flow reading can be used in conjunction with asthma action plans and are recommended for patients with moderate to severe asthma.

Pedigree: A diagram showing the genetic relationships between members of a family that is annotated with relevant medical information; used to visualize inheritance patterns and aid in diagnosis and risk assessment.

Peer Review: Peer review refers to a journal's policy of having experts in a given field examine a submitted article before accepting it for publication. This process assures that only high quality articles based on sound research that offer a significant contribution to the field are included for publication in the journal.

Penicillinase: An enzyme that deactivates penicillin.

Perceived Barriers: An individual's perception of the negative aspects of the behavior being required to reduce risk.

Perceived Behavioral Control: An individual's perception of their level of control of factors beyond their immediate control.

Perceived Benefits: An individual's perception of the positive aspects of the behavior being required to reduce risk.

Perceived Severity: An individual's perception of the seriousness of a disease and the consequences of having an illness.

Perceived Susceptibility: An individual's perception of the probability that he or she will acquire a disease or become ill.

Perinatal (also *Peripartum*)**:** Associated with pregnancy and childbirth.

Periodontitis: A more severe form of gum disease characterized by the breakdown of alveolar bone and connective tissues surrounding and supporting the teeth.

Persistent Infections:	Infection not cleared by the immune system.
Phagocytosis :	The process by which neutrophils and macrophages destroy microbes by engulfing them within a vacuole or phagosome formed by an in-folding of the plasma membrane within the cytoplasm
Phagosomal Antimicrobial Activity:	A potent mechanism of killing or inhibiting the growth of microbes which is stronger when oxygen is present.
Pharmacogenetics:	The study of genetic factors that directly influence a person's reaction to medications.
Pharmacogenomics:	The application of genomic information (all human genes and their interactions relevant to drug response) and technology in drug development and therapy.
Phenotype:	The physical expression of a trait or disease.
Phosphorus:	An essential element in the diet and a major component of bone. Phosphorus is also found in the blood, muscles, nerves, and teeth. It is a component of adenosine triphosphate (ATP), the primary energy source in the body.
Phytochemicals:	Naturally occurring plant chemicals that are not essential, but often aid in disease protection and maintaining health. Phytochemical compounds are intended to enhance the lives of plants themselves, but have recently been found to have benefits for humans as well.
Pineal Gland:	A small, cone-shaped organ of the brain that secretes the hormone melatonin into the bloodstream.
Plant Stanols/Sterols:	Naturally occurring substances found in plants, present in small quantities in many fruits, vegetables, vegetable oils, nuts, seeds, cereals and legumes. The sterols/stanols work by blocking the absorption of cholesterol in the small intestine, which lowers the low density cholesterol by 6 percent to 15 percent without lowering the high density cholesterol.
Plasmodium:	The genus of single-celled parasites that cause malaria. Four species—*Plasmodium falciparum, P. vivax, P. ovale,* and *P. malariae*—are the causative agents in human malaria.
Pneumonic or Pulmonary:	Relating to the lung, from inhalation of the biological agent (e.g., pneumonic plague results from inhalation of *Yersinia pestis*).
Polyp:	An abnormal tissue protuberance from a mucus membrane; can be found in the colon mucosa, nose, bladder, stomach, and uterus.
Polysomnography:	A diagnostic sleep test measuring several physiological variables including brain electrical activity, eye and jaw muscle movement, leg muscle movement, and airflow.
Postpartum:	After childbirth.
Precursor:	In nutrition, a component of a vitamin that, when combined with other components and processes in the body, will produce a full vitamin. Precursors are most often acquired from foods and are stored in the body so that the body can make whole vitamins as needed.
Prehypertension:	Precursor to high blood pressure where the systolic blood pressure is between 120 and 139 mm Hg and/or diastolic blood pressure is between 80 and 89 mm Hg in adults.
Prevalence:	The total number of existing cases of a disease in the population at a given time.
Prevention:	Any action to avoid an infectious process. Three types of preventive activities are: primary, which is the avoidance of disease; secondary, which interrupts any disease process before transmission to others is possible; and tertiary, which is the avoidance of disease sequelae or adverse effects of the disease process.
Primary Care (also, *Family Medicine, General Practice*)**:**	A type of healthcare where a provider (physician specializing in general medicine, physician assistant, nurse practitioner, chiropractor, etc.) acts as the first line of consultation about health for an individual in a long-term partnership, who provides medical care within the standards of the community and profession.
Primary Care Provider:	A physician who specializes in general and family practice, general internal medicine, or general pediatrics, or a nonphysician healthcare provider, such as a nurse practitioner, physician assistant, or certified nurse midwife.

Primary Prevention: Intervention to prevent a disease before it has occurred; includes efforts such as enhancing nutritional status, immunizing against communicable diseases, and eliminating environmental risks.

Prodrome: Early symptoms indicating development of a disease; in biological terrorism, the most common prodrome is a flu-like illness with fever, muscle pain, headache, and profound weakness.

Progression: Process by which a growing mass of initiated cells undergoes qualitative changes, potentially including a transition from benign to malignant behavior. This process is characterized by the accumulation of new genetic changes in and continued expansion of the tumor or disease.

Promotion: The process by which an initiated cell develops into an overt neoplasm; characterized by proliferation under permissive host conditions.

Prophylaxis: Medical intervention to prevent disease. Antibiotics and antivirals are chemoprophylactics (medications); vaccines are referred to as immunoprophylactics.

Protective Factors: Certain conditions that increase the health and well-being of an individual and decrease the likelihood of developing a disease or condition.

Provider Barriers: Any mental, physical, psychosocial, or environmental condition that prevents or discourages healthcare providers from offering preventive services. Examples include a poor practice environment, lack of knowledge, and lack of efficacy studies.

Public Health Genetics: The application of knowledge from genetics and genomics, in the context of the principles of public health, to improve the health of populations.

Pulmonary Tuberculosis: Active tuberculosis infection that is localized in the lungs.

Purpura Fulminans: A life-threatening condition involving cutaneous hemorrhage and necrosis, bacteremia, low blood pressure, and problems with the clotting system.

Quadriceps: Muscle in the front of the thigh that flexes (bends) the hip and extends (straightens) the knee.

Quadrivalent: A vaccine directed against four viral strains.

Quality: In medical practice, is a measure or the degree to which health systems, services, instrumentation, and standards for individuals, as well as populations, increases or elicits the likelihood for positive health outcomes and remain consistent with current professional knowledge.

Quarantine: Restriction of contacts between the uninfected and the infected until further assessment concludes the infected individual is not contagious or a danger to the spread of a disease.

Rapid Eye Movement (REM) Sleep: A recurring sleep state characterized by rapid eye movement and intense brain activity during which dreaming occurs.

Reabsorption: In the kidney, reabsorbed solutes are transported out of the fluid in the lumen of the nephron and returned to the blood.

Receptor: A molecular structure within a cell or on the surface characterized by selective binding of a specific substance and a specific physiological effect that accompanies the binding.

Reciprocal Determinism: The interaction of an individual's personal factors, actions, and environmental factors that help explain the overall behavior.

Rehabilitative Services: Activities, education, and exercises to restore specific skills in an impaired individual, including overall physical mobility and functional abilities.

Reinfection Rate: Number of times an individual is infected with a disease over a particular time period. In areas endemic with helminth infections, reinfection rates are high unless interventions (i.e., regular mass drug administrations, improved sanitation infrastructure, and health education) are implemented.

Reinforcement: A response to an individual's behavior that increases or decreases the repetition of that behavior.

Relapse: A second condition (e.g., infection) after the first one has occurred.

Relative Risk: The ratio of the risk of disease or death among the exposed to the risk among the unexposed.

Relaxation Therapy: A form of sleep behavioral therapy including muscle relaxation, biofeedback, meditation, and breathing techniques aimed at helping the patient fall asleep faster and stay asleep longer; also used for pain control and stress relief.

Resistive Strength Exercise: A type of physical activity that uses a force opposing the movement, such as a weight, to cause a strong muscle contraction. This type of exercise promotes low forces on bone that promotes healthy bone formation.

Restless Legs Syndrome: A sleep disorder primarily characterized by leg discomfort during sleep, which is only relieved by frequent movements of the legs.

Retroperitoneum: Area behind (posterior to) the abdominal cavity that contains the spinal column, kidneys, aorta, and inferior vena cava.

Retrovirus: A family of viruses that contain RNA and replicate through a DNA intermediate.

Reverse Transcriptase: A viral enzyme converting the RNA of a virus into double-stranded DNA.

Rheumatoid Arthritis (RA): Systemic inflammatory disease manifesting in multiple joints in the body, primarily affecting the lining of the joints and sometimes other organs.

Ribonucleic Acid (RNA): A group of nucleic acids that control several forms of cellular activity.

Risk Factor: An attribute or exposure that is causally associated with an increased probability of a disease or injury.

Screening: Efforts to detect illness in individuals before they are obviously sick or disordered, or when they have not sought care for a specific problem.

Search Engine: Used to find Internet and World Wide Web pages on a computer. Unlike a database, it is an unstructured environment (see *Internet*, *World Wide Web*).

Secondary Case: The same disease that occurs among close contacts of a primary patient ≥ 24 hours after onset of illness in the primary patient.

Secondary Prevention: Measures such as healthcare services designed to identify or treat individuals who have a disease or risk factors for a disease but who are not yet experiencing symptoms of the disease. Pap tests and high blood pressure screening are examples of secondary prevention.

Second-Degree Relatives: Grandparents, grandchildren, nieces, nephews, aunts, uncles, half siblings.

Second-Line Drugs: A group of medications that may be more toxic, less effective, have a longer response time, and/or are more expensive than first line medications; given to patients who cannot take first line medications (e.g., because of allergic or toxic reaction, expense, or availability). For example, antibiotics with anti-TB activity that are less potent, take longer to affect the disease, have serious side effects, and are more expensive than the first-line drugs may be the only treatment option for patients with MDR-TB.

Self-Efficacy: The confidence that an individual has in his or her ability to successfully carry out a certain behavior in order to produce a desired outcome.

Segregation: In genetics, the distribution of chromosomes during the formation of an egg or sperm. Each person has two versions of each chromosome, but can only contribute one of each pair to an egg or sperm cell.

Severe Malaria: Symptomatic malaria infection complicated by coma or recurrent seizures (i.e., cerebral malaria), severe anemia, respiratory distress, kidney or liver failure, systemic acidosis, or other associated life-threatening conditions.

SIRS (see *Systemic Inflammatory Response Syndrome*).

Sleep: A natural and periodic state during which consciousness of the environment is suspended.

Sleep Apnea: A serious, potentially life-threatening sleep disorder characterized by episodes of interrupted breathing during sleep.

Sleep Architecture: The predictable pattern of alternating REM and NREM sleep that occurs throughout the night and consists of four NREM phases and one REM phase.

Sleep Hygiene: Practices conducive to good sleep including maintaining the same sleep and wake patterns every day, avoiding stimulants late in the day, ensuring adequate exposure to natural daylight, and maintaining a cool, dark, and quiet sleep environment.

Sleep-Restriction Therapy: A form of sleep behavioral therapy that restricts the individual's time in bed, resulting in sleep deprivation that allows the individual to fall asleep.

Sleep-Wake Cycle: The biological pattern of alternating sleep and wakefulness in humans that is roughly eight hours of nocturnal sleep and 16 hours of daytime activity.

Smear Negative: Tuberculosis patients suffering from active pulmonary disease who produce, while coughing, less than 5,000 bacteria/mL of sputum that cannot be detected by microscopy.

Complementary diagnostic tests such as chest x-rays or culture must confirm tuberculosis. Smear negative patients are less infectious than smear positive ones.

Smear Positive: Tuberculosis patients suffering from active pulmonary disease who can produce, while coughing, more than 5,000 bacteria/mL of sputum that can be detected by microscopy. Smear positive patients are more infectious than those who are smear negative.

Smoking Cessation: An attempt to quit smoking, either unaided (*cold turkey*) or assisted by behavioral and/or pharmacological treatments.

Social Distancing: Removal of someone with an easily transmissible infection from normal situations in which they would potentially expose a large number of people (e.g., on the job site or attending school).

Sources: Data upon which analysis and dissemination of information are based. *Primary sources* are the raw data of public health research where data are collected on the population at all levels (individual, local, state, and national) to assess, assure, and plan for the health of the nation. *Secondary sources* are research reports (e.g., a published article on a specific topic). *Tertiary sources* are based on secondary sources and synthesize and explain research (e.g., a review article).

Spirometry: A diagnostic medical device used for pulmonary function testing (PFTs) that measures how much air can be breathed in or out (lung volumes) as well as how fast one is able to breathe air out (lung flow). Recommended use is to properly diagnose asthma and rule out any underlying condition, objectively measure a patient's response to treatment, and every one to two years to assess progressive decline in lung function.

Spleen: An organ of the immune system that resides in the left upper quadrant of the abdomen.

Standard Precautions: Measures that healthcare personnel take to reduce the risk of transmission of infection, including the donning of gown, gloves, mask, and eye protection during patient care involving bodily fluids.

Staphylococcus aureus: Gram-positive microorganism belonging to the genus *Staphylococcus*; the microorganism involved in MRSA infections (see *Methicillin-Resistant Staphylococcus aureus*).

Stimulus-Control Therapy: A form of sleep behavioral therapy that conditions the patient to associate the bed and bedroom with sleep.

Streptococcus mutans: Highly cariogenic microorganism involved in the breakdown of teeth, causing dental caries.

Stress: A condition in which the organism senses a challenge to physical or mental stability that leads to altered activities of body systems to meet that challenge.

Stroke: Sudden onset of persistent neurological deficits resulting from vascular causes in the brain.

Structural Changes: In reference to nutritional public health interventions, involves long-term adjustments to a population's behaviors and/or environment that allow them to better meet their nutritional needs.

Subjective Norms: An individual's belief about whether other people approve or disapprove of engaging in a certain behavior.

Supplementation: A direct dosage of a nutrient, often given as a vaccine or pill.

Suprachiasmatic Nucleus (SCN): A region in the hypothalamus that regulates circadian rhythms, acting as the body's sleep-wake center or "biological clock."

Surge Capacity: The amount of patients a given medical facility can accommodate in an emergency situation beyond its standard maximum amount, such as in a pandemic.

Surveillance: Continuous observation of a testing or procedure.

Sympathetic Nervous System: One of the main components of the autonomic nervous system, responsible for many automatic functions in the body (e.g., constriction of blood vessels when a person stands up).

Syndromic Surveillance: The use of certain symptom complexes and other health-related data to detect a potential outbreak or biological attack in its early phases so that public health measures may be rapidly mobilized to decrease morbidity and mortality. Examples of surrogate data sources include school absenteeism, sale of over-the-counter medications, and Emergency Department presenting complaints.

Systemic Inflammatory Response Syndrome (SIRS): A medical emergency characterized by a body-wide (system) inflammatory response that has no proven source. Some causes may be severe trauma, heart attack, drug overdose, or immunodeficiency (AIDS). Differentiated from sepsis, a systemic inflammatory response with a proven source.

Systolic Blood Pressure: The maximum pressure exerted when the heart contracts; top number is the systolic blood pressure reading (see *Blood Pressure*).

Targeted Prevention (also, *Selective* or *Secondary Prevention*): An intervention focused on individuals who are at risk for a disease or disorder aimed at arresting or alleviating its development.

Tau Protein: Major component of neurofibrillary tangles in Alzheimer's disease (see *Alzheimer's disease, neurofibrillary tangles*).

Temporality: Timing of exposure to the proposed causal agent must occur before the disease process begins.

Teratogen: Agent that causes birth defects, death, growth deficiency, and/or functional impairment.

Tertiary Prevention: Involves the management of individuals who have developed the disease with attempts made to restore to highest function, minimize the negative effects of disease, and prevent disease-related complications. Because the disease is now established, primary prevention activities may have been unsuccessful. Early detection through secondary prevention may have minimized the impact of the disease (see *Prevention*).

Therapeutic Drug Monitoring: A process where healthcare professionals monitor the patients' response to medications to ensure maximum efficacy and minimum toxicity by measuring drug concentrations in patient's blood to ensure a desire concentration has been achieved; usually only performed for those who need to be dosed to a certain narrow range of blood-drug concentrations in order to achieve the maximum efficacy versus toxicity ratio.

Third-Degree Relatives: First cousins, great-grandchildren, great-grandparents.

Tolerance: A state resulting from changes in the brain that occur in response to chronic exposure to an addictive substance. An individual exhibiting tolerance to a drug requires repeated and possibly increasing amounts of that substance to feel "normal."

Toxicity: Degree of effect an illness or damage produced by something has in the whole organism or its substructure (i.e., an organ or cell); also used metaphorically for negative emotional or behavioral effects in groups (i.e., family, community). The presence of too much of a single micronutrient in the body; each nutrient has a unique threshold for toxicity, and distinct harmful consequences from the ingestion of toxic amounts.

Toxic Shock Syndrome (TSS): A condition that is often associated with significant morbidity and mortality by inducing an overwhelming host immune response characterized by hypotension, fever, rash, and multi-organ involvement.

Toxoid: An altered toxin capable of inducing production of antibodies.

Transient Ischemic Attack (TIA): Sudden onset neurological deficits resulting from cessation of blood flow that recovers in less than 24 hours.

Triglycerides: The chief form of fat in the diet and the major storage form of fat in the body. People who have high levels of triglyceride often have a low level of "good" cholesterol (HDL) and a high level of "bad" cholesterol (LDL). Triglyceride levels of ≥150 mg/dL may have an increased risk for heart disease; those with heart disease, diabetes, or both also have high triglyceride levels.

Tuberculosis (TB) (also, *Consumption*): Caused by mycobacteria, a deadly infectious disease that most often attacks the lungs (75 percent) but can affect many other systems in the body. Only half of those who are untreated will survive. Symptoms of pulmonary TB include chest pain, prolonged (> 3 weeks) productive cough, and coughing up of blood; patients may experience fever, fatigue, chills, night sweats, appetite loss, weight loss, and pallor.

Type A Reactions: Responses to a medication that are generally an extension of the desired therapeutic effect (e.g., an agent used to treat hypertension might cause dizziness in a patient as a result of excess blood pressure lowering).

Type B Reactions: Responses to a medication that are not an extension of the normal therapeutic effect (e.g., allergic reactions associated with penicillin and other antibiotics).

Ulcer: An area of suppurative exudate (presence of pus) and liquefactive necrosis in a tissue or organ that extends into the body of the organ or tissue, but remains open at an outer or inner surface of that organ or tissue.

Uncomplicated Malaria: Symptomatic infection with the malaria parasite manifesting as fever, body aches, headache, diarrhea, and possibly other symptoms not associated with severe illness.

Universal Prevention (also, *Primary Prevention*): A strategy to avoid disease or infectious agents that targets the entire population (no-risk to high-risk individuals).

Uremia: The syndrome in chronic kidney disease stage 5, which includes lack of appetite, nausea, vomiting, pericarditis, peripheral neuropathy, and mental status changes (ranging from loss of concentration and lethargy to seizures and coma).

Vaccination: Injection of a vaccine in order to establish resistance to an infectious disease.

Vaccine: A preparation of antigenic material designed to induce an immune response and immunological memory when injected.

Vagotomy: The surgical division of the vagus nerve designed to reduce stomach acid secretion.

Vascular Adhesion and Leukocyte Emigration: The binding of leukocytes, most notably neutrophils and monocytes, to vascular endothelial cells in sites of tissue injury. A process that is stimulated by an up-regulation of selectins and integrins that cause adherence of the cell types to one another and hold the leukocytes in place long enough to come under the influence of chemo-attractants emanating from the site of injury. The chemo-taxins induce the leukocytes to move in an ameboid fashion between the endothelial cells and out of the vessel into the extravascular connective tissue and toward the site of greatest injury.

Vascular Response: In acute inflammation, the increase of blood flow and permeability that can occur within minutes in an area of injury or infection.

Vector-Borne Diseases: Infectious diseases, both bacterial and viral, that are transmitted via an arthropod.

Viremia: The presence of a viral load in the blood.

Virulence: Capacity of a pathogen to cause an infection.

Viscoelastic: Having both a relatively high resistance to flow and being capable of resuming its original shape after stretching or compression.

Vitamins: Organic compounds necessary for reproduction, growth, and maintenance of the body. Vitamins are required in miniscule amounts.

Vitamin D: A vitamin that is necessary for absorption of calcium and phosphorus and to maintain blood calcium and phosphorus within normal levels. Under normal conditions of sunlight exposure, dietary supplementation may not be necessary.

Vulnerable and At-Risk Populations: High-risk groups of people who have multiple health and social needs. Examples include pregnant women, people with human immunodeficiency virus infection, substance abusers, migrant farm workers, homeless people, poor people, infants and children, elderly people, people with disabilities, people with mental illness or mental health problems or disorders, and people from certain ethnic or racial groups who do not have the same access to quality healthcare services as other populations.

Waist Circumference: An anthropometric measurement used to assess a person's abdominal fat. Abdominal fat increases the risk of many of the serious conditions associated with obesity. Women's waist measurements should be less than 35 inches. Men's should be less than 40 inches.

Weight Bearing Activity: A type of physical exercise that applies pressure loads on bones through their length (e.g., when walking or running). This type of activity is essential for healthy bone formation.

Wikis: A type of Web site that allows visitors to easily add, remove, and otherwise edit and change available content. Any user can edit the site content, including other users' contributions, using a regular Web browser.

Withdrawal: Unpleasant adverse effects caused by abrupt cessation of a drug in an individual addicted to that drug.

World Wide Web (also, *WWW, Web*): One avenue of accessing information disseminated over the Internet by using a computer; a way of accessing information via the hypertext transfer protocol (http), utilizing browsers to access Web pages through hyperlinks. The simple act of "googling" (using a key word on a search engine) a term could result in thousands or even millions of results to sift through (see *Internet, Search Engine*).

Wound Organization: The process of healing through the formation of granulation tissue to the progressive accumulation of fibroblasts, collagen, and the formation of scar.

Written Action Plans: Directions from a healthcare provider to a patient or caregiver that instruct exactly what to do when patients are feeling well, when they are symptomatic, and when they are ill; usually involves which medications to take and when, types of side effects or triggers to avoid, and emergency contact information. An excellent communication tool between patients and providers, and recommended by national guidelines.

XDR-TB (see *Extensively Drug-Resistant Tuberculosis*).

Xenobiotic: Chemical substances foreign to the biological system; includes naturally occurring compounds, drugs, environmental agents, carcinogens, insecticides, etc.

X-Linked Trait: An inherited gene mutation from the X chromosome (that is, not on an autosome).

Yaw: To lean suddenly, unsteadily, and erratically from the vertical axis. When used in relationship to bullets, recall that bullets spin rapidly around their long axis; when bullets impact human tissue, this spinning is often partially disrupted.

Zoonosis (also, *Zoonotic Disease*): Infectious disease that can be transmitted from animals to humans (e.g., anthrax, plague, and tularemia).

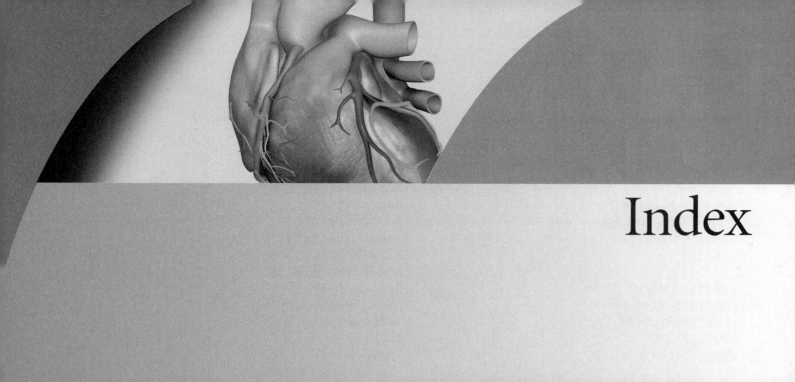

Index